D1377686

Childhood and Adolescent Diabetes

Childhood and Adolescent Diabetes

Edited by

Christopher J.H. Kelnar MA MD FRCP DCH
Consultant Pediatric Endocrinologist and Diabetologist,
Royal Hospital for Sick Children,
Edinburgh, and Senior Lecturer,
Department of Child Life and Health,
University of Edinburgh, Edinburgh, UK

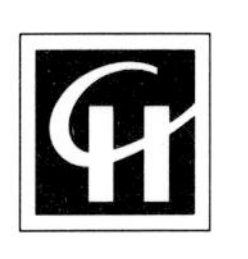

CHAPMAN & HALL MEDICAL
London · Glasgow · Weinheim · New York · Tokyo · Melbourne · Madras

Published by Chapman & Hall, 2–6 Boundary Row, London SE1 8HN, UK

Chapman & Hall, 2–6 Boundary Row, London SE1 8HN, UK

Blackie Academic & Professional, Wester Cleddens Road, Bishopbriggs, Glasgow G64 2NZ, UK

Chapman & Hall GmbH, Pappelallee 3, 69469 Weinheim, Germany

Chapman & Hall USA, One Penn Plaza, 41st Floor, New York NY 10119, USA

Chapman & Hall Japan, ITP-Japan, Kyowa Building, 3F, 2-2-1 Hirakawacho, Chiyoda-ku, Tokyo 102, Japan

Chapman & Hall Australia, Thomas Nelson Australia, 102 Dodds Street, South Melbourne, Victoria 3205, Australia

Chapman & Hall India, R. Seshadri, 32 Second Main Road, CIT East, Madras 600 035, India

First edition 1995

Typeset in 10/12 pt Palatino by Best-set Typesetter Ltd., Hong Kong
Printed in Great Britain at the University Press, Cambridge

ISBN 0 412 48610 5

A catalogue record for this book is available from the British Library

∞ Printed on acid-free text paper, manufactured in accordance with ANSI/NISO Z39.48-1992 (Permanence of Paper).

Contents

Colour plates appear between pages 314 and 315

PART TWO

PART THREE

Contributors

1
J.M. Hawdon
Neonatal Unit, Obstetric Hospital
University College Hospital
Huntley Street
London WC1E 6AU UK

M.P. Ward Platt
Neonatal Unit
Royal Victoria Infirmary
Newcastle Upon Tyne NE1 4LP UK

2
H.F. Stirling
Department of Child Life and Health
University of Edinburgh
20 Sylvan Place
Edinburgh EH9 1UW UK

C.J.H. Kelnar
as above

3
D.B. Dunger
Department of Paediatrics
John Radcliffe Hospital
Headington
Oxford OX3 9DU UK

J.A. Edge
as above

4
C.J.H. Kelnar
Department of Child Life and Health
University of Edinburgh
20 Sylvan Place
Edinburgh EH9 1UW UK

5
D.B. Dunger
Department of Paediatrics
John Radcliffe Hospital
Headington
Oxford OX3 9DU UK

6
D.H. Skuse
Behavioural Sciences Unit
Institute of Child Health
30 Guilford Street
London WC1N 1EH UK

7
B.J. Anderson
Mental Health Unit
The Joslin Diabetes Center
1 Joslin Place
Boston MA 02215 USA

8
C.J.H. Kelnar
Department of Child Life and Health
University of Edinburgh
20 Sylvan Place
Edinburgh EH9 1UW UK

9
D.I. Johnston
Children's Department
University Hospital
Queen's Medical Centre
Nottingham NG7 2UH UK

10
J.S. Dorman
Department of Epidemiology
Graduate School of Public Health
University of Pittsburgh
Pittsburgh PA 15261 USA

L.A. O'Leary
as above

A.N. Koehler
Children's Hospital of Pittsburgh
Department of Nutrition
Pittsburgh PA 15213 USA

11
J.M. Connor
Duncan Guthrie Institute of Medical Genetics
Yorkhill
Glasgow G3 8SJ UK

12
A.K. Foulis
Department of Pathology
Royal Infirmary
Glasgow G4 0SF UK

13
T. Mandrup-Poulsen
Steno Diabetes Center
2 Niels Steensensvej
DK-2820 Gentofte, Denmark

J. Nerup
as above

14
J.W. Gregory
Department of Child Health
University of Wales College of Medicine
Cardiff CF4 4XW UK

R. Taylor
Department of Medicine, Medical School
University of Newcastle upon Tyne
Newcastle upon Tyne NE2 4HH UK

15
S.J. Brink
New England Diabetes and Endocrine Center
(NEDEC)
25 Boylston Street
Suite 211
Chestnut Hill MA 02167 USA

16
J.P.H. Shield
Institute of Child Health
Hospital for Sick Children
St Michael's Hill
Bristol BS2 8BJ UK

J.D. Baum
as above

17
P.G.F. Swift
Children's Hospital
Leicester Royal Infirmary
Leicester LE1 5WW UK

18
S. Brenchley
Diet Information Service
British Diabetic Association
10 Queen Anne Street
London W1M 0BD UK

A. Govindji
as above

19
S.A. Greene
Department of Child Health
Ninewells Hopsital and Medical School
Dundee DD1 9SY UK

C. Thompson
as above

20
A.M. La Greca
Departments of Medicine, Psychology and Pediatrics
University of Miami School of Medicine
Coral Gables FL USA

J.S. Skyler
as above

21
M. Silink
Ray Williams Institute of Paediatric Endocrinology
Royal Alexandra Hospital for children
PO Box 34
Camperdown, NSW 2050 Australia

22
D.I. Johnston
Children's Department
University Hospital
Queen's Medical Centre
Nottingham NG7 2UH UK

23
S.C. Brown
Royal Hospital for Sick Children
Sciennes Road
Edinburgh EH9 1LF UK

S. Fallon
as above

L. Smith
as above

R.M. Mitchell
Lothian College of Health Studies
Edinburgh UK

24
R.M. Milaszkiewicz
Department of Anaesthetics
Edgware General Hospital
Edgware Middx UK

G.M. Hall
Department of Anaesthetics
St George's Hospital Medical School
Cranmere Terrace
London SW17 0RE UK

25
A.E. Gold
Department of Diabetes
Royal Infirmary of Edinburgh
1 Lauriston Place
Edinburgh EH3 9YW UK

B.M. Frier
as above

26
R.W. Newton
Department of Medicine
Ninewells Hospital and Medical School
Dundee DD1 9SY UK

S.A. Greene
Department of Child Health
Ninewells Hospital and Medical School
Dundee DD1 9SY UK

27
J.M. Steel
Department of Diabetes
Victoria Hospital
Kirkcaldy
Fife KY2 5AH UK

28
A.C. MacCuish
Diabetes Centre
Royal Infirmary
Glasgow G4 0SF Scotland UK

29
J.A. Batch
Royal Children's Hospital
Flemington Road
Parkville, Melbourne
Victoria 3052 Australia

G.A. Werther
as above

30
H.F. Stirling
Department of Child Life and Health
University of Edinburgh
20 Sylvan Place
Edinburgh EH9 1UW UK

C.J.H. Kelnar
as above

31
D.A. Hepburn
Diabetes Unit
Freeman Hospital
Newcastle upon Tyne NE7 7DN UK

J.M. Steel
Department of Diabetes
Victoria Hospital
Kirkcaldy
Fife KY2 5AH UK

32
G.M. Ingersoll
Department of Counseling and Educational Psychology
Indiana University
Bloomington Indiana 47405 USA

M.P. Golden
University of Washington
9805 21st Street
Bellevue WA 98004 USA

33
S. Strang
Department of Paediatrics
John Radcliffe Hospital
Headington
Oxford OX3 9DU UK

34
A. McEvilly
Diabetic Home Care Unit
The Institute of Child Health
The Children's Hospital
Ladywood Middleway
Birmingham B16 8ET UK

35
C. Waine
Director of Primary Care
Sunderland Health Commission
Durham Road
Sunderland SR3 4AF UK

E.A. Staveley
Chesterfield and North Derbyshire Royal Hospital NHS Trust
Calow
Chesterfield 544 58L UK

36
C. Thompson
Department of Medicine
Ninewells Hospital and Medical School
Dundee DD1 9SY Scotland UK

S.A. Greene
Department of Paediatrics
as above

R.W. Newton
Department of Medicine
as above

37
P.G.F. Swift
Children's Hospital
Leicester Royal Infirmary
Leicester LE1 5WW UK

J. North
BDA Health Education Consultant
c/o The British Diabetic Association
10 Queen Anne Street
London W1 0BD UK

S. Redmond
BDA Services Director
c/o The British Diabetic Association
10 Queen Anne Street
London W1 0BD UK

38
P.J. Bingley
Department of Diabetes and Metabolism
St Bartholomew's Hospital
London EC1A 7BE UK

E.A.M. Gale
as above

39
D.J. Becker
Division of Pediatric Endocrinology
Children's Hospital
3705 Fifth Avenue
Pittsburgh PA 15213 USA

T.J. Orchard
Graduate School of Public Health
Department of Epidemiology
University of Pittsburgh
Pittsburgh PA 15213

C.E. Lloyd
as above

40
B.F. Clarke
Department of Diabetes and University Department of Medicine
Royal Infirmary
Edinburgh EH3 9YW Scotland UK

41
R.J. Young
Diabetes and Endocrine Unit
Hope Hospital
Eccles Old Road
Salford
Manchester M6 8HD UK

42
A.B. Kurtz
University College
London Hospitals
NHS Trust
The Middlesex Hospital
Mortimer Street
London W1N 8AA UK

43
G.M. Danielsen
Diabetes Therapy
Novo Nordisk A/S
Novo Allé
2880 Bagsvaerd Denmark

K. Drejer
as above

L. Langkjær
as above

A. Plum
as above

44
J.C. Pickup
Division of Chemical Pathology
United Medical and Dental Schools
Guy's Hospital
London SE1 9RT UK

45
N.J.M. London
Leicester University Department of Surgery
Clinical Sciences Building
Leicester Royal Infirmary
Leicester LE2 7LX UK

G.S.M. Robertson
as above

D. Chadwick
as above

R.F.L. James
as above

P.R.F. Bell
as above

46
Z. Laron
Endocrinology and Diabetes Research Unit
Children's Medical Center of Israel (CMCI)
Beilinson Campus
14 Kaplan Street
Petah Tivka 49202
Sackler School of Medicine
Tel Aviv University
Tel Aviv, Israel

O. Kalter-Leibovici
as above

Foreword

Dr Kelnar and his co-authors have crafted a unique and highly important compendium covering all aspects of diabetes mellitus occurring in the child and adolescent. This is a big book, approximately 600 pages in length, comprising 46 separate chapters which are subdivided into 6 major areas of focus. This is predominantly a product of pediatric endocrinologists and diabetologists in the United Kingdom with 35 of the 46 chapters provided by authors located in the U.K. Eleven of the chapters, each multi-authored, are by prominent diabetes investigators in the United States, Denmark, Australia and Israel.

Part One of this imposing textbook has 7 chapters and covers energy homeostasis in the normal fetus and infant, the growing child and the adolescent. Endocrine alterations associated with the development of diabetes in childhood and adolescence receives special attention. Normal physical growth and development is very carefully reviewed. Two contributions on emotional growth and development complete this section: one chapter focuses on developmental trends in coping mechanisms in children and adolescents while the second specifically focuses on information that relates to the impact of diabetes mellitus on the psychological development of the child and adolescent.

Part Two is composed of 7 very important chapters which lay the groundwork for the understanding of diabetes mellitus. The chapters include an historical review of diabetes and an essential chapter on classification and diagnosis. The epidemiology of diabetes in childhood is covered in depth while the contribution on inheritance and genetics in childhood diabetes is quite brief and focused. The pathology of insulin dependent diabetes mellitus is covered in three chapters, including one on pancreatic morphology and pathology, a chapter on the current understanding of the pathogenesis of childhood diabetes and, finally, a comprehensive discussion of the biochemistry and intermediary metabolism as it relates to diabetes.

Part Three is in many respects the heart of this excellent contribution. In 17 chapters and approximately 250 pages of text this section definitively covers clinical aspects of diabetes in the child and adolescent. Clinical presentation and acute complications are covered in depth. General management issues receive definitive presentation. Special issues surrounding insulin types and regimens, dietary management and the integration of exercise as therapeutic modalities all stand alone in separate chapters. Behavioral issues are covered in two different contributions, one broadly directed to the psychological management of diabetes and the other sharply focused on eating disorders. Special issues like hospital nursing care, children's diabetes clinics, and perioperative management of the diabetic child are useful contributions that are rarely found in available publications. Three special chapters are also worthy of note, including a chapter on unusual forms of diabetes in childhood, neonatal diabetes and a valuable contribution on diabetes mellitus in the pregnant woman and its effect on the fetus and child.

Part Four comprises 6 chapters and provides uniquely important information on the child with diabetes in his society, in the home, in the school and at play, such as in special diabetes camping programs. A further look at mechanisms for care of the child with diabetes in the family are identified through three contributions on nursing care in the home, the importance of the primary care physician, that is, the pediatrician or family practitioner, and new approaches for self-help. All of these chapters are important contributions in an area that has not been well covered in the past.

Part Five is difficult to categorize but is nonetheless highly important. An excellent review of strategies for the prevention of IDDM will bring the reader completely up-to-date in terms of the difficult pragmatic and ethical issues surrounding intervention to prevent diabetes. This is followed by an excellent in-depth review of the interphase between diabetes control and outcome as it relates to the classical chronic vascular complications of diabetes. It is a well done and important review of a vast literature. A practical focus on mechanisms for screening for the evolution of complications in the young person with diabetes takes a practical clinical stand that can be adapted effectively by most practitioners and diabetes clinics. Finally, there is an interesting review of potential approaches to the prevention of complications.

Part Six is the closing section of this text and includes five chapters. A discussion of the new insulins, currently coming into the marketplace or anticipated in the foreseeable future opens this section. The second chapter focuses on imaginative and creative new routes for the delivery of insulin which we can expect to be introduced into management programs in the next decade. The third chapter is a valuable look at the present and future in terms of biosensors and mechanisms for feedback control of blood glucose. An up-to-date review of islet cell transplantation follows and the text is understandably closed with a review of current controversies in the management of the child and adolescent with diabetes.

There is repetition and overlap in this very long and definitive textbook. It is not objectionable: indeed, it is instructive to gain insights into behavioral aspects of childhood diabetes through the expertise of 7 behaviorists and clinicians in five separate contributions. Many of the same clinical care issues are covered in the several chapters in Part Three by different skilled clinicians focusing on different aspects of care and management. The problems of long-term management and complications are also covered in at least four chapters by investigators who bring very special qualifications and particular slants to the analysis and recommendations in this area.

The views of future therapeutic modalities provide encouragement and excitement while the possibility of the prevention of IDDM remains the goal of all of us.

This new textbook on diabetes mellitus in the child and adolescent is an important addition to this literature. It is clearly the most comprehensive text yet developed and covers essentially all significant investigative and clinical issues in a scholarly and up-to-date fashion. It is truly a compendium of information that will serve as a highly valuable resource for physicians working in the field. However, its value is not limited to physicians and diabetologists. Diabetes nurse educators, dietitians and behaviorists will find much of value here.

The field of diabetes mellitus is moving rapidly forward. The scientific and clinical advances that have occurred within the past decade have literally changed management and outcome. This book could not have been written ten years ago. Its publication at this critical point in history will ensure the wide distribution of current knowledge in the field and will lead to better care for children with diabetes mellitus around the world.

Dr Kelnar has produced the textbook that I envisaged was needed. It is a job well done.

Allan L. Drash, MD
Professor of Pediatrics and Epidemiology
University of Pittsburgh School of Medicine

Preface

Dispel not the happy illusions of childhood. – Goethe

At present we are inclined to the belief that more successful results are obtained with regard to the well-being of the patient when a normal blood sugar is aimed at.
Banting, 1923

A child who develops diabetes can now, potentially, lead a full, healthy and happy life with insulin therapy. Nevertheless, many still have a life expectancy reduced by 25% or more and many have a quality of life which is far from ideal and sometimes wretched even during childhood and adolescence let alone following the onset of disabling complications in young adulthood. The stresses and strains on family life can also be disastrous for parents and nondiabetic siblings.

Between 1914 and 1922 (the era of starvation therapy) the life expectancy of diabetic patients at the Joslin Clinic was 6.1 years. By 1950 to 1957, it had increased to 18.2 years. In young diabetics (<30 years old at onset) the 1.3 year life expectancy after diagnosis had increased to 2.9 years with the introduction of starvation therapy and by 1957, 35 years after the introduction of insulin, to 26.4 years.

There have been many less dramatic but important developments in recent years such as the concept of self-care, self-care aids such as home blood glucose monitoring sticks, objective measures of control such as glycosylated hemoglobin, new modes of insulin delivery such as infusion pumps and insulin pens, human insulin and insulin mixtures. Not all developments have been advances and beneficial. The diabetic 'way of life' still imposes great strain and discomfort on many children and their families.

In 1965, Sir Derrick Dunlop opening a diabetes mellitus symposium in Edinburgh asked 'Is the occurrence of these complications [retinopathy, nephropathy, neuropathy, coronary and peripheral angiopathy] to be regarded fatalistically as something inherent in the diabetic process . . . or can they be postponed by care and trouble directed to the control of the metabolic disturbance?'

It has taken nearly another 30 years to provide the answer. There is now irrefutable epidemiological evidence (at least in those aged 13 years or over) from the American 10-year prospective Diabetes Control and Complications Trial (DCCT) that if good glycemic control is achieved in the long term, the risks of microangiopathic complications (retinopathy, nephropathy and neuropathy) are greatly reduced. The question is not now why or whether to maintain good diabetic control but how.

Many other questions remain. Pediatricians seldom see the complications that they silently bequeath with their patients to adult diabetologists. What level of glycemic control in childhood and adolescence constitutes 'good' or 'good enough' control? Is the prevention of complications by the establishment of good control in childhood and adolescence a realistic goal? How is it to be achieved in the context of normal physical and emotional growth and 'normal' daily activities and family life-style? Will this be at the expense of more hypoglycemia? If so, how often must there be hypoglycemia and how low must the blood glucose be in children of different ages before is it damaging to long-term cognitive functioning? Does more education or learning new or improved skills by patients and clinicians necessarily lead to better control? The risks for macrovascular disease seem unaffected by tight glycemic control. The St Vincent and ISPAD Declarations (see Appendices) seek to achieve the maximum quality of life for our patients with diabetes through the efficient use of available resources. How is this to be done in the context of dwindling health care resources in many 'developed' countries, let alone in parts of the world (including even Eastern Europe) where insulin itself is unavailable.

Perhaps the single most important relevant message from the DCCT for children is that young people with diabetes and their families can work together in partnership with the support of a variety of health care professionals towards the shared aim of improving control in the context of improved quality of life.

There are many professionals whose skills are vital for supporting the efforts of the family in whom there is a boy or girl with diabetes, and encouraging the gradual and appropriate development of self-care by the child. This attempt to achieve optimal glycemic control in the context of normal physical and emotional growth must involve a multidisciplinary team of doctors, nurses and dieticians; this is reflected in the contributors represented in this volume.

There is specific and comprehensive coverage of:

- the background to childhood and adolescent diabetes in terms of normal childhood and pubertal growth, endocrine interactions and maturation during childhood (including a separate section on normal glycemic control), and normal psychological development – paying particular attention to the contexts in which diabetes impinges on childhood in growth, endocrine and psychological terms;
- the nature of insulin-dependent diabetes in terms of epidemiology, pathogenesis, immunopathology and biochemistry and intermediate metabolism;
- clinical presentation and all aspects of treatment and clinical care including chapters on associated disorders and unusual (including neonatal) diabetes;
- the child with diabetes in the context of the family, school, primary carers, liaison nursing team, and evaluation of diabetic camps and self-help groups;
- maternal diabetes and the fetus;
- epidemiological and clinical aspects of control and outcome in terms of complications and with screening;
- current controversies;
- future developments in terms of new insulins, new routes and means of insulin delivery, biosensors and biofeedback systems, the prevention of complications and progress in terms of preventing diabetes itself. The prevention of complications and even the prevention of diabetes are now moving from being inconceivable to realistically attainable future goals.

Contributors include pediatric diabetologists from the UK, the US, Israel and Australia and adult diabetologists from the UK and Scandinavia. There are contributions to specific sections from specialists in primary care, genetics, pathology, biochemistry, anesthesiology, liaison- and hospital-based nursing, dietetics and child and family psychology and psychiatry.

The varying perspectives of the contributors will inevitably lead to some overlap and also to differing opinions on particular topics. I have not tried to edit this into a spurious and anemic uniformity and have, on the contrary, encouraged the personal approach as well as the comprehensive review. Although terminology and spelling are, generally, according to American usage, Systems Internationale (SI) units have been used throughout. For convenience, 'conventional' units have been added in parentheses in Chapter 15.

I hope that this book will be a valuable resource for all who look after children and adolescents with diabetes. Whilst primarily intended for doctors – pediatric diabetologists, general pediatricians, adult diabetologists, general practitioners and child and family psychiatrists – I hope that it will be an important source of reference for others involved in diabetic care including dieticians and liaison nurse specialists both in the UK and internationally.

I am grateful to my many contributors, to Professor Allan Drash for writing the Foreword, and to Annalisa Page of Chapman & Hall who has guided and cajoled me (and them) to what I hope has been good effect. I could not have edited this multi-author international textbook without the support of my wife and children, in this as in everything that I undertake. To them a special thank you for their forbearance – and for making it all worthwhile.

Christopher J.H. Kelnar
Edinburgh
August 1994

PART ONE

1

Glucose homeostasis in the normal fetus and infant

J.M. HAWDON and M.P. WARD PLATT

1.1 INTRODUCTION

Glucose homeostasis is an ability which may normally be taken for granted in the adult and child and is only seriously disturbed by failure of insulin secretion in diabetes mellitus and in certain other rare metabolic and endocrine diseases. By contrast, this ability cannot be assumed in the newborn baby, which for a variety of reasons finds itself in a precarious metabolic state in the hours and days following birth. Babies born small for gestational age or more than 4 weeks early have even greater problems with blood glucose control.

An understanding of glucose homeostasis in the newborn infant requires first an appreciation of the homeostatic mechanisms in the fetus, and second, a knowledge of the relationships of glucose to the production and consumption of other fuels and substrates in infancy. The initiation of feeding and its metabolic and endocrine effects, mediated through the entero-insular and entero-hepatic axes, are unique physiologic events which are increasingly acknowledged to have profound and permanent effects on metabolism in later life (Lucas, 1991). However the mechanisms of this 'programming' are not fully understood and are beyond the scope of this chapter.

It is the intention in this chapter first to review fetal glucose homeostasis, then to describe the immediate adaptive changes consequent to birth, and finally to focus on the newborn infant in the early neonatal period, about which most is known. The emphasis will be upon glucose as an important, but not exclusive, element in infantile fuel metabolism, and the control of the fuel economy will be examined in terms of the influences of enzymes, hormones, and the substrates themselves.

1.2 FETAL BLOOD GLUCOSE HOMEOSTASIS

1.2.1 FETAL FUELS

During pregnancy, the fetus receives from the mother, via the placental circulation, a supply of substrates necessary for growth, for the deposition of fuel stores, and for energy to meet the basal metabolic rate and requirements for growth. Maternal hormonal changes in the second half of pregnancy ensure availability of such substrates. In the mother there is relative insulin resistance

Childhood and Adolescent Diabetes
Published in 1994 by Chapman & Hall, London
ISBN 0 412 48610 5

and increased secretion of hormones which antagonize insulin (human placental lactogen, estrogen, progesterone and cortisol) so that glucose is spared for fetal requirements; there is rapid maternal metabolism of fatty acids.

Studies of fetal metabolism have been hindered by the invasiveness of the necessary techniques, so that much information comes from the study of fetal animals. Some additional information is now available from clinical studies of the human fetus, using the methods of fetoscopy and fetal blood sampling. Interpretation of all these studies must take into account interspecies differences, variations with gestational age, and the effects of stress on fetal metabolism. However, it has been possible to gain some understanding of human fetal metabolism, as outlined below.

During pregnancy, the fetus deposits stores of glycogen and adipose tissue that can subsequently be mobilized when exogenous supplies do not meet energy requirements, notably in the period between birth and the first feed. Glycogen is deposited in the fetal liver such that the concentration at term is 80–100 mg/g liver and triglycerides are deposited in adipose tissue amounting to about 160 g/kg body weight by term (Adam, 1971).

At the same time as deposition of fuel stores occurs, the fetus has an ongoing energy requirement for growth and metabolism. This is supplied, in the healthy fetus, by aerobic metabolism, with glucose accounting for 65% of fetal oxygen consumption (Hay & Sparks, 1985). Fetal erythrocytes, renal cortex and adrenal medulla are obligate consumers of glucose, while it appears that the fetal brain can utilize glucose and ketone bodies (Adam *et al.*, 1975; Battaglia & Hay, 1984).

Glucose is transported across the placenta to the fetus, by facilitated diffusion, at a rate which is dependent on maternal blood glucose concentration, but independent of uterine blood flow (Hay *et al.*, 1984; Haugel *et al.*, 1986; Hay & Meznarich, 1989). Fetal glucose uptake, calculated to be 4–6 mg/kg/min, is similar to the glucose turnover rate of the neonate. The relationship between maternal and fetal blood glucose concentrations appears to vary with gestational age in the human fetus. At mid-term, there is a 1:1 relationship, while by late gestation, the maternal glucose concentration is higher than that of the fetus (Battaglia & Hay, 1984; Aynsley-Green *et al.*, 1985; Bozzetti *et al.*, 1988). Using stable isotope dilution techniques, it has been demonstrated that, under certain circumstances, when placental glucose transport may be reduced, there is glucose production from other substrates, such as glycerol, lactate and amino acids, by the human fetus (Hay *et al.*, 1983; Milner, 1984; Hay *et al.*, 1984; Hay & Sparks, 1985).

1.2.2 THE CONTROL OF FETAL METABOLISM

As in postnatal life, antenatal fetal metabolism is under hormonal control and, although there are some differences before and after birth, the fetus can regulate its own blood glucose concentration, independently of maternal hormones.

α and β cells are present in the human fetal pancreas from 9 and 10 weeks gestation, respectively (Van Assche *et al.*, 1984). Insulin and glucagon are present in human fetal plasma from 12 weeks gestation, and are thought to play a major role in stimulating growth. There is evidence that β-cell growth and insulin secretion occur in response to exogenous substrates such as amino acids and glucose (Adam, 1971; Milner, 1972; Van Assche *et al.*, 1984; Otonoski *et al.*, 1988). In early gestation, insulin has little apparent effect on glucose metabolism, and at 12–20 weeks gestation there is no relationship between circulating glucose and insulin levels. However, during the third trimester, circulating insulin levels and numbers of insulin receptors increase, in association with glycogen deposition in skeletal and cardiac muscle, and protein and fat synthesis (Shelley *et al.*, 1975). There is a relationship between human fetal glucose and insulin levels during fetal hyperglycemia at term, although the insulin response to hyperglycemia is blunted when compared to mature subjects (Obershain *et al.*, 1970).

Glucagon is present in the human fetal pancreas from 7 weeks gestation, and release occurs from 8–20 weeks (Milner, 1984). *In vitro* studies of fetal rat pancreas suggest that glucagon secretion is sensitive to exogenous amino acids and adrenaline, although *in vivo* studies suggest that fetal glucagon release is independent of blood glucose concentration, and is not stimulated by insulin (Shelley *et al.*, 1975; Ogata *et al.*, 1988). Studies in human fetal subjects provide evidence that fetal glucagon secretion, at term, occurs in response to exogenous amino acids. Like insulin, glucagon appears to have few metabolic effects in early fetal life. Fetal glucagon receptor numbers and affinity are less than for adults, and administration of high doses of glucagon is required to bring about fetal glucose mobilization. In addition, fetal glucagon administration does not induce ketone body production, as it does in mature subjects (Phillipps *et al.*, 1983; Sperling *et al.*, 1984). However, sensitivity to glucagon increases with gestational age.

Corticosteroids cross the placenta, and are manufactured by placental tissue. There is also an intact fetal pituitary-adrenal axis, with the secretion of glucocorticoids by fetal adrenals early in gestation, which increases markedly at term. However, fetal cortisol concentrations are not affected by blood glucose concentration (Solomon *et al.*, 1967; Shelley *et al.*, 1975). Glucocorticoids may be important in the regulation of glycogen synthesis by the fetal liver (Shelley *et al.*, 1975).

Finally, growth hormone is present in fetal plasma from 9 weeks of gestation, but is unlikely to play a major role in fetal glucose homeostasis (Adam, 1971; Browne & Thorburn, 1989). Fetal thyroid hormones are thought to have an indirect effect on metabolism by controlling enzyme synthesis at term (Shelley *et al.*, 1975; Browne & Thorburn, 1989).

1.3 METABOLIC CHANGES AT BIRTH

Multi-system changes must occur at birth to allow the infant's independent existence. Metabolic adaptation is important to preserve fuel supplies for vital organ function when the continuous flow of nutrients, mainly glucose, through the placenta is abruptly discontinued. In addition, infants must adapt to milk feeds, whose main caloric source is fat, and to the fast-feed cycle.

Animal studies have provided a model for the changes seen in human subjects at birth. After birth, before feeding is established, changes in insulin, glucagon and other counter-regulatory hormones allow substrates to be mobilized to sustain neonatal fuel supply (Blazquez *et al.*, 1974). Levels of glucagon and glucagon receptor numbers rise rapidly, while insulin levels and numbers of insulin receptors fall. In human subjects, the insulin:glucagon ratio falls rapidly at birth. There is a rapid rise in epinephrine and norepinephrine concentrations at birth, and these catecholamines appear to have both direct metabolic effects, and secondary effects via the release of glucagon from the pancreas (Shelley *et al.*, 1975). Cortisol and growth hormone levels also rise at birth, and may influence enzyme synthesis and lipid metabolism, while the catecholamines, glucagon and thyroid hormones provide the final stimulus for the induction of enzyme activity (Shelley *et al.*, 1975).

These hormonal changes control the metabolic changes which ensure fuel supply after birth. Glycogen is released from hepatic stores, lipolysis occurs in adipose tissue, and gluconeogenesis must occur to ensure glucose supply when hepatic glycogen is exhausted. During labor, the fetal organs, in particular the heart, have a limited capacity for anaerobic glycolysis, but the process is inefficient in terms of glucose utilization, and leads to lactate accumulation if hypoxia persists.

Catecholamines and glucagon activate the enzymes responsible for lipolysis, resulting in an early postnatal rise in levels of glycerol and free fatty acids, so that fat replaces glucose as the main energy source. These hormones also induce the enzymes of glycogenolysis. In order to enhance gluconeogenic capacity, glucagon also induces the enzymes of gluconeogenesis and fatty acid oxidation, the latter being an important source of energy and co-factors for gluconeogenesis.

1.4 NEONATAL BLOOD GLUCOSE HOMEOSTASIS

There is now an extensive knowledge, from the study of human neonates and those of other species, regarding the various factors which control neonatal blood glucose homeostasis. It has also become apparent that, unlike healthy adults, neonates may have labile blood glucose concentrations, even at full-term or when clinically stable. Low blood glucose concentrations are common in breast-fed term infants (Hawdon *et al.*, 1992). Many preterm infants, especially those who are very small or clinically stressed, become hyperglycemic, although this condition differs from the adult diabetic state in that it is transient, is not always associated with low plasma insulin levels, is usually rapidly responsive to reductions in glucose infusion rates, and is neither associated with ketosis nor an osmotic diuresis (Pagliara *et al.*, 1973; Lowick *et al.*, 1985; Stonestreet *et al.*, 1980).

The following discussion will focus on normal patterns of neonatal metabolic adaptation, but much of the present understanding of neonatal blood glucose homeostasis comes from the study of babies with disordered blood glucose homeostasis.

1.4.1 NEONATAL FUELS AND THEIR INTERRELATIONSHIPS

In the neonatal period, oxidation of glucose, fatty acids and ketone bodies provides energy for basal metabolism, physical activity, thermogenesis and continued growth. Milk feeds provide fatty acids, which are utilized as fuels, but, during periods of fasting, fuel availability must be maintained by the processes of glycogenolysis, gluconeogenesis, lipolysis and β-oxidation of fatty acids.

During the first few postnatal hours, breakdown of hepatic glycogen provides glucose at a rate of about 2 mg/kg/min (Bougneres, 1987). However, this is insufficient for the infant's needs, and hepatic glycogen stores, even in the healthy, well-grown, term infant, are soon exhausted. Therefore, gluconeogenesis must occur if hypoglycemia is to be avoided.

When exogenous sources of glucose are not available, the normal newborn infant has the capacity to produce glucose from carbon skeletons provided by lactate, pyruvate, amino acids (particularly alanine), and glycerol (Frazer *et al.*, 1981; Gleason *et al.*, 1985; Bougneres *et al.*, 1982; Snell & Walker, 1973) (Figure 1.1). It is thought that lactate is the precursor for 33% of glucose production, alanine for 5–10%, and glycerol for 5–7% (Bougneres, 1987). Data from studies which have calculated glucose production rates are shown in Table 1.1. The variation in results may be the consequence of variation in clinical status of the subjects, administration of enteral or parenteral feeds and fluids, or the use of different isotopes and analytical methods.

Neonatal glucose metabolism cannot be

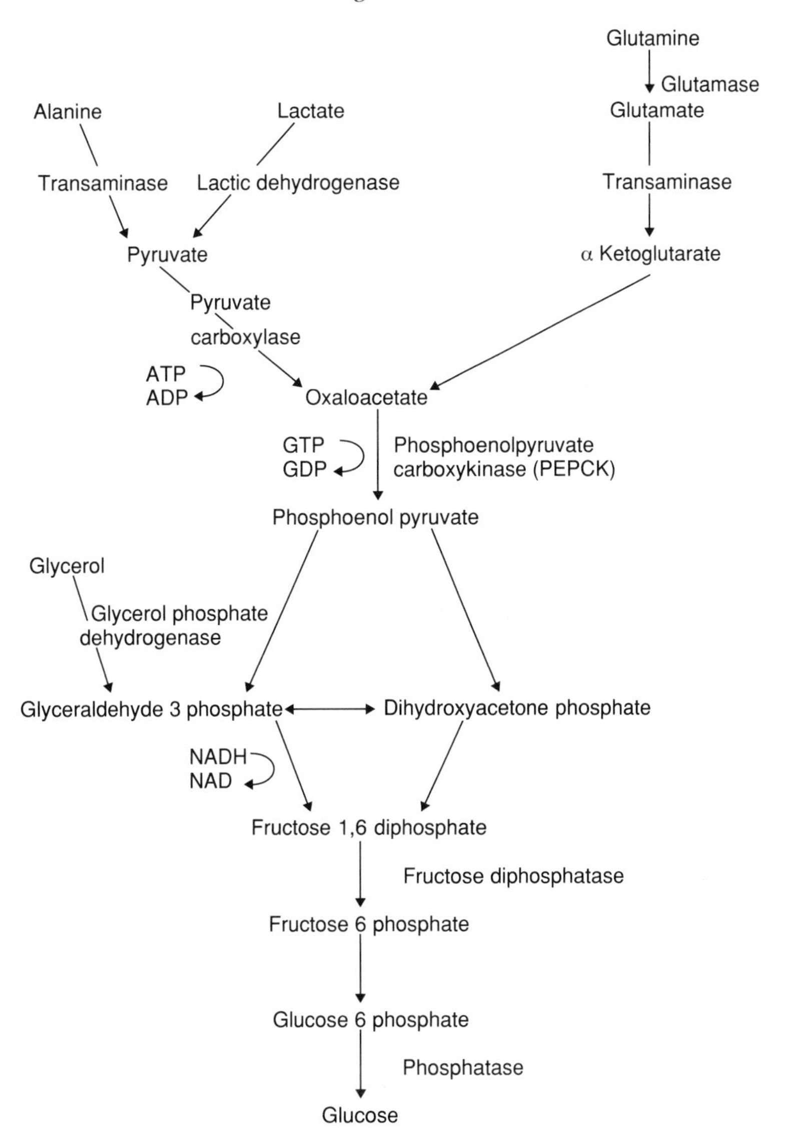

Figure 1.1 The gluconeogenic pathway.

considered in isolation. Fatty acid release from adipose tissue is controlled by the availability of glucose, and the provision of exogenous fat may increase blood glucose concentrations (Adam, 1971; Ferre *et al.*, 1978; Viliasis *et al.*, 1982; Savich *et al.*, 1985). The mechanism by which fatty acid oxidation supports gluconeogenesis is by the provision of energy and co-factors. Hepatic fatty acid oxidation provides energy for the conversion of pyruvate to glucose via the gluconeogenic pathway, acetyl CoA which activates pyruvate carboxylase, NADH which displaces the reversible glyceraldehyde-3-phosphate dehydrogenase reaction in the direction of gluconeogenesis, and carbon

Table 1.1 Calculated mean neonatal glucose production rates.

Author	Subjects	Rate (mg/kg/min)
Kalhan *et al.*,	Term 2 hours	4.4
1976	Term 1 day	3.8
Bier *et al.*,	Term	6.1
1977	Preterm	5.5
Kalhan *et al.*,	Term	4.5
1980		
Cowett *et al.*,	Term	7.7
1985	Preterm	8.1
Gilfillan *et al.*,	AGA fed	4.2
1985	AGA unfed	3.2
	SGA fed	3.2
Bougneres *et al.*, 1986	Term	6.5

AGA = appropriate for gestational age.
SEA = small for gestational age.

Table 1.2 Mean blood glucose and ketone body (KB) concentrations (mmol/l).

Author	Age	Glucose	KB
Term:			
Persson & Tunnell,	1 min	3.30	0.18
1971	120 mins	3.30	0.07
Stanley *et al.*, 1979	<8 hrs	3.17	0.34
Bougneres *et al.*, 1982	1 day	3.44	0.10
Hawdon *et al.*, 1992	<4 hrs	3.20	0.05
	12–24 hrs	3.50	0.25
	2 days	3.50	0.41
	3 days	3.40	0.43
	4 days	4.10	0.10
	5 days	4.0	0.08
Preterm:			
Stanley *et al.*, 1979	<8 hrs	2.06	0.31
Hawdon *et al.*, 1992	<4 hrs	2.50	0.05
	2 days	4.50	0.03
	3 days	4.10	0.04
	4 days	4.10	0.06
	5 days	5.70	0.04

atoms for the oxaloacetate-malate and dihydroxyacetone phosphate pools (Ferre *et al.*, 1979; Girard, 1986; Hay & Sparks, 1985) (Figure 1.1). Oxidation of medium chain fatty acids results in a high rate of ketogenesis and thus gluconeogenesis (Ferre *et al.*, 1981; Frost & Wells, 1981). In turn, ketone bodies are alternative fuels to glucose for neonatal metabolism, even in the absence of hypoglycemia (Edmond *et al.*, 1985; Bougneres *et al.*, 1986). Calculated neonatal ketone body turnover rates after a 4-hour fast, 13–22 μmol/kg/min, are the same as those achieved by adults after prolonged starvation, and, compared to adults, neonates have an increased capacity for ketone body utilization (Bougneres *et al.*, 1986).

It is clear that differences exist between the circulating concentrations and interrelationships of metabolic fuels in neonates and in adults and older children. Concentrations of glucose and ketone bodies found in various neonatal studies are shown in Table 1.2. The table demonstrates that the concentrations of these fuels, and their interrelationships, may vary with the gestational age, postnatal age and clinical status of the baby. In addition, since many of the older studies were performed, there have been changes in clinical practices, for example regarding infant feeding, which may influence results. The most recent study has examined the concentrations of metabolic fuels in a homogenous group of infants, managed according to current feeding practices, and has investigated variations with postnatal and gestational ages (Hawdon *et al.*, 1992). Blood glucose concentrations fall after birth, then rise gradually, even in infants who are fasted for up to 12 hours after birth (Table 1.2). Blood ketone body concentrations are also low after birth, even when blood glucose concentrations are low, but subsequently may be as high as those found in adults after prolonged fasting (Stanley *et al.*, 1979; Kraus *et al.*, 1974; Hawdon *et al.*, 1992).

The relationship between blood glucose and ketone body concentrations is important as an indicator of the ability of the infant to mount a counter-regulatory ketogenic response to low blood glucose concentrations. Table 1.2 demonstrates that many term neonates have blood glucose concentrations that would be considered 'hypoglycemic' by adult standards. However, it has been shown that like older subjects, healthy term infants have high blood ketone body concentrations when blood glucose levels are low, and this may be the protective mechanism whereby the cerebral function of these babies is not influenced by hypoglycemia (Hawdon *et al.*, 1992) (Figure 1.2). There is evidence from

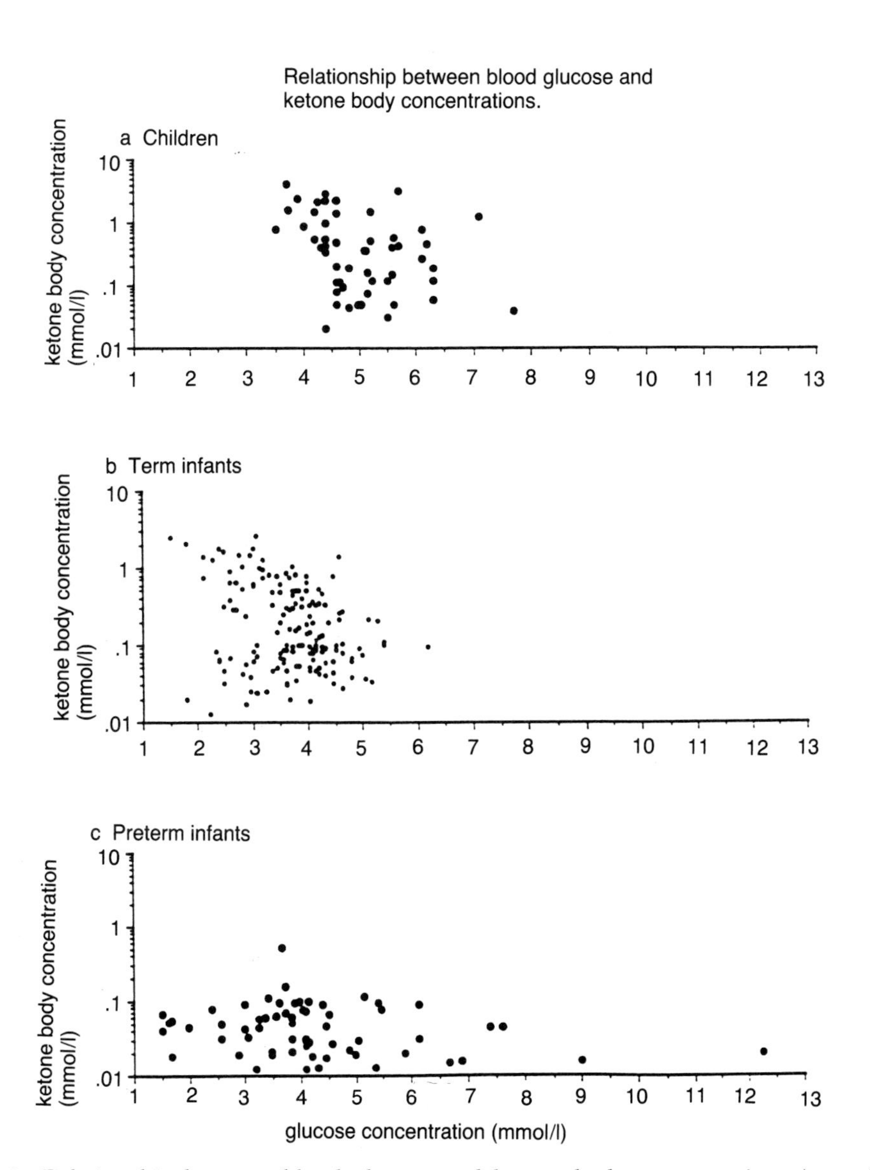

Figure 1.2 Relationship between blood glucose and ketone body concentrations (reproduced with permission of *Archives of Disease in Childhood*).

studies of human neonates, and those of other species, that ketone bodies are preferentially utilized by the neonatal brain (Settegren *et al.*, 1976; Kraus *et al.*, 1974; Levitsky *et al.*, 1973; Edmond *et al.*, 1985).

Therefore, for healthy, term babies who are capable of mounting a ketogenic response to low blood glucose concentrations, measuring blood glucose concentrations alone may give a misleading indication of fuel availability. However, it should be noted that some groups of infants, such as those who are preterm or small for gestational age, do not mount a counter-regulatory ketogenic response, and in these infants maintenance of adequate circulating blood glucose concentrations is likely to be of greater importance than for the term infant. This also demonstrates that a single definition for hypoglycemia cannot be widely applied in neonatal practice. However, discussion of neonatal hypoglycemia and failure of metabolic adaptation after birth is beyond the range of this chapter, which relates only to blood glucose homeostasis in healthy subjects.

1.4.2 THE CONTROL OF NEONATAL METABOLISM

1.4.2.1 Enzyme-mediated control

The processes of postnatal metabolic adaptation, whereby the infant generates glucose and alternative fuels, are influenced by changes in the levels and activities of the enzymes involved in metabolic pathways. Glycogenolysis, occurring almost immediately after birth, is the result of an increase in hepatic phosphorylase activity along with a decrease in the activity of glycogen synthetase D, both of which occur just before term (Hetenyi & Cowan, 1980).

Gluconeogenesis is influenced by the activity of many enzymes, including pyruvate carboxylase, phosphoenolpyruvate carboxykinase (PEPCK), glucose 6 phosphatase and fructose 1,6 diphosphatase (Figure 1.1). Aminotransferases provide carbon skeletons from amino acids. PEPCK is the rate-limiting enzyme for gluconeogenesis, both in adult and neonatal subjects (Hanson & Garber, 1972; Cake *et al.*, 1971).

It appears that both gestational maturity and the birth process itself affect the activity of these enzymes (Marsac *et al.*, 1976; Yeung & Oliver, 1968). In the human neonate, pyruvate carboxylase activity increases soon after birth and fructose diphosphatase activity doubles by the fifteenth postnatal day. PEPCK activity at birth is 0–25% adult values, and increases to a maximum at 4–5 postnatal days (Girard, 1986; Hetenyi & Cowan, 1980; Marsac *et al.*, 1976). Animal studies have demonstrated that, after birth, rates of gluconeogenesis parallel these changes in enzyme activity (Phillippidis & Ballard, 1970; Pearce *et al.*, 1974; Parameswaran & Arinze, 1981). However, there are no studies which relate enzyme activity to gluconeogenic capacity in human neonates.

Mitochondrial fatty acid oxidation depends upon carnitine and the carnitine acyl transferase enzymes for the transport of fatty acids into the cell and mitochondrion. Animal studies have demonstrated that the increased capacity for fatty acid oxidation after birth is not simply secondary to a reduction in lipogenesis, but also to increased activity of these enzymes (Ferre *et al.*, 1983; Bailey & Lockwood, 1973; Quant *et al.*, 1990; Prip-Buus *et al.*, 1990). Again, these relationships between enzyme activity and metabolism are still to be confirmed in human neonatal subjects.

1.4.2.2 Hormone-mediated control

The main glucoregulatory hormones in adult subjects are insulin and glucagon, but there is some disagreement over their relative roles in the neonatal period (Tse *et al.*, 1983; Blazquez *et al.*, 1974). Some authors maintain that insulin is the major glucoregulatory hormone, although this conclusion is based mainly on studies of neonatal animals, rather than human subjects (Susa *et al.*, 1979; Cowett & Tenenbaum, 1985). Others support the key role of glucagon in human neonatal metabolic adaptation (Sperling *et al.*, 1976). In truth, it is illogical to consider the actions of these hormones separately, and their concentrations relative to one another should be considered. The insulin : glucagon ratio falls from 10 in the fetus to 0.5 after birth, and this appears to be essential for the postnatal changes in gluconeogenic capacity (Girard, 1986). It should also be remembered that each of these hormones may influence the secretion of the other, and that other hormones, such as the catecholamines may also influence their secretion and activity. However, these interrelationships have not been explored fully in neonates.

There appear to be some differences between neonates and older subjects in terms of pancreatic structure, patterns of insulin secretion, and cellular response (Falorni *et al.*, 1974; Shelley *et al.*, 1975; Van Assche *et al.*, 1984, Gamara *et al.*, 1979; Gentz *et al.*, 1969). The relationships between insulin secretion and neonatal glucose homeostasis have recently been investigated more extensively (Hawdon *et al.*, 1993a & b). While a positive relationship between plasma insulin and blood glucose concentrations was demonstrated for healthy term and preterm infants, neonatal insulin levels were higher than those of older children, and were often unexpectedly high at low blood glucose concentrations (Figure 1.3). In another group of neonates, with disordered blood glucose homeostasis, there was no relationship between plasma insulin and blood glucose concentrations, nor between glucose production rates and plasma insulin concentrations. This suggests that insulin-mediated control of hepatic glucose production is lost in such infants.

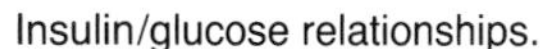

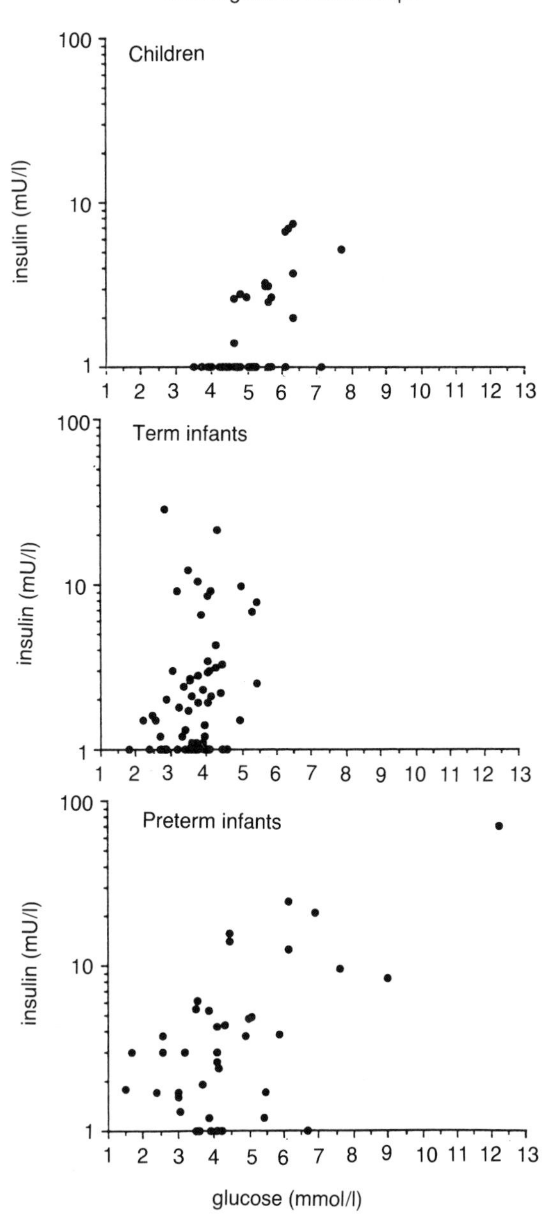

Figure 1.3 Insulin/glucose relationships.

Surges in plasma glucagon levels at birth and 2–3 days after birth have been demonstrated, attaining levels which are higher than those seen in adults. Neonatal glucagon secretion has been shown to increase in response to low blood glucose concentrations, enteral milk feeding and intravenous amino acid administration, although it is unclear whether secretion is suppressed by high blood glucose concentrations (Sperling *et al.*, 1974; Sann *et al.*, 1978; Fiser *et al.*, 1975; Sperling, 1982, Grasso *et al.*, 1983). A recent study of neonates with disordered blood glucose homeostasis has demonstrated that glucagon concentrations were higher during hypoglycemia than during hyperglycemia, suggesting an appropriate pancreatic glucagon secretory response to the extremes of blood glucose concentration (Hawdon *et al.*, 1993b).

There have been many animal studies which have demonstrated the mechanism of action of glucagon. The glycemic effect is the result partly of stimulation of glycogenolysis immediately after birth, and partly induction of gluconeogenic enzyme synthesis (Garcia-Ruiz *et al.*, 1978; Girard *et al.*, 1975; Beale *et al.*, 1984; Cimbala *et al.*, 1982; Lyonnet *et al.*, 1988). Glucagon also promotes substrate availability by releasing amino acids from muscle and stimulating lipolysis. Finally, glucagon may play a role in neonatal ketone body production (Schade & Eaton, 1975; Prip-Buus *et al.*, 1990). Although there have been no similar studies of the human neonate, it has been assumed that the same mechanisms apply.

Catecholamines are released in large quantities at birth, and to higher levels after complicated deliveries than after normal vaginal delivery or elective caesarean section (Sperling *et al.*, 1984; Leonetti *et al.*, 1980; Lagercrantz & Bistoletti, 1977; Padbury & Martinez, 1988). Catecholamines are thought to play a major role in the metabolic events after birth. They initiate glycogenolysis and lipolysis. However, it has recently been demonstrated that there is a reduced and poorly-coordinated catecholamine response to hypoglycemia in neonates, when compared to the adult counter-regulatory response, and animal studies have demonstrated that the neonatal glycemic response to these hormones is less than that of adults (Hawdon *et al.*, 1993c; Cowett, 1988).

Growth hormone levels are very high at birth, and fall gradually to basal levels by 6 days for term babies, and 24 days for preterm babies (Adrian *et al.*, 1983). Secretion increases postprandially and in response to hypoglycemia and hyperglycemia, but, unlike adults, neonates do not appear to have a growth hormone stress response (Milner & Wright, 1967; Adrian *et al.*, 1983; Shelley *et al.*, 1975; Stubbe & Wolfe, 1971).

The human neonate is capable of independently secreting glucocorticoids, with peak levels occurring a few hours after birth (Sippell *et al.*, 1978; Rokicki *et al.*, 1990). However, preterm neonates and some term babies, are unable to mount an appropriate coordinated cortisol secretory response to hypoglycemia or to other stresses (Anand *et al.*, 1984; Hughes *et al.*, 1987; Hawdon *et al.*, 1993c). Because there is a sequential maturation of the glucocorticoid synthesis pathways it is important to measure biologically active precursors as well as cortisol itself. Animal studies suggest that cortisol plays a role in the synthesis of aminotransferases and the initiation, but not maintenance, of neonatal gluconeogenesis, and administration of exogenous glucocorticoids to human neonates results in a small, unsustained rise in blood glucose concentration (Shelley *et al.*, 1975; Townsend *et al.*, 1989; Price *et al.*, 1976).

There is also a surge of thyroid-stimulating hormone secretion at birth. This results in high circulating levels of thyroid hormones, which persist for the first postnatal week. However, the specific role of thyroid hormones in neonatal metabolic adaptation is not known.

1.4.2.3 Substrate-mediated control

There is increasing evidence that, in addition to hormonal and enzymatic controls, the availability of metabolic substrates, administered enterally or intravenously, affects the metabolic changes seen in the neonatal period.

Milk feeds provide a limited supply of carbohydrate in the form of lactose which is hydrolyzed in the intestine to glucose and galactose. Glucose uptake from the portal circulation is low, so that it is spared for peripheral use, while galactose is completely taken up by the liver where it is converted to glucose or glycogen (Kliegman & Sparks, 1985). Breast milk contains lipase which enhances the conversion of triglycerides to non-esterified fatty acids, which will be transported preferentially to the liver for fatty acid oxidation and ketogenesis (Poland *et al.*, 1980). Thus, the major fuels provided by milk are fat-based. In particular, medium chain triglycerides are abundant in breast milk and some artificial formulae. Therefore, the ability of the neonate to utilize fatty fuels is an important part of neonatal metabolic adaptation.

Enteral feeding influences hormone secretion. First, there is a response to each feed, with postprandial surges in a number of hormones such as insulin, growth hormone, and the gut hormones, gastrin, enteroglucagon, secretin, motilin and neurotensin (Aynsley-Green, 1985). Second, enteral feeding itself may induce the mature pattern of gut hormone secretion. These responses are seen in the early postnatal period in term neonates, occur later in preterm neonates, and not at all in infants deprived of enteral nutrition (Lucas *et al.*, 1983). Third, different feeding methods and feed compositions affect gut hormone secretion (Lucas *et al.*, 1982; Aynsley-Green, 1985; Lucas *et al.*, 1985; Adrian *et al.*, 1983; Aynsley-Green *et al.*, 1979).

Feeding practices may also affect blood concentrations of glucose and other fuels, which, in turn, may be secondary to the effects of the gut hormones on glucoregulatory hormone secretion (the entero-insular axis). Cyclical changes are seen in blood glucose concentrations in response to feeding (Aynsley-Green *et al.*, 1977; Siegel *et al.*, 1988). Our recent study has shown that breast-fed infants have lower blood glucose concentrations than formula-fed infants in the first postnatal week, but that breast-fed infants have higher ketone body concentrations, and a greater ketogenic response to low blood glucose concentrations (Hawdon *et al.*, 1992).

1.5 SUMMARY

Despite total dependence on fuel supply via the placental circulation, the fetus exerts considerable control over its own metabolism, apportioning fuels and energy for growth and for organ function. Although the emphasis is on anabolism, the fetus is capable of releasing fuel from stores if exogenous supply fails, and thus maintains glucose homeostasis. This metabolic homeostasis is achieved by fetal hormone secretion.

At birth, there is a reversal of this situation. There are no immediate exogenous fuel sources, and to maintain organ function, the neonate must generate fuels for itself. Subsequently, the healthy neonate must adapt to the fast-feed cycle, and to the provision of fat-based fuels, as opposed to glucose which was the main fuel supplied to the fetus. These changes are mediated by alterations in enzyme activity, which are themselves under hormonal control.

Neonatal glucose homeostasis appears to differ from that of adults and children in that circulating blood glucose concentrations are lower. However, it has been demonstrated that glucose is not the sole source of energy for the neonate, and some organs, such as the brain, preferentially utilize ketone bodies. Therefore, in the healthy term neonate, low blood levels of glucose may be of less clinical significance than in older individuals. Neonatal glucose homeostasis must therefore be considered in the context of the many processes of metabolic adaptation which occur after birth.

REFERENCES

Adam, P.A.J. (1971) Control of glucose metabolism in the human fetus and newborn infant. *Adv. Metab. Disord.*, **5**, 183–275.

Adam, P.A.J., Raiha, N., Rahiala, E.L. *et al.* (1975) Oxidation of glucose and β-hydroxybutyrate by the early human fetal brain. *Acta Paed. Scand.*, **64**, 17–24.

Adrian, T.E., Lucas, A., Bloom, S.R. *et al.* (1983) Growth hormone response to feeding in term and preterm neonates. *Acta Paed. Scand.*, **72**, 251–54.

Anand, K.J.S., Brown, M., Bloom, S.R. *et al.* (1984) The metabolic and endocrine response of neonates to surgical stress. *Ped. Res.*, **18**, 1207.

Aynsley-Green, A. (1985) Metabolic and endocrine interrelationships in the human fetus and neonate. *Am. J. Clin. Nutr.*, **41** (suppl. 2), 399–417.

Aynsley-Green, A., Lucas, A., Bloom, S.R. *et al.* (1977) Endocrine and metabolic response in the newborn to the first feed of human milk. *Arch. Dis. Child.*, **52**, 291–95.

Aynsley-Green, A., Lucas, A. and Bloom, S.R. (1979) The effects of feeds of differing composition on entero-insular hormone secretion in the first hours of life in human neonates. *Acta Paed. Scand.*, **68**, 265–70.

Anysley-Green, A., Soltesz, G., Jenkins, P.A. *et al.* (1985) The metabolic and endocrine milieu of the human fetus at 18–21 weeks gestation. II. Blood glucose, lactate, pyruvate and ketone body concentrations. *Biol. Neonate*, **47**, 19–25.

Bailley, E. and Lockwood, E.A. (1973) Some aspects of fatty acid oxidation and ketone body formation and utilization during development of the rat. *Enzyme*, **15**, 239–53.

Battaglia, F.C. and Hay, W.W. (1984) 'Energy and substrate requirements for fetal and placental growth and metabolism', in R.W. Beard and P.W. Nathanieesz (eds). *Fetal Physiology and Medicine*. Marcell Decker, New York.

Beale, E., Andreone, T., Kock, S. *et al.* (1984) Insulin and glucagon regulate cytosolic phosphoenolpyruvate carboxykinase (GTP) mRNA in rat liver. *Diabetes*, **33**, 328–32.

Bier, D.M., Leake, R.D., Haymond, W.H. *et al.* (1977) Measurement of true glucose production rates in infancy and childhood with 6,6 dideuteroglucose. *Diabetes*, **26**, 1016–23.

Blazquez, E., Sugase, M., Blazquaez, M. *et al.* (1974) Neonatal changes in the concentration of liver cAMP and of serum glucose, FFA, insulin pancreatic and total glucagon in man and in the rat. *J. Lab. Clin. Med.*, **83**, 957–67.

Bougneres, P.F. (1987) Stable isotope tracers and the determination of fuel fluxes in newborn infants. *Biol. Neonate*, **52** (suppl. 1), 87–96.

Bougneres, P.F., Karl, I.E., Hillman, L.S. *et al.* (1982) Lipid transport in the human newborn. Palmitate and glycerol turnover and the contribution of glycerol to neonatal hepatic glucose output. *J. Clin. Invest.*, **70**, 262–70.

Bougneres, P.F., Zemmel, C., Ferre, P. *et al.* (1986) Ketone body transport in the human neonate and infant. *J. Clin. Invest.*, **77**, 42–48.

Bozzetti, P., Buscaglia, M., Marconi, A.M. *et al.* (1988) The relationship of maternal and fetal glucose concentrations in man from mid gestation until term. *Metab.*, **37**, 358–63.

Browne, C.A. and Thorburn, G.D. (1989) Endocrine control of fetal growth. *Biol. Neonate*, **55**, 331–46.

Cake, M.H., Yeung, D. and Oliver, I.T. (1971) The control of postnatal hypoglycaemia. *Biol. Neonate*, **18**, 183–92.

Cimbala, M.A., Lamers, W.H., Nelson, K. *et al.* (1982) Rapid changes in the concentration of phosphoenolpyruvate carboxykinase mRNA in rat liver and kidney. Effects of insulin and cyclic AMP. *J. Biol. Chem.*, **257**, 7629–36.

Cowett, R.M. (1988) α-adrenergic agonists stimulate neonatal glucose production less than β-adrenergic agonists in the lamb. *Metabolism*, **37**, 831–36.

Cowett, R.M. and Tenenbaum, D.G. (1985) Insulin is the primary hormone for control of neonatal glucose homeostasis. *Ped. Res.*, **19**, 311A.

Cowett, R.M., Wolfe, M.H. and Wolfe, R.R. (1985) Lactate turnover is increased in the neonate relative to the adult. *Ped. Res.*, **19**, 311A.

Edmond, J., Auestad, N., Robbins, R.A. *et al.* (1985) Ketone body metabolism in the neonate: development and the effect of diet. *Fed. Proc.*, **44**, 2359–64.

Falorni, A., Fracassini, F., Massi-Benedetti, F. *et al.* (1974) Glucose metabolism and insulin secretion in the newborn infant. *Diabetes*, **23**, 172–78.

Ferre, P., Pegorier, J.P. and Girard, J.R. (1978) Influence of exogenous fat and gluconeogenic substrates on glucose homeostasis in the newborn rat. *Am. J. Physiol.*, **234**, E129–E136.

Ferre, P., Pegorier, J.P., Williamson, D.H. *et al.* (1979) Interactions *in vivo* between oxidation of non-esterified fatty acids and gluconeogenesis in the newborn rat. *Biochem. J.*, **182**, 593–98.

Ferre, P., Satabin, P., El Monouli, L. *et al.* (1981) Relationship between ketogenesis and gluconeogenesis in isolated hepatocytes from newborn rats. *Biochem. J.*, **200**, 429–33.

Ferre, P., Satabin, P., Decause, J.F. *et al.* (1983) Development and regulation of ketogenesis in hepatocytes isolated from newborn rats. *Biochem. J.*, **214**, 937–42.

Fiser, R.H., Williams, P.R., Fisher, D.A. *et al.* (1975) The effect of oral alanine on blood glucose and glucagon in the newborn infant. *Pediatr.*, **56**, 78–81.

Frazer, T.E., Karl, I.E., Hillman, L.S. *et al.* (1981) Direct measurement of gluconeogenesis from (2,3-$^{13}3C_2$) alanine in the human neonate. *Am. J. Physiol.*, **240**, E615–E621.

Frost, S.C. and Wells, M.A. (1981) A comparison of the utilisation of medium and long chain fatty acids for ketogenesis in the suckling rat: *in vivo* and *in vitro* studies. *Arch. Biochem. Biophys.*, **211**, 537–46.

Gamara, E., Monitte, G. and Relier, J.P. (1979) Response of insulin and glucagon to a routine constant rate infusion (CII) in very low birth weight infants (LBW) during the first 4 days of life. *Ped. Res.*, **13**, 474.

Garcia-Ruiz, J.D., Ingram, R. and Hanson, R.W. (1978) Changes in hepatic messenger RNA for phosphoenolpyruvate carboxykinase (GTP) during development. *Proc. Natl. Acad. Sci.*, **75**, 4189–93.

Gentz, J.C.H., Warrner, R., Persson, B.E.H. *et al.* (1969) Intravenous glucose tolerance, plasma insulin, free fatty acids and β-hydroxybutyrate in underweight newborn infants. *Acta Paed. Scand.*, **58**, 481–90.

Gilfillan, C.A., Tseng, K.-Y. and Kalhan, S.C. (1985) Glucose-lactate relation in the human newborn. *Ped. Res.*, **19**, 312A.

Girard, J. (1986) Gluconeogenesis in the late fetal and early neonatal life. *Biol. Neonate*, **50**, 237–58.

Girard, J.R., Guillet, I., Marty, J. *et al.* (1975) Plasma amino acid levels and development of hepatic gluconeogenesis in the newborn rat. *Am. J. Physiol.*, **229**, 466–73.

Gleason, C.A., Roman, C. and Rudolph, A.M. (1985) Hepatic oxygen consumption, lactate uptake and glucose production in neonatal lambs. *Ped. Res.*, **12**, 1235–39.

Grasso, S., Fallucca, F., Mazzone, D. *et al.* (1983) Inhibition of glucagon secretion in the human newborn by glucose infusion. *Diabetes*, **32**, 489–92.

Hanson, R.W. and Garber, A.J. (1972) Phosphoenolpyruvate carboxykinase I: Its role in gluconeogenesis. *Am. J. Clin. Nutr.*, **25**, 1010–21.

Hauguel, S., Desmaizieras, V. and Challier, J.C. (1986) Glucose uptake, utilisation and transfer by the human placenta as functions of maternal glucose concentration. *Ped. Res.*, **20**, 269–73.

Hawdon, J.M., Ward Platt, M.P. and Aynsley-Green, A. (1992) Patterns of metabolic adaptation for preterm and term infants in the first postnatal week. *Arch. Dis. Child.*, **67**, 357–65.

Hawdon, J.M., Aynsley-Green, A., Alberti, K.G.M.M. *et al.* (1993a) The role of pancreatic insulin secretion in neonatal glucoregulation. I: Healthy term and preterm infants. *Arch. Dis. Child.*, **68**, 274–79.

Hawdon, J.M., Aynsley-Green, A., Bartlett, K. *et al.* (1993b) The role of pancreatic insulin secretion in neonatal glucoregulation. II: Infants with disordered blood glucose homeostasis. *Arch. Dis. Child.*, **68**, 280–85.

Hawdon, J.M., Weddell, A., Aynsley-Green, A. *et al.* (1993c) The hormonal and metabolic response to hypoglycaemia in small for gestational age infants. *Arch. Dis. Child.*, **68**, 269–73.

Hay, W.W. and Meznarich, H.K. (1989) Effect of maternal glucose concentration on uteroplacental glucose consumption and transfer in pregnant sheep. *Proc. Soc. Exp. Biol. Med.*, **190**, 63–69.

Hay, W.W. Jr. and Sparks, J.W. (1985) Placental, fetal and neonatal carbohydrate metabolism. *Clin. Obstet. Gynaecol.*, **28**, 473–85.

Hay, W.W., Sparks, J.W., Wilkening, R.B. *et al.* (1983) Partition of maternal glucose production between conceptus and maternal tissues in sheep. *Am. J. Physiol.*, **245**, E347–E350.

Hay, W.W., Sparks, J.W., Wilkening, R.B. *et al.* (1984) Fetal glucose uptake and utilisation as functions of maternal glucose utilisation. *Am. J. Physiol.*, **246**, E237–E242.

Hetenyi, G. and Cowan, J.S. (1980) Glucoregulation in the newborn. *Can. J. Physiol. Pharmacol.*, **58**, 879–88.

Hughes, D., Murphy, J.F., Dyas, J. *et al.* (1987) Blood spot glucocorticoid concentrations in ill preterm infants. *Arch. Dis. Child.*, **62**, 1014–18.

Kalhan, S.C., Savin, S.M. and Adam, P.A.J. (1976) Measurement of glucose turnover in the human newborn with glucose-1-^{13}C. *J. Clin. End. Metab.*, **43**, 704–707.

Kalhan, S.C., Bier, D.M., Savin, S.M. *et al.* (1980) Estimation of glucose turnover and ^{13}C recycling in the human newborn by simultaneous [1-^{13}C] glucose and [6,6-$^{2}H_2$] glucose tracers. *J. Clin. End. Metab.*, **50**, 456–60.

Kliegman, R.M. and Sparks, J.W. (1985) Perinatal galactose metabolism. *J. Pediatr.*, **107**, 831–41.

Kraus, H., Schlenker, S. and Schwedesky, D. (1974) Developmental changes of cerebral ketone body utilisation in human infants. Hoppe-seyler's Z. *Physiol. Chem.*, **355**, 164–70.

Lagercrantz, H. and Bistoletti, P. (1977) Catecholamine release in the newborn infant at birth. *Ped. Res.*, **11**, 889–93.

Leonetti, G., Bianchini, C., Picotti, G.B. *et al.* (1980) Plasma catecholamines and plasma renin activity at birth and during the first days of life. *Clin. Sci.*, **59**, 319s–321s.

Levitsky, L.L., Paton, J.B. and Fisher, D.B. (1973) Cerebral utilisation of alternative substrates to glucose: an explanation for asymptomatic neonatal hypoglycaemia. *Ped. Res.*, **7**, 418.

Lowick, C., Mitchell, A.A., Epstein, M.J. *et al.* (1985) Risk factors for neonatal hyperglycaemia associated with 10% dextrose infusion *Am. J. Dis. Child.*, **139**, 783–86.

Lucas, A. (1991) 'Programming by early nutrition in man', in *The childhood environment and adult disease*. John Wiley & Sons, Chichester.

Lucas, A., Bloom, S.R. and Aynsley-Green, A. (1982) Postnatal surges in plasma gut hormones in term and preterm infants. *Biol. Neonate*, **41**, 63–67.

Lucas, A., Bloom, S.R. and Aynsley-Green, A. (1983) Metabolic and endocrine consequences of depriving preterm infants of enteral nutrition. *Acta Paed. Scand.*, **72**, 245–49.

Lucas, A., Bloom, S.R. and Aynsley-Green, A. (1985) Gastrointestinal peptides and the adaptation to extrauterine nutrition. *Can. J. Physiol. Pharmacol.*, **63**, 527–37.

Lyonnet, S., Coupe, C., Girard, J. *et al.* (1988) *In vivo* regulation of glycolytic and gluconeogenic enzyme gene expression in newborn rat liver. *J. Clin. Invest.*, **81**, 1682–89.

Marsac, C., Saudubray, J.M., Mancion *et al.* (1976) Development of gluconeogenic enzymes in the liver of newborns. *Biol. Neonate*, **28**, 317–25.

Milner, R.D.G. (1972) Neonatal hypoglycaemia – a critical reappraisal. *Arch. Dis. Child.*, **47**, 679.

Milner, R.D.G. (1984) 'Fetal fat and glucose metabolism', in R.W. Beard and P.M. Nathanielsz (eds). *Fetal Physiology and Medicine*. Marcel Decker, New York.

Milner, R.D.G. and Wright, A.D. (1967) Plasma glucose, non-esterified fatty acids, insulin and growth hormone response to glucagon in the newborn. *Clin. Sci.*, **32**, 249–55.

Obershain, S.S., Adam, P.A.J., King, K.C. *et al.* (1970) Human fetal response to sustained maternal hyperglycaemia. *N. Engl. J. Med.*, **283**, 566–72.

Ogata, E.S., Collins, J.W. Jr and Finley, S. (1988) Insulin injection in the fetal rat: accelerated intrauterine growth and altered fetal and neonatal glucose homeostasis. *Metab.*, **37**, 649–55.

Otonoski, T., Andersson, S., Knip, M. *et al.* (1988) Maturation of insulin response to glucose during human fetal and neonatal development. Studies with perifusion of pancreatic islet cell-like clusters. *Diabetes*, **37**, 286–91.

Padbury, J.F. and Martinez, A.M. (1988) Sympathoadrenal system activity at birth: integration of postnatal adaptation. *Semin. Perinatol.*, **12**, 164–72.

Pagliara, A.S., Karl, I.E. and Kipnis, D.B. (1973) Transient neonatal diabetes: delayed maturation of pancreatic β cell function. *J. Pediatr.*, **82**, 97–101.

Paramesweran, M. and Arinze, I.J. (1981) Relationship of mitochondrial phosphoenolpyruvate carboxykinase to neonatal gluconeogenesis. *Biol. Neonate*, **39**, 260–65.

Pearce, P.H., Buirchell, B.J. and Weaver, P.K. (1974) The development of phosphopyruvate carboxylase and gluconeogenesis in the neonatal rat. *Biol. Neonate*, **24**, 320–29.

Persson, B. and Tunnell, R. (1971) Influence of environmental temperature and acidosis on lipid mobilisation in the human infant in the first two hours after birth. *Acta Paed. Scand.*, **60**, 385–98.

Phillippidis, H. and Ballard, F.J. (1970) The development of gluconeogenesis in rat liver. *Biochem. J.*, **120**, 385–92.

Phillipps, A.F., Dubin, J.W., Motty, P.J. *et al.* (1983) Influences of exogenous glucagon on fetal glucose metabolism and ketone production. *Ped. Res.*, **17**, 51–56.

Poland, R.L., Schultz, G. and Garg, G. (1980) High milk lipase activity associated with breast milk jaundice. *Ped. Res.*, **14**, 1328.

Price, H.V., Courley, T. and Cameron, E.H.D. (1976) Neonatal hydrocortisone administration: effect on cortisol and glucose levels. *Biol. Neonate*, **30**, 138–41.

Prip-Buus, C., Pegorier, J.P., Duee, P.H. *et al.* (1990) Evidence that the sensitivity of carnitine-palmitoyl transferase I to malonyl CoA inhibition is the major site of regulation of fatty acid oxidation in the rabbit liver during the fetal-neonatal transition. *Biochem. J.*, **269**, 409–415.

Quant, P.A., Robin, D., Robin, P. *et al.* (1990) Control of hepatic mitochondrial 3-hydroxy-3-methyl glutaryl CoA synthase during the fetal-neonatal and suckling-weaning transitions in the rat. *Eur. J. Biochem.*, **187**, 169–74.

Rokicki, W., Forest, M.G., Loras, B. *et al.* (1990) Free cortisol of human plasma in the first three months of life. *Biol. Neonate*, **57**, 21–29.

Sann, L., Ruitton, A., Mathieu, M. *et al.* (1978) Effect of intravenous L-alanine administration on plasma glucose, insulin and glucagon, blood pyruvate, lactate and β-hydroxybutyrate concentrations in newborn infants. Study in appropriate and preterm newborn infants. *Acta Paed. Scand.*, **67**, 297–302.

Savich, R.D., Finley, S., Bussey, M.E. *et al.* (1985) Lipid infusion enhances gluconeogenesis from amino acids in premature infants. *Ped. Res.*, **19**, 312A.

Schade, D.S. and Eaton, R.P. (1975) Glucagon regulation of plasma ketone body concentration in human diabetes. *J. Clin. Invest.*, **56**, 1340–44.

Settegren, G., Linblad, B.S. and Persson, B. (1976) Cerebral blood flow and exchange of oxygen, glucose, ketone, bodies, lactate, pyruvate and amino acids in infants. *Acta Paed. Scand.*, **65**, 343–53.

Shelley, H.J., Bassett, J.M. and Milner, R.D.G. (1975) Control of carbohydrate metabolism in the fetus and newborn. *Br. Med. Bull.*, **31**, 37–43.

Siegel, C.D., Sparks, J.W. and Battaglia, F.C. (1988) Patterns of serum glucose and galactose concentrations in term newborn infants after milk feeding. *Biol. Neonate*, **54**, 301–306.

Sippell, W.G., Becker, H., Versmold, H.T. *et al.* (1978) Longitudinal studies of plasma aldosterone, corticosterone, deoxycorticosterone, progesterone, 17 hydroxy progesterone, cortisol and cortisone determined simultaneously in mother and child at birth and during the early neonatal period. I: Spontaneous delivery. *J. Clin. End. Metab.*, **46**, 971–85.

Snell, K. and Walker, D.G. (1973) Glucose metabolism in the newborn rat. *Biochem. J.*, **132**, 739–52.

Solomon, S., Baird, C.E., Ling, W. *et al.* (1967) Formation and metabolism of steroids in the fetus and placenta. *Recent Prog. Horm. Res.*, **23**, 297–347.

Sperling, M.A. (1982) Integration of fuel homeostasis by insulin and glucagon in the newborn. *Monogr. Pediatr.*, **16**, 39–58.

Sperling, M.A., De Lameter, P.V., Phelos, D. *et al.* (1974) Spontaneous and amino acid stimulated glucagon secretion in the immediate postnatal period. *J. Clin. Invest.*, **53**, 1159–66.

Sperling, M.A., Grajwer, L.A., Leake, R. *et al.* (1976) Role of glucagon in perinatal glucose homeostasis. *Metabolism*, **25** (suppl. 1), 1385–86.

Sperling, M.A., Ganguli, S., Leslie, N. *et al.* (1984) Fetal-perinatal catecholamine secretion: Role in perinatal glucose homeostasis. *Am. J. Physiol.*, **247**, E69–E74.

Stanley, C.A., Anday, E.K., Baker, L. *et al.* (1979) Metabolic fuel and hormone responses to fasting in newborn infants. *Pediatr.*, **64**, 613–19.

Stonestreet, B.S., Rubin, L., Pollack, A. *et al.* (1980) Renal function of low birthweight infants with hyperglycaemia and glucosuria produced by glucose infusion. *Pediatrics*, **66**, 561–67.

Stubbe, P. and Wolfe, H. (1971) The effect of stress on growth hormone, glucose and glycerol levels in newborn infants. *Horm. Metab. Res.*, **3**, 175–79.

Susa, J.B., Cowett, R.M. and Oh, W. (1979) Suppression of gluconeogenesis and endogenous glucose production by exogenous insulin administration in the newborn lamb. *Ped. Res.*, **13**, 594–99.

Townsend, S.F., Rudolph, C.D. and Rudolph, A.M. (1989) Cortisol induces perinatal hepatic gluconeogenesis. *Ped. Res.*, **25**, 298.

Tse, T.F., Clutter, W.E., Shah, S.D. *et al.* (1983) Mechanisms of postprandial counterregulation in man. Physiologic role of glucagon and epinephrine *vis-à-vis* insulin in the prevention of hypoglycaemia late after glucose ingestion. *J. Clin. Invest.*, **72**, 278–86.

Van Assche, F.A., Hoet, J.J. and Jack, P.M.B. (1984) 'Endocrine pancreas of the pregnant mother, fetus and newborn', in R.W. Beard, P.W. Nathanielsz (eds). *Fetal Physiology and Medicine*. Marcel Decker, New York.

Viliasis, R., Cowett, R.M. and Oh, W. (1982) Glycaemic response to lipid infusion in the premature neonate. *J. Pediatr.*, **100**, 108–112.

Yeung, D. and Oliver, I.T. (1968) Factors affecting the premature induction of phosphopyruvate carboxylase in neonatal rat liver. *Biochem. J.*, **108**, 325–31.

2

Glucose homeostasis in the normal child

H.F. STIRLING and C.J.H. KELNAR

In a healthy child, blood glucose levels are normally carefully controlled between 4 and 7 mmol/l. The maintenance of a 'normal' plasma glucose level is a balance between the amount of glucose entering the bloodstream and the amount leaving it. This balance is affected by nutritional state, is controlled predominantly by hormone release, and is designed to meet the demands put on it, particularly by the growing brain of the child (Figure 2.1).

2.1 FACTORS CONTRIBUTING TO GLUCOSE HOMEOSTASIS

2.1.1 DIETARY INTAKE

This is a principal determinant of the amount of glucose entering the blood stream. The maximal rate of glucose absorption from the intestine is about 120 g/h (adult man). Children have nutritional needs which will provide sufficient energy for normal growth and development without promoting obesity. It is recommended that children should obtain 45–50% of their total energy intake from carbohydrate. When less carbohydrate is taken then more fat will be required for energy.

In adult men, approximately 5% of ingested glucose is converted into glycogen in the liver, and 30–40% is converted into fat. The remainder is metabolized in brain, muscle and other tissues.

2.1.2 ENDOCRINE FACTORS

Insulin is a major anabolic hormone. It is one of four hormones secreted by the pancreas (the others being pancreatic polypeptide, somatostatin, and glucagon), which, together with other hormonal influences, have roles to play in glucose homeostasis.

Pancreatic hormone secretion is influenced by vagal and sympathetic nervous input, the pericellular concentrations of nutrients (especially glucose and amino acids) and extra-pancreatic hormones in addition to the pancreatic hormones themselves.

After eating, blood glucose and amino acid concentrations rise and stimulate insulin secretion from the pancreatic β cells. This release is controlled by pancreatic arterial nutrient concentrations, neural influences on the pancreas (Woods and Porte Jr, 1974) and the secretion of insulinogenic factors from the gastro-intestinal mucosa. These gastro-intestinal humoral factors which promote insulin release have been called 'incretins'. Gastric inhibitory polypeptide (GIP) and gastrin are the only gut hormones released by carbohydrate in the gut, but gastrin is not re-

Childhood and Adolescent Diabetes
Published in 1994 by Chapman & Hall, London
ISBN 0 412 48610 5

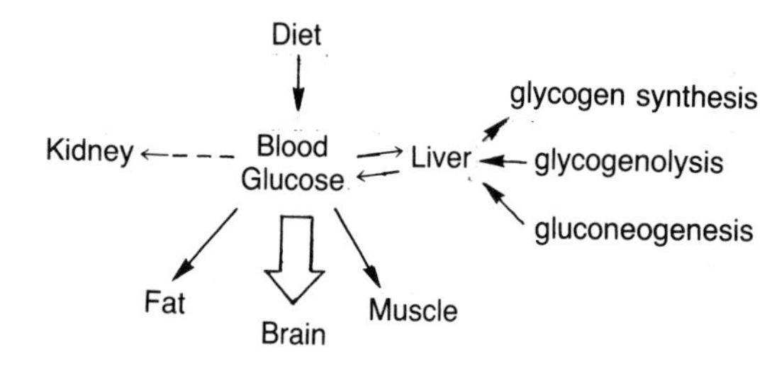

Figure 2.1 Relationships between dietary intake, plasma glucose and glucose utilization.

leased by exogenous glucose. GIP is released only by absorption of carbohydrate rather than just its presence in the gut (which may be protective against hypoglycemia) and there is feedback control present on GIP by insulin. Thus GIP is the strongest 'incretin' candidate though other factors may have a role (Creutzfeldt, 1979). The gastro-intestinal neural system may participate in the entero-insular axis in two ways: firstly by the release of an incretin (probably via β-adrenergic receptors), and secondly by direct stimulation of the islets by neural pathways.

Insulin stimulates the movement of glucose into muscle and adipose tissue and the conversion of glucose into glycogen and triglycerides. Thus the disappearance of glucose from the blood is accelerated. Muscle breakdown and fat lipolysis are inhibited thus decreasing the release of fatty acids and the supply of gluconeogenic precursors (glycerol and amino acids). In animal studies, insulin reduces the basal rate of both fatty acid and glycerol release from isolated fat cells in starved rats, and also blocks the stimulatory effects of growth hormone and dexamethasone on fatty acid and glycerol release. Low concentrations of insulin have potent effects in decreasing this lipolysis and protein catabolism with the insulin effects on fat seen at concentrations well below that required to stimulate glucose metabolism (Fain *et al.*, 1966).

Insulin also stimulates hepatic glycogen synthesis and decreases glycogenolysis and gluconeogenesis via its effects on hepatic enzymes (see below).

Thus insulin decreases plasma glucose through a variety of mechanisms. In states of relative insulin dominance there are low levels of circulating ketone bodies, free fatty acids and branched chain amino acids.

Glucagon, a polypeptide containing 29 amino acid residues produced by the α cells of the pancreas, has a major role in raising and maintaining blood glucose in states of relative starvation or hypoglycemia. Secretion of glucagon is increased by stimulation of the sympathetic nerves to the pancreas, mediated via β-adrenergic receptors and cyclic AMP.

During starvation the balance between insulin and glucagon secretion changes, with a fall in insulin levels to very low concentrations and a rise in glucagon concentrations. In 15 obese adult subjects fasted for six weeks without calories, there was a significant rise in glucagon levels to a maximum by day three, followed by a gradual return to pre-fast levels. There was a concomitant fall in insulin levels during the fast. The early rise in plasma glucagon seemed to correspond to the period of increased hepatic gluconeogenesis (Marliss *et al.*, 1970). Unger *et al.* (1969) suggested that the relative levels of insulin and glucagon are important during fasting – elevated plasma glucagon levels in the presence of lowered insulin levels having a synergistic effect on hepatic glucose release.

Although glucagon is glycogenolytic, it only acts on glycogen stores in the liver and does not cause muscle glycogenolysis.

Glucagon can also stimulate gluconeogenesis (Sokal, 1966). In animal studies in isolated rat liver there is increased incorporation of alanine into glucose in the presence of glucagon (Garcia *et al.*, 1966), elevation of the metabolic rate, and lipolytic activity which increases ketogenesis. In humans, it increases lipolysis and ketogenesis, particularly in states of relative insulin deficiency (Johnston & Alberti, 1982). The half-life of glucagon in the circulation is 5–10 minutes. It is degraded particularly by the liver and, since it is secreted into the portal vein and reaches the liver before it reaches the peripheral circulation, peripheral blood levels are relatively low.

Falling blood glucose levels are also detected by the hypothalamus and, in addition to the effects on insulin and glucagon, there are effects on other 'counter-regulatory hormones' – notably catecholamines, growth hormone and, via ACTH, on cortisol. These counter-regulatory hormones act in a variety of ways:

- Epinephrine, cortisol and growth hormone inhibit glucose uptake by muscle, stimulate the production of gluconeogenic precursors (gluconeogenic amino acids from muscle and glycerol from adipose tissue), and induce hepatic enzyme activity for glycogenolysis (glycogen phosphorylase) and gluconeogenesis (Cahill, 1971).
- Epinephrine also inhibits insulin release from the pancreas. After a 24-hour fast, in children there is a negative correlation between blood glucose levels and cortisol levels (Chaussain *et al.*, 1974, Chaussain *et al.*, 1977) demonstrating an adrenal response to fast-induced hypoglycemia.

The main metabolic markers for counter-regulation are increased levels of fatty acids and blood ketone bodies due to lipolysis and β-oxidation, and of branched chain amino acids from protein catabolism.

During acute insulin-induced hypoglycemia, glucagon appears to play the major role in recovery with adrenal-derived catecholamines providing a secondary role (Gerich *et al.*, 1979). However children produce an exaggerated epinephrine response to hypoglycemia compared to adults (Amiel *et al.*, 1987), although their growth hormone and cortisol responses are similar. Adrenalectomized subjects can cope with insulin-induced hypoglycemia as long as they are able to produce glucagon normally. Epinephrine will compensate largely for deficient glucagon secretion, but counter-regulation will fail in the absence of both hormones.

Growth hormone and cortisol, while not as important in the immediate recovery from a hypoglycemic insult, are necessary for the maintenance of recovery from the episode. After a 24-hour fast, children with growth hormone deficiency have fasting blood glucose concentrations that are lower than those seen in normal children. There is relatively poor production of ketones with lower concentrations of hydroxybutyrate (Wolfsdorf *et al.*, 1983). This is also seen after insulin-induced hypoglycemia and at the end of a normal night's fast (Stirling *et al.*, 1991). These children are susceptible to hypoglycemia and this is an important reason for the early initiation of growth hormone therapy in growth hormone deficient children. Children with isolated ACTH deficiency (and hence cortisol deficiency) are also likely to become hypoglycemic at times of stress, for example during fasting or illness.

Somatostatin is present in D-cells of the pancreas. It has a major role in controlling the entry of nutrients from the gastrointestinal tract by direct action – suppressing the gastrointestinal hormones gastrin, cholecystokinin and secretin, and also suppressing pancreatic exocrine secretion (Raptis *et al.*, 1978). It delays gastric emptying, alters splanchnic blood flow and decreases duodenal motility. It also has effects on other hormone levels inhibiting (via β-adrenergic stimulation) basal and stimulated release of glucagon, insulin and pancreatic polypeptide by direct action on the alpha, beta and pancreatic polypeptide cells. It also suppresses TSH and growth hormone release from the pituitary (Arimura *et al.*, 1978).

The precise function of human pancreatic polypeptide is unclear but there is a rapid

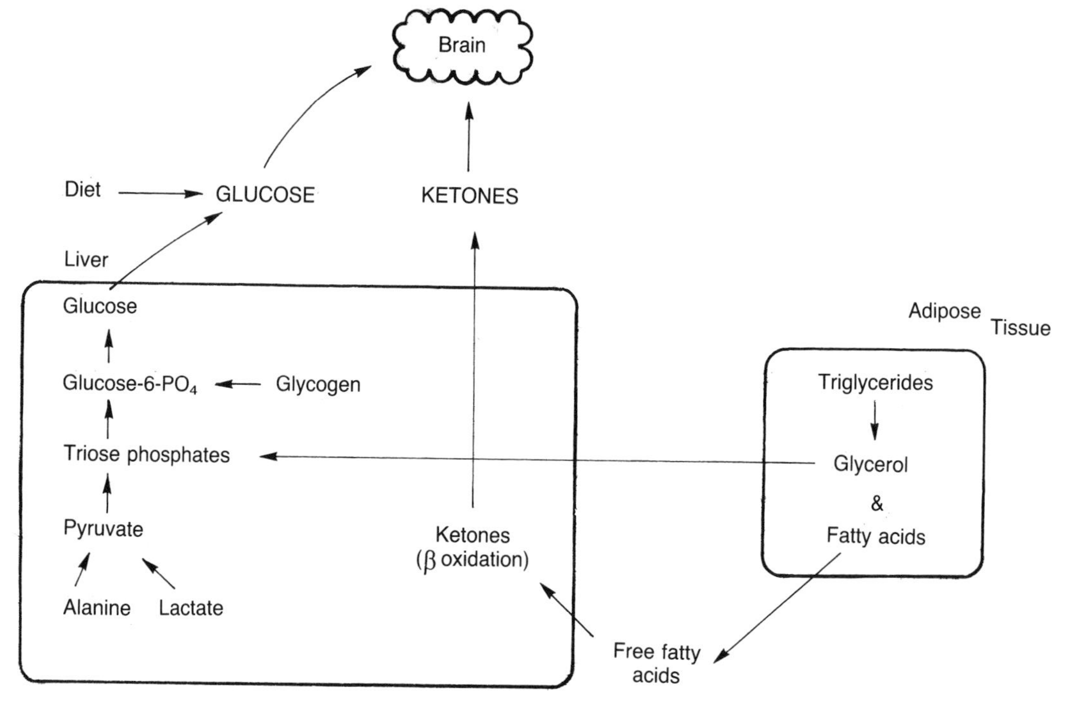

Figure 2.2 Maintenance of energy supply to the brain.

and considerable rise after a meal (Adrian *et al.*, 1981). In healthy adult volunteers, it is actively secreted for several hours after a meal, but there does not appear to be significant effects on circulating metabolites or the pancreatic hormones glucagon and insulin.

2.1.3 HEPATIC METABOLISM

The liver is the most important single organ for maintenance of glucose homeostasis and ensuring a constant supply of metabolic fuel for the brain and other tissues (Figure 2.2).

When blood glucose levels are high, there is a net uptake of glucose by the liver, and net release of glucose from the liver when glucose levels are low. Glucose uptake and release from the liver are under hormonal control (as described above). The liver plays a key role in the maintenance of a normal blood sugar by two major mechanisms:

- glycogen synthesis and glycogenolysis
- gluconeogenesis

2.1.3.1 Glycogen synthesis and glycogenolysis

Glycogen, the storage form of glucose is present in most body tissues, but the major stores are in liver and skeletal muscle. Hepatic glycogen synthesis is regulated by the enzyme glycogen synthetase, and glycogen breakdown is regulated by the enzyme phosphorylase. The two are inversely co-ordinated – as one becomes active the other becomes relatively inactive. These enzymes are themselves controlled by an enzyme cascade involving kinases and phosphatases. The various hormones discussed above exert their effects on glycogen production and breakdown via this enzyme cascade.

After a meal, the increase in blood glucose

and plasma insulin stimulates glycogen production and inhibits glycogenolysis.

During glycogen formation glucose enters the hepatocyte and is converted to uridine diphosphate glucose (UDPG) under the influence of hexokinase and phosphoglucomutase. Glycogen synthetase then causes transfer of glucose residues to an outer chain of the glycogen molecule. Following this there is further build-up of the glycogen molecule, under the control of brancher enzymes.

Three to four hours after a meal the liver begins to release glucose into the circulation. At this stage, the majority of this glucose release is accounted for by glycogenolysis (Wahren *et al.*, 1971). During glycogen breakdown, debranching must first occur (under the influence of 'debrancher' enzymes) before phosphorylase can release units from the glycogen molecule in the form of glucose-1-phosphate. Phosphorylase is the rate-limiting enzyme. Glucose-1-phosphate is then converted to glucose-6-phosphate by phospho-glucomutase, and subsequently dephosphorylated to free glucose by glucose-6-phosphatase. It is only as free glucose that the sugar can diffuse out of the cell. Glucagon and adrenalin initiate a cascade of reactions which regulate the relative amounts of active and inactive phosphorylase present and hence have an important role in controlling glycogenolysis.

Other tissues can store glycogen to a greater or lesser extent, but can only use it locally as they do not contain glucose-6-phosphatase and so cannot liberate free glucose into the circulation. Thus they do not play a role in maintaining plasma glucose levels. Muscle glycogen, although greater in content than hepatic glycogen, is mobilized by exercise or anoxia rather than by periods of relative starvation.

Hypoglycemia may result from defects in glycogen synthesis or release of glucose from stored glycogen. Glycogen synthesis is impaired in hepatic glycogen synthetase deficiency (Aynsley-Green *et al.*, 1977). In the glycogen storage diseases impairment of glycogenolysis occurs at various levels. For example, in type I glycogenosis there is glucose-6-phosphatase deficiency, in type III glycogenosis there is inactivity of the debranching enzyme, and in type IV defects of the hepatic phosphorylase system are present.

2.1.3.2 Gluconeogenesis

The term 'gluconeogenesis' is commonly used to describe the formation of glucose from any substrate other than monosaccharides and glycogen. Formation of new glucose molecules from non-carbohydrate precursors (protein and fat), must be distinguished from the process of glucose generation through recycling of pyruvate, lactate and alanine. The major part of the glucose output from the liver is from recycling.

Various substrates are used for gluconeogenesis in the liver: glycerol, amino acids especially alanine and glutamine (Felig, 1973), lactate and pyruvate. Amino acids are derived from protein catabolism in skeletal muscle. Alanine can be derived directly from muscle breakdown, or be formed indirectly from other amino acids. Alanine has a central role as the key protein-derived gluconeogenic precursor. The alanine released from extrahepatic tissues consists not only of preformed alanine derived by catabolism of cellular proteins, but also includes peripherally synthesized alanine formed by *in situ* transamination of glucose-derived pyruvate – the glucose-alanine-glucose cycle (Felig, 1973; Garber *et al.*, 1976) (Figure 2.3).

Glucose released by the liver is taken up by muscle, where it is converted to pyruvate and transaminated to form alanine. This can be released by muscle and taken up by the liver where its carbon skeleton is reconverted to glucose.

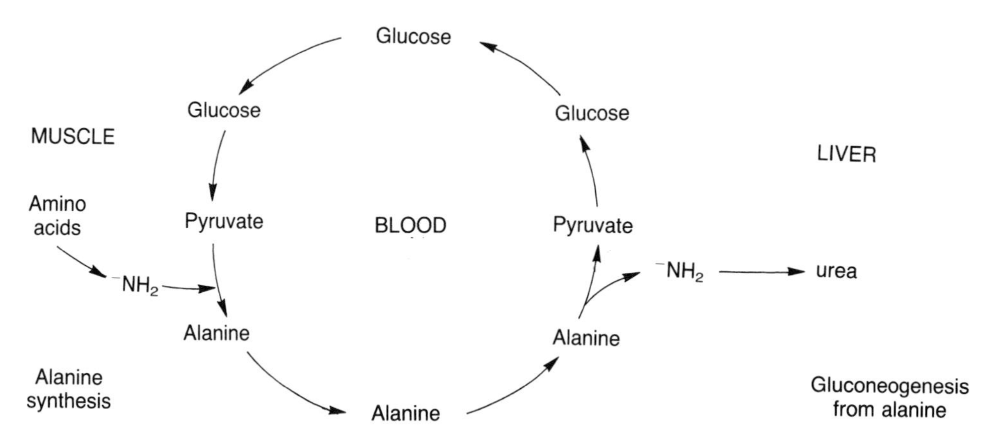

Figure 2.3 The glucose-alanine-glucose cycle.

Alanine is quantitatively the most important amino acid released by muscle and extracted by the splanchnic bed. The hepatic capacity for conversion of alanine to glucose exceeds that of all other amino acids.

Insulin inhibits gluconeogenesis by reducing hepatic alanine uptake. In states of prolonged fasting, gluconeogenesis is reduced because of diminished alanine release. In circumstances where alanine is deficient, fasting hypoglycemia is accentuated.

Exogenous insulin, or stimulation of endogenous insulin secretion, leads to a reduction in the total plasma amino acid content, most consistently the branched amino acids, tyrosine and phenylalanine. Alanine itself is unique in that its levels do not fall in these circumstances. Insulin increases muscle uptake of circulating alanine but this is counterbalanced by augmented intracellular production and release. As insulin does not cause a net decrease in circulating alanine, its effects on the reduction of hepatic gluconeogenesis must depend on a hepatic rather than a peripheral effect (Felig & Wahren, 1971). Thus insulin appears to have a direct hepatic effect on regulating gluconeogenesis.

Lactate and pyruvate are derived from glycolysis in erythrocytes and leucocytes with skeletal muscle contributing little to these under normal resting conditions (Kreisberg, 1972). The amino acids (predominantly alanine) and lactate are converted to pyruvate and thence to oxaloacetate via the citric acid cycle in order to act as substrates for gluconeogenesis.

The main source of glycerol is adipose tissue and adipose tissue contains the most important long-term energy store in the body. During periods of fasting, lipolysis of adipose tissue triglycerides not only yields glycerol which can be used for gluconeogenesis, but also free fatty acids. These fatty acids undergo β-oxidation in the liver to produce ketone bodies (acetyl CoA, acetoacetic acid, β-hydroxybutyric acid and acetone) which are alternative metabolic fuels, particularly in the brain (Owen *et al.*, 1967). Fatty acid oxidation provides the energy necessary for gluconeogenesis. Ketones are the only non-glucose energy source that can be utilized by the brain, and hence any insult to the brain may be less in episodes of hypoglycemia when ketones are present compared to insulin-induced hypoglycemia in which ketones will be absent. Ketone utilization relates directly to their concentration. The younger children who produce higher concentrations of ketones after a fast (Saudubray *et al.*, 1981) oxidize the most ketones with a proportionate diminution in the oxidation of glucose. By conserving glucose they sustain normoglycemia. This younger age group are particularly vulnerable to a shortage of ketones, compromising their ability to conserve glucose and pre-disposing them to hypoglycemia.

In the post-absorptive state, the liver is essentially the sole source of glucose production. 70–80% of glucose production is from glycogenolysis, with the remaining 20–30% from gluconeogenesis. 10–15% of total glucose production is from uptake and utilization of lactate, 1–2% from pyruvate and glycerol and 5–12% from uptake of alanine. Although alanine only accounts for 5–12% of total glucose production from the liver, it does account for 25% of gluconeogenesis. As fasting extends, gluconeogenesis rather than glycogenolysis becomes the dominant mode of glucose formation. After a 48–72 hour fast in an adult, alanine uptake accounts for approximately 26% of hepatic glucose production.

The endocrine changes described above during relative starvation (low insulin levels and increased counter-regulatory hormones) are essential for the mobilization of these gluconeogenic substrates. The enzymes involved in gluconeogenesis involving these substrates are stimulated by the counter-regulatory hormones and their effects diminished by raised plasma insulin levels.

Adequate supplies of the substrates themselves are necessary for gluconeogenesis to occur and may be limited in certain inborn errors of metabolism. Alanine levels in children with ketotic hypoglycemia have been reported to be reduced by 30% after an overnight fast, and fall to lower levels than observed in normal children during ingestion of a provocative low-carbohydrate diet. Infusion of exogenous alanine, or administration of cortisone acetate (which raises alanine levels) restores blood glucose levels to normal in such children (Pagliara *et al.*, 1972).

Many other inborn errors of metabolism can lead to hypoglycemia due to defects in hepatic gluconeogenesis. The enzyme glucose-6-phosphatase is not only involved in glycogenolysis but is also necessary to liberate free glucose during gluconeogenesis. Therefore an abnormality of this enzyme affects both glycogenolysis and gluconeogenesis and can cause profound hypoglycemia.

Glycerokinase deficiency and fructose 1.6. diphosphatase deficiency result in impaired conversion of glycerol to glucose. Impaired recycling of lactate to glucose occurs in pyruvate carboxylase deficiency, phosphoenolpyruvate carboxykinase deficiency as well as in fructose 1.6. diphosphatase deficiency.

Signs which suggest gluconeogenic enzyme defects include hypoglycemia, metabolic acidosis, hepatomegaly and neurological symptoms.

In fructosemia and galactosemia, diminished output of glucose occurs with ingestion of the particular sugar rather than with fasting. The enzyme defects in these conditions interfere with the normal metabolic disposal of fructose or of galactose, and ingestion of the offending sugar causes a decline in the level of plasma glucose.

Defects in conservation of glucose by failure of ketone production for example in the acyl-CoA dehydrogenase deficiencies (Gregersen, 1985) can lead to profound hypoglycemia. The most common of these metabolic defects is medium chain acyl-CoA dehydrogenase deficiency. A quarter of these children present with a Reye-like illness and/or sudden death with crises being induced by a fast or viral illness (Touma & Charpentier, 1992).

2.1.4 GLUCOSE UTILIZATION

The bulk of glucose produced is used by the brain, with smaller amounts of glucose taken up by obligate glycolytic tissues such as the formed elements of blood, and renal medulla. Red blood cells are dependent on glucose for energy, but as they lack mitochondria, breakdown of glucose proceeds only as far as lactate which returns to the liver for resynthesis to glucose. In the fed state, liver and muscle are the main glucose consumers – replenishing glycogen stores. Four to six hours after a meal the brain is the main glucose consumer. The estimated rate of cerebral glucose uptake in an adult man is 125–150 gm/day (Reinmuth *et al.*, 1965). Glucose uptake into muscle, liver and adipose tissue requires insulin, but this is not necessary for transport into the brain.

Using techniques that allow carbohydrate metabolism to be studied *in vivo* with stable isotopically-labelled glucose, studies of the quantitative and dynamic aspects of glucose production and utilization are possible in young children. Bier *et al.* (1977) studied 35 children, aged four months to 14 years, after an 8-hour fast. Total glucose production increased in a curvilinear fashion from 1 kg body weight up to 25 kg body weight (age approximately 6 years), when it reached a maximum of 140 mg/min, only slightly less than the adult average of 173 mg/min.

Expressed in terms of body weight, glucose production in the neonate and young child (up to the age of approximately 6 years) is in the order of 5–8 mg/kg/min, compared to the adult values of 2–3 mg/kg/min. The main consumer of energy is the brain (60–80% of total daily glucose consumption) and in young children the brain is relatively heavy compared to body mass, and is growing rapidly. There is a significant correlation between glucose production and estimated brain weight. This accounts for the increased energy demands of the young child compared to the adult. By the age of 6 years when brain weight approaches 90% of that of the adult brain, glucose demands fall to nearer those of the adult.

2.1.5 RENAL HANDLING OF GLUCOSE

Glucose is freely filtered in the kidney and at normal blood glucose levels all but a very small amount is reabsorbed in the proximal tubules. There is a maximum amount of glucose the tubules can reabsorb, and when this is exceeded glycosuria occurs. The renal threshold for glucose is reached when the venous blood concentration is about 10 mmol/l. Glycosuria can occur because of diabetes mellitus or because of excessive glycogenolysis after physical or emotional trauma. In some individuals the glucose transport mechanism in the tubules is congenitally defective so that glycosuria is present at normal blood glucose levels (renal glycosuria).

2.2 ADAPTATION DURING STARVING IN THE CHILD

After an overnight fast in adults the liver contains 40–50 gm of glucose stored as glycogen (Nilsson & Hultmann, 1973), but if the fast is continued for a further 24–36 hours these glycogen stores are virtually depleted and gluconeogenesis is the main source of glucose.

The liver in young children is relatively small compared to that of an adult, and hence the amount of stored glycogen is less. Glycogen reserves may only last for 12 hours in the absence of exogenous input. The amount of glycogen stored will depend on the amount of glycogen synthesized over the preceding day, i.e. on energy intake. Quanitative data concerning the amount of glycogen stored in the liver of normal children are scarce. Indirect information from the glucose response to glucagon or epinephrine after varying periods of fasting is available. Pagliara *et al.* (1972) showed that 14 children aged three to five years were able to mount a significant increase in plasma glucose in response to glucagon after 12–15 hours of fasting, suggesting adequate glycogen is maintained for at least this period of time (Figure 2.4).

Thereafter the child is dependent on gluconeogenesis for maintenance of blood glucose. A child who has a low adipose tissue mass and low protein mass relative to body mass may have decreased gluconeogenic

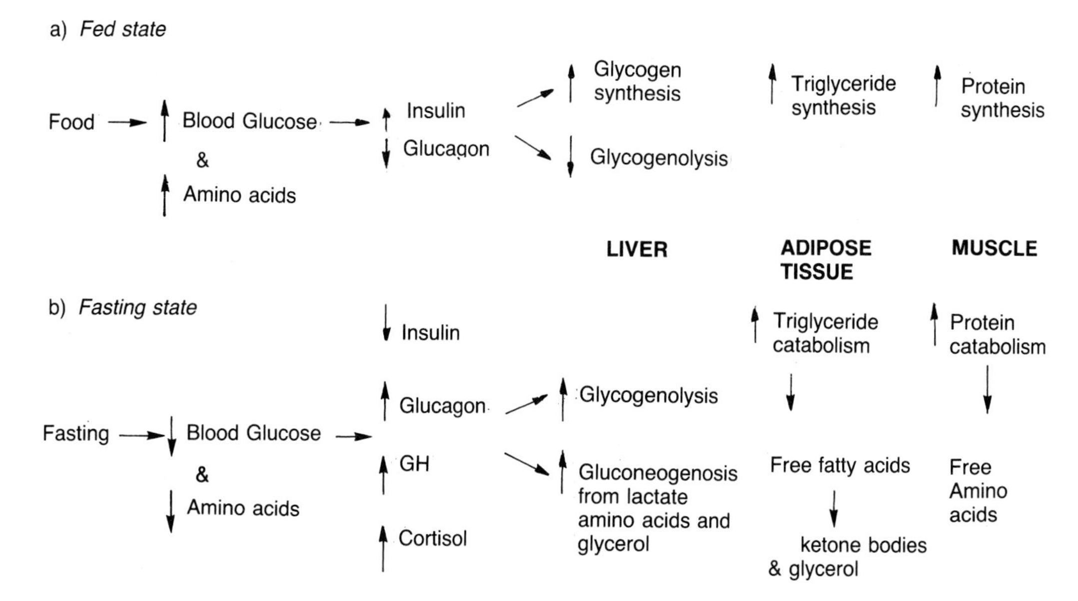

Figure 2.4 Comparison of fed and fasted states.

capabilities compared to an adult. In adults almost a third of glucose production is derived from amino acids with muscle being the major source of these. The child has a relatively small muscle compared to body mass, and this therefore limits the amount of substrates available for gluconeogenesis. Thus both the rates of change and absolute gluconeogenic substrate concentrations are very different in the child compared to the adult, with overall decreased availability of gluconeogenic substrates in the child.

Haymond *et al.* (1982) showed that in the postprandial state circulating concentrations of glucose, ketone bodies, potential gluconeogenic substrates and glucoregulatory hormones are similar in adults and children. However, after 30 hours of fasting, children had lower glucose (2.9 mmol/l compared to 4.0 mmol/l), lower alanine (167 μmol cf. 279 μmol) but higher betahydroxybutyrate (3.7 mmol cf. 0.9 mmol) compared to adult men. Plasma cortisol levels were higher than in adult men, but there were no differences in growth hormone, glucagon or insulin concentrations.

Glucose sparing by ketone production may be relatively more important in children than adults, as in young children the brain has an increased demand for fuel compared to body mass of the child, and ketone bodies are the only alternative energy source that can be utilized instead of glucose. Young children who have defects of fatty acid oxidation e.g., medium chain acyl-CoA dehydrogenase deficiency, are at grave risk of life-threatening hypoglycemia during periods of fasting or intercurrent illness. Their inability to make ketones renders them more susceptible to neurological damage during hypoglycemia.

There is relatively poor toleration of fasting in young children compared to the adult. Whereas adults rarely become hypoglycemic even after several days of starvation, children are much more prone to develop hypoglycemia after 20–24 hours of fasting even in the absence of any underlying metabolic problems (Chaussain *et al.*, 1974, 1977; Haymond *et al.*, 1984). Great care must be exercised in fasting even normal children prior to routine surgery as prolonged periods of pre-operative fasting may precipitate hypoglycemia (Kelnar,

1976). Chaussain *et al.* (1977) studied 28 children aged 2–17 years, during a 24-hour fast and found a progressive increase in fasting blood sugar with age. They demonstrated that after the age of 10 years the fasting blood sugar levels were not dissimilar to those seen in adults. A negative correlation was seen between cortisol levels and fasting blood sugar.

Chaussain also showed an age-related increase in fasting blood glucose and fall in free fatty acids after a 24-hour fast in normal children (Chaussain *et al.*, 1977), and Saudubray (1981) demonstrated an inversely age-related increase in fatty acid oxidation in young children after a prolonged period of fasting. Stirling *et al.* (1991) have shown similar results with an age-related increase in plasma glucose, and an inverse fall in fasting beta-hydroxybutyrate (a marker of fatty acid metabolism), not after a prolonged fast but simply after a 'normal' night's sleep in a group of short but otherwise normal healthy children. Young children show definite evidence of fatty acid oxidation (increased β-hydroxybutyrate levels) by the end of a normal (8–10 hour) fast overnight. Thus normal young children are switching over to ketone production to maintain energy supplies to the brain by the end of a night's sleep.

2.3 CONCLUSION

The maintenance of a normal blood glucose level is dependent on an adequate supply of gluconeogenic substrates, intact hepatic glycogenolytic and gluconeogenic enzyme systems, and a normal endocrine system to integrate the entire process. Childhood places increased demands on the system, and failure of any component can have devastating consequences.

REFERENCES

Adrian, T.E., Greenberg, G.R. and Bloom, S.R. (1981) 'Actions of pancreatic polypeptide in man', in S.R. Bloom and J.M. Polak (eds). *Gut Hormones*. Churchill Livingstone, London.

Amiel, S.A., Simonson, D.C., Sherwin, R.S. *et al.* (1987) Exaggerated epinephrine responses to hypoglycaemia in normal and insulin-dependent diabetic children. *J. Pediatr.*, **110**, 832–37.

Arimura, A., Coy, D.H., Chihara, M. *et al.* (1978) Somatostatin, in S.R. Bloom and J.M. Polak (eds). *Gut Hormones*. Churchill Livingstone, London.

Aynsley-Green, A., Williamson, D.M. and Gitzelmann, R. (1977) Hepatic glycogen synthetase deficiency. Definition of a syndrome from metabolic and enzyme studies in a 9 year old girl. *Arch. Dis. Child*, **52**, 573–79.

Bier, D.M., Leake, R.D., Haymond, M.W. *et al.* (1977) Measurement of 'true' glucose production rates in infancy and childhood with 6,6-dideuteroglucose. *Diabetes*, **26**, 1016–23.

Cahill, G.F. (1971) 'Action of adrenal cortical steroids on carbohydrate metabolism', in N.P. Christy (ed.). *The Human Adrenal Cortex*, pp. 205–240. Harper and Row, New York.

Chaussain, J.L., Georges, P., Olive, G. *et al.* (1974) Glycemic response to 24-hour fast in normal children and children with ketotic hypoglycaemia: II. Hormonal and metabolic changes. *J. Pediatr.*, **85**, 776–81.

Chaussain, J.L., Georges, P., Calzada, L. *et al.* (1977) Glycemic response to 24-hour fast in normal children: III. Influence of age. *J. Pediatr.*, **91**, 711–14.

Creutzfeldt, W. (1979) The incretin concept today. *Diabetologia*, **16**, 75–85.

Cryer, P.E., Tse, T.F., Clutter, W.E. *et al.* (1984) Roles of glucagon and epinephrine in hypoglycaemic and nonhypoglycaemic glucose counter-regulation in humans. *Am. J. Physiol.*, **247**, E198–E205.

Fain, J.N., Kovacev, V.P. and Scow, R.O. (1966) Antilipolytic effect of insulin in isolated fat cells of the rat. *Endocrinology*, **78**, 773–78.

Felig, P. (1973) The glucose-alanine cycle. *Metabolism*, **22**, 179–207.

Felig, P. and Wahren, J. (1971) Influence of endogenous insulin on splanchnic glucose and amino acid metabolism. *J. Clin. Invest.*, **50**, 1702.

Garber, A.J., Karl, I.E. and Kipnis, D.M. (1976) Alanine and glutamine synthesis and release from skeletal muscle. *J. Biol. Chem.*, **251**, 836–43.

Garcia, A., Williamson, J.R. and Cahill, G.F. Jr. (1966) Studies on the perfused rat liver. II. Effect of glucagon on gluconeogenesis. *Diabetes*, **15**, 188.

Gerich, J., Davis, J., Lorenzi, M. *et al.* (1979) Hormonal mechanisms of recovery from insulin-induced hypoglycaemia in man. *Am. J. Physiol.*, **236**:4, E380–E385.

Gregersen, N. (1985) The acyl CoA dehydrogenase deficiencies. *Scand. J. Clin. Lab. Invest.*, **45** (suppl. 174), 1–60.

Haymond, M.W., Karl, I.E., Clarke, W.L. *et al.* (1982) Differences in circulating gluconeogenic substrates during short-term fasting in men, women and children. *Metabolism*, **31**, 33–42.

Johnston, D.G. and Alberti, K.G.M.M. (1982) Hormonal control of ketone body metabolism in the normal and diabetic state. *Clinics in Endocrinology and Metabolism*, **11**, 329–61.

Kelnar, C.J.H. (1976) Hypoglycaemia in children undergoing tonsillectomy. *Brit. Med. J.*, **1**, 751–52.

Kreisberg, R. (1972) Glucose-lactate inter-relationships in man. *New Eng. J. Med.*, **287**, 132–37.

Marliss, E.B., Aoki, Th. T., Unger, R.H. *et al.* (1970) Glucagon levels and metabolic effects in fasting man. *J. Clin. Invest.*, **49**, 2256–70.

Nilsson, L., Hultman, E. (1973) Liver glucose in man – the effect of total starvation on a carbohydrate-poor diet followed by carbohydrate refeeding. *Scand. J. Clin. Lab. Invest.*, **32**, 325–30.

Owen, O.E., Morgan, A.P., Kemp, H.G. *et al.* (1967) Brain metabolism during fasting. *J. Clin. Invest.*, **46**, 1589–95.

Pagliara, A.S., Karl, I.E., DeVivo, D.C., *et al.* (1972) Hypoalaninaemia: a concomitant of ketotic hypoglycaemia. *J. Clin. Invest.*, **51**, 1440–49.

Raptis, S., Schlegal, W. and Pfeiffer, E.F. (1978) 'Effects of somatostatin on gut and pancreas', in S.R. Bloom and J.M. Polak (eds). *Gut Hormones*. Churchill Livingstone, London.

Reinmuth, O., Scheinberg, P. and Bourne, B. (1965) Total cerebral blood flow and metabolism. *Arch. Neurol.*, **12**, 49.

Saudubray, J.M., Marsac, C., Limal, J.M. *et al.* (1981) Variation in plasma ketone bodies during a 24-hour fast in normal and hypoglycemic children: relationship to age. *J. Pediatr.*, **98**, 904–908.

Sokal, J. (1966) Glucagon – an essential hormone. *Am. J. Med.*, **41**, 331.

Stirling, H.F., Darling, J.A.B. and Kelnar, C.J.H. (1991) Nocturnal glucose homeostasis in normal children. *Hormone Research*, **35** (suppl. 2), 54.

Touma, E.H. and Charpentier, C. (1992) Medium chain acyl-CoA dehydrogenase deficiency. *Arch. Dis. Child.*, **67**, 142–45.

Unger, R.H., Ohneda, A., Aguliar-Parada, E. *et al.* (1969) The role of aminogenic glucagon secretion in blood gluose homeostasis. *J. Clin. Invest.*, **48**, 810–22.

Wahren, J., Felig, P.H., Ahlborg, G. *et al.* (1971) Glucose metabolism during leg exercise in man. *J. Clin. Invest.*, **50**, 2715–25.

Wolfsdorf, J.I., Sadeghi-Nejad, A. and Senior, B. (1983) Hypoketonemia and age-related fasting hypoglycaemia in growth hormone deficiency. *Metabolism*, **32**, 457–62.

Woods, S.C. and Porte, Jr. (1974) Neural control of the endocrine pancreas. *Physiol. Rev.*, **54**, 596–619.

3

Glucose homeostasis in the normal adolescent

D.B. DUNGER and J.A. EDGE

3.1 INTRODUCTION

The adolescent years are characterized by rapid growth and profound changes in diet and lifestyle. The pubertal growth spurt results in an almost doubling of lean body mass and an increase in height of, on average, 20 cm in girls and 23 cm in boys. Dietary habits of adolescents are poorly characterized but total energy intake increases, reflecting the need for rapid growth. Where nutrition is inadequate, or the normal endocrine changes which regulate glucose homeostasis are impaired, growth may be blunted and pubertal development will be delayed. The appropriate interplay between glucose homeostasis and growth is a fundamental part of normal pubertal development.

3.2 THE RELATIONSHIP BETWEEN PLASMA GLUCOSE AND INSULIN LEVELS

Fasting plasma glucose levels are maintained within a very narrow range at all ages, but the relationship with fasting insulin levels is not constant. Cross-sectional data indicate that fasting insulin levels increase between age 10–20 (Grant, 1967; Smith *et al.*, 1988) and then return to levels comparable to those noted in early childhood during early adult life (Figure 3.1a). Further analysis indicates that these changes are more closely correlated with puberty than with age (Smith *et al.*, 1988, 1989; Laron *et al.*, 1988). The changes in the two sexes are remarkably similar with maximal fasting plasma insulin levels being observed at around Tanner stage 3–4 for genital or breast development. A consistent finding has been that fasting insulin levels tend to be higher in females than in males (Figure 3.2). These differences do not always reach statistical significance, and may reflect anomalies in the interpretation of cross-sectional data. There is a strong relationship between fasting plasma insulin concentration and height velocity in normal children (Hindmarsh *et al.*, 1988) and the higher levels in girls may reflect their earlier maturation and pubertal growth spurt.

Stimulated insulin concentrations are also greater during puberty (Figure 3.1b). Adolescents have greater insulin responses to both oral and intravenous glucose tolerance, when compared with younger children and adults (Rosenbloom *et al.*, 1975; Bloch *et al.*, 1987; Smith *et al.*, 1988). These changes in fasting and stimulated insulin concentrations

Childhood and Adolescent Diabetes
Published in 1994 by Chapman & Hall, London
ISBN 0 412 48610 5

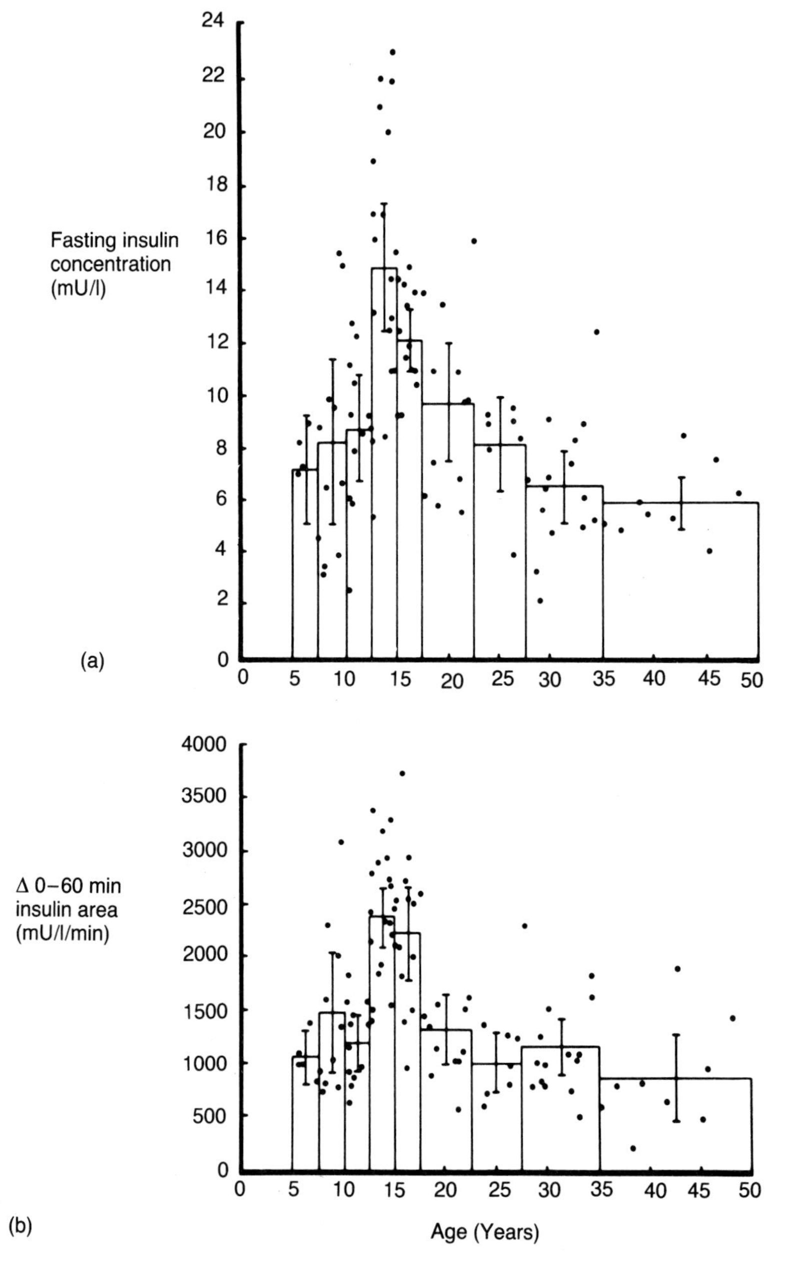

Figure 3.1 (a) Fasting plasma insulin concentrations and (b) insulin responses to IV glucose, in relation to age. The bars indicate the mean values, with 95% confidence intervals for different age groups (Smith *et al.*, 1989).

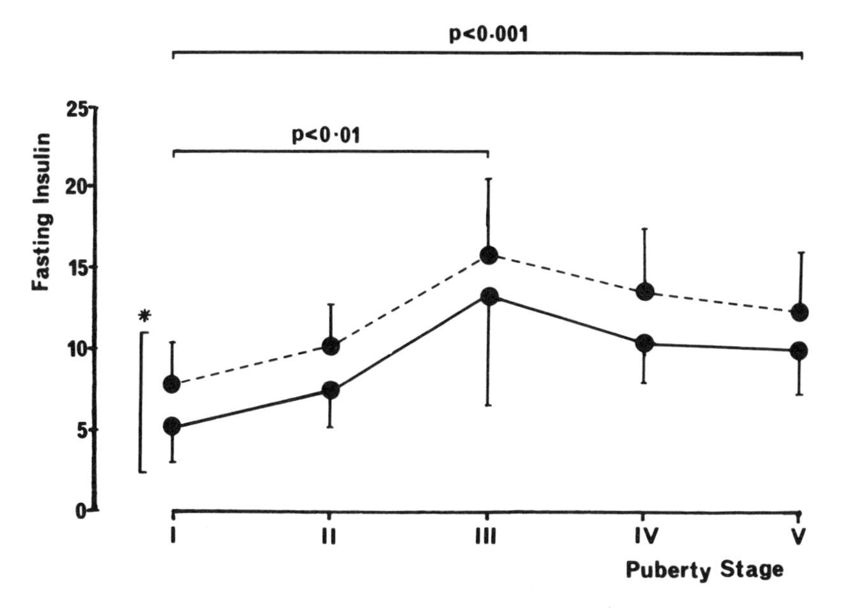

Figure 3.2 Fasting insulin levels during puberty in females (------) and males (——).

are accompanied by similar changes in C-peptide levels (Ludvigsson & Heding, 1977; Ratzmann *et al.*, 1986; Laron *et al.*, 1988), reflecting a profound change in endogenous insulin secretion during puberty. Evidence has accumulated which indicates that these increases in basal and stimulated insulin concentrations occur to compensate for a reduction in insulin sensitivity during puberty.

3.3 CHANGES IN INSULIN SENSITIVITY DURING ADOLESCENCE

Several recent studies, some using the euglycemic clamp technique, have shown that normal puberty is associated with an alteration in insulin-stimulated glucose metabolism (Amiel *et al.*, 1986; Bloch *et al.*, 1987; Caprio *et al.*, 1989). Amiel *et al.* (1986) demonstrated a reduction of between 34–42% in insulin-stimulated glucose metabolism in pubertal when compared with prepubertal and adult subjects (Figure 3.3). As would be predicted

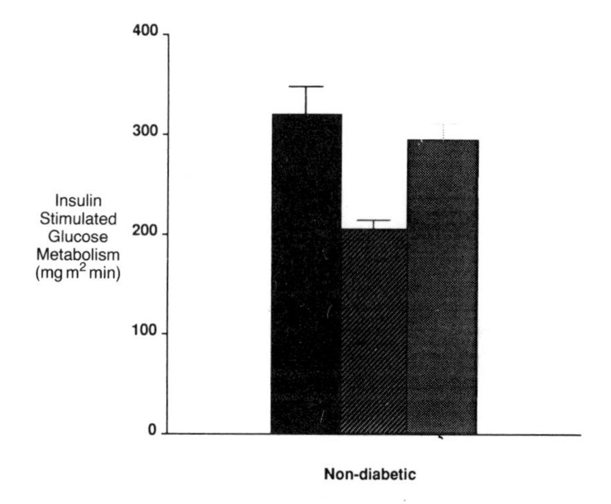

Figure 3.3 Effect of puberty on insulin-stimulated glucose metabolism in nondiabetics (redrawn from Amiel *et al.*, 1986). Tanner I: ■; Tanner II–IV: ▨; Adult: ▩.

from the fasting insulin data, these changes are more closely related to puberty than age. Changes in insulin sensitivity parallel those of fasting insulin concentrations and peak at around puberty stage 3–4 in both sexes. Whereas sex differences in the levels of fasting insulin have been observed, there are no comparable data concerning differences in insulin sensitivity. Arslanian *et al.* (1991) were able to show sexual dimorphism in the insulin sensitivity of adolescents with IDDM, but control data were not reported.

The site of insulin resistance during puberty has also been studied by the euglycemic clamp technique. A decrease in insulin-stimulated glucose disposal might arise from either a reduction in peripheral glucose disposal or impaired suppression of hepatic glucose production. Hepatic glucose production rates tend to be high in neonates and infants (Bier *et al.*, 1977; Kalhan *et al.*, 1980), but thereafter they remain stable throughout childhood. In studies using euglycemic clamps with sequential 8 and 40 ml/m^2/min insulin infusions, Amiel *et al.* (1991) were able to show that hepatic glucose production remained remarkably stable during puberty and that the impaired insulin-stimulated glucose disposal was a defect restricted to peripheral glucose metabolism.

From these data we can conclude that the increased insulin secretion during puberty can be seen as a compensatory response to reductions in insulin sensitivity which are restricted to peripheral glucose metabolism. These changes in insulin sensitivity are very closely related to the other changes of puberty, particularly growth, and we might expect that they may be directly related to the other endocrine changes of puberty.

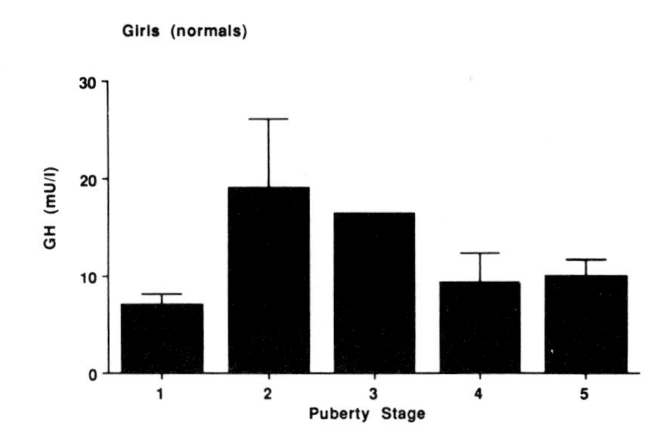

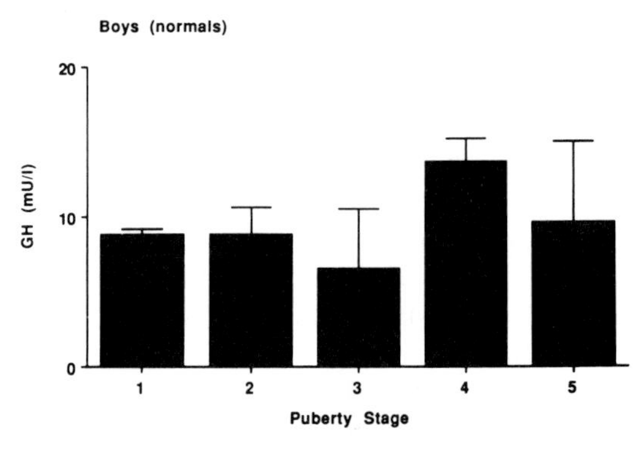

Figure 3.4 Mean overnight growth hormone levels of normal subjects according to puberty stage.

3.4 THE RELATIONSHIP BETWEEN INSULIN RESISTANCE AND GROWTH HORMONE SECRETION DURING PUBERTY

Growth hormone levels increase dramatically during normal puberty (Zadik *et al.*, 1985; Hindmarsh *et al.*, 1988). The transition through puberty is characterized by an increase in growth hormone pulse amplitude, particularly at night, whereas pulse frequency remains unchanged. An earlier increase in mean growth hormone levels is noted in girls (Figure 3.4) corresponding with their earlier growth spurt and maturation (Edge *et al.*, 1990a).

It has long been recognized that short-term increases in growth hormone concentrations lead to impaired suppression of hepatic glucose production and reduced insulin-stimulated glucose utilization (Rizza *et al.*, 1982; Bratusch-Marrain *et al.*, 1982). Further, in normal subjects, the metabolic effects of growth hormone are limited by a compensatory increase in plasma insulin levels such as those observed in normal adolescents during puberty. Amiel *et al.* (1986) in their studies of insulin sensitivity in pubertal and prepubertal children were able to show a correlation between 24-hour mean growth hormone levels and insulin-stimulated glucose metabolism. The results of several other studies have also suggested that the puberty-associated rise in plasma growth hormone concentrations may be responsible for the insulin resistance during adolescence (Smith *et al.*, 1988; Bratush-Marrain *et al.*, 1982; Hindmarsh *et al.*, 1988).

Growth hormone secretion is pulsatile and during early puberty the majority of secretion occurs during the night. Recent studies indicate that it is the growth hormone pulse amplitude rather than baseline concentrations which lead to changes in insulin sensitivity (Fowelin *et al.*, 1991; Pal *et al.*, 1992). Studies of the effects of growth hormone pulse administration on forearm substrate fluxes demonstrate a change in glucose uptake which is maximal 120 minutes after GH administration and is sustained for 240 mins (Moller *et al.*, 1990). Fowelin *et al.* (1991) demonstrated that the duration of insulin resistance following a growth hormone pulse is dependent on the peak growth hormone levels: levels in excess of 50 mU/l, which are often encountered during puberty, might be expected to lead to sustained changes in insulin sensitivity lasting 6–7 hours. The effects of overnight growth hormone secretion might therefore be expected to result in a 'dawn phenomenon' of increasing insulin resistance overnight as has been demonstrated in adolescents with IDDM (Beaufrere *et al.*, 1988; Edge *et al.*, 1990b; Perriello *et al.*, 1990). However, it has proved surprisingly difficult to confirm the existence of a dawn phenomenon in normal subjects. Paradoxically, in some studies a very slight fall in blood glucose concentration overnight has been observed in normal children but not in adults (Marin *et al.*, 1988). Bolli *et al.* (1984), using a continuous infusion of a cold isotope of glucose, were able to show that rates of glucose production, glucose utilization and insulin secretion all increased after 03.00 hours in normal volunteers. Schmidt *et al.* (1984) using a continuous blood sampling technique were also able to show an increase in plasma insulin concentrations at dawn. Early methodological problems complicated many of these studies, but even some recent studies have proposed that the observed 'dawn' changes in insulin requirements in normals and adolescents with IDDM may reflect changes in insulin clearance unrelated to growth hormone secretion (Arslanian *et al.*, 1992).

One may conclude that although there is compelling evidence that growth hormone may be a major factor responsible for the insulin resistance at puberty, other factors may also play a part.

3.5 THE RELATIONSHIP BETWEEN SEX STEROIDS AND INSULIN RESISTANCE DURING PUBERTY

There is a temporal relationship between changes in the levels of sex steroids and the development of insulin resistance during puberty. However, whereas insulin resistance declines during early adult life, levels of sex steroids remain elevated. Further, it has not been possible to demonstrate any changes of insulin-mediated glucose disposal during the phases of the normal menstrual cycle despite large changes in sex steroid levels (Yki-Jarvinen, 1984; Toth *et al.*, 1987). Nevertheless, sex steroids may play a role in the early development of insulin resistance during puberty by modulating the changes in growth hormone pulse amplitude (Ho *et al.*, 1987; Mauras *et al.*, 1987).

There has been considerable interest in a possible link between the early rises in adrenal androgens and the development of insulin resistance during puberty. Several syndromes of hyperandrogenemia are associated with insulin resistance (Richards *et al.*, 1985) and Bloch *et al.* (1987) found a negative correlation between insulin sensitivity and DHEAS concentrations. One might conclude that adrenarche may be an important factor for the decline in insulin sensitivity during adolescence. However, these conclusions may have been biased by the inclusion of pubertal children in the analysis, for when Smith *et al.* (1989) compared rising DHEAS levels and insulin sensitivity in prepubertal children no relationship could be identified.

A role for sex steroids in determining changes in insulin sensitivity during puberty cannot be entirely ruled out. The circulating levels of sex steroids may not accurately reflect the availability of free hormone to tissue receptor sites. Sex hormone binding globulin (SHBG) binds testosterone and estradiol with high affinity and it is considered to be an important factor in determining the fraction of hormone which is free and available for receptor binding (Anderson, 1974). In cross-sectional studies of normal adolescents, SHBG levels fall in both sexes throughout puberty and regression analysis reveals a close correlation with insulin in both sexes (Holly *et al.*, 1989a). It has yet to be determined whether changes in 'free' as opposed to bound sex steroid concentrations may play a part in the insulin resistance of puberty. Suffice it to say that a temporal relationship does not necessarily imply causality.

3.6 THE RELATIONSHIP BETWEEN THE INSULIN-LIKE GROWTH FACTORS AND INSULIN RESISTANCE DURING PUBERTY

The relationship between changes in fasting insulin and insulin-like growth factor-I (IGF-I) concentrations is particularly striking and it remains constant throughout childhood,

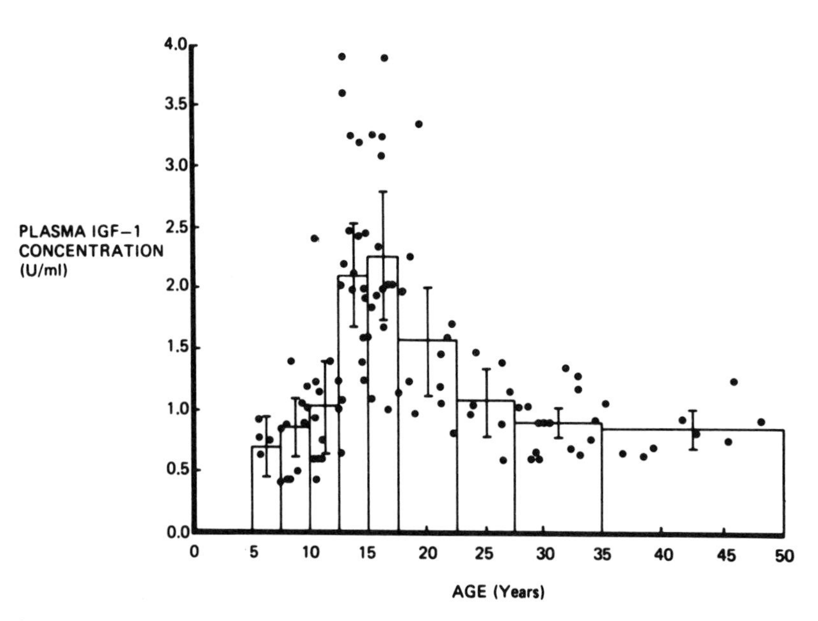

Figure 3.5 Plasma IGF-I concentrations in relation to age. The bars indicate the mean values, with 95% confidence intervals for the different age groups (Smith *et al.*, 1989).

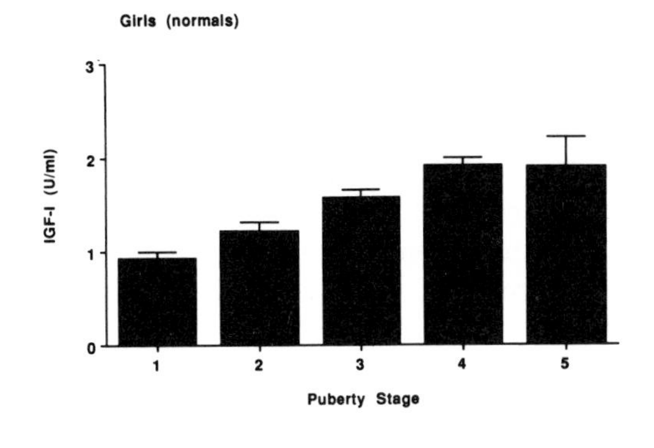

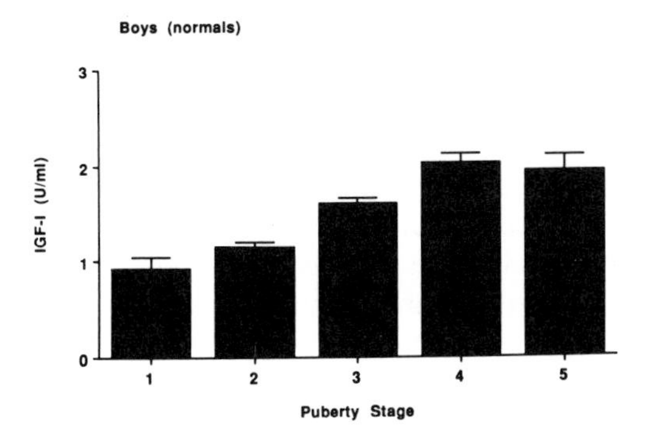

Figure 3.6 IGF-I levels of normal subjects according to puberty stage.

puberty and adult life (Figure 3.5). IGF-I levels show a similar pattern of change during puberty to that observed with insulin (Figure 3.6). IGF-I concentrations are growth hormone dependent and it could be argued that any effects of growth hormone on insulin resistance might be achieved via paracrine production of IGF-I. It was observed that in IGF-I deficient subjects such as the African Pygmy who have normal growth hormone levels, growth hormone administration fails to alter IGF-I or insulin levels, whereas in subjects who have low levels of growth hormone and IGF-I, this treatment results in an increase in IGF-I and a change in insulin levels (Merimee *et al.*, 1982). However, in diabetic subjects where there is also partial growth hormone resistance at the liver receptor leading to a subnormal IGF-I response and elevated growth hormone levels (Dunger *et al.*, 1991), the growth hormone excess still results in profound insulin resistance.

The availability of recombinant IGF-I has permitted further evaluation of the metabolic effects of IGF-I both *in vitro* and *in vivo*. Studies suggest that IGF-I causes *increased* insulin sensitivity in isolated rat muscle (Dimitriadis *et al.*, 1992) and it will lower blood glucose concentrations when IV-administered in man (Guler *et al.*, 1987). However, it may be difficult to extrapolate directly from these observations, as they are largely related to IGF-I concentrations which exceed the binding capacity of the plasma, for unlike insulin, IGF-I circulates bound to a series of binding proteins. Levels of IGF-I in the plasma during puberty are most closely related to those of the larger binding protein IGFBP-3 (Baxter & Martin, 1986). Thus IGF-I circulating bound to IGFBP-3 provides a reservoir of available peptide whereas the smaller binding proteins and in particular, IGFBP-1, may act as 'delivery' proteins which have an important role in the regulation of IGF bioactivity (Holly & Wass, 1989; Taylor *et al.*, 1990). Injections of recombinant IGFBP-1 have been shown to have dramatic effects on blood glucose concentrations in the rat and the availability of 'free' IGF-I may be an important determinant of insulin sensitivity. The insulin and IGF-I receptors share a high degree of sequence homology (Rechler & Nissley, 1986) and a hybrid receptor has been described. The interrelationships between IGF-I, insulin, IGF-II (a peptide which as yet has no important physiologic role) and the IGFBPs at the receptor level is likely to be complex and may yet yield important insights into the regulation of glucose metabolism. Whereas there is no direct evidence for a role of IGF-I in the development of insulin resistance during normal puberty, the very high levels of IGFBP-1 in IDDM may contribute to the insulin resistance encountered during puberty in those subjects (Baxter & Martin, 1986).

The close relationship between insulin and the levels of IGF-I point towards a role for insulin in the regulation of IGF bioactivity and thus indirectly in the control of growth. We can therefore with justification ask the question, 'Do the changes in insulin sensitivity during puberty play a role in normal pubertal development?'

3.7 THE ROLE OF CHANGES IN INSULIN SENSITIVITY DURING PUBERTY

It has become clear from studies of prepubertal children receiving growth hormone treatment that changes in growth hormone concentrations and improved growth are associated with a rise in insulin production rates as a compensation for decreased insulin sensitivity. Insulin is an important anabolic hormone, and at first sight it appears paradoxical that the development of insulin resistance should occur at a time of rapid growth during normal pubertal development. Several lines of enquiry suggest that increased insulin production may in fact have an essential role in normal pubertal growth and development.

3.7.1 ANABOLIC EFFECTS OF INSULIN

Insulin-stimulated glucose uptake may be impaired during puberty but pubertal subjects are just as sensitive to the suppressive effects of insulin on circulating free fatty acid and β-hydroxybutyrate levels as prepubertal children. Fasting free fatty acid and β-hydroxybutyrate concentrations show a negative correlation with fasting insulin levels and show a progressive fall with advancing puberty (Edge *et al.*, 1993). Under euglycemic hyperinsulinemic conditions, Amiel *et al.* (1991) were able to demonstrate a similar fall in branch chain amino acids in both prepubertal and pubertal subjects. They argued that this was the result of inhibition of protein breakdown (Fukagaura *et al.*, 1985) and that the insulin resistance of puberty was selective. Insulin resistance which selectively affects peripheral glucose but not amino acid metabolism has also been observed in normal adult subjects during fasting (Jensen *et al.*, 1988). These data would imply that the hyperinsulinemia resulting from impaired peripheral glucose uptake, might result in a greater fall in branch chain amino acids and enhanced protein anabolism during puberty.

3.7.2 INSULIN REGULATION OF IGF-I

As was discussed briefly in the previous section, insulin and IGF-I are closely related during puberty independently of growth hormone. *In vitro* studies suggest that insulin enhances IGF-I production (Daughaday *et al.*, 1976) by either direct regulation of the growth hormone receptor (Baxter *et al.*, 1980) or a permissive effect on post-growth hormone receptor events (Maes *et al.*, 1986). It could be argued that the hyperinsulinemia during puberty has a direct or permissive role in the generation of IGF-I. However, insulin also plays a more subtle role in the regulation of IGF bioactivity. Insulin regulates the circulating levels of the low MW IGFBP-1 (Sui *et al.*, 1988; Holly *et al.*, 1988a) and inhibits the production of IGFBP-1 by a human hepatoma cell line (Cotterill *et al.*, 1989). Recent reports suggest that insulin might also facilitate transcapillary transport of IGFBP-1 (Bar *et al.*, 1990). IGFBP-1 levels show a marked circadian rhythm reflecting changes in insulin concentrations (Holly *et al.*, 1988a). During normal puberty, fasting levels of IGFBP-1 progressively decline with increasing concentration of insulin (Holly *et al.*, 1989b) (Figure 3.7). As IGFBP-1 levels tend to inhibit IGF bioactivity (Taylor *et al.*, 1990) this reduction in IGFBP-1 may lead to enhanced IGF bioactivity during puberty.

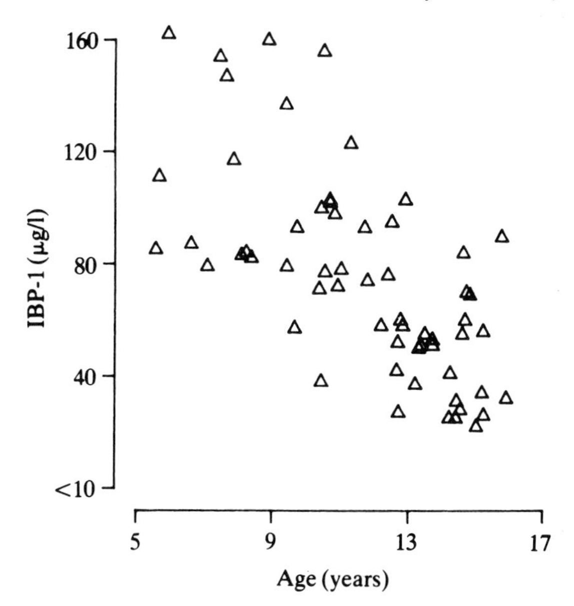

Figure 3.7 Relationship between fasting levels of insulin-like growth factor-binding protein (IGFBP-1) and age (Holly *et al.*, 1989b).

Thus the hyperinsulinemia of puberty may have a dual role in promoting IGF-I production and reducing levels of the inhibitory IGFBP-1. In many conditions where insulin levels are reduced, such as diabetes (Taylor *et al.*, 1988) and fasting (Busby *et al.*, 1988) IGF-I levels and IGF bioactivity are reduced. The hyperinsulinemia of puberty can be seen as having a facilitatory role in the promotion of growth during puberty and also providing a 'physiologic brake' to growth at times of nutrient and insulin deficiency.

3.7.3 INSULIN AND THE REGULATION OF SEX HORMONE BINDING GLOBULIN

In cross-sectional studies, sex hormone binding globulin levels (SHBG) fall in both males and females throughout the pubertal period (Holly *et al.*, 1989a). SHBG levels show a remarkable correlation with the small MW IGFBP-1 which led to the suggestion that SHBG like IGFBP-1 might be regulated by insulin. *In vitro* studies have shown that insulin inhibits SHBG production in human hepatoma cell lines (Plymate *et al.*, 1988). A role for insulin in the regulation of SHBG and thus levels of free sex steroids, might also contribute to the nutritional regulation of growth and sexual development, adequate nutrition and normal portal insulin delivery being necessary for the appropriate suppression of SHBG and IGFBP-1 during puberty.

3.7.4 ROLE OF INSULIN IN OVARIAN GROWTH AND MATURATION

There is considerable evidence that insulin and IGF-I may play an important role in ovarian physiology (Adashi *et al.*, 1985; Poretsky & Kalin, 1987). A full discussion of the possible mechanisms is beyond the scope of this chapter but includes the effects of insulin on the paracrine production of IGF-I and IGFBP-1 in the ovary and regulation of free sex steroid levels by suppression of SHGB. Insulin may have an important role in both growth and genital development during puberty.

3.8 ESTIMATION OF INSULIN REQUIREMENTS DURING PUBERTY IN CHILDREN WITH DIABETES

The dramatic changes in insulin sensitivity during puberty have important implications for the management of adolescents with diabetes. Studies of insulin sensitivity during normal puberty would predict that insulin requirements in the diabetic child might increase two-fold between the beginning of puberty and the attainment of genital stage 4 in boys and breast stage 4 in girls. However, it is not necessarily possible to extrapolate directly from these data to determine insulin requirements in adolescents with diabetes.

Direct measurements of insulin require-

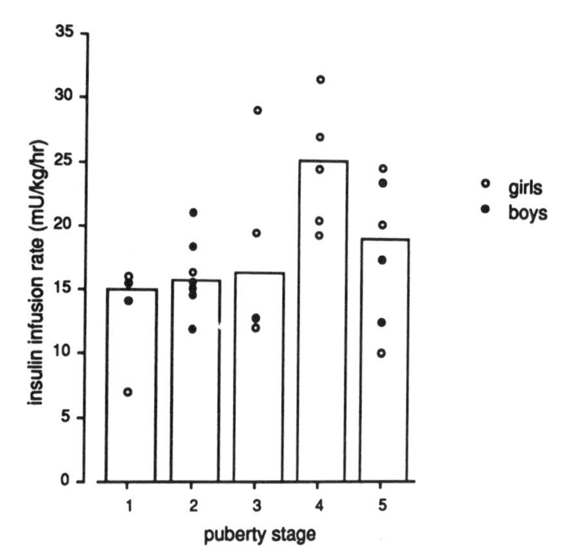

Figure 3.8 Insulin infusion rates during the euglycemic part of the night (01.00–08.00 h) per kilogram of lean body mass (LBM). Histogram shows median value at each puberty stage.

Table 3.1 Suggested daily basal insulin doses required for normoglycaemia at different puberty stages, calculated from requirement during the overnight glucose clamp from 01.00–08.00 h.

	Median (range) basal insulin dose Units/kg/day		
Puberty Stage	Girls	Boys	All
1	0.21 (0.13–0.29)	0.29 (0.28–0.29)	0.29 (0.13–0.29)
2	0.29	0.29 (0.23–0.38)	0.29 (0.23–0.38)
3	0.37 (0.22–0.52)	0.28	0.32 (0.22–0.52)
4	0.40 (0.38–0.56)	–	0.40 (0.38–0.56)
5	0.33 (0.18–0.44)	0.36 (0.27–0.47)	0.35 (0.18–0.47)

ments in subjects with diabetes are possible using closed loop systems, where insulin is given in direct response to a measured concentration of glucose (Clemens *et al.*, 1974). Early use of artificial systems such as the 'Biostator' were troubled by aggregation of insulin in the infusion system. However, the addition of albumin or the patient's own blood may overcome these problems. Matthews *et al.* (1990) developed a direct insulin-varying infusion system which overcame some of these difficulties in order to measure insulin requirements during adolescence. The overall median insulin requirements during puberty were in the order of 13 mU/kg/hr which corresponds well with data reported in adults of 7–20 mU/kg/hr (Clarke *et al.*, 1980; White *et al.*, 1982). An increase in insulin requirements was observed during puberty which was most significant when related to lean body mass rather than body weight (Figure 3.8). The estimated

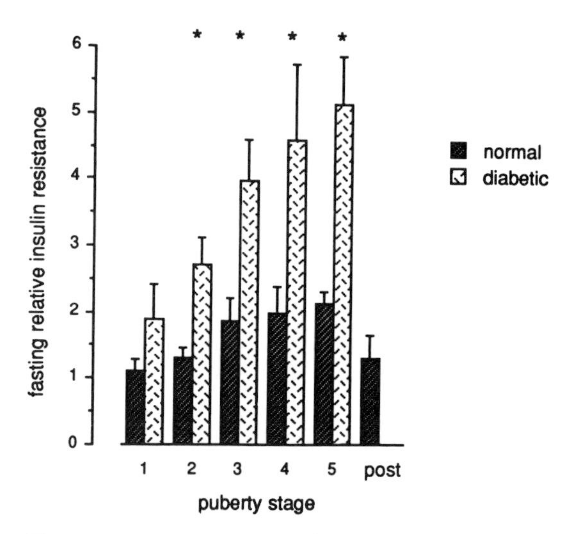

Figure 3.9 Comparison of mean ± SEM fasting relative insulin resistance in the diabetics at the end of the clamp study, and the normal adolescents. During puberty, the diabetics were more insulin resistant than the normal adolescents at every stage. * = $p < 0.02$.

changes in basal insulin requirements increasing from 0.21 units/kg/day at breast stage 1 to 0.40 units/kg/day at breast stage 4 and from 0.29 at genital stage 1 to 0.36 units/kg/day at genital stage 5 in boys (Table 3.1).

As one would have predicted from the normal data, there was a two-fold increase in insulin requirement in girls and a smaller increment in boys. However, direct assessment of insulin sensitivity from reported data indicate that the change in insulin resistance is up to two-fold greater in diabetic than in normal subjects during puberty (Figure 3.9). Variations in insulin sensitivity between normals and diabetics are but one of a number of problems which limit our ability to predict insulin requirements during puberty in adolescents with diabetes.

3.8.1 VARIATIONS IN INSULIN SENSITIVITY AND THE DAWN PHENOMENON

Insulin resistance is far greater in diabetics than in normal subjects during adolescence, and this may be directly attributable to variations in growth hormone secretion as discussed earlier in this chapter.

Insulin sensitivity may also vary within individuals according to physical fitness, meals or exercise, and prevailing overall glycemic control. Overnight insulin requirements in diabetic subjects are also affected by the dawn phenomenon. The dawn decrease in insulin sensitivity is thought to be due to nocturnal surges of growth hormone secretion (Campbell *et al.*, 1985; Edge *et al.*, 1990b), and the dawn increase in insulin requirements changes during puberty in direct relation to the growth hormone secretion (Edge *et al.*, 1990b). Whereas during early childhood and adult life the dawn change in insulin requirements may be relatively trivial compared with other determinants of insulin requirements (such as physical fitness), during puberty it may be critical to successful control of blood glucose overnight.

3.8.2 INSULIN DELIVERY

Endogenous insulin secretion is associated with less insulin resistance than exogenous insulin delivery, and portal delivery may be superior to subcutaneous delivery of insulin (Shisko *et al.*, 1992). Thus the efficacy of basal insulin delivery depends not only on the dose but also the mode of administration. Long-acting insulin given either twice daily or late at night as part of multiple injection therapy may not provide adequate insulin delivery overnight. Whether the long-acting insulin is an isophane, lente or ultralente preparation, free insulin levels tend to wane overnight. As a consequence, insulin levels tend to be higher during the early part of the night, with a high incidence of nocturnal hypoglycemia at around 4 a.m. and low during the latter part of the night which leads to an accelerated rise in blood glucose during the morning (Edge *et al.*, 1990c). Standard subcutaneous insulin delivery will not produce insulin profiles comparable with those obtained with continuous SC or IV insulin.

Finally, we have to consider whether glucose homeostasis is the only consideration when striving for good diabetic control. Even intravenous clamping of glucose within the normal range will not adequately suppress intermediate metabolites or free fatty acid levels overnight in adolescents with diabetes. Portal venous delivery of insulin may be superior but not entirely practical (Shisko *et al.*, 1992). It has to be recognized that standard insulin therapy in IDDM will not correct all of the metabolic abnormalities.

3.9 CONCLUSIONS

The regulation of glucose homeostasis undergoes profound changes during adolescence which have enormous implications for the management of diabetes mellitus. Whereas glucose levels remain stable, fasting insulin levels in normal children rise steadily until midpuberty. These changes relate to increases in insulin resistance which result from the increases in growth hormone secretion during puberty. Growth hormone secretion in adolescents with diabetes is increased over and above that encountered in normal subjects. The increased insulin resistance overall during puberty, provides problems in targeting insulin therapy since standard insulin therapy may not appropriately deal with changing insulin sensitivity overnight and subcutaneous rather than portal delivery overnight may not correct all of the metabolic abnormalities.

The appropriate and adequate delivery of insulin during puberty not only ensures glucose homeostasis, but also promotes normal pubertal growth and development. Persisting abnormalities of the growth hormone/IGF-I and gonadal axis may not only interfere with normal development but also lead to deterioration in glucose homeostasis, by increases in insulin resistance.

REFERENCES

Adashi, E.Y., Resnick, C.E., E'Ercole, A.J. *et al.* (1985) Insulin-like growth factors as intra-ovarian regulators of granulosa cell growth and function. *Endocrin. Rev.*, **6**, 400–420.

Amiel, S.A., Caprio, S., Sherwin, R.S. *et al.* (1991) Insulin resistance of puberty: a defect restricted to peripheral glucose metabolism. *J. Clin. Endocrin. Metab.*, **72**, 277–82.

Amiel, S.A., Sherwin, R.S., Simonson, D.V. *et al.* (1986) Impaired insulin action in puberty. A contributing factor to poor glycaemic control in adolescents with diabetes. *N. Eng. J. Med.*, **315**, 215–19.

Anderson, D.C. (1974) Sex hormone binding globulin. *Clin. Endocrin.*, **3**, 69–96.

Arslanian, S.A., Heil, B.V., Becker, D.T. *et al.* (1991) Sexual dimorphism in insulin sensitivity in adolescents with insulin-dependent diabetes mellitus. *J. Clin. Endocrin. Metab.*, **71**, 920–26.

Arslanian, S., Ohki, Y., Becker, D.J. *et al.* (1992) The dawn phenomenon: Comparison between normal and insulin-dependent diabetic adolescents. *Ped. Res.*, **31**, 203–206.

Bar, R.S., Boes, M., Clemmons, D.R. *et al.* (1990) Insulin differentially alters trans-capillary movement of intravascular IGFBP-1, IGFBP-2 and endothelial cell IGF-binding proteins in the rat heart. *Endocrinology*, **127**, 497–99.

Baxter, R.C., Bryson, J.M. and Turtle, J.R. (1980) Somatogenic receptors of rat liver: regulation by insulin. *Endocrinology*, **107**, 1176–81.

Baxter, R. and Martin, J.L. (1986) Radioimmunoassay of growth hormone dependent insulin-like growth factor binding protein in human plasma. *J. Clin. Invest.*, **78**, 1504–12.

Beaufrere, B., Beylot, M., Metz, C. *et al.* (1988) Dawn phenomenon in Type 1 (insulin-dependent) diabetic adolescents: Influence of nocturnal growth hormone secretion. *Diabetologia*, **31**, 607–611.

Bier, D.M., Leake, R.D., Haymond, M.W. *et al.* (1977) Measurement of 'free' glucose production rate in infancy and childhood with G-6 dideulerolglucose. *Diabetes*, **26**, 1016–23.

Bloch, C.A., Clemons, P. and Sperling, M.A. (1987) Puberty decreases insulin sensitivity. *J. Pediatr.*, **110**, 481–87.

Bolli, G.B., Defreo, P., De Cosmo, S. *et al.* (1984) Demonstration of a dawn phenomenon in normal human volunteers. *Diabetes*, **33**, 1150–53.

Bratusch-Marrain, P.R., Smith, D. and De Fronzo, R.A. (1982) The effects of growth hormone on glucose metabolism and insulin secretion in man. *J. Clin. Endocrin. Metab.*, **55**, 973–82.

Busby, W.H., Snyder, D.K. and Clemmons, D.R. (1988) Radioimmunoassay of a 26 000-dalton plasma insulin-like growth factor binding protein control by nutritional variables. *J. Clin. Endocrin. Metab.*, **67**, 1225–30.

Campbell, P.J., Bolli, G.B., Cryer, P.E. *et al.* (1985) Pathogenesis of the dawn phenomenon in patients with insulin-dependent diabetes mellitus. Accelerated glucose production and impaired glucose utilisation due to nocturnal surges in growth hormone secretion. *N. Eng. J. Med.*, **312**, 1473–79.

Caprio, S., Plewe, G., Diamond, M.P. *et al.* (1989) Increased insulin secretion during puberty: A compensatory response to reductions in insulin sensitivity. *J. Pediatr.*, **114**, 963–67.

Clarke, W.L., Haymond, M.W. and Santiago, J.V. (1980) Overnight basal insulin requirements in fasting insulin-dependent diabetes. *Diabetes*, **29**, 78–80.

Clemens, A.H., Chang, P.H. and Myers, R.W. (1977) The development of the Biostator, a glucose controlled insulin infusion system (GCIIS). *Horm. Metab. Res.*, **7** (Suppl.), 23–33.

Cotterill, A.M., Cowell, C.J. and Silink, M. (1989) Insulin and variation in glucose levels modify the secretion rates of growth hormone independent insulin-like growth factor binding protein-I in the human hepatoblastoma cell line Hep G2. *Endocrinology*, **123**, R17.

Daughaday, W.H., Phillips, L.S. and Mueller, M.S. (1976) The effects of insulin and growth hormone on the release of somatomedin by the isolated rat liver. *Endocrinology*, **98**, 1214–19.

Dimitriadis, G., Parry-Billings, M., Dunger, D.B. *et al.* (1992) The effect of *in vivo* administration of insulin-like growth factor-I (IGF-I) on the sensitivity of glucose utilisation to insulin the soleus muscle of rat. *J. Endocrin.*, **133**, 37–43.

Dunger, D.B., Edge, J.A., Pal, R. *et al.* (1991) The impact of increased growth hormone secretion on carbohydrate metabolism in the adolescent diabetic. *Acta Paed. Scand.*, **377** (Suppl.), 69–77.

Edge, J.A., Dunger, D.B., Matthews, D.R. *et al.* (1990a) Increased overnight growth hormone concentrations in diabetic compared with normal adolescents. *J. Clin. Endocrin. Metab.*, **71**, 1356–62.

Edge, J.A., Matthews, D.R. and Dunger, D.B. (1990b) The dawn phenomenon is related to overnight growth hormone release in adolescent diabetics. *Clin. Endocrin.*, **33**, 729–37.

Edge, J.A., Matthews, D.R. and Dunger, D.B. (1990c) Failure of current insulin regimes to meet the overnight insulin requirements of adolescent diabetics. *Diabetes Res.*, **15**, 109–112.

Edge, J.A., Harris, D.A., Phillips, P.E. *et al.* (1993) Evidence for a role for insulin and growth hormone in the overnight regulation of 3-hydroxybutyrate in normal and adolescents with diabetes. *Diabetes Care*, **16**, 1011–19.

Fowelin, J., Attoal, S., Van Schenck, H. *et al.* (1991) Characterisation of the insulin-dependent effect of growth hormone in man. *Diabetologia*, **34**, 500–506.

Fukagaura, N.K., Minaker, K.L., Rowe, J.W. *et al.* (1985) Insulin-mediated reduction of whole body protein breakdown: dose response effects on leucrine metabolism in post-absorptive man. *J. Clin. Invest.*, **76**, 2306–11.

Grant, D.B. (1967) Fasting serum insulin levels in childhood. *Arch. Dis. Child.*, **375**, 378.

Guler, H.P., Zapf, J. and Froesch, E.R. (1987) Short-term metabolic effects of recombinant human insulin-like growth factor-I in healthy adults. *N. Eng. J. Med.*, **317**, 137–40.

Hindmarsh, P.C., Matthews, D.R. and Brook, C.D.G. (1988) Growth hormone secretion in children determined by time series analysis. *Clin. Endocrin.* (Oxford), **29**, 35–44.

Ho, K.Y., Evans, W.S., Blizzard, R.M. *et al.* (1987) Effects of sex and age on 24-hour profiles of growth hormone secretion in man: importance of endogenous oestradiol concentrations. *J. Clin. Endocrin. Metab.*, **64**, 51–58.

Holly, J.M.P., Biddlecombe, R.A., Dunger, D.B. *et al.* (1988a) Circadian variation of GH-Independent IGF binding protein in diabetes mellitus and its relationship to insulin: A new role for insulin? *Clin. Endocrin.* (Oxford), **29**, 667–75.

Holly, J.M.P., Amiel, S.A., Sandhu, R.R. *et al.* (1988b) The role of growth hormone in diabetes mellitus. *J. Endocrin.*, **118**, 353–64.

Holly, J.M.P. and Wass, J.A.H. (1989) Insulin-like growth factors: Autocrine paracrine or endocrine? New perspectives of the somatomedin hypothesis in the light of recent developments. *J. Endocrin.*, **122**, 611–18.

Holly, J.M.P., Smith, C.P., Dunger, D.B. *et al.* (1989a) Relationship between the pubertal fall in sex hormone binding globulin and insulin-like growth factor binding protein-I. A synchronised approach to pubertal development. *Clin. Endocrin.* (Oxford), **31**, 277–84.

Holly, J.M.P., Smith, C.P., Dunger, D.B. *et al.* (1989b) Levels of the small MW IGF-I binding protein are strongly related to those of insulin in prepubertal and pubertal children but weakly so after puberty. *J. Endocrin.*, **121**, 383–87.

Jensen, M.D., Miles, J.M., Gerich, J.E. *et al.* (1988) Preservation of insulin effects on glucose production and proteolysis during fasting. *Am. J. Physio.*, **254**, E700–E707.

Kalhan, S.C., Bier, D.M., Savin, S.M. *et al.* (1980) Estimation of glucose turnover with 13-carbon recycling in human newborn by simultaneous [1-13C] Glucose and [66-2H2] glucose tracer. *J. Clin. Endocrin. Metab.*, **50**, 456–60.

Laron, Z., Aurbarch-Klipper, Y., Flasterstein, B. *et al.* (1988) Changes in endogenous insulin secretion during childhood as expressed by plasma and urinary C-peptide. *Clin. Endocrin.*, **29**, 625–32.

Ludvigsson, J. and Heding, L.G. (1977) C-peptide in juvenile diabetics. *Acta Paed. Scand.*, **270** (Suppl.), 53–60.

Maes, M., Underwood, L.E. and Ketelslegers, J.-M. (1986) Low serum somatomedin-C in insulin dependent diabetes: evidence for a post receptor mechanism. *Endocrinology*, **118**, 377–82.

Marin, G., Rose S.R., Kebarian, M. *et al.* (1988) Absence of dawn phenomenon in normal children and adolescents. *Diabetes Care*, **11**, 393–96.

Matthews, D.R., Edge, J.A. and Dunger, D.B. (1990) An unbiased glucose clamp method using a variable insulin function: Its application in adolescents. *Diabetic Med.*, **7**, 246–51.

Mauras, N., Blizzard, R.M., Link, K. *et al.* (1987) Augmentation of growth hormone secretion during puberty: evidence for a pulse amplitude-modulated phenomenon. *J. Clin. Endocrin.*, **64**, 596–601.

Merimee, T.S., Zapf, F. and Froesch, E.R. (1982) Insulin-like growth factors in pygmies and subjects with pygmy trait. Characterisation of the metabolic actions of IGF-I and IGF-II in man. *J. Clin. Endocrin. Metab.*, **55**, 1081–88.

Moller, N., Jorgensen, J.O.L., Schmitz, O. *et al.* (1990) Effects of a growth hormone pulse on total and forearm substrate fluxes in humans. *Am. H. Physiol.*, **258**, E86–E91.

Pal, B.R., Phillips, P.E., Matthews, D.R. *et al.* (1992) Contrasting metabolic effects of continuous and pulsatile growth hormone administration in young adults with Type 1 (insulin-dependent) diabetes mellitus. *Diabetologia*, **35**, 542–49.

Perriello, G., Defeo, P., Torlone, E. *et al.* (1990) Nocturnal spikes of growth hormone secretion cause the dawn phenomenon in Type 1 (insulin-dependent) diabetes mellitus by decreasing hepatic (and extrahapatic) sensitivity to insulin in the absence of insulin waning. *Diabetologia*, **33**, 52–59.

Plymate, S.R., Matej, L.A., Jones, R.E. *et al.* (1988) Inhibition of sex hormone-binding globulin production in the human (Hep G2) cell line by insulin and prolactin. *J. Clin. Endocrin. Metab.*, **67**, 460–64.

Poretsky, L. and Kalin, M.F. (1987) The gonadotrophic function of insulin. *Endocrin. Rev.*, **8**, 132–41.

Ratzmann, K.P., Strese, J., Kohnert, M.D. *et al.* (1986) Age-dependent relationship of fasting C-peptide concentration and insulin secretion in non-obese subjects with normal glucose tolerance. *Exp. Clin. Endocrin.*, **88**, 57–63.

Rechler, M.M. and Nissley, S.P. (1986) Insulin-like growth factor (IGF)/somatomedin receptor subtypes; structure, function and relationships to insulin receptors and IGF carrier proteins. *Horm. Res.*, **24**, 152–59.

Richards, G.E., Caralles, A., Meyer III, W.J. *et al.* (1985) Obesity, acanthosis nigricans, insulin resistance and hyperandrogenemia: pediatric perspective and natural history. *J. Pediatr.*, **107**, 893–97.

Rizza, R.A., Mandarino, L. and Gerich, J.E. (1982) Effects of growth hormone on insulin action in man: mechanisms of insulin resistance impaired suppression of glucose production and impaired stimulation of glucose utilisation. *Diabetes*, **31**, 663–69.

Rosenbloom, A.L., Wheeler, L., Biachi, R. *et al.* (1975) Age-adjusted analysis of insulin responses during normal and abnormal glucose tolerance tests in children and adolescents. *Diabetes*, **24**, 820–28.

Schmidt, M.I., Lin, Q.X., Gwynne, J.T. *et al.* (1984) Fasting early morning rise in peripheral insulin: evidence of the dawn phenomenon in non-diabetics. *Diabetes Care*, **7**, 32–35.

Shisko, P.I., Kovaler, P.A., Goncharov, V.G. *et al.* (1992) Comparison of peripheral and portal (via the umbilical vein) routes of insulin infusion in IDDM patients. *Diabetes*, **41**, 1042–49.

Smith, C.P., Archibald, H.R., Thomas, J.M. *et al.* (1988) Basal and stimulated insulin levels rise with advancing puberty. *Clin. Endocrin.* (Oxford), **28**, 7–14.

Smith, C.P., Dunger, D.B., Williams, A.J.K. *et al.* (1989) Relationship between insulin, insulin-like growth factor-I and dehydroepiandrosterone sulphate concentrations during childhood, puberty and adult life. *J. Clin. Endocrin. Metab.*,

68, 932–37.

Sui, K., Kari, A.M., Kovisto, V.A. *et al.* (1988) Insulin regulates the serum levels of low molecular weight insulin-like growth factor-binding protein. *J. Clin. Endocrin. Metab.*, **66**, 266–72.

Taylor, A.M., Dunger, D.B., Grant, D.B. *et al.* (1988) Somatomedin-C/IGF-I measured by radioimmunoassay and somatomedin bioactivity in adolescents with insulin-dependent diabetes mellitus compared with puberty matched controls. *Diabetes Res.*, **9**, 177–81.

Taylor, A.M., Dunger, D.B., Preece, M.A. *et al.* (1990) The growth hormone independent insulin-like growth factor-I binding protein BP-28 is associated with serum insulin-like growth factor-I inhibitory bioactivity in adolescent insulin-dependent diabetics. *Clin. Endocrin.*, **32**, 229–39.

Toth, E.L., Suthijumroon, A., Crockford, P.M. *et al.* (1987) Insulin action does not change during the menstrual cycle in normal women. *J. Clin. Endocrin. Metab.*, **64**, 74–80.

White, N.H., Skor, D. and Santiago, J.V. (1982) Practical closed-loop insulin delivery: a system for the maintenance of overnight euglycaemia and the calculation of basal insulin requirements in insulin-dependent diabetics. *An. Int. Med.*, **97**, 210–13.

Yki-Jarvinen, H. (1984) Insulin sensitivity during the menstrual cycle. *J. Clin. Endocrin. Metab.*, **59**, 350–53.

Zadik, Z., Chalew, S.A., MacCarter, J. *et al.* (1985) The influence of age on the 24-hour integrated concentration of growth hormone in normal individuals. *J. Clin. Endocrin. Metab.*, **60**, 513–16.

4

Normal childhood and pubertal growth and hormonal maturation

C.J.H. KELNAR

For a comprehensive background to childhood and pubertal growth see also the reviews by Tanner (1989, 1992) and Kelnar (1992a, 1992b), Kelnar (1993a) and Brook (1989). Useful reference manuals of normal physical measurements and characteristics are Buckler (1979) and Hall *et al.* (1989). US and UK growth charts are readily available (e.g., Tanner, 1992).

4.1 INTRODUCTION

4.1.1 THE IMPORTANCE OF GROWTH ASSESSMENT

Somatic growth is intrinsic to childhood and a healthy, adequately nourished and emotionally secure child grows at a normal rate. Thus an understanding of, and the ability to assess, childhood and pubertal growth and maturation is crucial for the early detection of disease in children and of particular value in detecting a wide variety of chronic childhood disorders in which poor growth may be the earliest, or only, sign that there is something wrong.

Growth velocity represents the current dynamics of growth much better than does a single measurement of stature which merely reflects previous growth (Brook, 1983). A slowly-growing child has a pathological disorder requiring diagnosis, and if possible, treatment. With conditions of recent onset, slow growth may not have occurred for sufficient time to cause short stature.

4.1.2 NORMAL GROWTH RATES

From the fifth month of prenatal life, rapid growth decelerates markedly over 3–4 years. Subsequently growth decelerates steadily, but more slowly, and is interrupted in most children by a phase of slight growth acceleration at 6–8 years (the mid-childhood growth spurt) which is synchronous with increasing adrenal androgen secretion (adrenarche). Prepubertal height velocities are similar in both sexes.

There is an approximately four year difference between the earliest 3% of normal children who enter puberty and the 3% in whom puberty is most delayed. In early puberty, leg growth predominates because of increasing growth hormone secretion. As puberty progresses, the secretion of sex steroids (testosterone in boys and estradiol in girls) increases and these primarily stimulate spinal growth. Both types of hormone act

Childhood and Adolescent Diabetes
Published in 1994 by Chapman & Hall, London
ISBN 0 412 48610 5

synergistically to stimulate overall growth at puberty. There is wide individual variation in the duration of the pubertal growth spurt which is unrelated to age at onset. The 14 cm difference between the 50th centile heights of men and women (as shown in the new UK growth standards which are becoming available during 1994) largely reflects the greater pubertal growth spurt in boys, which is on average around 20 cm. Boys do not reach maximal height velocity until late puberty (10–12 ml volume testes). The onset of rapid growth in girls sometimes even precedes breast development and menarche always occurs after peak height velocity is passed and growth is decelerating. Pubertal growth is discussed in more detail below.

The ability to measure a child accurately and reproducibly is indispensable for growth assessment. Height measurements are often valueless or misleading because of inadequate apparatus and careless techniques. Measuring techniques eliminating postural drops and positional errors are readily learned (Tanner, 1992). Suitably cheap and portable apparatus for primary carers to obtain accurate measurements in all age groups is now available (for the UK, see addresses at the end of this section).

Weight is a poor guide to obesity which is best assessed using skinfold calipers which measure directly the thickness of subcutaneous fat. Slow growth with >50th centile skinfold measurements are characteristic of an endocrine disorder in childhood. In severe growth hormone insufficiency, there is often a characteristic puckered or marbled appearance and texture to the abdominal fat.

A child's growth is remarkably regular over months or years, but variations occur seasonally and with, for example, episodes of intercurrent mild illness. Under normal circumstances, growth is regulated so that temporary periods of slow growth are com-

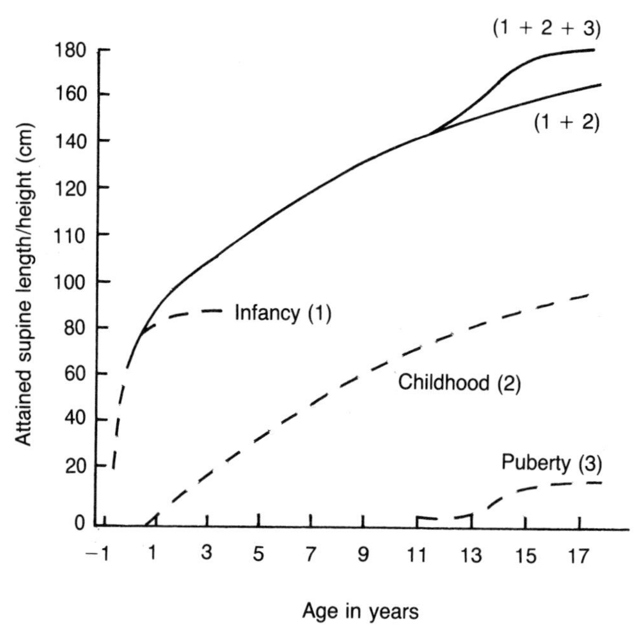

Figure 4.1 ICP (infancy–childhood–puberty) growth chart (boys) (Karlberg *et al.*, 1987a; 1987b).

pensated for (catch-up growth, see below), height velocity over a year is normal and a normal adult stature is achieved.

Mathematical models of the human growth curve have been descriptive (Preece & Hendrich, 1981; Stuetzle *et al.*, 1980) but models relating to possible underlying dynamics of hormonal (and other) control have more recently been proposed (Karlberg *et al.*, 1987). The infancy-childhood-puberty (ICP) growth model (Figure 4.1) suggests that the infancy component (which is a continuation of fetal growth) is primarily determined by nutritional factors, the childhood component by growth hormone and the puberty component by sex steroids. Thus the infancy component is initially rapid but decelerates as the influence of growth hormone (GH) appears by the end of the first year. The effect of GH is sustained but in the absence of adequate sex steroid secretion the pubertal growth spurt is blunted or absent. The combined input of the three components results in the normal pattern of growth until final height is achieved. Such a conceptual model, though simplistic if taken literally (see above), does allow the effects of different insults and treatments that could affect growth to be studied more effectively.

With accurate measurements, information on the normality of growth can be obtained over three months. Nevertheless, not every child grows at a consistent rate month by month and measurement over one year may be necessary before growth velocity can be clearly seen to be abnormal. In addition, there is recent evidence which suggests that a) normal growth may be cyclical with the rate varying over two to three years (Butler *et al.*, 1989a) and b) there may be short-term variations in growth velocity over quite short periods. Information relating to this latter phenomenon has been derived from knemometric measurement of lower leg length changes. The technique of knemometry (Hermanussen *et al.*, 1988a & 1988b), measuring the length of the lower limb from knee to heel, is also capable of detecting short-term fluctuations in growth, for example, during intercurrent illness or when daily (Wolthers & Pedersen, 1990) or alternate day (Wales & Milner, 1988) steroids are administered therapeutically.

4.1.3 CATCH-UP AND CATCH-DOWN GROWTH

Catch-up growth still remains a poorly understood phenomenon and the overall mechanisms by which physiologic states, growth hormone regulation and the genetic determination of growth potential are integrated to achieve appropriate stature are largely unknown. Increased understanding of these mechanisms is crucial to the scientific application of growth-promoting therapies in various clinical contexts. The concept of a 'sizostat', and the occurrence of 'catch-up' (Prader *et al.*, 1963) and 'catch-down' growth make it uncertain, on theoretical grounds, that exogenous hormone therapy in various categories of short children will necessarily increase final height and this is proving to be the case in many such situations (Kelnar, 1993b).

It has been proposed (Tanner, 1963) that the CNS contains a 'sizostat'. The rate of synthesis or release of a specific molecule could decrease as maturity increases and another molecule could be synthesized in proportion to the amount of growth. A 'mismatch' would be sensed by the sizostat and growth adjusted accordingly. Recent evidence from infusing dexamethasone into the proximal tibial growth plate of rabbits suggests that catch-up growth, rather than being entirely central nervous system dependent, could be intrinsic to the growth plate at least in part (Baron *et al.*, 1993).

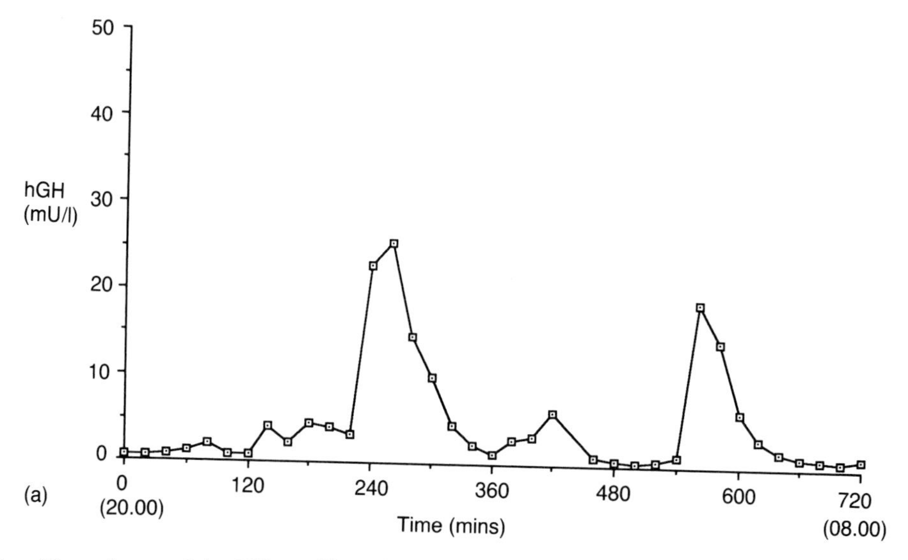

Figure 4.2a Normal overnight GH profile in late prepuberty (height velocity 4.5 cm/year).

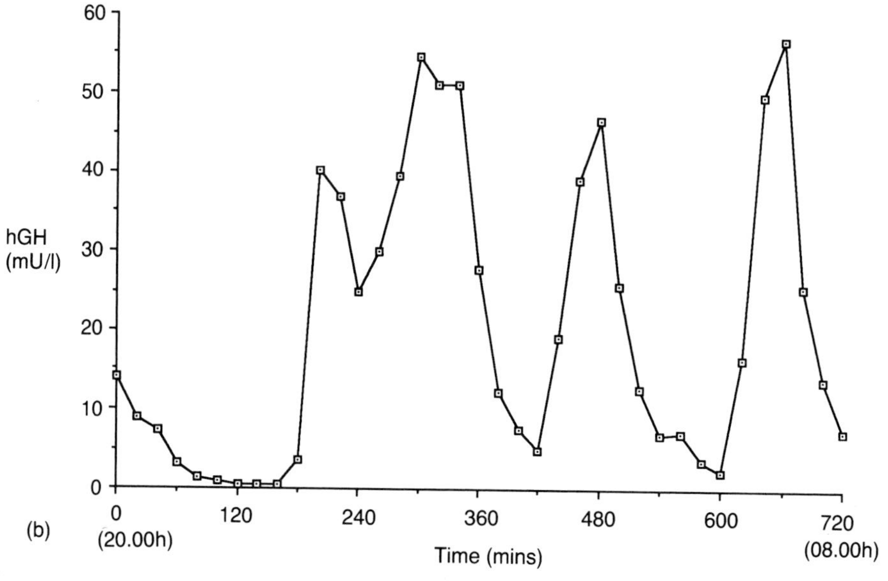

Figure 4.2b Overnight GH secretion in a boy growing rapidly (10 cm/year) in mid/late puberty (10 ml testicular volumes).

4.1.4 SKELETAL MATURATION – 'BONE AGE'

Bone age is computed from the maturity of bones in radiographs of the left hand and wrist by comparison with normal population standards. The child's 'bone age' is that chronological age for which the maturity score is at the 50th centile. Bone age, whether delayed or advanced in relation to chrono-

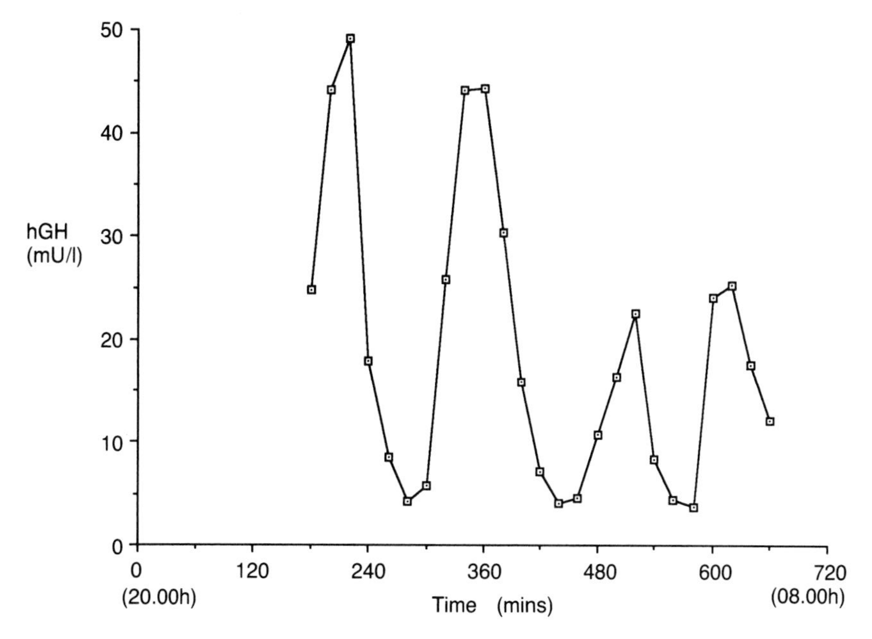

Figure 4.3 Overnight GH profile: poor growth despite high pulse amplitude – failure to return to baseline.

logical age, is seldom helpful diagnostically. It estimates the percentage of completed growth more accurately than does chronological age and is useful in the prediction of final height assuming growth is normal and the child does not have significant bone abnormalities. This has implications not only for management of the individual child but for the interpretation of the changes in height prognosis predicted following a treatment intervention in specific disorders. As with height measurements, bone age must be accurately assessed if it is not to be seriously misleading to the clinician and computerized assessments are being developed (Tanner *et al.*, 1993).

4.2 GROWTH HORMONE (GH) AND GROWTH REGULATION

4.2.1 CONTROL OF GH SECRETION

GH is of cardinal importance in the control of growth in childhood. GH is a 191 amino acid anterior pituitary polypeptide. It is secreted episodically throughout 24 hours but predominantly at night during slow wave sleep (Figures 4.2a, 4.2b) during which there are usually 3–5 discrete pulses (Hunter *et al.*, 1966; Finkelstein *et al.*, 1972). Release is mediated by the two hypothalamic peptides: growth hormone releasing hormone (GHRH) (Guillemin *et al.*, 1982; Rivier *et al.*, 1982; Frohman & Jansson, 1986) which is stimulatory and somatostatin which is inhibitory (Wass, 1983). Tall children secrete more growth hormone than their short peers (Albertsson-Wikland *et al.*, 1983) and GH secretory pulse amplitude correlates with growth velocity although not very strongly (see below). For growth to be normal it seems important that GH levels become undetectable between pulses (normal somatostatin tone) (Figure 4.3).

Dopaminergic, serotonergic and noradrenergic pathways all impinge on the GH regulatory neurone system, but cholinergic neurotransmitter pathways seem particularly important in controlling GHRH and somatostatin release. Hippocampal impulses, perhaps related to sleep, are stimulatory whilst impulses from the amygdala may be either stimulatory or inhibitory. Somatostatin secretion seems to be mediated via the hypothalamic ventromedial nucleus.

A number of drugs induce changes in GH secretion via specific neurotransmitter pathways: clonidine is stimulatory via alpha-adrenergic and diazepam via GABA pathways; bromocriptine, propranalol and cholinergic agents probably inhibit somatostatin release. This is relevant in understanding pharmacological stimulation tests and, potentially, for therapy that might stimulate GH secretion.

Growth hormone is unusual in being species specific. Two forms of growth hormone are present in humans and it is secreted as a heterogeneous molecular species. The predominant, and presumably more bioactive, form is of 22 000 molecular weight (22 K). A smaller (approximately 20 K) form is present in smaller amounts. Structurally abnormal growth hormone variants with varying bioactivity could be important in the etiology of growth failure in certain rare conditions but are unlikely to be common reasons for poor growth in the population as a whole.

Peptides are also important in the regulation of GH secretion: endorphins, neurotensin and vasoactive intestinal peptide (VIP) are stimulatory whilst substance P and central TRH pathways are inhibitory.

GH is not inhibited by feedback from peripheral endocrine glands although thyroxine and glucocorticoids influence its secretion. Regulation seems to be by GH itself (at hypothalamic and pituitary levels), peripheral GH-dependent growth factors (e.g., IGF-1), GHRH and somatostatin and metabolic factors such as free fatty acids and glucose. The integration of this control with physiologic states such as sleep, exercise, appetite and nutrition is presumably via the monoaminergic and peptide systems described above. For a review of the neuroregulation of GH in health and disease, see Dieguez *et al.* (1988).

4.2.2 GH ACTION – INSULIN-LIKE GROWTH FACTORS

The plasma half-life of exogenously administered GH is 20–25 minutes and that of endogenous GH is thought to be similar or shorter although this remains controversial (Faria *et al.*, 1989; Hindmarsh *et al.*, 1989). GH partly effects linear growth directly by stimulating early epiphyseal growth plate precursor cell differentiation. However, it is thought that the predominant mechanism of GH action works by inducing tissue differentiation allowing the expression of insulin-like growth factor (IGF) receptors and local IGF-1 production. IGFs are polypeptides which share some sequence homology and biological properties with insulin. Circulating IGF-1 is mainly produced in the liver but IGF-1 is also produced in virtually all tissues and its synthesis is regulated in many organs by GH. IGFs are not stored and are secreted continuously. The high circulating levels are almost completely bound to specific binding proteins (IGF BPs). The predominant mechanism of GH action is thus by inducing tissue differentiation allowing expression of IGF-1 receptors and local (paracrine/autocrine) IGF-1 production. Locally produced IGF-1 in, for example, the proliferating chondrocytes of the growth plate requires the synergistic action of liver-derived circulation IGF-1 to induce target tissue differentiation and growth. Insulin, sex steroids and nutritional status also influence IGF-1 levels. IGF-2 shares 65% structural homology with IGF-1.

The *in vivo* metabolic actions of recombinant IGF-1 (Zapf *et al.*, 1993) include insulin-like and complex GH-like and GH-opposite metabolic effects of IGF-1 on protein (reduced plasma urea), glucose and fat (reduced serum triglycerides, and cholesterol) metabolism. Although bolus I/V injections cause sustained hypoglycemia, during prolonged S/C administration the hypoglycemic effect is blunted by the generation of specific IGF IGFBPs which sequester circulating IGF-1 into a large molecular weight (150 K) metabolically inactive complex. IGF-1 also increases renal glomerular filtration and suppresses both insulin and GH secretion. More recent studies in normal subjects, GH-deficient adults, type 2 diabetics and patients with type A insulin resistance suggest that IGF-1 may turn out to have a therapeutic role in catabolic situations such as severe injury or burns and in insulin resistant states.

Recombinant IGF-1 is becoming available for the treatment of those (rare) children who have GH receptor disorders such as GH insensitivity syndrome (GHIS, Laron-type dwarfism) (Savage *et al.*, 1993; Laron & Klinger, 1993). Their height velocity improves significantly over at least 12 months on recombinant IGF-1 therapy but side effects, especially hypoglycemia, are a major problem in some. Endogenous IGF-1 production is enhanced as a protective mechanism following neuronal injury and exogenous IGF-1 could have a future role in the treatment of asphyxial injury (Gluckman *et al.*, 1993) with important implications in the fields of neurology and neonatology.

4.2.3 THE GH RECEPTOR

In the interaction between GH and tissue growth, it is becoming clearer that the GH receptor is of crucial importance and in recent years there have been major advances in understanding the structure and functional analysis of the human GH receptor (Wood, 1993) and the molecular basis of GH action (Carter-Su *et al.*, 1993). The GH receptor was cloned by 1987 and consists of a 620 amino acid (AA) peptide situated astride the target cell membrane with a single trans-membrane domain. At the time it was a newly discovered type of receptor. The extra-cellular hormone-binding domain consists of around 245 AAs and there is a cytoplasmic region of 350 residues. 85% of the cytoplasmic domain is not required for signal transduction. Overall there is 24% homology to the prolactin receptor but some sections are strikingly similar. Defects in the gene encoding the receptor have been identified in GHIS (Laron-type dwarfism) indicating that the receptor is required for normal growth. The extracellular component circulates as a high affinity GH binding protein (i.e., GHBP). One molecule of GH binds to and dimerizes two molecules of receptor; thus there are two binding sites on the GH molecule with the second near the N terminus. This dimerization of the receptor is the first step in the GH signaling pathway. A prediction of the model is that high levels of circulating GH or GH with one abnormal binding site should have antagonist rather than agonist activity. This is true of site 2 GH mutants although site 1 GH mutants show poor antagonism. GH:receptor concentrations of 1:1 show antagonism as predicted.

A current model of GH signal transduction involving the membrane bound receptor and tyrosine kinase (Carter-Su *et al.*, 1993) hypothesizes that activation by GH of a GH receptor-associated tyrosine kinase (GHRTK) is an important early (and perhaps initiating) step in signal transduction. This is supported by the finding that GHRTK is stimulated within less than 30 seconds of GH binding to the receptor, that it is stimulated by very low GH concentrations and that it is likely to have a role in stimulation by GH of a variety of cellular responses including kinase activity and gene expression. In particular, GH stimulates tyrosyl phosphorylation and kinase activity of a GH receptor-associated kinase JAK 2 (one of a family of Janus kinases) which is GH dependent. It is probable that JAK 2 serves as a signaling molecule for multiple members of a cytokine/ hematopoietin family which includes GH, prolactin, erythropoietin, interleukin-3, etc. It is likely that GHRTK functions both to activate other proteins by phosphorylation and to phosphorylate tyrosyl residues in itself and the GH receptor. These phosphorylated tyrosines may serve as docking sites for proteins in other signalling pathways. Such studies should lead to the identification of new cellular actions for GH.

It is likely that the acuteness or chronicity of exposure to GH profoundly influences the rate of GH receptor turnover. This has potentially far-reaching implications: circulating levels of GH as measured by even sophisticated frequent sampling techniques can only be expected to have a relatively poor correlation with growth; GH receptor numbers and turnover may be equally if not more important factors in the growth equation and are much less easily studied *in vivo* in humans.

4.3 GH SECRETORY ABILITY AND BIOCHEMICAL GROWTH MARKERS

4.3.1 GH MEASUREMENT

Random determination of serum GH levels is unhelpful in assessing poor growth – pulsatile release and short serum half-life often result in low levels in normal children. All GH provocation tests may give false-negative and false-positive responses. Screening tests (e.g., exercise) are difficult to standardize and response is variable. The insulin hypoglycemia test remains the 'gold standard'. Adequate (symptomatic) hypoglycemia must be obtained if results are to be meaningful (blood glucose less than 2.2 mmol/l). It is safe only if adequately supervised by staff who perform it regularly (there must be reliable I/V access, hydrocortisone and 10% glucose immediately available). As with other pharmacological GH provocation tests (particularly if there is rebound hypoglycemia, e.g., following glucagon) it should only be carried out in a specialist (tertiary referral) growth center.

All such tests are unpleasant for the child

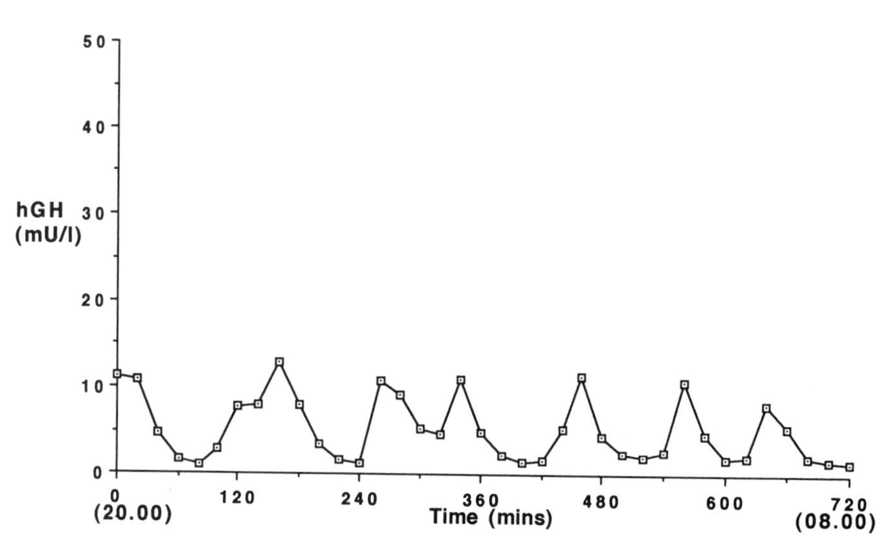

Figure 4.4 Overnight GH profile: neurosecretory dysfunction.

and their interpretation can be difficult: the time of the last spontaneous pulse is unknown and will influence responsiveness; there is complex heterogeneity of circulating GH forms (Baumann, 1990) and GH assay variability and non-specificity (Chatelain *et al.*, 1990; Granada *et al.*, 1990; Stahnke & Jenke, 1993); inadequate GH secretion may be physiological or secondary to other pathology; some short, slowly-growing children have an abnormal pattern of GH pulsatile release (Figure 4.4) but normal responses to pharmacological tests – 'neurosecretory dysfunction'. Nevertheless, following adequate hypoglycemia, 85% of 'normal' children will produce a serum GH level of over 15 mU/l (usually after 30–60 minutes).

Some centers now measure spontaneous nocturnal pulsatile GH release to provide greater insight into secretory control mechanisms (Adlard *et al.*, 1987; Hindmarsh *et al.*, 1987; Butler *et al.*, 1989b). Their relevance to short stature assessment or as a predictor of response to therapy remains controversial, although there may be a relationship between the amplitude of GH pulses and growth velocity (Hindmarsh *et al.*, 1987; Butler *et al.*, 1989b). Such tests are impracticable for 'screening' large numbers of children. Overall, the measurement of spontaneous nocturnal pulsatile GH release provides insight into pathophysiology but is only sometimes helpful in individual patients and remains a research tool.

4.3.2 BIOCHEMICAL GROWTH MARKERS

There is much current interest in biochemical markers of growth in the contexts of understanding pathophysiology in different growth disorders, aiding diagnosis and identifying predictive markers for response to growth promoting therapies.

Recent studies (Crofton *et al.*, 1992, 1993) evaluating a number of biochemical growth markers including total and bone alkaline phosphatase (bALP), procollagen type 1 propeptide (P1CP, a marker of bone growth) and procollagen type 111 propeptide (P111P, a marker of soft tissue collagen growth) in groups of short normal children taking part in trials of growth-promoting therapies (placebo, GH, the anabolic steroid oxandrolone, testosterone), showed that for all treatment groups (combined), the increment in each biochemical marker at three months was significantly correlated with the increment in height velocity after one year. The best overall predictor of response was bALP. Within the GH (alone) treated group, P111P, intriguingly a marker of soft tissue growth, was the best predictor of growth response at one year. Pre-treatment height velocity was of no significant predictive value. IGFBP-3 may turn out to have a useful role as a growth marker and predictor as it has virtually no circadian fluctuation during GH therapy (Blum *et al.*, 1993).

Urinary GH measurements could become a useful, non-invasive, repeatable and inexpensive way of assessing physiologic GH secretion (Albini *et al.*, 1988). Unfortunately, GH levels in urine are of the order of 1000-fold lower than in plasma and some currently available assay methods leave much to be desired in terms of accuracy and reproducibility (Girard *et al.*, 1990). Nevertheless, assays for urinary GH measurement are becoming sufficiently sensitive and could provide a useful noninvasive ('screening') assessment of physiologic GH secretion. In a study (Stirling *et al.*, 1993) of the relationship between overnight (12-hour) plasma growth hormone profiles and simultaneous nocturnal timed urinary GH excretion in a group of 100 patients (mean age 11.0 years, range 3.4–33.9) undergoing investigation of GH secretion, there were highly significant correlations between urinary GH concentration and mean pulse amplitude (Figure 4.5), mean

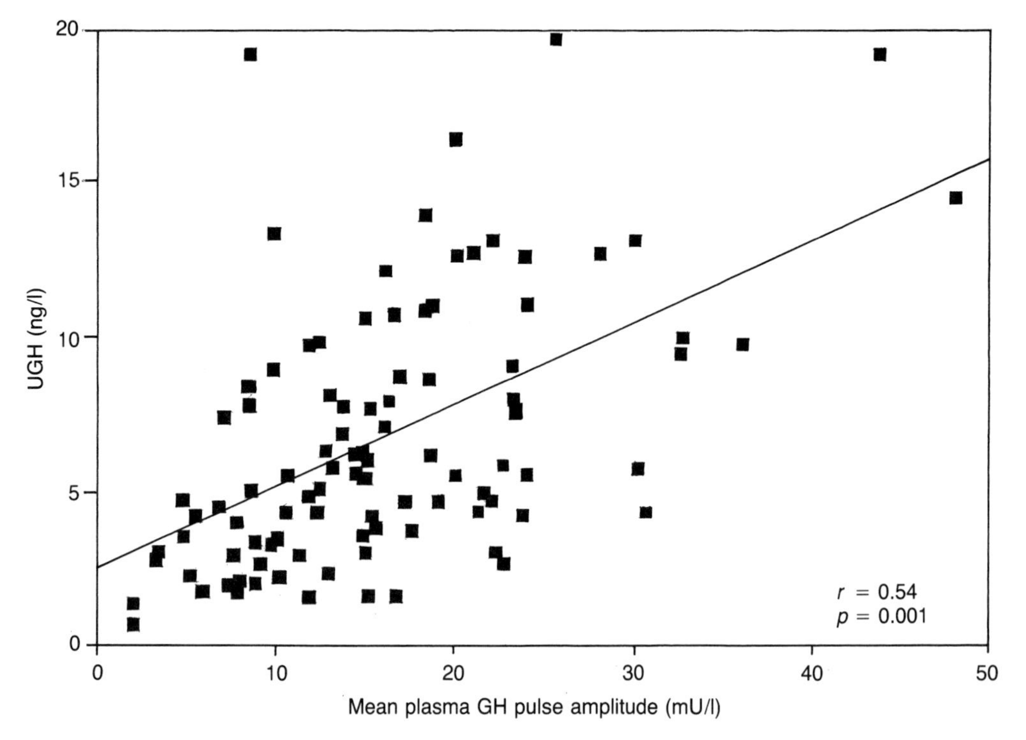

Figure 4.5 Relationship between mean pulse amplitude and overnight urinary growth hormone concentration (from Stirling *et al.*, 1993).

overnight plasma GH level, sum of pulse amplitude and sum of pulse area.

Comparing prepubertal children with severe GH insufficiency (low overnight plasma GH secretion and GH response to insulin hypoglycemia <10 mU/ml) with prepubertal children with 'normal variant short stature (NVSS)' (familial stature +/− growth delay, with normal overnight and stimulated GH levels) (Table 4.1) showed that although the growth rates of the two groups are not significantly different, mean urine GH levels are significantly lower in the GH 'deficient' children compared to those with NVSS (Stirling *et al.*, 1993). However there is a degree of overlap between the two groups, reflecting the continuum of GH secretory ability. The measurement of overnight

Table 4.1 Growth and GH secretion in GH 'deficiency' and normal variant short stature (Stirling *et al.*, 1993).

	GH 'deficiency'	NVSS	
number of children	5	58	
height velocity (cm/yr)	3.9	4.2	p = NS
mean plasma pulse amplitude (mU/l) (range)	3.5 (1.9–7.7)	15.2 (4.6–32.6)	p = 0.001
mean urinary GH (ng/l) (range)	1.9 (0.6–2.9)	6.9 (1.5–19.7)	p = 0.015

urinary GH excretion may prove to be a useful screening test in short children.

4.4 THE SHORT OR SLOWLY-GROWING CHILD

4.4.1 GROWTH ASSESSMENT

The 'normality' of a child's height is determined by reference to growth charts showing population norms. Ideally each country and ethnic group should have its own growth standards. In practice, UK charts serve well even in developing countries and for ethnic minorities within the UK as differences in final stature reflect minor differences in growth velocity over the whole growing period. Nevertheless, available UK growth charts have, over the last 30 years, reflected the growth pattern of children living in southern England in the mid-1960s. Coordinated efforts have now been made to update the standards, taking account of data from different regions of the UK and these have just become available. Growth standards are now also available for a variety of growth disorders – e.g., Turner syndrome (e.g., Lyon *et al.*, 1985), Down syndrome (Cronk *et al.*, 1988) and achondroplasia (Horton *et al.*, 1978). They are particularly valuable in enabling the additional effect on growth of a separate condition to be suspected from recognition of deviations from the growth norm for the underlying condition. The differential diagnosis in a child presenting with slow growth or short stature is summarized in Table 4.2.

The parental genetic contribution reduces the population standard deviation of height by about 30%. 95% of the children of given parents will have a height prognosis within ±8.5 cm of the mid-parental centile. Children also 'inherit' an environment from their parents. A child's shortness, whilst 'appropriate' for his short parents, may reflect poor nutrition or emotional deprivation continuing

Table 4.2 Differential diagnosis of short stature or slow growth.

Short with currently normal growth velocity

Constitutional short stature, short normal parent(s)

Previous problem affecting growth, now cured or no longer operative
- Prolonged intrauterine growth retardation – light for gestational age, low birth length and head circumference, difficult feeders in infancy, Silver-Russell syndrome – triangular facies, clinodactyly, facial and limb length asymmetry
- Congenital heart disease

Physiologic growth delay (delayed bone age, normal height prognosis)
Growing slowly (whether already short or still of normal stature)

With increased skinfold thicknesses
- Endocrine disease
  (e.g., panhypopituitarism, severe growth hormone insufficiency – idiopathic or secondary to tumour or irradiation, hypothyroidism, pseudohypoparathyroidism, Cushing's syndrome)

Disproportionate
- Short limbs for spine (the dyschondroplasias) (e.g., achondroplasia, hypochondroplasia, multiple epiphyseal dysplasia)
- Short limbs and spine (spine relatively shorter) (e.g., mucopolysaccharidoses, metatrophic dwarfism)

Often without other obvious signs of disease (see text)
- Malnutrition
- Psychosocial deprivation
- Unrecognized asthma (may be misdiagnosed)
- Chromosomal abnormalities (e.g., Turner syndrome – other signs variable)
- Malabsorption due to celiac disease, ulcerative colitis, Crohn's disease (bowel habit may be normal)
- Cardiovascular or renal disease

down the generations with no family member achieving their true genetic height potential. The mean height of children from social class IV and V families remains significantly less than that of those from social classes I and II in Britain in the 1980s as it did in the 1870s despite the secular trend to increasing height in both groups (Kelnar, 1990).

3% of normal children will, by definition, be below the third centile on a distance (height × age) chart yet a child with a growth disorder of recent onset will be of normal stature. Only serial measurements and calculation of growth velocity will distinguish normality from abnormality.

4.4.2 CAUSES OF GH INSUFFICIENCY

A few children lack the gene for making GH (Illig *et al.*, 1971; Phillips *et al.*, 1986), demonstrate prenatal GH deficiency, respond to GH therapy with the major antibody response expected to a foreign protein and cannot be treated with any form of GH. Otherwise there is a wide spectrum of GH secretory ability (Albertsson-Wikland *et al.*, 1983), which, within the normal population, is likely to be largely genetically determined. At one end of the spectrum are children, perhaps 1 in 4000 (Vimpani *et al.*, 1977), with severe GH insufficiency ('GH deficiency'). They grow slowly and often demonstrate characteristic clinical features (truncal obesity with characteristic 'marbling' of the fat, crowding of facial features to the center with an immature facial appearance and, in the male, small genitalia with micropenis) and show an inadequate (<7 mU/l) response to a pharmacological stimulus to GH secretion (such as insulin-induced hypoglycemia – see above).

There is a continuum from them through moderate GH insufficiency (so-called 'partial' GH deficiency with GH responses in the 7–15 mU/l range) and through short normal, averagely tall to tall normal individuals and those with gigantism (Figure 4.6). The question as to whether GH therapy could increase the height of the normally growing short child is being actively investigated in a number of centers.

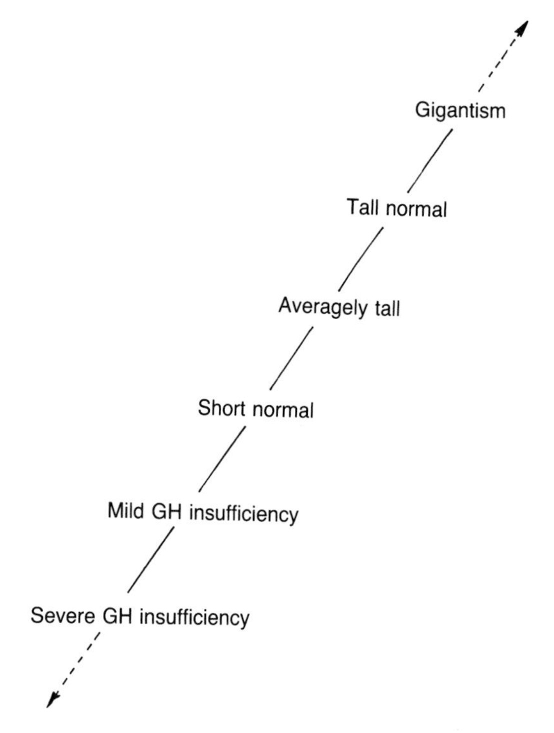

Figure 4.6 The spectrum of growth hormone secretory ability.

Some short, slowly-growing children have what is considered to be an abnormal pattern of GH pulsatile release (see Figure 4.4) but normal GH responses to provocative (pharmacological) tests – 'neurosecretory dysfunction' – see above (Spiliotis *et al.*, 1984).

Temporary GH deficiency is seen in children with psychosocial deprivation (Figure 4.7) and occurs physiologically in late prepuberty and in early male puberty. GH biosynthesis and release is also impaired in other conditions (e.g., primary hypothyroidism or celiac disease) and secretion returns to normal with treatment of the underlying disorder.

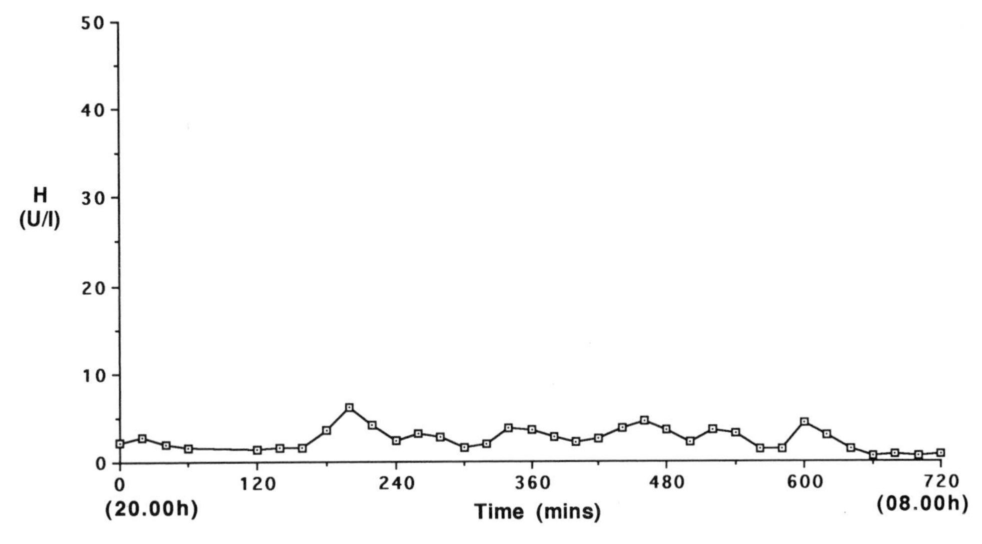

Figure 4.7 Overnight GH profile: reversible severe GH insufficiency in a girl with Munchausen syndrome by proxy and severe psychosocial deprivation.

Careful growth assessment will often detect chronic disorder long before there are more specific symptoms or signs. Poor growth is often the major diagnostic clue to psychosocial deprivation (see below), unrecognized or undertreated asthma, renal tubular acidosis and malabsorption syndromes such as celiac disease (Ashkenazi, 1989) and chronic inflammatory bowel disease (Barton & Ferguson, 1990; Kirschner, 1990) – Crohn's disease (Kanof *et al.*, 1988) or ulcerative colitis, or poorly controlled diabetes mellitus. Emotional individual and family stresses in the context of chronic disease may also be important factors in sub-optimal growth in these contexts.

Psychosocial deprivation in itself often causes poor growth (Annecillo & Money, 1985), may mimic idiopathic hypopituitarism in terms of GH responses to conventional stimuli (Powell *et al.*, 1967a, 1967b) and abnormal overnight GH secretory profiles may return to normal rapidly following admission to hospital (Stanhope *et al.*, 1988; Thomas *et al.*, 1993). Any child who grows poorly at home but who thrives when in hospital or fostered should be suspected of being emotionally deprived and accurately maintained growth data are increasingly accepted as evidence in British courts. Severe growth failure may result from Munchausen syndrome by proxy (see Figure 4.7, Lyall *et al.*, 1992).

4.5 THE ENDOCRINE BACKGROUND TO NORMAL PUBERTY

For a recent review, see Stirling & Kelnar (1992). The physical changes of puberty are well-known (see Brook & Stanhope, 1989; Tanner, 1962, 1992; Tanner & Whitehouse, 1976). Individual secondary sexual characteristics result from different hormonal events and must be assessed independently. The timing and duration of puberty are very variable in the normal population but pubertal development is an harmonious process and marked discrepancies from the normal sequence of events (loss of 'consonance' – Stanhope & Brook, 1989) should lead to suspicion of pathology. In contrast, adolescence is sometimes far from harmonious and social pressures and emotional problems may be particularly marked in those with age of onset of puberty at either end of the normal spectrum or in those with underlying chronic disease. Emotional and psychiatric aspects of adolescence are considered elsewhere in this volume.

4.5.1 EVOLUTION OF ENDOCRINE CONTROL

Changes in the fetus, infant and child could all be relevant to the initiation of puberty. Fetal gonadotrophin production occurs from about the fifth week of development and rises until 20 weeks. Levels are higher in the female (Kaplan *et al.*, 1976) perhaps because of feedback inhibition by fetal testosterone in the male. However placental chorionic gonadotrophin is secreted from implantation onwards and is the major stimulus to fetal Leydig cell testosterone production. Thus it seems unlikely that the fetal hypothalamo-pituitary-gonadal axis is fully functional by postpubertal standards. After delivery, there is a rise in gonadotrophin levels which persists for several months in both sexes. Total testosterone levels are high in the male partly due to high SHBG levels (Forest *et al.*, 1973; Anderson *et al.*, 1976).

During the first year, the axis becomes quiescent. It has been postulated that specific inhibitory hormones may be involved but there is little evidence for the existence of such mechanisms although central nervous system inhibitory influences may still be important (precocious puberty is a common sequel to cranial irradiation for acute lymphoblastic leukemia).

The pineal gland could be of relevance, however, although its role in humans remains speculative. At one time thought to be the seat of the soul (Descartes), seen as guiding the cerebral hemispheres (Voltaire), it may, more mundanely, be important in the control of the onset of human puberty. Pineal tumors may be associated with precocious, delayed or absent puberty. Pineal destruction is usually associated with precocious puberty (Kitay, 1954). Pinealocytes convert tryptophane via serotonin to melatonin. It had been conjectured that the endocrine events of puberty were held in check prepubertally by melatonin following reports that its concentration falls abruptly between pubertal stages G1 and G2 (Tanner, 1962) from age 11.5 to 14 years (Silman *et al.*, 1979) and that melatonin inhibits gonadal development in some males (Wurtman & Moskowitz, 1977).

Other studies have not confirmed the results of Silman *et al.* (Lenko *et al.*, 1982) and have demonstrated no inhibitory effect of melatonin on gonadotrophin secretion (Weinberg *et al.*, 1980). 24-hour melatonin profiles are the same in prepuberty, puberty and adult males (with low levels by day and high levels at night) and levels in precocious puberty are similar to those in normal puberty (Ehrenkranz *et al.*, 1982) implying that melatonin has no major role in normal or precocious puberty, although blindness, which would upset the pineal circadian clock, is associated with early menarche (Zacharias & Wurtman, 1964). Hypogonadal children with the Prader-Willi syndrome also have normal plasma melatonin rhythms (Tamarkin *et al.*, 1982) and a study of urinary melatonin metabolite excretion during childhood and puberty found children to resemble adults with no marked changes of rhythm during puberty apart, surprisingly, from a rise in urinary 6-hydroxymelatonin excretion at the onset of breast development (Tanner stage 2) in girls (Tetsuo *et al.*, 1982).

More recent evidence, however, suggests that melatonin may have some role as an inhibitor of gonadal development. For a recent review, see Sizonenko & Lang (1988). There is evidence for a decline in the day-to-night increment of serum melatonin concentrations from infancy to childhood, that children with early puberty have lower melatonin day-to-night increments than age-matched controls, and that those with constitutionally delayed puberty show increments comparable to those of preschool children (Attanasio *et al.*, 1983). This implies a relationship between maturation and the mechanisms controlling pineal gland secretion whether or not melatonin plays any significant role in the onset of puberty. Using what is claimed to be a sensitive and specific assay, with frequent nighttime sampling, melatonin nighttime levels decrease significantly with sexual maturation and age (Waldhauser *et al.*, 1984). However, the greatest fall in mean nocturnal melatonin levels was between prepubertal children under and over 7 years which does not support the hypothesis that it is that fall which might trigger the events of puberty.

4.5.2 ADRENARCHE

However, there are other important changes taking place at around this age. During mid-childhood there is a steep rise in adrenal androgen secretion ('adrenarche') (Figure 4.8) coincident with the development of the adrenal zona reticularis. This adrenal androgen rise is not accompanied by any significant increase in intermediate metabolites in cortisol or corticosterone biosynthesis when related to body surface area (Kelnar & Brook, 1983; Kelnar, 1985).

In the present context adrenarche may be of importance from several points of view: a) the mechanisms underlying it and its relation to the subsequent rises in gonadotrophins and gonadal steroids at the clinical onset of puberty ('gonadarche') are controversial but of potential relevance to the understanding of the triggering of normal human puberty; b) the etiology of the mid-childhood growth spurt; c) possible abnormalities of adrenarche in a number of disease states (e.g., asthma and diabetes).

The role of adrenarche in humans remains controversial (Stirling & Kelnar, 1990). It is difficult to extrapolate from pathological situations to the normal control of gonadarche. Adrenarche may be delayed in children with constitutional delay of gonadarche and isolated GH deficiency but not in hypergonadotrophic hypogonadism (e.g., Turner syndrome – Lee *et al.*, 1975). Children with

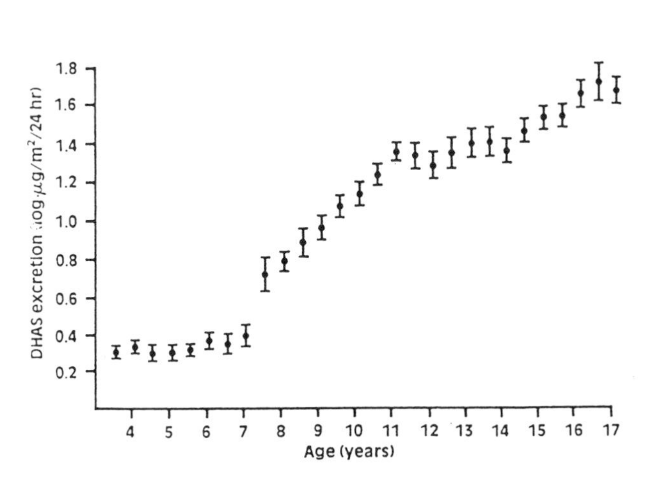

Figure 4.8 Urinary excretion of dehydroepiandrosterone sulphate (DHAS) in childhood (from Kelnar, 1985).

Addison's disease enter puberty normally (Grumbach *et al.*, 1978) and in diabetic adolescents gonadarche may proceed normally despite delayed adrenarche (Cohen *et al.*, 1984) (Chapter 5, p. 83). Children with congenital adrenal hypoplasia all have hypogonadotrophic hypogonadism and therefore do not enter puberty normally (Hay *et al.*, 1981). It is possible that the adrenals may have a much earlier priming effect on gonadarche analogously to the situation in the rat (but rats do not have an adrenarche) but a causal role for adrenarche in gonadarche in humans seems unlikely.

Adrenarche is coincident with the preadolescent fat spurt (Stolz & Stolz, 1951; Tanner & Whitehouse, 1976) and with the mid-childhood growth spurt (Tanner, 1962; Molinari *et al.*, 1980). The latter could reflect a bone and muscle response to adrenal androgens either directly or indirectly by influencing GH secretion – androgens are important in determining the pulsatile nature of GH secretion in rats (Millard *et al.*, 1986) and at about age 7 years a change in GH secretion with the development of the dominant periodicity of about 200 minutes has been observed in humans (Hindmarsh & Brook, 1989).

It is possible that adrenarche may simply be a by-product of the need of the inner fetal adrenal cells to respond to the hormonal milieu of pregnancy by developing an androgen (i.e., estrogen precursor) synthesizing zone (Anderson, 1980). Other than humans, only the chimpanzee has an adrenarche (Cutler *et al.*, 1978; Albertson *et al.*, 1984). Thus adrenarche occurs in the two species which have the most prolonged interval between birth and puberty. It is conceivable that adrenarche is merely revealed by such an interval. However, the more complex the organism the greater the advantage in prolonging the period between birth and reproductive activity to allow brain growth and childhood learning to take place. If during that period androgens are required for continuing skeletal and muscular growth, this could be achieved by transferring androgen biosynthesis from gonad to adrenal – adrenarche (Tanner, 1981).

4.5.3 GONADARCHE

It has been clear since the work of Knobil (1980) in rhesus monkeys that pulsatile secretion of GnRH is of paramount importance in primate sexual maturation but the initiation of puberty (gonardarche) does not simply result from the sudden activation of hypothalamic gonadotrophin releasing hormone (GnRH) secretion. There is increasing biochemical and ultrasound evidence for activity well before the onset of clinical gonadarche. During childhood, there appears to be a gradual amplification of GnRH signals and occasional random and short-lived bursts of secretory activity (Brook & Stanhope, 1989) or pulses of low frequency and amplitude (Wu *et al.*, 1991) may be seen in the young child. From well before the clinical onset of puberty, (and around the time of adrenarche), nocturnal pulsatile GnRH secretion is detectable with increasing pulse frequency (Wu *et al.*, 1989, 1990a) and this is associated with a multicystic appearance in the prepubertal ovary on ultrasound. This normal stage of ovarian development (characterized by the presence of more than 6 follicles of diameter greater than 4 mm) is associated with activation of the axis resulting in nocturnal pulsatile GnRH secretion (Boyar *et al.*, 1972) without (as yet) estrogen-mediated positive feedback (Stanhope *et al.*, 1985).

Modulation of pituitary luteinising hormone (LH) secretion resulting from an increase in the frequency of GnRH secretion is an important characteristic of the transition between juvenile and peripubertal stages in humans (Figures 4.9 & 4.10) (Wu *et al.*, 1990a). Biochemical assessment in prepuberty has

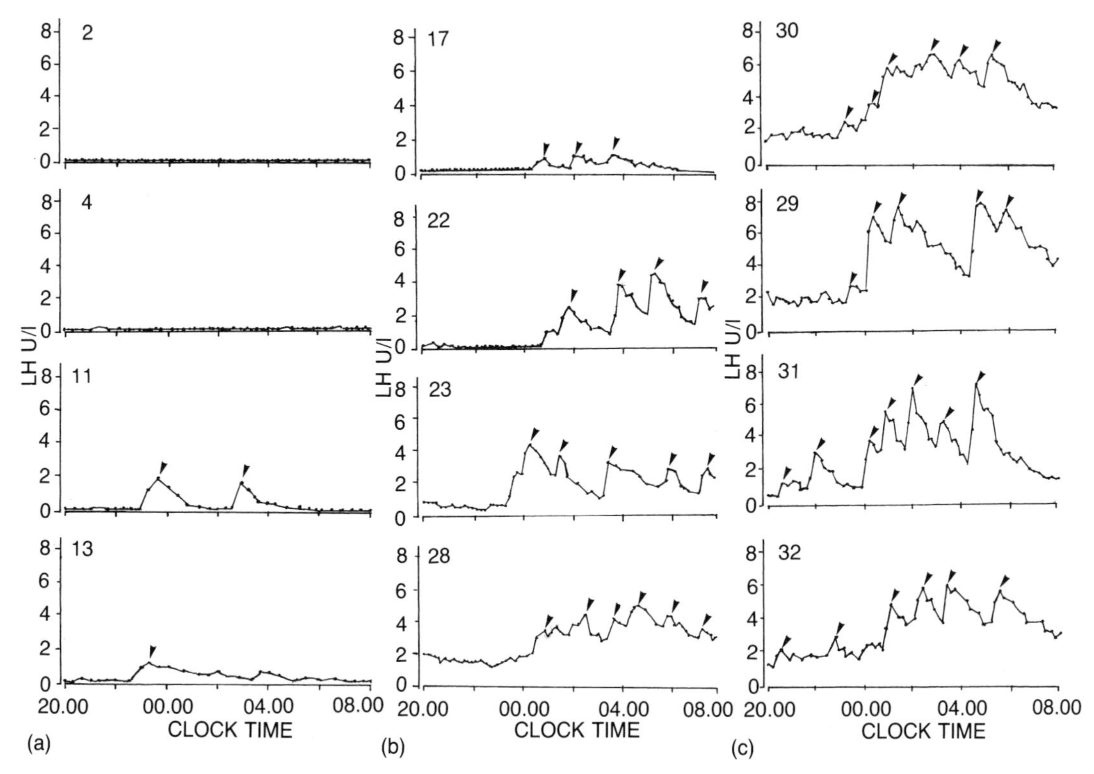

Figure 4.9 Evolution of gonadotrophin (GT) secretory profiles (1). Profiles of plasma LH between 20.00 and 08.00 h in (a) four young prepubertal subjects (G1 PH1 testicular volume ≤2 ml); arrowheads indicate a significant LH pulse; none of these patients progressed into puberty during the following 12 months; (b) four peripubertal subjects: two with G1 PH1 testicular volume ≤2 ml at time of study, but progression into puberty with testicular volume ≥4 ml within 12 months (subjects 15 and 19); two in early puberty at study (G1 PH1–2 testicular volume 3–4 ml); (c) four pubertal subjects (G2 PH1–3 testicular volume 6–10 ml) (from Wu *et al.*, 1990).

been helped by the development of sensitive LH radiometric assays (Butler *et al.*, 1987, 1988) although the bioactivity of what is measured is not beyond question. Using a recently developed ultrasensitive immunofluorometric assay (IFA), pulsatile LH and follicle stimulating hormone (FSH) fluctuations can be seen even in Kallman syndrome patients (see below) (Wu *et al.*, 1991). However, in contrast to normal late prepubertal children, there is poor synchronization between LH and FSH pulses and an absence of entrainment to nocturnal sleep. It may be, therefore, that a crucial condition for normal pubertal development may involve organization of neuronal circuits which not only maintain synchronized pulsatile GnRH release but enable their incorporation into the daily sleep-wake rhythm (Wu *et al.*, 1991). It is likely that the ongoing pubertal transition to adult pituitary-gonadal function involves the gradual further recruitment, organization and synchronization of GnRH neuronal discharge over an increasing proportion of the evening/night and a resetting of gonadal negative feedback (Wu *et al.*, 1990b, 1991).

For normal ranges of ovarian and uterine size during childhood see Adams (1989). As

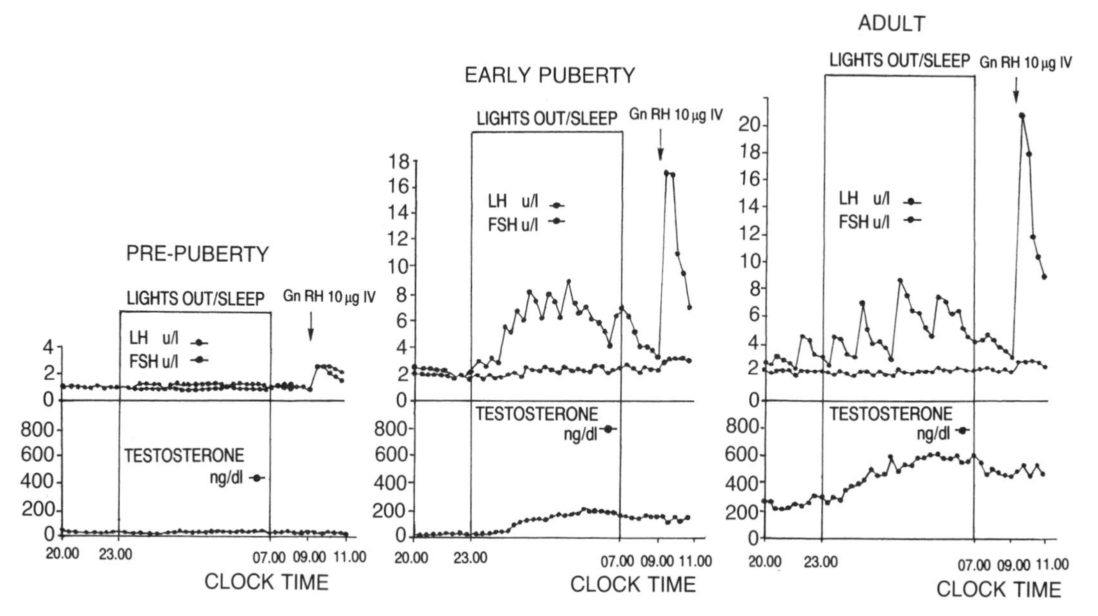

Figure 4.10 Evolution of GT secretory profiles (2) and response to exogenous GnRH at different stages of pubertal development (data by courtesy of Dr F.C.W. Wu).

puberty progresses, the pulse frequency of GnRH (and thus gonadotrophin) secretion remains at about 2 hours (Jakacki *et al.*, 1982) but there is increasing pulse amplitude and the occurrence of daytime as well as nocturnal pulses (Penny *et al.*, 1977). 24-hour pulsatile release is necessary for full pubertal development, menarche and ovulation (Boyar *et al.*, 1972). In the follicular phase of the cycle in girls, GnRH pulse frequency increases to about every hour and falls to every 3 hours in the luteal phase (Brook & Stanhope, 1989). Increasing sex steroid secretion resulting from the increasing pulsatile secretion of GnRH produces the physical changes of puberty and all the events of puberty can be induced by the pulsatile administration of exogenous GnRH (Brook *et al.*, 1987; Stanhope *et al.*, 1987; Wu *et al.*, 1987) – even if this is a cumbersome way to do so in clinical practice (see below).

Further experiments in the rhesus monkey (Wilson *et al.*, 1984) suggest the presence in the hypothalamus of a GnRH pulse generator but its site and nature are unknown. A pulse of GnRH is associated with a burst of electrical activity and results in a pulse of LH secretion. There appears to be no other modulation of LH secretion but the inhibin/activin system (de Jong, 1988) is important in modulating FSH secretion which could theoretically explain the dissociation of LH and FSH secretion found in a condition such as isolated premature thelarche.

4.5.4 NUTRITION, METABOLIC SIGNALS AND PUBERTY

Although in pathological situations (e.g., anorexia nervosa, excessive exercise) nutritional factors are important for pubertal development and the onset of menarche, there is no evidence for the hypothesis (Frisch & Revelle, 1970) that menarche depends on the attainment of a critical weight for height. For a given body weight, the proportion of girls reaching menarche increases with age (Billewicz *et al.*, 1976) and the relative weight (weight as a percentage of standard weight) at 11 years explains less than 5% of the variation in the age of menarche (Stark *et al.*, 1989). It is likely that in normally nourished populations, genetic factors are of paramount importance in the timing of menarche and this is probably true of pubertal onset and events in general.

This does not mean that metabolic factors and signals are unimportant for pubertal development. From experiments in the rat (Harris & Jacobsohn, 1952) and rhesus monkey (Wilson *et al.*, 1984) and non-human primates (Steiner *et al.*, 1983) and circumstantial evidence in the human (see above), there is no doubt that it is brain (rather than pituitary) maturation which is of primary importance for the onset of puberty. Are there simply genetically-determined biological clocks which, in the absence of pathological modulators, trigger puberty or could there be metabolic or other cues which signal into the central nervous system? In anorexia nervosa or severe malnutrition there are low gonadotrophin levels, menstruation ceases and puberty regresses as a way of conserving energy – the likely outcome of maintenance of reproductive capacity in such circumstances would be disastrous for mother and fetus. But whereas anorexics who regain about 75% of ideal body weight resume menstrual cycling with normal pituitary responsiveness to GnRH (Warren *et al.*, 1975), leanness alone cannot account for the reproductive disturbances. Sustained exercise (in female distance runners) affects the amplitude of pulsatile GnRH secretion (Veldhuis *et al.*, 1985) and amenorrheic ballet dancers who stop training resume normal menstruation within a few months without detectable changes in body weight or composition (Warren & Van de Wiele, 1973) suggesting that metabolic signals could be important in controlling reproductive function in these situations and, more speculatively, in the control of normal pubertal development.

There are increases in basal insulin levels associated with puberty in primates (Steiner *et al.*, 1983) and humans (Hindmarsh *et al.*, 1988) which may simply be secondary to changes in growth hormone secretion, but insulin does enhance basal and GnRH-stimulated gonadotrophin (GT) release by pituitary cells *in vitro* (Adashi *et al.*, 1981) and also affects brain neurotransmitter activity by regulating precursor availability (Fernstrom, 1979). Thus both direct humoral stimuli and metabolic factors such as amino acids acting as neurotransmitter precursor substrates could influence the GnRH pulse generator. A combined CHO/amino acid infusion in *Macaca fascicularis* monkeys produces dramatic increases in bioassayable plasma LH levels whereas CHO alone has no effect (Steiner *et al.*, 1983) but much more work is needed before the role of metabolic factors in the initiation of normal puberty in humans becomes clear (Brown *et al.*, 1992a).

4.6 DELAYED SEXUAL MATURATION

4.6.1 DIFFERENTIAL DIAGNOSIS

Distinguishing physiologic delay from pathology may not be possible clinically. The appropriateness or otherwise of height velocity can only be determined in the context of the stage of pubertal development – e.g., growth should be accelerating in a girl with stage 2 breast development but slow growth is normal in a boy until testes are 8–10 ml in volume. A simplified classification of puberty disorders is shown in Table 4.3.

Virtually any chronic systemic disease in childhood may be associated with both growth retardation and pubertal delay (Preece *et al.*, 1986), not least diabetes mellitus. Although other and specific symptoms or signs may be obvious (e.g., cystic fibrosis), they may be

Table 4.3 A simplified classification of disorders of puberty (see text).

Precocious puberty:
Consonance:
Idiopathic central precocious puberty
Central precocious puberty due to, e.g.,
intracranial tumors
cranial irradiation
raised intracranial pressue
Gonadotrophin-independent precocious puberty (GIPP, testotoxicosis)
Loss of consonance (pseudopuberty):
Isolated premature thelarche
Adrenal causes
premature pubarche
congenital adrenal hyperplasia
Cushing's syndrome
adrenocortical tumors
Gonadal causes
ovarian cysts
ovarian or testicular tumors
Ingestion of sex steroid (accident or child abuse)
Primary hypothyroidism
McCune-Albright syndrome
Extrapituitary tumors (e.g., hepatoblastoma)
Delayed puberty:
Consonance:
Constitutional delay of growth and puberty
Chronic systemic disease
Idiopathic hypogonadotrophic hypogonadism
Hypogonadotrophic hypogonadism due to, e.g.,
Kallmann's syndrome
craniopharyngioma
cranial irradiation
Panhypopituitarism
Primary hypothyroidism
Loss of consonance:
Turner syndrome
Ovarian agenesis with normal karyotype
Polycystic ovaries
Anorchia (1ry or 2ry to testicular irradiation)

misinterpreted (e.g., the chronic nocturnal cough of asthma treated with courses of antibiotics), masked (anorexia normalizing bowel habit in chronic inflammatory bowel disease), difficult to assess (e.g., emotional deprivation, anorexia nervosa) or absent. Early testicular enlargement is often overlooked by the patient and referring physician. An assessment of skeletal maturity may indicate the likely delay before puberty starts spontaneously (if it will do so) but seldom distinguishes underlying pathology from physiologic delay.

Children with loss of consonance should be investigated at any age as should those with signs or symptoms attributable to an underlying pathological process (Wu, 1993). Where height and degree of skeletal maturational delay seem appropriate for the family in terms of final height prediction, the delay is probably physiologic. In the UK, 3% of normal boys and girls will have no signs of puberty by around 13.8 and 13.4 years respectively and it is reasonable to investigate those presenting after this. Even if delay is physiologic it is unkind (in emotional and psychological terms) and inappropriate (in growth terms) to allow too much delay in relation to the child's peers and pubertal induction is often indicated (see below).

The imminence of puberty can be assessed by measuring GT pulsatile release during sleep – pulsatile nocturnal GnRH release will be observed before the clinical onset of puberty is detectable – or more practically by measuring the GT response to a small (0.25 mcg/kg I/V) dose of GnRH. If puberty is imminent, the LH response will exceed that of FSH and a significant rise will be seen. Where available, skilled ultrasound assessment is the most helpful and least invasive technique (Adams, 1989). There is recent evidence that an 8 a.m. plasma testosterone level may be a useful simple guide to the clinical imminence of pubertal development in boys (Wu *et al.*, 1993) and that a 6-hour overnight LH profile can sensitively distinguish pubertal delay from (permanent) idiopathic hypogonadotrophic hypogonadism (Brown *et al.*, 1992b, 1993; Kelnar *et al.*, 1993).

If pathology is suspected, investigations should be carried out urgently (treatment of the underlying condition or lesion may be necessary) and puberty induced at a normal time and tempo. Otherwise, although much can be learnt over a period of months by observation of growth and for the first signs of pubertal development, the psychological pressures on individuals at school can be enormous (Kelnar, 1990). The short, undeveloped and poorly-qualified 16-year-old school leaver may, in addition, find it particularly hard to obtain employment.

Pelvic ultrasound examination in girls is a sensitive guide to the etiology of pubertal delay and the imminence of the clinical onset of puberty. Sex steroid measurements provide no additional information to the clinical staging of breast or genital maturation and uterine growth (in response to exogenous or endogenous estrogen) is best assessed ultrasonically. Raised GT levels are diagnostic of primary gonadal failure but are not elevated before about 10 years. In males (in whom there is no comparable technique to the ultrasonic assessment of ovarian function), GnRH tests are of little value in distinguishing constitutional pubertal delay from hypogonadotrophic hypogonadism, but, when available, assessment of the overnight GT profile using immunoradiometric (Butler *et al.*, 1987, 1988) or immunofluorometric (Wu *et al.*, 1991) assays may be valuable.

There is physiologic blunting of GH secretion in late prepuberty in both sexes and in early male puberty so that, if pharmacological testing of GH secretion is deemed necessary and is to be interpreted correctly, priming with sex steroid is necessary. Stilboestrol is the drug of choice in both sexes but depot testosterone or oral estrogen may be used in boys and girls respectively.

4.6.2 CONSTITUTIONAL DELAY OF GROWTH AND PUBERTY

Constitutional delay of growth and puberty is the likely diagnosis in a healthy adolescent in whom stature is currently short for the family but appropriate for the stage of puberty and skeletal maturation giving a normal height prognosis for the family. There is often a family history of similar delay in parents or siblings (mother usually remembers her age at menarche, father is more likely to remember whether he was still growing after leaving school than when he started shaving) but its presence does not make the diagnosis and its absence does not exclude it. The problem is both commoner and more stressful in a boy – the growth spurt occurs late and is blunted in relation to his more average peers (Prader, 1975). The emotional, psychological and social consequences may be severe despite the absence of underlying pathology. Potential aspects of treatment which require consideration are puberty induction, growth stimulation and emotional support (see below). Individual treatment modalities interact with each other in terms of their psychological and physical effects (Kelnar, 1994).

4.6.3 CHRONIC SYSTEMIC DISEASE

Chronic systemic disease may cause slowing of growth which may or may not be reversible. Such growth delay is often associated with subsequent maturational delay in pubertal terms or even with failure to enter puberty. The association with diabetes mellitus is discussed by Dunger (p. 75). The signs of the underlying disorder usually allow diagnosis of such conditions as severe or undertreated chronic asthma, cystic fibrosis, heart disease or chronic renal failure. However abnormal signs or symptoms may be absent in gastrointestinal disease such as celiac disease, Crohn's disease or ulcerative colitis. Anorexia with a 'normal' bowel habit should lead to suspicion of such a diagnosis and anorexia nervosa also classically presents with lack of onset of puberty or pubertal arrest. Anorexia nervosa itself results in secondary endocrine disturbances whilst growth and maturational delay causes secondary psychological disturbances. Liaison with a sympathetic child psychiatrist is often necessary and extremely helpful in seeking evidence of underlying emotional problems and in their management.

The causes of growth and maturational delay or failure in these conditions may be explicable in nutritional, secondary hormonal, metabolic or therapeutic (e.g., glucocorticoid treatment) terms. However in many conditions the etiology is both multifactorial and poorly understood. For a useful review, see Preece *et al.* (1986).

4.6.4 NUTRITION

Undernutrition is the commonest cause of growth failure and pubertal delay worldwide and may occur in 'developed' countries, for example, because of inappropriate faddish diets, a desire of diabetic adolescent girls to remain slim (see Steel, p. 375) or in association with emotional deprivation. Whatever the specific relevance of metabolic signals for the onset of puberty, it is likely that growth retardation and pubertal delay or failure are a secondary adaptation to the need to conserve energy and to prevent reproduction in suboptimal circumstances. Undernutrition or malabsorption is likely to be important in the growth and pubertal failure in a number of the chronic diseases mentioned above.

REFERENCES

Adams, J. (1989) 'The role of pelvic ultrasound in the management of paediatric endocrine disorders', in C.G.D. Brook (ed.). *Clinical Paediatric Endocrinology*, 2nd edn, pp. 675–91. Blackwell Scientific Publications, Oxford.

Adashi, E.Y., Hsueh, A.J. and Yen, S.S. (1981) Insulin enhancement of luteinising hormone and follicle-stimulating hormone release by cultured pituitary cells. *Endocrinology*, **108**, 1441–49.

Adlard, P., Buzi, F., Jones, J. *et al.* (1987) Physiological growth hormone secretion during slow-wave sleep in short prepubertal children. *Clin. Endocrin.*, **27**, 355–61.

Albertson, B.D., Hobson, W.C., Burnett, B.S. *et al.* (1984) Dissociation of cortisol and adrenal androgen secretion in the hypophysectomised, adrenocorticotropin-replaced chimpanzee. *J. Clin. Endocrinol. Metab.*, **59**, 13–18.

Albertsson-Wikland, K., Rosberg, S., Isaksson, O. *et al.* (1983) Secretory pattern of growth hormone in children of differing growth rates. *Acta Endocrinologica*, **103** (suppl. 256), 72.

Albini, C.H., Quattrin, T., Vandlen, R.L. *et al.* (1988) Quantitation of urinary growth hormone in children with normal and abnormal growth. *Pediatr. Res.*, **23**, 89–92.

Anderson, D.C. (1980) The adrenal androgen-stimulating hormone does not exist. *Lancet*, **ii**, 454–56.

Anderson, D.C., Lasley, B.L., Fisher, R.A. *et al.* (1976) Transplacental gradients of sex-hormone-binding-globulin in human and simian pregnancy. *Clin. Endocrin.*, **5**, 657–59.

Annecillo, C. and Money, J. (1985) Abuse or psychosocial dwarfism: an update. *Growth, Genetics and Hormones*, **1**:4, 1–4.

Ashkenazi, A. (1989) Occult celiac disease: a common cause of short stature. *Growth, Genetics and Hormones*, **5**:2, 1–3.

Attanasio, A., Borelli, P., Marina, R. *et al.* (1983) Serum melatonin in children with early and delayed puberty. *Neuroendocrinology Letters*, **5**, 387–92.

Baron, J., Oerter, K.E., Yanovski, J.A. *et al.* (1993) Catch-up growth is intrinsic to the epiphyseal growth plate. *Pediatr. Res.*, **33** (suppl. 41), (abstract 224).

Barton, J.R. and Ferguson, A. (1990) Clinical features, morbidity and mortality of Scottish children with inflammatory bowel disease. *Qu. J. Med.*, **75**, 423–39.

Baumann, G. (1990) Growth hormone binding proteins and various forms of growth hormone: implications for measurements. *Acta Paed. Scand.*, **370** (Suppl.), 72–80.

Billewicz, W.Z., Fellowes, H.M. and Hytten, C.H. (1976) Comments on the critical metabolic mass and the age at menarche. *Ann. Hum. Biol.*, **3**, 51–59.

Blum, W.F., Rosberg, S., Ranke, M.B. *et al.* (1993) The short-term increases of IGF-1 and IGF-BP3 during GH treatment predict the long-term growth response in short children. *Pediatr. Res.*, **33** (Suppl.), 48 (abstract 271).

Boyar, R.M., Finkelstein, J., Roffwarg *et al.* (1972) Synchronisation of augmented luteinising hormone secretion with sleep during puberty. *N. Eng. J. Med.*, **287**, 582–86.

Brook, C.G.D. (1983) Earlier recognition of abnormal stature. *Arch. Dis. Child.*, **58**, 840.

Brook, C.G.D. and Stanhope, R. (1989) 'Normal puberty: physical characteristics and endocrinology', in C.G.D. Brook (ed.). *Clinical Paediatric Endocrinology*, 2nd edn, pp. 169–88. Blackwell Scientific Publications, Oxford.

Brook, C.G.D., Jacobs, H.S., Stanhope, R. *et al.* (1987) Pulsatility of reproductive hormones: applications to the understanding of puberty and the treatment of infertility. *Bailliere's Clinics in Endocrinology and Metabolism*, **1**, 23–41.

Brown, D.C., Stirling, H.F., Butler, G.E. *et al.* (1992b) Predicting male clinical pubertal onset – comparison of testosterone, overnight LH and LHRH-stimulated LH measurement. *Eur. J. Paediatr.*, **151**, 925 (abstract).

Brown, D.C., Wu, F.C.W. and Kelnar, C.J.H. (1992a) Does pubertal progress affect basal metabolic rate independent of body weight? *Eur. J. Paediatr.*, **151**, 923 (abstract).

Buckler, J.M.H. (1979) *A Reference Manual of Growth and Development*. Blackwell Scientific Publications, Oxford.

Butler, G.E., Kelnar, C.J.H. and Wu, F.C.W. (1988) Pituitary responsiveness in prepuberty and hypogonadotrophic hypogonadism is related to endogenous LHRH secretion. A study using a highly selective immunoradiometric assay. *J. Endocrin.*, **117** (Suppl.), A277.

Butler, G.E., McKie, M. and Ratcliffe, S.G. (1989a) 'An analysis of the phases of mid-childhood growth by synchronisation of the growth spurts', in J.M. Tanner (ed.). *Auxology '88: Perspectives in the science of growth and development*. Smith-Gordon, London.

Butler, G.E., Sellar, R.E., Kelnar, C.J.H. *et al.* (1987) A sensitive immunoradiometric assay (RMA) for luteinising hormone (LH) in the assessment of prepubertal males with idiopathic hypogonadotrophic hypogonadism (IHH), and constitutional delayed puberty. *J. Endocrin.*, **112** (Suppl.), A243.

Butler, G.E., Stirling, H.F., Wu, F.C.W. *et al.* (1989b) Do growth hormone secretory patterns relate to growth velocity in both prepubertal and pubertal children? *Horm. Res.*, **31** (Suppl.), A109.

Carter-Su, C., Wang, X., Campbell, G.S. *et al.* (1993) Molecular basis of growth hormone action. *Pediatr. Res.*, **33** (Suppl.), 8 (abstract 34).

Chatelain, P., Bouillat, B., Cohen, R. *et al.* (1990) Assay of growth hormone levels in human plasma using commercial kits: analysis of some factors influencing the results. *Acta Paed. Scand.*, **370** (Suppl.), 56–61.

Cohen, H.N., Paterson, K.R., Wallace, A.M. *et al.* (1984) Dissociation of adrenarche and gonadarche in diabetes mellitus. *Clin. Endocrinol.*, **20**, 717–24.

Crofton, P.M., Schönau, E., Stirling, H.F. *et al.* (1993) Can biochemical markers predict response to growth-promoting treatments in short normal children? *Pediatr. Res.*, **33** (Suppl.), 35 (abstract 193).

Crofton, P.M., Stirling, H.F. and Kelnar, C.J.H. (1992) Rise in bone alkaline phosphatase (bALP) can be used to predict responses to growth promoting treatments. *Acta Paed. Scand.*, **379** (Suppl.), 181.

Cronk, C.E., Crocker, A.C., Pueschel, S.M. *et al.* (1988) Growth charts for children with Down's syndrome: 1 month to 18 years of age. *Pediatrics*, **81**, 102–110.

Cutler, G.B. Jr., Glenn, M., Bush, M. *et al.* (1978) Adrenarche: a survey of rodents, domestic animals and primates. *Endocrinology*, **103**, 2112–18.

De Jong, F.H. (1988) Inhibin. *Physiol. Rev.*, **68**, 555–607.

Dieguez, C., Page, M.D. and Scanlon, M.F. (1988) Growth hormone neuroregulation and its alteration in disease states. *Clin. Endocrin.*, **28**, 109–143.

Ehrenkranz, J.R.L., Tamarkin, L., Comite, F. (1982) Daily rhythm of plasma melatonin in normal and precocious puberty. *J. Clin. Endocrinol. Metab.*, **55**, 307–310.

Faria, A.C., Veldhuis, J.D., Thorner, M.O. *et al.*

(1989) Half-time of endogenous growth hormone disappearance in normal man after stimulation of growth hormone secretion by growth hormone-releasing hormone and suppression with somatostatin. *J. Clin. Endocrin. Metab.*, **68**, 535–41.

Fernstrom, J.D. (1979) In D.T. Kreiger. *Endocrine Rhythms*. Raven Press, New York, 89–122.

Finkelstein, J.W., Roffwarg, H.P., Boyar, R.M. *et al.* (1972) Age-related change in the twenty four hour spontaneous secretion of growth hormone. *J. Clin. Endocrin. Metab.*, **35**, 665–70.

Forest, M.G., Cathiard, A.M. and Bertrand, J.A. (1973) Evidence of testicular activity in early infancy. *J. Clin. Endocrin. Metab.*, **37**, 148–51.

Frisch, R.E. and Revelle, R. (1970) Height and weight at menarche and a hypothesis of critical body weights and adolescent events. *Science*, **169**, 397–99.

Frohman, L.A. and Jansson, J.-O. (1986) Growth hormone-releasing hormone. *Endocrine Rev.*, **7**, 223–53.

Girard, J., Celniker, A., Price, D.A. *et al.* (1990) Urinary measurement of growth hormone secretion. *Acta Paed. Scand.*, **366** (Suppl.), 149–54.

Gluckman, P., Guan, J., Beilharz, E. *et al.* (1993) A role for IGF-1 and its binding proteins in neuronal rescue following asphyxial injury. *Pediatr. Res.*, **33** (Suppl.), 37 (abstract 203).

Granada, M.L., Sanmarti, A., Lucas, A. *et al.* (1990) Assay-dependent results of immunoassayable spontaneous 24-hour growth hormone secretion in short children. *Acta Paed. Scand.*, **370** (Suppl.), 63–70.

Grumbach, M.M., Richards, G.E., Conte, F.A. *et al.* (1978) 'Clinical disorders of adrenal function and puberty: an assessment of the role of the adrenal cortex in normal and abnormal puberty in man and evidence for an ACTH-like pituitary adrenal androgen stimulating hormone', in V.H.T. James, M. Serio, G. Giusti *et al.* (eds). *The Endocrine Function of the Human Adrenal Cortex*, pp. 583–612. Academic Press, New York.

Guillemin, R., Brazeau, P., Bolan, P. *et al.* (1982) Growth hormone releasing factor from a human pancreatic tumour that caused acromegaly. *Science*, **218**, 585–87.

Hall, J.G., Froster-Iskenius, V.G. and Allanson, J.E. (1989) *Handbook of Normal Physical Measurements*. Oxford Medical Publications, Oxford.

Harris, G.W. and Jacobsohn, D. (1952) Functional grafts of anterior pituitary gland. *Proceedings of the Royal Society, London*, **139**, 263–76.

Hay, I.D., Smail, P.J. and Forsyth, C.C. (1981) Familial cytomegalic adrenocortical hypoplasia: an X-linked syndrome of pubertal failure. *Arch. Dis. Child.*, **56**, 715–21.

Hermanussen, M., Geiger-Benoit, K., Burmeister, J. *et al.* (1988a) Knemometry in childhood: accuracy and standardization of a new technique of lower leg measurement. *An. Hum. Biol.*, **15**, 1–16.

Hermanussen, M., Geiger-Benoit, K., Burmeister, J. *et al.* (1988b) Periodical changes of short-term growth velocity (mini-growth spurts) in human growth. *An. Hum. Biol.*, **15**, 103–111.

Hindmarsh, P.C. and Brook, C.G.D. (1989) 'Normal growth and its endocrine control', in C.G.D. Brook (ed.). *Clinical Paediatric Endocrinology*, pp. 57–73. Blackwell Scientific Publications, Oxford.

Hindmarsh, P.C., Matthews, D.R., Brain, C.E. *et al.* (1989) The half-life of exogenous GH after suppression of endogenous GH secretion with somatostatin. *Clin. Endocrin.*, **30**, 443–50.

Hindmarsh, P.C., Matthews, D.R., di Silvio, L. *et al.* (1988) Relation between height velocity and fasting insulin concentrations. *Arch. Dis. Child.*, **63**, 665–66.

Hindmarsh, P.C., Smith, P.J., Brook, C.G.D. *et al.* (1987) The relationship between height velocity and growth hormone secretion in short prepubertal children. *Clin. Endocrin.*, **27**, 581–91.

Horton, W.A., Rotter, J.I., Rimoin, D.L. *et al.* (1978) Standard growth curves for achondroplasia. *J. Pediatr.*, **93**, 435–38.

Hunter, W.M. and Rigal, W.M. (1966) The diurnal pattern of plasma growth hormone concentration in adults. *J. Endocrin.*, **34**, 147–53.

Illig, R., Prader, A., Ferrandez, A. *et al.* (1971) Hereditary prenatal growth hormone deficiency with increased tendency to growth hormone antibody formation ('A type' isolated growth hormone deficiency). *Acta Paed. Scand.*, **60**, 607.

Jakacki, R.J., Kelch, R.P., Sauder, S.E. *et al.* (1982) Pulsatile secretion of luteinising hormone in children. *J. Clin. Endocrin. Metab.*, **55**, 453–58.

Kanof, M.E., Lake, A.M. and Bayless, T.M. (1988) Decreased height velocity in children and adolescents before the diagnosis of Crohn's disease. *Gastroenterology*, **95**, 1523–27.

Kaplan, S.L., Grumbach, M.M. and Aubert, M.L. (1976) The ontogenesis of pituitary hormones and hypothalamic factors in the human fetus: maturation of central nervous system regulation of anterior pituitary function. *Rec. Prog. Horm. Res.*, **32**, 161–234.

Karlberg, J., Engstrom, I., Karlberg, P. *et al.* (1987a) Analysis of linear growth using a mathematical model. 1. From birth to three years. *Acta Paed. Scand.*, **76**, 478–88.

Karlberg, J., Fryer, J.G., Engstrom, I. *et al.* (1987b) Analysis of linear growth using a mathematical model. 2. From 3 to 21 years of age. *Acta Paed. Scand.* (Suppl.), **337**, 12–29.

Kelnar, C.J.H. (1985) *Adrenal Steroids in Childhood* (MD Thesis, University of Cambridge).

Kelnar, C.J.H. (1990) Pride and prejudice – stature in perspective. *Acta Paed. Scand.*, **370** (Suppl.), 5–15.

Kelnar, C.J.H. (1992a) 'Endocrine gland disorders' (chapter), in A.G.M. Campbell, and N. McIntosh. *Forfar and Arneil's Textbook of Paediatrics*, 4th edition, pp. 1085–171. Churchill Livingstone, Edinburgh.

Kelnar, C.J.H. (1992b) 'Physical growth and development – endocrinological aspects of puberty and adolescence' (chapter), in A.G.M. Campbell and N. McIntosh. *Forfar and Arneil's Textbook of Paediatrice*, 4th edn, pp. 424–45. Churchill Livingstone, Edinburgh.

Kelnar, C.J.H. (1993a) Growth. *Medicine International* **21**:6, 217–23.

Kelnar, C.J.H. (1993b) Growth hormone (GH) therapy in the normal short child. *Proc. Eur. Soc. Paediatr. Res.*, 135 (abstract).

Kelnar, C.J.H. (1994) Does the short, sexually immature adolescent boy need treatment and what form should it take? *Arch. Dis. Child.* (in press).

Kelnar, C.J.H. and Brook, C.G.D. (1983) A mixed longitudinal study of adrenal steroid excretion in childhood and the mechanism of adrenarche. *Clin. Endocrinol.*, **19**, 117–29.

Kelnar, C.J.H., Wu, F.C.W., Brown, D.C. *et al.* (1993) Differentiation between normal prepuberty and hypogonadotrophism in boys: consideration of hourly mean LH concentrations. *Pediatr. Res.*, **33** (Suppl.), 84 (abstract 484).

Kirschner, B.S. (1990) Growth and development in chronic inflammatory bowel disease. *Acta Paed. Scand.*, **366** (Suppl.), 98–104.

Kitay, J.I. (1954) Pineal lesions and precocious puberty: a review. *J. Clin. Endocrin. Metab.*, **14**, 622–25.

Knobil, E. (1980) The neuroendocrine control of the menstrual cycle. *Rec. Prog. Horm. Res.*, **36**, 53–88.

Laron, Z. and Klinger, B. (1993) One year treatment with IGF-1 of children with Laron syndrome (LS). *Pediatr. Res.*, **33** (Suppl.), 5 (abstract 18).

Lee, P.A., Kowarski, A., Migeon, C.J. *et al.* (1975) Lack of correlation between gonadotrophin and adrenal androgen levels in agonadal children. *J. Clin. Endocrinol. Metab.*, **40**, 664–69.

Lenko, H.L., Lang, V., Aubert, M.L. *et al.* (1982) Hormonal changes in puberty vii: Lack of variation of daytime plasma melatonin. *J. Clin. Endocrinol. Metab.*, **54**, 1056–58.

Lyall, E.G.H., Crofton, P.M., Stirling, H.F. *et al.* (1992) Albuminuric growth failure. A case of Munchausen syndrome by proxy. *Acta Paed.*, **81**, 373–76.

Lyon, A.J., Preece, M.A. and Grant, D.B. (1985) Growth curve for girls with Turner syndrome. *Arch. Dis. Child.*, **60**, 932–35.

Millard, W.J., Politch, J.A., Martin, J.B. *et al.* (1986) Growth hormone secretory patterns in androgen resistant (testicular feminised) rats. *Endocrinology*, **119**, 2655–60.

Molinari, L., Largo, R.H. and Prader, A. (1980) Analysis of the growth spurt at age seven (midgrowth spurt). *Helvetica Paed. Acta*, **35**, 325–34.

Penny, R., Olambiwannu, N.O. and Frasier, S.D. (1977) Episodic fluctuations of serum gonadotrophins in pre- and post-pubertal girls and boys. *J. Clin. Endocrinol. Metab.*, **45**, 307–311.

Phillips, J.A. III, Ferrandez, A., Frisch, H. *et al.* (1986) 'Defects of growth hormone genes – clinical syndromes', in S. Raiti and R.A. Tolinan (eds). *Human Growth Hormone*, pp. 211–26. Plenum, New York.

Powell, G.F., Brasel, A. and Blizzard, R.M. (1967a) Emotional deprivation and growth retardation simulating idiopathic hypopituitarism. I. Clinical evaluation of the syndrome. *New Eng. J. Med.*, **276**, 1271–78.

Powell, G.F., Brasel, A., Raiti, S. *et al.* (1967b) Emotional deprivation and growth retardation simulating idiopathic hypopituitarism. II. Endocrinologic evaluation of the syndrome. *New Eng. J. Med.*, **276**, 1279–83.

Prader, A. (1975) Delayed adolescence. *Clinics in Endocrinology and Metabolism*, **4**, 143–55.

Prader, A., Tanner, J.M. and von Harnack, G.A. (1963) Catch-up growth following illness or starvation. *J. Pediatr.*, **62**, 646–59.

Preece, M.A. and Hendrich, I. (1981) Mathematical modelling of individual growth curves. *Brit. Med. Bull.*, **37**, 247–52.

Preece, M.A., Law, C.M. and Davies, P.S.W. (1986) 'The growth of children with chronic paediatric disease', in M.O. Savage and R.A. Randall (eds). Growth Disorders. *Clinics in Endocrinology and Metabolism*, **15**, 453–77.

Rivier, J., Speiss, J., Thorner, M. *et al.* (1982) Characterisation of a growth hormone releasing factor from a human pancreatic islet cell tumour. *Nature*, **300**, 276–78.

Savage, M.O., Wilton, P., Ranke, M.B. *et al.* (1993) Therapeutic response to recombinant IGF-1 in thirty two patients with growth hormone insensitivity. *Pediatr. Res.*, **33** (Suppl.), 5 (abstract 17).

Silman, R.E., Leone, R.M., Hopper, R.J.L. *et al.* (1979) Melatonin, the pineal gland and human puberty. *Nature*, **282**, 301–303.

Sizonenko, P.C. and Lang, U. (1988) 'Melatonin and human reproductive function', in A. Miles, D.R.S. Philbrick and C. Thompson (eds). *Melatonin – Clinical Perspectives*, pp. 62–78. Oxford University Press, Oxford.

Spiliotis, B.E., August, G.P., Hung, W. *et al.* (1984) Growth hormone neurosecretory dysfunction. A treatable cause of short stature. *J. Am. Med. Ass.*, **251**, 2223–30.

Stahnk, N. and Jenke, I. (1993) Comparing apples with pears. *Pediatr. Res.*, **33** (Suppl.), 68 (abstract 386).

Stanhope, R. and Brook, C.G.D. (1989) 'Disorders of puberty', in C.G.D. Brook (ed.). *Clinical Paediatric Endocrinology*, 2nd edn, pp. 189–212. Blackwell Scientific Publications, Oxford.

Stanhope, R., Adlard, P., Hamill, G. *et al.* (1988) Physiological growth hormone secretion during the recovery from psychosocial dwarfism: a case report. *Clin. Endocrin.*, **28**, 335–40.

Stanhope, R., Brook, C.G.D., Pringle, P.J. *et al.* (1987) Induction of puberty by pulsatile gonadotrophin-releasing hormone. *Lancet*, **ii**, 552–55.

Stanhope, R., Pringle, P.J., Adams, J. *et al.* (1985) Spontaneous gonadotrophin pulsatility and ovarian morphology in girls with central precocious puberty treated with cyproterone acetate. *Clin Endocrin.*, **23**, 547–53.

Stark, O., Peckham, C.S. and Moynihan, C. (1989) Weight and age at menarche. *Arch. Dis. Child.*, **64**, 383–87.

Steiner, R.A., Cameron, J.L., McNeill, T.H. *et al.* (1983) *Metabolic signals for the onset of puberty. Neuroendocrine Aspects of Reproduction*, pp. 183–227. Academic Press, New York

Stirling, H.F. and Kelnar, C.J.H. (1990) Adrenarche. *Growth matters*, **1**:4, 6–8.

Stirling, H.F. and Kelnar, C.J.H. (1992) Puberty. *Curr. Paediatr.*, **2**, 131–36.

Stirling, H.F., Seth, J., Sturgeon, C.M. *et al.* (1993) The relationship between plasma overnight growth hormone profiles and nocturnal urinary growth hormone excretion. *Pediatr. Res.*, **33** (Suppl.), 40 (abstract 222).

Stolz, H.R. and Stolz, L.M. (1951) *Somatic development of adolescent boys. A study of the growth of boys during the second decade of life*. Macmillan, New York.

Stuetzle, W., Gasser, T.H., Molinari, L. *et al.* (1980) Shape-invariant modelling of human growth. *An. Hum. Biol.*, **7**, 507–528.

Tamarkin, L., Abastillas, P., Chen, H.-C. *et al.* (1982) The daily profile of plasma melatonin in obese and Prader-Willi syndrome children. *J. Clin. Endocrinol. Metab.*, **55**, 491–95.

Tanner, J.M. (1962) *Growth at Adolescence*, 2nd edn. Blackwell Scientific Publications, Oxford.

Tanner, J.M. (1963) The regulation of human growth. *Child Dev.*, **34**, 817–47.

Tanner, J.M. (1981) 'Endrocrinology of puberty', in C.G.D. Brook (ed.). *Clinical Paediatric Endocrinology*, pp. 207–223. Blackwell Scientific Publications, Oxford.

Tanner, J.M. (1989) *Foetus into Man*, 2nd edition. Castlemead Publications, Ware.

Tanner, J.M. (1992) 'Physical growth and development', in A.G.M. Campbell and N. McIntosh (eds). *Forfar and Arneil's Textbook of Paediatrics*, 4th edn, pp. 389–424. Churchill-Livingston, Edinburgh.

Tanner, J.M., Gibbons, R.D. and Bock, R.D. (1993) Advantages of the computer-aided image analysis system for estimating TW skeletal maturity:

increased reliability and a continuous scale. *Pediatr. Res.*, **33** (Suppl.), 35 (abstract 189).

Tanner, J.M. and Whitehouse, R.H. (1976) Clinical longitudinal standards for height, weight, height velocity and weight velocity and the stages of puberty. *Arch. Dis. Child.*, **51**, 170–79.

Tetsuo, M., Poth, M. and Markey, S.P. (1982) Melatonin metabolite excretion during childhood and puberty. *J. Clin. Endocrinol. Metab.*, **55**, 311–13.

Thomas, B.C. and Stanhope, R. (1993) Long-term growth data and growth hormone secretion in 65 patients with psycho-social dwarfism. *Pediatr. Res.*, **33** (Suppl.), 312 (abstract).

Veldhuis, J.D., Evans, W.S., Demers, L.M. *et al.* (1985) Altered neuroendocrine regulation of gonadotrophin secretion in women distance runners. *J. Clin. Endocrin. Metab.*, **61**, 557–63.

Vimpani, G.V., Vimpani, A.F., Lidgard, G.P. *et al.* (1977) Prevalence of severe growth hormone deficiency. *Brit. Med. J.*, ii, 427–30.

Waldhauser, W., Weiszenbacher, G., Frisch, H. *et al.* (1984) Fall in nocturnal serum melatonin during prepuberty and pubescence. *Lancet*, **i**, 362–65.

Wales, J.K.H. and Milner, R.D.G. (1988) Variation in lower leg growth with alternate day steroid treatment. *Arch. Dis. Child.*, **63**, 981–83.

Warren, M.P. and Van de Wiele, R.L. (1973) Clinical and metabolic features of anorexia nervosa. *Am. J. Obst. Gyn.*, **117**, 435–49.

Warren, M.P., Jewelewicz, R., Dyrenfurth, I. *et al.* (1975) The significance of weight loss in the evaluation of pituitary responsiveness to LH-RH in women with secondary amenorrhea. *J. Clin. Endocrin. Metab.*, **40**, 601–611.

Wass, J.A.H. (1983) Growth hormone neuroregulation and the clinical relevance of somatostatin. *Clinics in Endocrinology and Metabolism*, **12**, 695–724.

Weinberg, V., Weitzman, E.D., Fukushima, D.K. *et al.* (1980) Melatonin does not suppress the pituitary luteinizing hormone response to luteinizing hormone-releasing hormone in men. *J. Clin. Endocrinol. Metab.*, **51**, 161–62.

Wilson, R.C., Kesner, J.S., Kaufman, J.M. *et al.* (1984) Central electrophysiologic correlates of pulsatile luteinising hormone secretion in the rhesus monkey. *Neuroendocrinology*, **39**, 256–60.

Wood, W.I. (1993) Structure and functional analysis of the human growth hormone receptor. *Pediatr. Res.*, **33** (Suppl.), 9 (abstract 35).

Wolthers, O.D. and Pedersen, S. (1990) Short term linear growth in asthmatic children during treatment with prednisolone. *Brit. Med. J.*, **301**, 145–48.

Wu, F.C.W. (1993) Delayed puberty. *Medicine International*, **21**: 6, 224–28.

Wu, F.C.W., Borrow, S.M., Nicol, K. *et al.* (1989) Ontogeny of pulsatile gonadotrophin secretion and pituitary responsiveness in male puberty in man – a mixed longitudinal and cross-sectional study. *J. Endocrin.*, **123**, 347–59.

Wu, F.C.W., Butler, G.E., Brown, D.C. *et al.* (1993) Early morning testosterone is a useful predictor of the imminence of puberty. *J. Clin. Endocrin. Metab.*, **76**, 26–31.

Wu, F.C.W., Butler, G.E., Kelnar, C.J.H. *et al.* (1990a) Patterns of pulsatile LH secretion before and during the onset of puberty in boys – a study using an immunoradiometric assay. *J. Clin. Endocrin. Metab.*, **70**, 629–37.

Wu, F.C.W., Butler, G.E. and Kelnar, C.J.H. (1990b) Pulsatile LH secretion during male puberty – a longitudinal study in patients with and without testosterone treatment for induction of sexual maturation. *J. Endocrin.*, **124** (Suppl.), A182.

Wu, F.C.W., Butler, G.E., Kelnar, C.J.H. *et al.* (1991) Patterns of pulsatile luteinizing hormone and follicle stimulating hormone secretion in prepubertal (midchildhood) boys and girls and patients with idiopathic hypogonadotrophic hypogonadism (Kallmann's syndrome): a study using an ultrasensitive time-resolved immunofluorometric assay. *J. Clin. Endocrin. Metab.*, **72**, 1229–37.

Wurtman, R.J. and Moscowitz, M.A. (1977) The pineal organ. *N. Eng. J. Med.*, **296**, 1329–33 and 1383–86.

Zacharias, L. and Wurtman, R. (1964) Blindness: its relation to age of menarche. *Obstetr. Gynaecol.*, **30**, 507–509.

Zapf, J., Hussain, M. and Froesch, E.R. (1993) *In vivo* metabolic actions of IGF-1. *Pediatr. Res.*, **33** (Suppl.), 4 (abstract 15).

APPENDIX: USEFUL ADDRESSES FOR UK READERS

The Child Growth Foundation
2 Mayfield Avenue, London W4 1PW
As well as providing parental support also runs seminars and information programmes to increase awareness of growth and its disorders amongst health care professionals. They also supply a wide selection of measuring equipment.

Castlemead Publications
Swains Mill, 4a Crane Mead
Ware, Herts SG12 9PY
Supplies a wide range of UK growth charts including Tanner/Whitehouse height and height velocity normal standards, height velocity screening charts, charts for Turner and Down syndromes, etc.

5

Endocrine evolution, growth and puberty in relation to diabetes

D.B. DUNGER

5.1 INTRODUCTION

In the years immediately following the introduction of insulin therapy, short stature was consistently reported in patients with insulin-dependent diabetes mellitus (IDDM) (Joslin *et al.*, 1925; Wagner *et al.*, 1942). In 1930 Mauriac described a 10-year-old, poorly-controlled girl with hepatomegaly, protuberant abdomen, dwarfism, moon-shaped face and fat deposition about the shoulders and abdomen. She suffered recurrent ketoacidosis and her puberty was delayed (Mauriac, 1934). These features were later encapsulated into the **Mauriac syndrome** and this condition was reasonably common even in 1953 (Guest, 1953). Less severe abnormalities of growth and sexual maturation were also common and in 1973 Tattersall and Pyke reported a mean difference of 2.5 inches in the final adult height and a 4–5 year difference in the age at menarche between identical twins with and without diabetes.

Fortunately the Mauriac syndrome is now rare, but delayed puberty and reductions in adult height in children developing diabetes are still reported even in apparently well-controlled subjects (Jivani & Rayner, 1973; Petersen *et al.*, 1978; Hjelt *et al.*, 1983; Herber & Dunsmore, 1988). Childhood growth and pubertal development in subjects with IDDM has been the subject of extensive study over the last 50 years and the data that have accumulated are summarized in the first part of this chapter. The chapter concludes with a description of reported endocrine abnormalities in IDDM and their impact on growth and development.

5.2 GROWTH AND PUBERTAL DEVELOPMENT IN CHILDREN WITH IDDM

5.2.1 HEIGHT AT DIAGNOSIS

It is perhaps remarkable that after almost 20 years of study, there should still be controversy about the height at diagnosis of children with diabetes. Some studies have reported that children are taller than controls at diagnosis (Jivani & Rayner, 1973; Edelsten *et al.*, 1981; Hjelt *et al.*, 1983; Salardi *et al.*, 1987; Songer *et al.*, 1986; Drayer, 1974; Lee *et al.*, 1984) whereas others have refuted these observations (Tattersall & Pyke, 1973; Hoskins *et al.*, 1985; Petersen *et al.*, 1978; Evans *et al.*, 1972; Emmerson & Savage, 1988). Much of the debate has centered on the choice of

Childhood and Adolescent Diabetes
Published in 1994 by Chapman & Hall, London
ISBN 0 412 48610 5

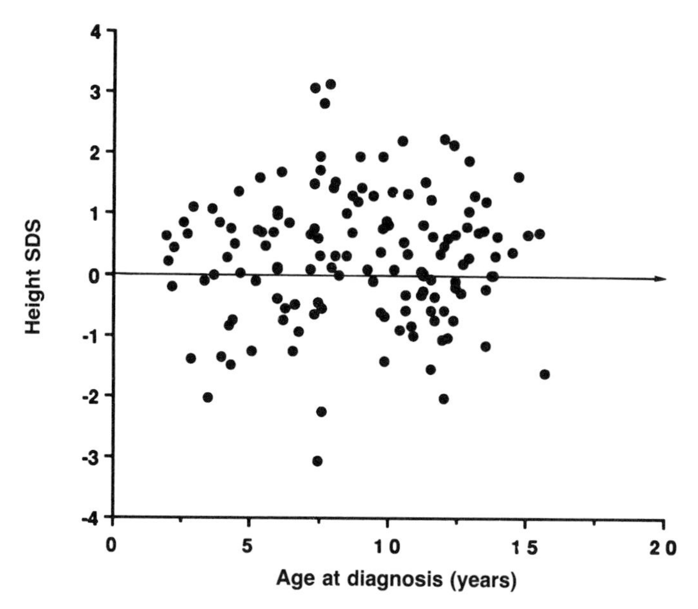

Figure 5.1 Height at diagnosis of children with insulin-dependent diabetes mellitus (Brown *et al.*, 1994).

control data, which must reflect any possible secular trend in growth and the social class distribution of the control subjects. There was a suggestion in some early studies that there was a bias towards the upper social classes in populations of children with IDDM (Lee *et al.*, 1984) but this was not confirmed by subsequent studies. Recent data collected in the Oxford district concerning the growth of 140 children with diabetes diagnosed between 1969 and 1990 showed an identical social class distribution to national census data for that area. Mean height standard deviation score (SDS) at diagnosis of these children calculated from the normal data of Tanner *et al.*, 1966, was +0.29 and this is not dissimilar from the mean height SDS of controls in Oxford who have followed the secular trend towards increased stature over the years since the Tanner data were first compiled. Detailed analysis revealed however, that those children diagnosed between the ages of 5 and 10 were taller than Oxford controls (+0.46 v. +0.24), particularly the girls studied (Figure 5.1).

The issue of height at diagnosis remains perplexing as is evident from several recent studies reporting growth of children with IDDM prior to diagnosis. In the studies reported by Hoskins *et al.* (1985), and Leslie *et al.* (1991), the growth of a twin who did not develop diabetes was compared with that of the twin who did develop diabetes. A reduction in growth velocity was observed over 1–2 years before the development of diabetes with significant loss of stature. However, in a large epidemiological study carried out in Sweden, Blom *et al.* (1992) demonstrated that high linear growth was positively associated with the risk of diabetes particularly in boys. A similar conclusion was drawn by Price and Burden (1992) who reported increased growth in diabetic children but not their siblings at diagnosis.

This confusing array of data may in fact reflect a more profound heterogeneity in children with IDDM. In a recent study, comparing heights at diagnosis in Japan and Pittsburgh, the respective research groups showed a remarkable discrepancy (Japan & Pittsburgh, 1989). Songer *et al.* (1986) demonstrated that children diagnosed between 5–9 years were taller at diagnosis but they also noted that nondiabetic siblings at high risk for the disease were closer in height to the diabetic siblings than were the low-risk siblings. Genetic variation may thus explain much of the discrepant data in the literature.

It is perhaps easier to explain loss of height prior to diagnosis than a gain in height. It could be argued that variations in nutrition might predispose to both tall stature and the development of diabetes. Obesity is clearly related to tall stature during childhood (Frisch & Revelle, 1969) and children destined to develop IDDM may weigh more during infancy (Baum *et al.*, 1975). Alternatively the tall stature may reflect a period of excessive insulin production prior to diagnosis although the loss of height in the twin studies would not support this.

5.2.2 GROWTH AFTER DIAGNOSIS

Fortunately there is a greater consensus concerning the effects of diabetes on growth after diagnosis. Several studies have reported a reduction in height SDS over the first 3–4 years from diagnosis (Hjelt *et al.*, 1983; Petersen *et al.*, 1978; Jivani & Rayner, 1973; Lee *et al.*, 1984; Thon *et al.*, 1992). As with height at diagnosis, the age at diagnosis is more closely related to loss of height SDS than the duration of diabetes. Ironically the greatest loss of height is often seen in those children who were tallest at diagnosis, i.e., those diagnosed between the ages of 5–10 years. In the Oxford studies the loss of height SDS between diagnosis and the onset of puberty averaged 0.06 SDS per year (Brown *et al.*, 1994).

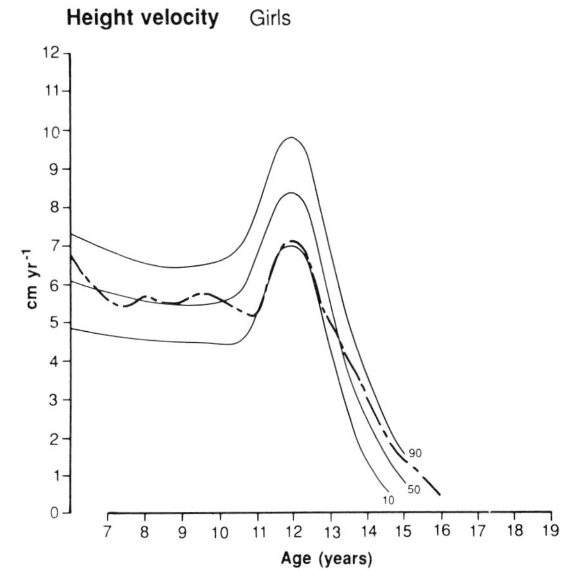

Figure 5.2 Height velocity in girls with IDDM. The dotted line represents the mean growth velocity of girls with IDDM studied in Oxford.

5.2.3 GROWTH AT PUBERTY

The pubertal growth spurt is invariably blunted in girls with IDDM (Salardi *et al.*, 1987; Tattersall & Pyke, 1973; Jivani & Rayner, 1973; Lee, 1984; Stewart-Brown *et al.*, 1985) (Figure 5.2) whereas pubertal growth may be normal in boys. The timing of peak height velocity was delayed in the studies reported by Lee *et al.* (1984) and Jivani & Rayner (1973) but recent data from the Oxford group indicates a normal timing and duration of pubertal growth. Nevertheless, the peak height velocity SDS was -1.09 (± 1.02) in the girls and -0.5 (± 1.14) in the boys studied in Oxford, observed irrespective of the age at onset of diabetes. However, Salardi *et al.* (1987) reported the poorest pubertal growth in those girls diagnosed just prior to the onset of puberty whereas the Oxford data suggested that the greatest loss of height during puberty was observed in those diagnosed under the age of 5 years.

5.2.4 FINAL HEIGHT OF CHILDREN WITH DIABETES

It is clear from the previous discussions that some loss of height occurs in children with diabetes but because of variations in height at diagnosis this may not be always evident in population studies of final height. While some studies have shown that subjects with IDDM attain a normal adult stature (Birkbeck, 1972; Jackson, 1984) others have shown that in apparently well-controlled patients final height may still be less than in normals (Knowles *et al.*, 1965; Sterky, 1967; Tattersall & Pyke, 1973). The final adult heights of 80 children studied in Oxford over the last 10 years was −0.06 SDS, which did not differ significantly from the mid-parental height SDS. Table 5.1 demonstrates the relationship between height at diagnosis and final height in this cohort. Despite loss of height after diagnosis, those subjects diagnosed between the ages of 5 and 10 years, achieved respectable final heights because they were tall at

Table 5.1 Height at diagnosis and final height SDS according to age at diagnosis in children with IDDM.

Age at diagnosis	Height SDS at diagnosis	Final height SDS
All	0.29 n = 140	−0.06 n = 80
<5 years	0.02 n = 22	−0.74 n = 10
5–10 years	0.46 n = 57	0.00 n = 36
>10 years	0.22 n = 61	0.09 n = 34

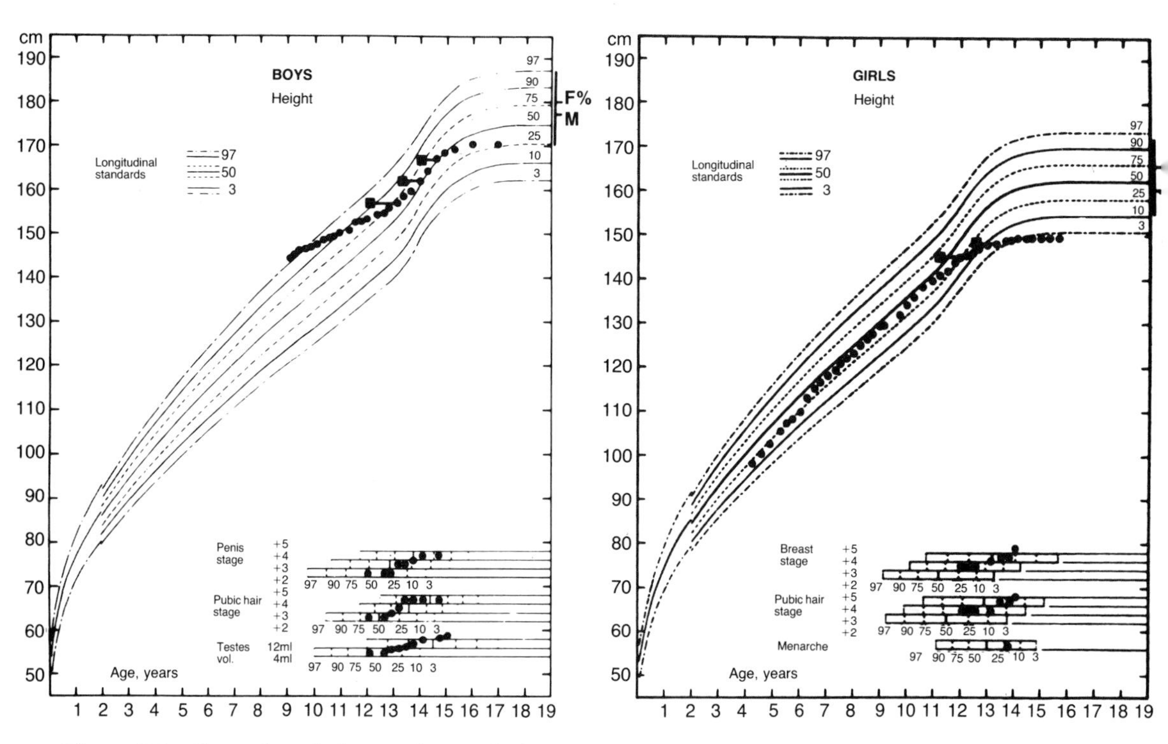

Figure 5.3 Examples of abnormal growth during puberty in adolescents with IDDM.

diagnosis. Those diagnosed under the age of 5 years showed similar loss of height but were not tall at diagnosis. In some individuals, the loss of the pubertal growth spurt may lead to severe growth impairment. This is most likely to occur in those diagnosed under the age of 5 years, who were not tall at diagnosis and have the longest duration of diabetes at the onset of puberty (Figure 5.3).

5.2.5 WEIGHT GAIN IN CHILDREN WITH IDDM

The weight of children with IDDM has been less often studied than stature but generally the range of body weight falls into the normal age-related distributions (Petersen *et al.*, 1978; Evans *et al.*, 1972; Clarson *et al.*, 1985). Nevertheless, a recent study from Germany indicated that over the first three years from diagnosis there was a tendency towards a greater increase in weight and a relative reduction in length when compared with controls (Thon *et al.*, 1992). Interestingly, the same study reported that weight gain was not associated with accelerated skeletal maturity as is reported in simple obesity. These observations require further confirmation.

Excess weight gain is, however, frequently encountered in girls with IDDM during puberty (Evans *et al.*, 1972) and during late adolescence the body mass index is significantly greater than in normal puberty and social class matched controls (Peveler *et al.*, 1992).

5.2.6 PUBERTAL DEVELOPMENT IN IDDM

Delayed sexual maturation was invariably reported in early studies of children with IDDM, but this has become less common in more recent reports. Lee *et al.* (1984) reported that menarche was delayed by on average 0.5 years but in the recent Oxford data the timing of the menarche was identical to that reported by Tanner *et al.* (1966). There are no detailed studies of the timing and sequence for the development of secondary sexual characteristics in IDDM, but clinical observation would suggest that these are not markedly different from normal.

Abnormalities of the menstrual cycle are, however, more common in girls with IDDM than in normal controls (Table 5.2). In a recent study where the menstrual histories of 24 post-menarchal girls with IDDM were compared with 24 age, puberty and social class-matched controls, the age at menarche was similar in the two groups as were the number of years post-menarche (Adcock *et al.*, 1994). Yet the numbers of girls who had experienced an irregular cycle or prolonged periods of amenorrhoea were considerably greater in the group with diabetes (54% v. 21%). Data from young adult women with IDDM indicate a greater incidence of secondary amenorrhoea and reduced fertility compared with controls (Trzeciak, 1978; Djursing *et al.*, 1985).

5.2.7 THE RELATIONSHIP BETWEEN GLYCEMIC CONTROL GROWTH AND PUBERTAL DEVELOPMENT IN IDDM

The outcome with respect to growth and pubertal development in subjects with IDDM has improved dramatically over the last 50 years, and this must reflect improvements in diabetic management. However, the relationship between 'good and bad' glycemic control and the growth of children with IDDM has proved to be difficult to define. If one uses glycosylated hemoglobin as an index of metabolic control in IDDM then there seems to be no relationship with growth (Jivani & Rayner, 1973; Hjelt *et al.*, 1983; Clarson *et al.*, 1985; Salardi *et al.*, 1987; Herber & Dunsmore, 1988; Thon *et al.*, 1992). It is evident from even a cursory examination of any clinic population that there are some subjects who have very poor glycemic control as judged by HbA_1 or

Table 5.2 Abnormalities of the menstrual cycle: a comparison of subjects with IDDM and controls (from Adcock *et al.*, 1994).

	IDDM n = 24	Controls n = 24	Significance p value
Age [yrs]	15.8 ± 0.4	15.9 ± 0.2	NS
Age at menarche [yrs]	12.9 ± 0.2	12.8 ± 0.2	NS
BMI [kg/m^2]	22.3 ± 0.5	20.7 ± 0.6	<0.05
Menstrual cycle			
Regular*	11 [45%]	19 [79%]	<0.01
Irregular	13 [54%]	5 [21%]	<0.01
Amenorrhea**	5 [21%]	1 [4%]	<0.01

NS Not Significant.
BMI Body Mass Index.
* A regular cycle was defined as lasting no more than 35 days with less than a 6-day variation in length between cycles.
** Amenorrhea for 3 months or more after the first post-menarchal year.

HbA_1c who nevertheless grow normally, yet others with only modestly poor control, grow badly. Genetic factors may play a part but this alone would not explain the improvements in growth observed over the last few decades.

The Mauriac syndrome can be seen as one extreme of the spectrum of growth abnormalities seen in IDDM but the relationship with glycemic control, even in that condition may be difficult to discern. In two recently reported cases the HbA_1c values were 12 and 15.9% compared with diabetic control values of 10.7% (Mauras *et al.*, 1991). Investigation of these subjects highlighted the abnormalities of the growth hormone/insulin-like growth factor-I axis. That axis is highly dependent on the appropriate delivery of insulin and it is perhaps in this area that improvements have occurred since the first attempts at insulin therapy. An increase in insulin dose and caloric intake may be sufficient to improve growth in some children with the Mauriac syndrome (Figure 5.4). In keeping with these observations intensive insulin treatment alone may accelerate linear growth in children who were previously thought to be growing normally (Rudolf *et al.*, 1982).

5.3 ENDOCRINE ABNORMALITIES IN CHILDREN AND ADOLESCENTS WITH IDDM

5.3.1 THE GROWTH HORMONE/INSULIN-LIKE GROWTH FACTOR-I AXIS IN DIABETES

Childhood growth, and to some extent the pubertal growth spurt, are thought to be growth hormone dependent. Growth hormone (GH) has direct effects on cartilage growth but it also acts through the paracrine production of insulin-like growth factor-I (IGF-I). Circulating levels of IGF-I reflect the growth hormone status of the individual and thus, generally, growth hormone deficiency is associated with low levels of IGF-I, and growth hormone excess, such as that seen in acromegaly, is associated with high circulating IGF-I levels. In subjects with IDDM however, there is often a discrepancy between GH levels and IGF-I production.

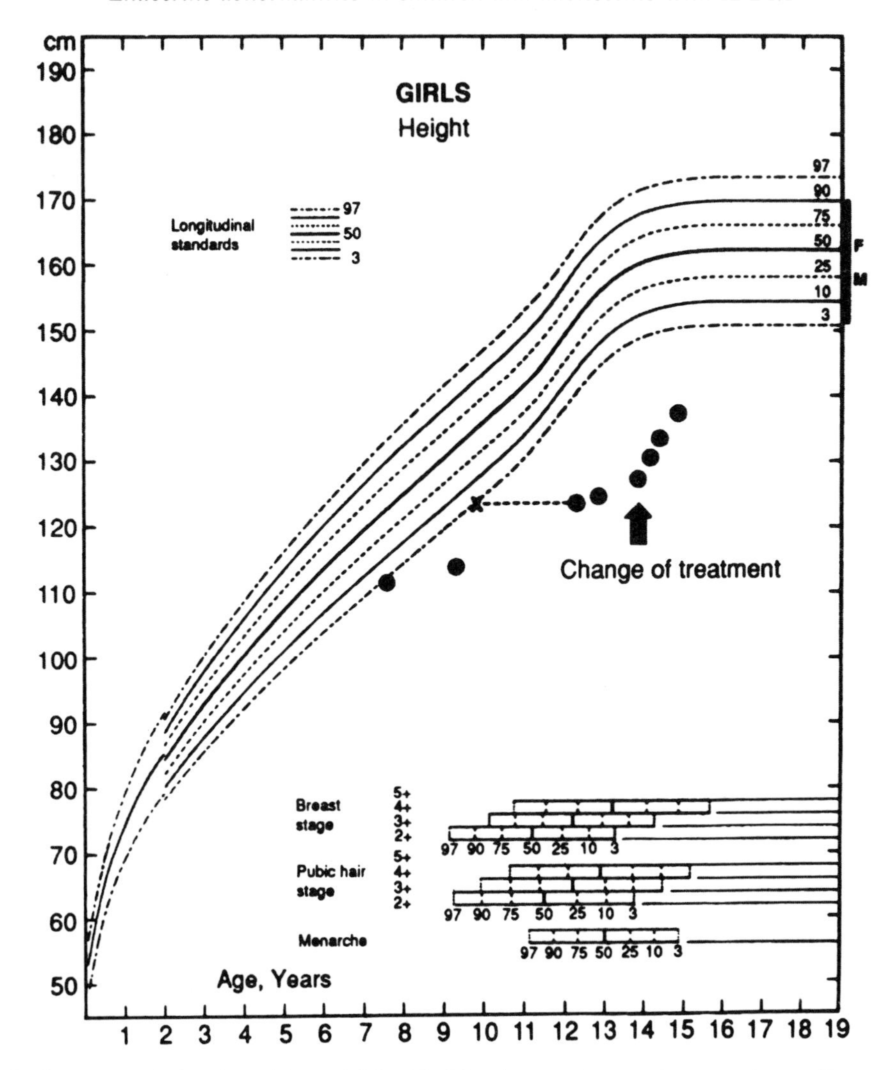

Figure 5.4 Response to treatment in a child with Mauriac syndrome. Improved growth resulted from an increase in carbohydrate intake and insulin dose.

Spontaneous growth hormone secretion has been extensively studied in adolescents with IDDM and the plasma growth hormone profiles are characterized by an increase in both pulse amplitude and baseline concentrations (Edge *et al.*, 1990) (Figure 5.5). There is evidence that growth hormone clearance may be delayed in IDDM (Mullis *et al.*, 1992) but even allowing for this, deconvolution analysis indicates that growth hormone secretion is grossly elevated throughout puberty in males and females with IDDM (Pal *et al.*, 1992). A number of hypotheses have been proposed to explain these high levels of growth hormone, including resetting of a putative glucose sensitive mechanism for growth hormone secretion within the hypothalamus (Press *et al.*, 1984) or a direct sup-

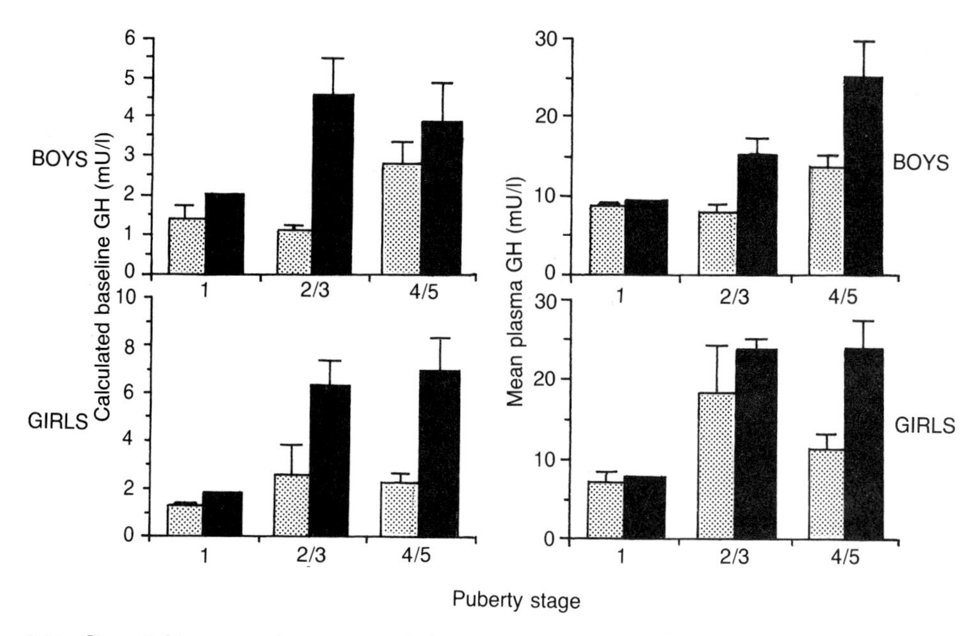

Figure 5.5 Overnight mean plasma growth hormone concentrations and calculated baseline growth hormone concentrations in normal ▩ and diabetic ■ adolescents (Edge *et al.*, 1990).

pressive effect of glucose on somatostatin release at the level of the hypothalamus (Lewis *et al.*, 1987). Animal and human studies indicate that excess growth hormone secretion is associated with reduced somatostatin tone in the hypothalamus. The regulation of hypothalamic growth hormone releasing hormone and somatostatin is complex, but in diabetic subjects, the imbalance may result as a direct or indirect effect of reduced circulating levels of IGF-I (Holly *et al.*, 1988a).

Whereas growth hormone levels are invariably elevated in IDDM those of IGF-I are generally low or in the low normal range (Yde, 1969; Winter *et al.*, 1979; Amiel *et al.*, 1984; Taylor *et al.*, 1988; Tamborlane *et al.*, 1981). A reduced IGF-I response to exogenous growth hormone administration has been reported in diabetic children (Lanes *et al.*, 1985) and there is a resistance to the effects of growth hormone at the hepatic growth hormone receptor. In animals rendered diabetic using streptozotocin there is evidence of a post-receptor defect in growth hormone action. However, recent studies of the growth hormone binding protein in humans may suggest a decrease in growth hormone receptor numbers. This circulating binding protein has proved to be identical to the extracellular domain of the growth hormone receptor (Leung *et al.*, 1987); levels may therefore reflect receptor numbers. In adolescents with IDDM, growth binding protein levels are low at all stages of puberty when compared with controls (Menon *et al.*, 1992).

It seems likely that the abnormalities of growth hormone function and thus circulating IGF-I levels result from inadequate portal delivery of insulin. *In-vitro* studies suggest that insulin enhances IGF-I production (Daughaday *et al.*, 1976) by either direct regulation of the GH receptor (Baxter *et al.*, 1980) or a permissive effect on post-GH receptor events (Maes *et al.*, 1986). Failure to provide adequate portal delivery of insulin will thus result in reduced GH receptor

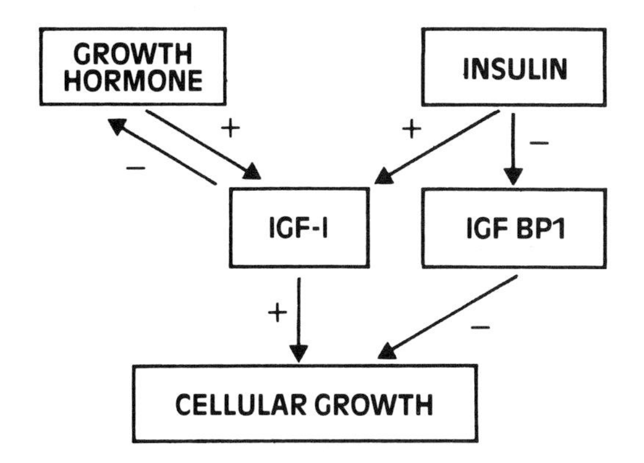

Figure 5.6 Cellular growth hypothesis: the GH/IGF-I/IGF-BP1 axes.

function and low circulating IGF-I levels. Improved insulin delivery during intensified treatment invariably leads to improved circulating levels of IGF-I (Amiel *et al.*, 1984; Rudolf *et al.*, 1982).

Insulin also has an important role in the regulation of IGF bioactivity as it controls the levels of one of the small MW binding proteins of IGF-I, IGFBP-I (Holly *et al.*, 1988b). This binding protein is closely related to IGF bioactivity (Taylor *et al.*, 1988) and levels are invariably high in poorly controlled subjects with IDDM (Holly *et al.*, 1992a). It can be postulated that the low IGF-I bioactivity is one of the major determinants of poor growth in IDDM (Figure 5.6).

Reduced circulating levels of IGF-I and IGF bioactivity lead to elevated GH levels, and these have a major impact on the metabolic control of diabetes particularly during puberty (Dunger *et al.*, 1991). Resistance to the effects of GH is confined to the generation of IGF-I in IDDM, and the effects of high levels of GH at the insulin receptor result in an exaggeration of the normal insulin resistance of puberty.

The relationship between these abnormalities of the GH/IGF-I axis and growth in IDDM is still to be clarified although there is convincing evidence from animal data that low IGF bioactivity is largely responsible for the poor growth. In prepubertal children with diabetes, Salardi *et al.* (1987) noted a reasonable correlation between IGF bioactivity and height velocity SDS. It is likely that the C-peptide status of these younger children will be important, for residual endogenous insulin production may be more effective at maintaining normal IGF-I levels and IGF bioactivity. During puberty when growth is frequently impaired in children with IDDM, abnormalities of the GH/IGF-I axis are more profound. Although firm data are lacking, a direct relationship between appropriate insulin delivery, the abnormality of the GH/IGF-I axis and growth in IDDM seems likely.

5.3.2 THE GONADOTROPHIN/GONADAL AXIS AND ADRENAL SEX STEROID PRODUCTION IN DIABETES

Although puberty is not severely delayed in the majority of children with diabetes, abnormalities of gonadal and adrenal sex steroid secretion have been reported.

A dissociation between pubarche and adrenarche was reported by Cohen *et al.* (1984). In a study of diabetic males they found lower levels of DHEAS compared with controls who had similar levels of testosterone, and identical bone ages at the same stage of pubertal development. Diminished urinary DHA excretion has also been observed in adults with IDDM of both sexes (Alesandro *et al.*, 1982). The significance of these observations is unclear and as yet there are no published longitudinal studies comparing the changes in sex steroid in normals and subjects with diabetes.

Cross-sectional data concerning levels of sex hormone binding globulin (SHBG) and sex steroids were reported by Holly *et al.* (1992b). They noted comparable levels of testosterone in males and females with diabetes and normal controls at all puberty stages, but levels of SHBG were lower in subjects with diabetes. This could result in higher levels of 'free testosterone' in the diabetic subjects, but these observations require confirmation by longitudinal study.

Menstrual irregularities are more common in post-menarchal girls with diabetes, and this group of subjects has been studied in more detail. Adcock *et al.* (1994) reported lower SHBG, higher androstenedione, and an elevated LH/FSH ratio in diabetic girls who had an irregular cycle. Djursing *et al.* (1985), in a study group of regularly menstruating girls with IDDM found raised levels of testosterone but noted suppression of androgens in amenorrheic patients. Menstrual irregularity in the diabetic subjects studied by Adcock *et al.* (1994) was associated with low levels of IGF-I and higher levels of IGFBP-I, highlighting the importance of the IGFs and their binding proteins in normal ovarian maturation (see Chapter 3). These observations require further confirmation as does the suggestion that girls with IDDM have a higher incidence of polycystic ovarian change on pelvic ultrasound (Adcock *et al.*, 1994).

Menstrual irregularity in IDDM may be associated with poor control, weight gain and the early development of microangiopathic complication. Further study of these associations is of great importance.

5.4 CONCLUSIONS

Over the last 50 years the prognosis for growth and pubertal development in children with IDDM has improved considerably, but subtle abnormalities and occasionally severe growth arrest such as that reported by Mauriac (1934) can still be observed. The relationship between abnormalities of growth and development and metabolic control is difficult to define. There may be no correlation between growth rates and glycemic control as judged by the glycosylated hemoglobin.

Evidence is accumulating that it is the failure of current insulin regimens, leading to derangements of the growth hormone/IGF-I axis which determine the rate of growth and maturation in IDDM. The C-peptide status may have an important protective role, and intensification of insulin therapy will result in an elevation of serum IGF-I levels and improved growth.

Endocrine abnormalities involving the growth hormone/IGF-I and gonadal axis are common in IDDM. Although their impact on growth and pubertal development has been minimized over recent years with improved insulin delivery, they still contribute to morbidity in IDDM. The high levels of growth hormone during adolescence may lead to a deterioration in glycemic control, and abnormalities in the regulation of gonadal steroids may be associated with weight gain, insulin resistance and menstrual irregularities. These endocrine abnormalities may also predispose to the early development of microangiopathic complications.

REFERENCES

Adcock, C., Perry, L.A., Lindsell, D.R.M., *et al.* (1994) Menstrual irregularities are more common in adolescents with Type I diabetes: association with poor glycaemic control and weight gain. *Diabetic Med.*, **11**, 465–70.

Alesandro, M., Wesler, D., Rhodes, G. *et al.* (1982) Quantitative alterations of steroid urinary profiles associated with diabetes mellitus. *Clinica Chimica Acta*, **126**, 243–55.

Amiel, S.A., Sherwin, R.S., Hintz, R.L. *et al.* (1984) Effects of diabetes and its control on insulin-like growth factors in the young subject with type 1 diabetes. *Diabetes*, **33**, 1175–79.

Baum, J.D., Ounsted, M. and Smith, M.A. (1975) Weight gain in infancy and subsequent development of diabetes mellitus in childhood. *Lancet*, **ii**, 866.

Baxter, R.C., Bryon, J.M. and Turtle, J.R. (1980) Somatogenic receptors of rat liver: regulation by insulin. *Endocrinology*, **107**, 1176–81.

Birkbeck, J.A. (1972) Growth in juvenile diabetes mellitus. *Diabetologia*, **8**, 221–24.

Blom, L., Persson, L.A. and Dalquist, G. (1992) A high linear growth is associated with an increased risk of childhood diabetes mellitus. *Diabetologia*, **35**, 528–33.

Brown, M., Ahmed, M.L., Clayton, K.L. *et al.* (1994) Growth during childhood and final height in type 1 diabetes. *Diabetic Med.*, **11**, 182–87.

Clarson, C., Daneman, D. and Ehrlich, R.M. (1985) The relationship of metabolic control to growth and pubertal development in children with insulin-dependent diabetes. *Diabetes Res.*, **2**, 237–41.

Cohen, H.N., Paterson, K.R., Wallace, A.M. *et al.* (1984) Dissociation of adrenarche and gonadarche in diabetes mellitus. *Clin. Endocrin.*, **20**, 717–24.

Daughaday, W.H., Phillips, L.S. and Mueller, M. (1976) The effects of insulin and growth hormone on the release of somatomedin by the isolated rat liver. *Endocrinology*, **98**, 1214–19.

Djursing, H., Hagen, C., Anderson, A.N. *et al.* (1985) Serum sex hormone concentrations in insulin dependent women with and without amenorrhoea. *Clin. Endocrin.*, **23**, 147–54.

Drayer, N.M. (1974) Height of diabetic children at onset of symptoms. *Arch. Dis. Child.*, **49**, 616–62.

Dunger, D.B., Edge, J.A., Pal, R. *et al.* (1991) Impact of increased growth hormone secretion on carbohydrate metabolism in adolescents with diabetes. *Acta Paed. Scand.*, **377** (Suppl.), 69–77.

Edelsten, A.D., Hughes, I.A., Oakes, S. *et al.* (1981) Height and skeletal maturity in children with newly diagnosed juvenile-onset diabetes. *Arch. Dis. Child.*, **56**, 40–44.

Edge, J.A., Dunger, D.B., Matthews, D.R. *et al.* (1990) Increased overnight growth hormone concentrations in diabetic compared with normal adolescents. *J. Clin. Endocrin. Metab.*, **71**, 1356–62.

Emmerson, A.J.B. and Savage, D.C.L. (1988) Height at diagnosis in diabetics. *Eur. J. Pediatr.*, **147**, 319–21.

Evans, N., Robinson, V.P. and Lister, J. (1972) Growth and bone age of juvenile diabetics. *Arch. Dis. Child.*, **47**, 589–93.

Frisch, R.E. and Revelle, R. (1969) The height and weight of adolescent boys and girls at the time of peak velocity of growth in height and weight: Longitudinal data. *Hum. Biol.*, **41**, 531–39.

Guest, G.M. (1953) The Mauriac Syndrome: dwarfism, heptomegaly and obesity with juvenile diabetes mellitus. *Diabetes*, **2**, 4–15.

Herber, S.M. and Dunsmore, I.R. (1988) Does control affect growth in diabetes mellitus? *Acta Paed. Scand.*, **77**, 303–305.

Hjelt, K., Braendholt, V., Kamper, J. *et al.* (1983) Growth in children with diabetes mellitus. *Dan. Med. Bul.*, **30**, 28–33.

Holly, J.M.P., Amiel, S.A., Sandhu, R.R. *et al.* (1988a) The role of growth hormone in diabetes mellitus. *J. Endocrin.*, **118**, 353–64.

Holly, J.M.P., Biddlecombe, R.A., Dunger, D.B. *et al.* (1988b) Circadian variation of GH-Independent IGF binding proteins in diabetes mellitus and its relationship to insulin: A new role for insulin? *Clin. Endocrin.*, **29**, 667–75.

Holly, J.M.P., Dunger, D.B., Edge, J.A. *et al.* (1992a) Insulin-like growth factor binding protein-I (IGFBP-1) levels in diabetic adolescents and their relationship to metabolic control. *Diab. Med.*, **7**, 618–23.

Holly, J.M.P., Dunger, D.B., Edge, J.A. *et al.* (1992b) Sex hormone binding globulin levels in adolescents with insulin dependent diabetes mellitus. *Diab. Med.*, **9**, 371–74.

Hoskins, P.J., Leslie, R.D.G. and Pyke, D.A. (1985) Height at diagnosis of diabetes in children: a study in identical twins, *Brit. Med. J.*, **290**, 278–80.

Jackson, R.L. (1984) Growth and maturation of children with insulin-dependent diabetes mellitus. *Pediatr. Clin. N. America*, **31**, 545–67.

Japan and Pittsburgh Childhood Diabetes Research Groups (1989) Height at onset of insulin-dependent diabetes mellitus in high- and low-risk countries. *Diabetes Res. Clin. Prac.*, **6**, 173–76.

Jivani, S.K.M. and Rayner, P.H.W. (1973) Does control influence growth of diabetic children? *Arch. Dis. Child.*, **48**, 109–115.

Joslin, E.P., Root, H.F. and White, P. (1925) The growth, development and prognosis of diabetic children. *J. Am. Med. Assoc.*, **85**, 420–22.

Knowles, H.C., Guest, G.M., Lampe, J. *et al.* (1965) The course of juvenile diabetes treated with unmeasured diet. *Diabetes*, **14**, 239–73.

Lanes, R., Recker, B., Fort, P. *et al.* (1985) Impaired somatomedin generation test in children with insulin-dependent diabetes mellitus. *Diabetes*, **34**, 156–60.

Lee, T.J., Stewart-Brown, S., Wadsworth, J. *et al.* (1984) 'Growth in children with diabetes', in J. Borms (ed.). *Human growth and development*, pp. 613–18. Plenum Press, New York.

Leslie, R.D., Lo, S., Millward, B.A. *et al.* (1991) Decreased growth velocity before IDDM onset. *Diabetes*, **40**, 211–16.

Leung, D.W., Spencer, S.A., Cochranes, G. *et al.* (1987) Growth hormone receptor and serum binding protein: purification, cloning and expression. *Nature*, **330**, 537–43.

Lewis, B.M., Deiguez, C., Inglesias, R. *et al.* (1987) Effects of glucose on somatostaton and TRH release in the phpothalamus. *J. Endocrin. Invest.*, **10** (suppl. 3), 31.

Maes, M., Underwood, L.E. and Ketelslegers, J.-M. (1986) Low serum somatomedin-C in insulin-dependent diabetes: evidence for a post receptor mechanism. *Endocrinology*, **118**, 377–82.

Mauras, N., Merimee, T. and Rogol, A.D. (1991) Function of the growth hormone-insulin-like growth factor I axis in the profoundly growth-retarded diabetic child: Evidence for defective target organ responsiveness in the Mauriac syndrome. *Metabolism*, **40**, 1106–1111.

Mauriac, P. (1934) Heptomegalies de l'enfants avec troubles de la croissance et de la metabolisme des glucides. *Paris Med.*, **2**, 525–28.

Menon, R.K., Arslanian, S., May, B. *et al.* (1992) Diminished growth hormone-binding protein in children with insulin-dependent diabetes mellitus. *J. Clin. Endocrin. Metab.* **74**, 934–38.

Mullis, P.E., Pal, B.R., Matthews, D.R. *et al.* (1992) Half life of exogenous growth hormone following suppression of endogenous growth hormone secretion with somatostatin in type 1 (insulin-dependent) diabetes mellitus. *Clin. Endocrin.*, **36**, 255–63.

Pal, B.R., Matthews, D.R., Edge, J.A. *et al.* (1992) The frequency and amplitude of growth hormone secretory episodes as determined by deconvolution analysis are increased in adolescents with insulin dependent diabetes mellitus and are unaffected by short term euglycaemia. *Clin. Endocrin.*, **38**, 93–100.

Petersen, H.D., Korsgaard, B., Deckert, T. *et al.* (1978) Growth, body weight and insulin requirements in diabetic children. *Acta Paed. Scand.*, **67**, 453–57.

Peveler, R.C., Fairburn, E.C., Boller, I. *et al.* (1992) Eating disorders in adolescents with insulin-dependent diabetes mellitus: A controlled study. *Diabetes Care*, **15**, 1–5.

Press, M., Tamborlane, M.V., Thorner, M.O. *et al.* (1984) Pituitary response to growth hormone-releasing factor in diabetes failure of glucose mediated suppression. *Diabetes*, **33**, 804–806.

Price, D.E. and Burden, A.C. (1992) Growth of children before diabetes. *Diabetes Care*, **15**, 1393–95.

Rudolf, M.C.J., Sherwin, R.S., Markowitz, R. *et al.* (1982) Effect of intensive insulin treatment on linear growth in the young diabetic patient. *J. Pediatr.*, **101**, 333–39.

Salardi, S., Tonioli, S., Tassoni, P. *et al.* (1987) Growth and growth factors in diabetes mellitus. *Arch. Dis. Child.*, **62**, 57–62.

Songer, T.J., LaPorte, R.E., Tajima, N. *et al.* (1986) Height at diagnosis of insulin dependent diabetes in patients and their non-diabetic family members. *Brit. Med. J.*, **292**, 1419–22.

Sterky, G. (1967) Growth pattern in juvenile diabetes. *Acta Paed. Scand.*, **56** (suppl. 177), 80–82.

Stewart-Brown, S.L., Lee, T.J. and Savage, D.C.L. (1985) Pubertal growth in diabetics. *Arch. Dis. Child.*, **60**, 768–69.

Tamborlane, W.V., Hintz, R.L., Bergman, M. *et al.* (1981) Insulin-infusion-pump treatment of diabetes. Influence of improved metabolic control on plasma somatomedin levels. *N. Eng. J. Med.*, **305**, 303–307.

Tanner, J.M., Whitehouse, R.H. and Takaishi, M. (1966) Standards from birth to maturity for height, weight, height velocity and weight velocity: British Children 1965. Part I, *Arch. Dis. Child.*, **41**, 454–71. Part II, *Arch. Dis. Child.*, **41**, 613–35.

Tattersall, R.B. and Pyke, D.A. (1973) Growth in diabetic children: studies in identical twins. *Lancet*, **II**, 1105–1109.

Taylor, A.M., Dunger, D.B., Preece, M.A. *et al.* (1990) The growth hormone independent insulin-like growth factor-I binding protein BP-28 is associated with serum insulin-like growth factor-I inhibitory bioactivity in adolescent insulin-dependent diabetics. *Clin. Endocrin.*, **32**, 229–39.

Taylor, A.M., Dunger, D.B., Grant, D.B. *et al.* (1988) Somatomedin-C /IGF-I measured by radioimmunoassay and somatomedin bioactivity in adolescents with insulin dependent diabetes mellitus compared with puberty matched controls. *Diabetes Res.*, **9**, 177–81.

Thon, A., Heinze, E., Feilen, K.D. *et al.* (1992) Development of height and weight in children with diabetes mellitus: report on two prospective multicentre studies, one cross-sectional, one longitudinal. *Eur. J. Pediatr.*, **151**, 258–62.

Trzeciak, B. (1978) The effect of diabetes mellitus on the incidence of abnormal genital bleeding in women. *Ginecologia Polska*, **49**, 119.

Wagner, R., White, P. and Bogan, I. (1942) Diabetic dwarfism. *Arch. Dis. Child.*, **63**, 667–727.

Winter, R.J., Phillips, L.S., Klein, M.N. *et al.* (1979) Somatomedin activity and diabetic control in children with insulin-dependent diabetes mellitus. *Diabetes*, **28**, 952–54.

Yde, H. (1969) The growth hormone dependent sulfation factor in serum from patients with various types of diabetes. *Acta Med. Scand.*, **186**, 293–97.

6

Developmental trends in coping in childhood and adolescence

D.H. SKUSE

6.1 INTRODUCTION

Children who have insulin-dependent diabetes mellitus (IDDM) often experience difficulties coping with this chronic disorder; the success with which they manage in terms of psychological adjustment and physical health, must reflect both their individual resilience and adaptation, as well as the empathy, understanding and support they obtain from their families, friends and relations. Although early psychological research tended to focus on the assumption that there might be some form of relatively specific and homogeneous 'diabetic personality' which would predispose an individual to develop the disease, subsequent research has failed to support that view (Johnson, 1980). Accordingly, current concepts on the functioning of children with chronic diseases such as IDDM view them as a heterogeneous population of individuals. Each child with the disorder possesses a unique range of personality and other characteristics. If psychological influences are important in determining which children are better able to cope with their disorder, how might knowledge of the processes by which this happens influence pediatric management of the condition? Some broad issues which are relevant to an understanding of developmental trends in coping are presented. Not all have been investigated in relation to chronic disease or disorder, let alone IDDM in particular. However, they are potentially of great relevance and, in years to come, may well assume greater importance in a 'holistic' approach to the condition.

Over the years, various attempts have been made to devise theoretical 'models' which incorporate what are believed to be the most important of the psychological and other variables which might influence adjustment to IDDM, in order to predict outcome. These models are necessarily complex (Johnson, 1988). Relationships between patients, their environmental contexts and their health status are assumed to be bidirectional. In other words, at any one point in time the child's overall state of adjustment to the disease will be influenced by, for example, the emotional atmosphere in their home or by their relationships at school. But children's relationships with their family and school friends will also be influenced by their state of health. The two are intimately interrelated, and if we just take a 'snapshot' of that interaction at one point in time it is quite impossible to decide whether health is influencing relationships or vice versa. Alternatively, if

Childhood and Adolescent Diabetes
Published in 1994 by Chapman & Hall, London
ISBN 0 412 48610 5

we study development longitudinally we are likely to find that there are a number of ways by which an influence at one point in time can have consequences some considerable time later; an acute early experience may produce a contemporaneous disorder which then persists if untreated. For example, children may develop a needle phobia as a consequence of their experience of venepuncture or injections at the time the diagnosis of IDDM is first made. Alternatively, patterns of parent–child interaction might be set in motion as a consequence of IDDM which appear to be adaptive at one point in time but which, if they persist until they are developmentally inappropriate, constitute a reason for intervention. For example, parents might respond to an initial life-threatening episode of ketoacidosis by becoming over-protective of their child, thereby hindering that child's proper socioemotional development in areas such as independence, self-confidence and the development of friendships outside the immediate family. Finally, changes within the family, such as the exit of a parent by divorce or the entry of a step-parent or sibling, may also have longlasting consequences in virtue of their impact upon the family system.

Studies of how successfully children manage to adapt to living with a chronic illness have devoted a great deal of attention to their social and emotional adjustment, and behavioral competence (Drotar, 1981; Perrin *et al.*, 1987; Wallander *et al.*, 1988). Two broad approaches are taken to measuring psychological adjustment. By far the most commonly encountered method is the use of a checklist, to be completed by parents and/or a teacher, or by the child him or herself, of symptoms that are indicative of emotional or behavioral problems. Almost ubiquitous in research of this nature, especially with children of school age, are the Child Behavior Checklist (CBCL), the Teacher's Report Form (TRF) and the Youth Self Report (YSR) developed by Achenbach and Edelbrock (Achenbach, 1991a,b,c). Each measure has been standardized separately within each gender group for children aged 4–18 years. The scales can be scored by a simple computer program which generates a profile of subscale scores and a total problem score. These can then be compared with norms within each age and gender group. The CBCL scales were however not designed for use with children suffering from chronic physical disorders and concerns have been raised about their appropriateness for the measurement of this subject group (Perrin *et al.*, 1991). Potential problems with the interpretation of findings include a) a possible bias in interpreting data concerning physical symptoms because questions asking about such symptoms contribute toward the total score, b) a limited sensitivity to identify minor adjustment problems of the sort most often encountered in children with chronic physical illnesses, and c) superficial and potentially misleading questions on the subject of social competence. Little is asked about areas of competence such as positive social behavior, altruism, or empathy. Rather, there is an emphasis on social and school activities such as sports which are not necessarily accessible to a child with a chronic illness.

An alternative approach to measuring the influence of chronic illness on psychological adjustment is the assessment of health-related quality of life. In recent years there has been increasing interest in the use of quality-of-life measures to evaluate the benefits of treatment. Such measures can be seen as an attempt to describe the impact an illness has on a child's everyday life. A limited amount of work has been undertaken in assessing the quality of life of children with chronic physical conditions (Ditesheim & Templeton, 1987; Walker & Rosser, 1990); most investigations have been carried out with adult patients. Those which have involved children usually obtained ratings made by a third party and the child's subjective assessment was not included. The relative paucity of relevant studies of children is largely due to the lack of suitable measures.

A chronic disorder such as IDDM possesses significance for children and their families because it is either directly or indirectly a source of stress, both in terms of daily hassles and in terms of major episodes such as life-threatening exacerbations of illness and associated hospitalizations. A developmental perspective will be taken on the matter, with childhood broadly divided into three periods. Firstly, infancy and the preschool phase of development. Secondly, middle childhood which covers the period during which children are normally attending elementary school. Finally, adolescence, which as clinicians well recognize is a time when the management of chronic disorders such as IDDM can become exceptionally difficult for a whole variety of reasons. Within each period of development the most important sources of vulnerability to the various stresses associated with the disorder will be considered. Also, the current state of knowledge on how children in general learn to cope with stress will be reviewed.

6.1.1 THE CONCEPT OF STRESS

Although most lay persons would have little or no difficulty in giving examples of their feelings in response to stress, and recognizing it when they are experiencing it, the concept has proved elusive for researchers to pin down and define satisfactorily. Stress is part of our everyday lives, and we all have to cope with it. We start learning at a very early age, and learning how to cope with stress successfully is an important aspect of every child's developmental agenda.

Stressful events in general make us feel bad. In psychological jargon we refer to this as a 'negative affective state', a state of mind which puts us at risk of a poorer state of physical and psychological health. An adverse event does not always trigger severe psychological discomfort; the degree of distress will be much greater if the pressures associated with the adversity in question exceed a child's or a family's ability to cope. If it does do so, and the consequence is an emotional or behavioral disturbance severe enough to warrant treatment, we say the stressor has 'pathological singificance' (Lazarus & Folkman, 1984). Although it is clear that major life stressors such as bereavement (Van Eerdewegh *et al.*, 1982) or divorce (Block *et al.*, 1988; Wallerstein, 1991) are important influences upon children's health (Johnson, 1986; Goodyer, 1990), major life events of this nature are low frequency occurrences for most families. In other words, children are likely to encounter, at the most, only one divorce or bereavement; these are not, for the great majority, recurrent events (Crnic & Greenberg, 1990). On the other hand, it is likely that for families of children with a chronic illness which is not immediately life-threatening, the cumulative impact of relatively minor daily hassles will be of more salience. Lazarus (1984) and Lazarus *et al.* (1985) have hypothesized that the way in which an individual interprets the significance of life events for their own well-being is likely to be the main predictor of the impact of such stressors upon mental health. For example, a hospitalization might for most children be an unpleasant and unwelcome event. But, if a child with uncontrolled diabetes is admitted, feeling lethargic and ill, and as a consequence of that admission rapidly recovers equilibrium, he or she might well regard it overall as a positive experience.

Hassles are those irritating, frustrating, annoying and distressing demands that are part of everyone's life, but which may be rather more frequent, or of a different quality, in the lives of children who have a chronic physical disorder. Some may be situation-specific and infrequent, such as attendance at the outpatient clinic. Others may be a persistent source of annoyance on a daily basis (for example, remembering to stick to a diet, remembering to give the insulin injection), and arise from the fact the child is growing up within a particular context, with consistent predictable demands. Belsky (1984) proposed that everyday stressors can also be a major influence upon the parenting a child receives, thereby directly and indirectly influencing a child's development by means of that route too. Dealing with the ramifications of their child's chronic physical illness is likely to constitute an important source of stress to any parents, but it may present particular problems to those who are already living in difficult circumstances because of poverty (Werner & Smith, 1982), single parenthood (Weinraub & Wolf, 1983) or who are themselves suffering from a psychiatric disorder such as depression (Downey & Coyne, 1990).

The impact of major discrete stressors upon a child's mental and physical equilibrium may not have the same consequence those same stressors would have upon an adult. Although it is often assumed children are more vulnerable than adults, there are counterbalancing influences to be taken into account. For example, young children cannot be upset by events whose implications they do not understand so they might be buffered against the impact of an adverse event, at least in the short term. So far as young children are concerned, an admission to hospital with a life-threatening complication of their illness may be important only insofar as they are separated for a time from their family and friends. The fact that the illness was life threatening may not be appreciated by them, but even if it is, young children's attitudes towards death are quite different to those of adolescents and adults (e.g., Orbach *et al.*, 1985). The ultimate impact of the stress might well only become clear if one takes into account its indirect consequences upon important aspects of the child's life. For example, parental divorce is not a truly discrete event. There will usually be longlasting economic, social and emotional consequences upon the child's immediate environment (Wallerstein, 1991).

The way in which a child perceives and reacts to certain sorts of threat, and thereby experiences an associated degree of stress, changes through early life according to a developmental timetable. One of the major stressors experienced by a child of a year or so of age is separation from their parents, even for very brief periods (Klagsburn & Bowlby, 1976; Shouldice & Stevenson-Hinde, 1992; Main & Cassidy, 1988). Older children are usually able to cope with brief separations, secure in the knowledge they have not been abandoned. When a little older, children may be frightened, and experience as stressful, encounters with unfamiliar large animals whether or not those animals (such as a dog, pony or cow) constitute a genuine threat (Marks, 1987). In general, the younger the child the greater the importance of environmental structure in reducing that child's vulnerability to emotional and behavioral disruption in potentially stressful circumstances. By environmental structure is meant the presence of a familiar family routine, together with predictable and comprehensible physical surroundings and social milieu (Maccoby, 1983).

6.1.2 THE CONCEPTS OF COPING AND RESILIENCE

6.1.2.1 Coping

Because not every individual with a chronic illness has a poor psychological outcome, considerable efforts have been expended over the years to try and improve the prospective identification of those children who will do well, as opposed to those who will not do so. Obviously if it was possible to demonstrate that one's predictions were consistently successful it would be reasonable to conclude that one had picked a valid set of predictor variables. The way would then be open to attempt to modify the most important influences upon children who were believed to be at high risk in order to enhance their ability to cope and consequently to improve their outcomes, through some form of therapeutic intervention.

Throughout our lives we are developing coping strategies which permit us to get on with the necessary business of living without being thrown off-course. Coping consists of cognitive and behavioral efforts to manage specific external demands we perceive as likely to tax, or even exceed, our mental resources (Folkman & Lazarus, 1988). We are constantly making cognitive and behavioral efforts of this sort. In other words, we plan, we work out strategies to manage stressful events we anticipate, and then we enact them. For example, some children who cannot face the idea of injecting their own insulin will get a parent to do it for them and close their eyes or look away when the needle is inserted into their skin. Our tactics change and evolve as a consequence of repeated reappraisals of our relationship to the environment in which we live. But that, of course, is also developing and changing over time. Coping is therefore a process of adjustment. Researchers can only learn about it by observing what people actually do in real stressful situations. Coping must imply a conscious response, involving effort, to a psychologically stressful situation. In general, coping strategies include a whole range of potential behaviors and thoughts, some of which may be successful in reducing stress but others of which may turn out not to have any benefit at all. Coping is not quite the same thing as mastery, a term to which we shall return.

Some coping strategies we use are aimed at altering the situation that is causing us distress. This is known as **problem-focused coping** and is evidently accessible only to those who have sufficient cognitive maturity to employ it. It entails making plans in order to solve the stress-producing problem. Problem-focused forms of coping are likely to be used if the outcome of the encounter with the stressor appears to be amenable to change. For instance, a child might want to find out whether there is a less painful way of giving daily injections, or of avoiding unsightly lipolysis. In contrast there is **emotion-focused coping**, which means the way in which we attempt to regulate the distress itself. Emotion-focused forms of coping are more likely to be used if the outcome appears to be inevitable, for example, the realization that diabetes is a lifelong illness with potential detriment to a whole variety of bodily symptoms. It includes methods of dealing with stress by seeking social support from family and friends, accepting responsibility or blame for the stressful circumstances (whether this is justified or not), or otherwise exerting self-control over the expression of feelings, such as avoiding thinking about the source of distress. Adults normally rely upon both emotion-focused and problem-focused coping strategies, but the extent to which they apply in children has not been fully evaluated and is not known in any detail.

6.1.2.2 Resilience

It is a common experience that, when faced with apparently equivalent degrees and forms of stress, some individuals seem to cope relatively well while others fail to do so successfully. Presumably the capacity to cope with a persistent stressor such as a chronic illness reflects in some way the individual's resilience. The term 'resilience' usually means a repertoire of individual or personal stress-resistant traits or skills, and is acquired from a process of interaction between relatively more 'internal' qualities and relatively 'external' influences (Masten & Garmezy, 1985). Some sources of resilience have been outlined by Garmezy (1985). They include, firstly, stable 'internal' individual traits such as temperament, which have been most comprehensively studied in infancy and may be determined largely by genetic influences. In older children, relevant individual traits include cognitive dispositions such as locus of control, perceived self-competence and attributional style (Rae-Gant *et al.*, 1989). Secondly, resilience arises as a consequence of the history of children's dynamic interactions with their family and peers. Important influences include social support (Pellegrini *et al.*, 1986; Greenberg & Crnic, 1988), social integration, and family cohesion (Seifer *et al.*, 1992; Wahler & Zigler, 1991). Specific influences upon a child's behavioral adjustment which have wide-ranging significance include the quality of the mother-child relationship (Werner & Smith, 1982), and the quality of the father-child relationship (Phares & Compas, 1992). In a recent study by Jenkins and Smith (1990), children who had poor relationships with their parents were at risk of developing emotional and behavioral problems even if their parents had a harmonious marriage, but not surprisingly such relationships were more common in families in which the quality of the marriage was poor. The presence of a best friend and the general quality of children's friendships with their peer group are also very important, poor peer relations being a potent sign of disordered social and emotional development (Newcomb *et al.*, 1993).

Actually, we are probably not justified in attempting to draw a clear distinction between children's 'internal' vulnerabilities (such as a temperamental or cognitive disposition) and 'external' protective factors (such as the parenting style they experience) because one will influence the other over time (Rutter, 1987). For example, what we might term 'true' protective influences may come into play only when the risk is highest. In other words, their presence does not exert any significant influence upon a child's functioning when that child is in a supportive non-threatening environment, because there is nothing to 'protect' the child from in those circumstances. In their investigation of children living in dysharmonious homes, Jenkins and Smith (1990) found that a close relationship with an adult outside the family, or engaging in an activity which gained the child positive recognition, or having close sibling relationships, all served to protect children from the adverse consequences of serious marital conflict. However, the influence of these relationships and activities did not seem to have much impact upon adjustment in the absence of marital conflict. In other words, children who were not living in dysharmonious homes but who had good relationships with their siblings, adult friends outside the family and so on were no better adjusted than other children living in similar circumstances, Accordingly, perhaps we should think of vulnerability and protection as different aspects of a single dimension, which influences how children respond to risk, and put the emphasis of research upon the process of functional adaptation to stress (Masten, 1989).

6.2 INFANCY AND EARLY CHILDHOOD

Two of the most important factors which are likely to be relevant to the impact of a chronic illness upon the psychological adjustment of infants and young children are temperamental disposition and security of attachment. The major sources of stress during this period, which are related to the diagnosis of IDDM, are likely to be hospitalizations and painful procedures. Of course, hospitalization is one of the most common stressful events experienced during childhood; the impact of the event and the child's capacity to cope with it are closely related to the child's age at the time. Distress is most marked in those aged between 6 months and 4 years (Illingworth & Holt, 1955; Schaffer & Callender, 1959). This is the age at which 'selective attachments' are first forming, yet when children are just beginning to maintain the sense of how a relationship can survive a period of separation. Interference with the attachment relationship is implicit in the hospital admission, and this is one important aspect of that admission which makes it a disturbing experience for the young child.

6.2.1 ATTACHMENT

In the terminology of developmental psychology **attachment** has a rather specific meaning. Attachment theory suggests that children (and indeed adults too) have mental constructs of relationships (Bretherton, 1985). Based upon their previous interactions with their caregivers, children are assumed to develop expectations about how those 'attachment figures' will continue to relate to them in the future. A 'selective attachment' is a relationship with just one (rarely more than two or three) individual with whom the child is in frequent contact, is dependent upon for nurture, and from whom separation is distressing. Methods have been developed to allow the objective categorization of such attachments (Ainsworth *et al.*, 1978) both in infancy and in later childhood (Shouldice & Stevenson-Hinde, 1992; Cassidy, 1988). Amongst a randomly selected group of young children we would expect roughly one-half clearly to be securely attached but about 10% or so who would have what has been termed an 'insecure attachment', characterized by anxiety, ambivalence or disorganization. Research has suggested that insecure attachment results largely from relative neglect or maltreatment within the family (e.g., Crittenden & Ainsworth, 1989). Security of attachment may predict the degree of distress provoked by separations such as hospitalizations.

6.2.2 TEMPERAMENT

The suggestion has been made that a greater attention to the concept of temperament (i.e., individual differences in behavioral style) could prove illuminating in clinical work within pediatric medicine (Carey & McDevitt, 1989). A variety of studies have looked specifically at temperamental attributes in relation to the management of children with IDDM (e.g., Rovet & Ehrlich, 1988; Garrison *et al.*, 1991).

But what is temperament, and how is it measured? The notion is commonly understood to mean a stable, consistent 'behavioral disposition' (Bates, 1989a; Campos *et al.*, 1983) or a characteristic style of emotional and behavioral responses of the individual to situations. Temperamental patterns which are discernible early in life have powerful effects on the reactions of other people to the individual (Prior, 1992). Unfortunately, as in the case of stress, although there is a lay consensus as to what the term means, researchers who work in the area have found it difficult, if not impossible, to agree on a definition (Bates, 1989a; Goldsmith *et al.*, 1987). However, similar debates rage about the meaning of terms in everyday parlance such as intelligence (De la Bruyere, 1991). So lack of agreement on a definition should not prevent us acquiring an understanding of the nature of operations of individual characteristics and how they impinge on current and future behavioral adaptation (Rutter, 1987).

The literature on temperament is vast so this review will consider briefly just two aspects; its structure and its clinical significance (see also Prior, 1992).

One of the earliest studies on the nature of temperament in infancy and early childhood was that of Thomas *et al.* (1968) who intuitively derived nine dimensions including activity, mood, intensity (of response to stimulation), threshold of response, persistence, approach and withdrawal to new stimuli, adaptability over time to new experiences, distractibility, and rhythmicity (or the regularity of biological functions). Subsequently, Buss and Plomin (1984) argued for just three heritable factors which have considerable generality: sociability, emotionality, and activity. There is rather greater consensus on the existence of these very broad dimensions than on the more discrete temperamental traits described by Thomas and his colleagues. The most common method of measuring temperament is by questionnaire, relying largely on parental impressions, usually maternal ratings. There is of course the risk that such ratings will be biased by parental attitudes which have little to do with the child's objective characteristics, even if the scale does seek accounts of specific everyday behaviors rather than broad impressions of behavioral styles (Lancaster *et al.*, 1989; Bates & Bailes, 1984).

Other approaches to delineating temperamental attributes have included direct observation of children's behavior (e.g., Hinde *et al.*, 1985; Matheny *et al.*, 1987). Such observations may prove useful in validating the data gathered by questionnaire, but usually a large number of observations will be needed over an extended period of time in order to satisfy reliability criteria (Bates, 1989a). Caretakers are, after all, summarizing the results of a lifetime's observation, and draw upon extensive knowledge of their child in response to direct questions about that child's habitual behaviors.

Because by the term 'temperament' we generally mean to imply a largely stable characteristic, the establishment of patterns of continuity, stability and change over time is critical to the validity of the concept, as is a lack of contextual specificity. In other words, we should expect to find the temperamental characteristics of an individual persist, at least over the short to medium term, and the same set of characteristics will be manifest across a variety of interpersonal and other encounters. Thus Thomas and Chess (1977) assumed there would be a fair degree of continuity, in the nine dimensions they described, over the lifespan (Lerner *et al.*, 1982). Although older children's temperamental traits do show modest stability over relatively brief time intervals, there is little if any continuity within the first year. Stability increases to a maximum correlation of about 0.8 between 5–7 years of age (Prior, 1992). Certain clusters of attributes, such as irritability, negative emotionality or shyness (inhibitedness) show better stability than others such as sociability (Plomin & DeFries, 1985). Interestingly, stability seems to be higher for children who score at the extreme of temperamental factors or dimensions than for those who score in the middle ranges (Sanson *et al.*, 1990).

Although gender differences in temperament appear to be minimal during infancy they become increasingly important from toddlerhood onwards and different degrees of stability may be found in boys and girls (Earls & Jung, 1987).

From a clinical point of view more attention has been paid to clusters of temperamental characteristics, than to discrete elements of behavioral styles. The most widely researched cluster of attributes comprises so-called 'difficult' temperament (e.g., Thomas *et al.*, 1982). 'Difficult' in this context usually means the combination of a behavioral style which is unadaptable to new situations, slow to warm up, emotionally negative, intense in emotional and behavioral expression and irregular in terms of biological rhythms such as sleep. A great deal of work has gone into investigating the relationship between dimensions of temperament and the development of psychiatric disorder in childhood. On the whole, it seems temperaments which are 'difficult' render children more vulnerable to poor outcomes. Those which are positive, or 'easy', may protect a child against psychiatric maladjustment in situations of adversity (Werner & Smith, 1982; Maziade *et al.*, 1985; Sanson *et al.*, 1990). Difficult children are more likely to be singled out for parental criticism and irritability (Graham *et al.*, 1973). On the other hand, timid children may be more prone to illnesses, worries and fears (Stevenson-Hinde & Simpson, 1982).

Temperament is generally considered to be a style of responsiveness which is not consciously motivated (Thomas & Chess, 1989). The concept has been most extensively studied in children who have yet to develop language. By the time a child reaches school age the term 'temperament' is not so commonly applied; instead we speak about children's 'personality' characteristics. The extent to which the dimensions of behavioral style known as 'temperament' and 'personality' blend into one another is not really clear. This state of affairs raises questions as to whether it is meaningful to try and draw a distinction between the two. The former is commonly thought to represent a style of responding which is largely constitutionally determined and the latter a more diffuse behavioral disposition, which has been modified by cognitions and the individual's interaction with the environment over time (Matheny, 1989; Bates, 1989b).

6.3 MIDDLE CHILDHOOD

To date, most studies on how subjects in middle childhood cope with medical procedures and other medical situations have been concerned simply with providing broad descriptions (e.g., Brown *et al.*, 1986; Curry & Russ, 1985; Peterson & Toler, 1986) or have focused upon other aspects of their everyday lives (Band & Weisz, 1988; Compas *et al.*, 1988; Blanchard-Fields & Irion, 1988). However, it is of interest to know which coping strategies are more or less successful with specific medical events, because there might be scope for intervention to assist children who are having difficulties in these circumstances. We have already discussed the distinction which was made by Lazarus & Folkman (1984) between problem-focused coping strategies and emotion-focused strategies. Problem-focused coping (planning, and thinking out solutions) may not be the ideal solution to the difficulties posed by a chronic illness for a young child. On the other hand, emotion-focused strategies, which can entail avoidance of the stressful situation (such as turning a blind eye to it) might offer a range of more appropriate and potentially useful solutions (Kliewe, 1991).

The way in which children think about themselves and their social environment has long been of interest to those researchers who seek to understand why some children in middle childhood manage to cope well with a chronic illness such as IDDM whereas others do not. Measures have included locus of control, attributional style and self-concept (Brown *et al.*, 1991). Other factors which are believed to be important, in determining how children of this age cope, include social competence and family influences such as supportiveness and cohesion (Kager & Holden, 1992).

6.3.1 LOCUS OF CONTROL

The concept of **locus of control** is intimately related to the idea that reinforcement is a major determinant of behavior. If we are rewarded for a certain desired behavior we are more likely to do it again, especially if we believe there has been a causal relationship between our behavior and getting the reward. A corollary of that idea is the notion that the more steadfastly we believe that events which follow our actions are in some way contingent upon our behavior, or upon some aspect of our personality or whatever, the more we are likely to believe we have those events within our control. This is known as an internal locus of control. On the other hand, if we perceive ourselves to be at the mercy of events, and believe they happen to us as the result of luck, or chance, or fate, and are relatively unpredictable, then we see ourselves as subject to forces outside our sphere of influence. In other words, we have a belief in an external locus of control (Rotter, 1966; Nowicki & Strickland, 1973). Studies of the association between locus of control and coping have yielded equivocal results in children (e.g., Blanchard-Fields & Irion, 1988; LaMontagna, 1984). There is some evidence that children who have an internal locus of control, who tend to see themselves in control of events rather than otherwise, engage in more cognitive avoidance (Kliewe, 1991). Cognitive avoidance is a passive coping response which entails efforts to avoid thinking about the problem and finding ways to ignore it, such as wishing it had never happened (an emotion-focused rather than a problem-focused coping strategy).

6.3.2 ATTRIBUTIONAL STYLE

The idea of locus of control is closely linked to that of **attributional style**. Substantial evidence exists to suggest that a knowledge of the beliefs that a person holds about the causes of events, which are termed 'causal attributions', can inform us about a range of significant aspects of how they live their lives (Garber & Seligman, 1980; Antaki & Brouwen, 1982; Stratton *et al.*, 1986).

Brouwen and Shapiro (1984) have been critical of locus-of-control measures, on the grounds that they usually fail to distinguish between attributions for positive and negative outcomes. The essential problem is that locus-of-control measures tend to treat both positive and negative outcomes as equivalent. Take, for example, a widely-used scale which measures children's locus of control devised by Nowicki and Strickland (1973). The scale treats as indicative of an external locus of control a positive answer to the question 'Do you feel that when a kid your age decides to hit you, then there's little you can do to stop him/her?' (a negative outcome is implied) and a positive answer to the question 'Do you feel that most problems will solve themselves if you just don't fool with them?' (in which a positive outcome is implied). Another question on this scale, 'Do you usually feel that it's almost useless to try in school because most other kids are just plain smarter than you are?' relates to yet another issue, that of self-esteem or self-concept (Harter, 1982). There is evidence that children who tend to hold themselves responsible for events which are likely to have a negative outcome (i.e., believe they can exert some control over them) have better metabolic control of their diabetes (Brown *et al.*, 1991). Such children do not necessarily hold themselves responsible for positive events. In other words, they may ascribe positive events to chance, rather than believing they can by their own efforts bring positive or desired outcomes about.

6.3.3 LEARNED HELPLESSNESS

Linked to the notion of attributional style is that of **learned helplessness**, which has also been studied in relation to diabetic control (Kuttner *et al.*, 1990). Learned helplessness is a term which was originally coined by Seligman (1975) and Abramson *et al.* (1978) following a series of ingenious, albeit unpleasant, experiments with animals. The concept implies that individuals suffering from learned helplessness tend to attribute negative events to internal, global and stable causes. They are thereby susceptible to a sense of hopelessness and depression (Seligman *et al.*, 1984). The acquisition of learned helplessness is linked to three main factors: the extent to which individuals anticipate a positive outcome in response to their actions; the extent to which they perceive a positive outcome is within their control; and the extent to which their own failures are attributed to unalterable faults in themselves, rather than to behaviors which they can modify, or external circumstances which they can change. For example, children who do a task and fail, and then go on to fail subsequent tasks with a deterioration in their performance, are often found to have attributed the initial failure to their innate lack of ability. They have effectively 'given up trying' right at the outset. Yet they might, in actuality, be capable of succeeding in that later series of tasks. A similar process could occur to diabetic patients who repeatedly perceive a lack of association between their attempts to manage their diet and insulin dosage, and the degree of metabolic control they achieve. If they come to attribute their failure to attain good metabolic control to internal, global and stable causes their self-care performance might be expected to deteriorate. This in turn would lead to poorer metabolic control. A vicious cycle would be set up which could ultimately result in hospitalization. On the other hand, children who persist in the face of failure, and eventually master a task, even if their initial efforts were unsuccessful, may attribute their initial failure to their own lack of effort (that is to say, they have internal, unstable and specific attributes). Such children subsequently exercise mastery over the situation and do not show a deteriorating performance over time. Note that there may not be a simple cause-and-effect relationship operating here; the degree to which children feel helpless to control their diabetes will not correlate precisely with their metabolic control. There is likely to be a disordinal interaction; so long as things are going reasonably well the disposition to this attributional style may not be important. Then, when the child is faced with an unanticipated stressor, perhaps an intercurrent infection, control goes awry. From knowledge of the child's attributional style, the prediction can be made that in certain circumstances their diabetic control is likely rapidly to deteriorate. A measure of the degree to which a diabetic child expresses learned helplessness at one point in time can be shown to account for 10% of the variance in mean HbA_1 over the previous year (Kuttner *et al.*, 1990). The concept certainly has potential significance for the effective management of diabetic control in children.

Another term which has gained currency in the literature on stress in young children concerns the distinction between controllable and uncontrollable stressors. A chronic physical disorder is a cause of both of these. It has recently been suggested that controllable stressors may most effectively be handled by 'approach (monitoring) strategies', whereas uncontrollable stressors may be handled by an 'avoidance strategy' known as 'blunting' (Miller & Green, 1985; Altshuler & Ruble, 1989). For example, an effective means of dealing with a controllable stressor such as poor performance at school would be to focus on the problem in order to change the situation, probably by studying harder (Lazarus & Folkman, 1984). In contrast, an uncontrollable stressor such as an incurable illness is something a child has got to learn to live with, and calls for strategies to manage the situation as it already exists (Band & Weisz, 1988). We have seen that an emotion-focused response, such as avoiding thinking about the situation, may be the only feasible coping tactic in an uncontrollable situation where no direct action mode of coping is possible (e.g., Brown *et al.*, 1986). However, such a tactic may be especially difficult for children under the age of 7 years or so, because of their relative cognitive immaturity. When they are faced with contemplating an uncontrollable situation, whether it is going to be a positive event (e.g., waiting for a present), or a negative event (such as waiting for an injection) they will in general tend to use behavioral rather than cognitive strategies (Altshuler & Ruble, 1989; Kliewe, 1991). Behavioral distractions include tactics such as fidgeting, staring around, looking at a book, whereas cognitive strategies include emotion-focused distraction techniques, such as thinking about something else.

6.4 ADOLESCENCE

There is substantial evidence that the management of a chronic disorder such as IDDM becomes especially difficult for children at the time of adolescence (e.g., Tattersall & Lowe, 1981). To some extent difficulties in management of IDDM at this time might be related to metabolic changes associated with maturation (e.g., Amiel *et al.*, 1986). A comprehensive recent review considered whether adolescents were merely victims of their 'raging hormones' (Buchanan *et al.*, 1992). The traditional view is that adolescents' mood and behavior does differ from that of younger children and adults in some general way; they experience more swings in mood, more intense moods, lower or more variable energy levels and more restlessness than do people at other stages of development. The degree to which mood states vary, and the extent to which they become more negative with increasing age, has been studied using a novel technique of self-monitoring by Larson and Lampman-Petraitis (1989). Anxiety and self-consciousness may be heightened during adolescence, but parents are not reliable sources of information on adjustment difficulties in their offspring at this time. An accurate picture would most probably be obtained by coordinating the findings from a variety of sources; for example, some aspects of antisocial behaviour may be seen only by teachers. Reliance upon self-report data alone is likely to underestimate the adolescent's degree of psychological disturbance insofar as he or she is probably unwilling readily to admit involvement in activities of which society would disapprove (Offer & Schonert-Reichl, 1992).

Although historically adolescence has been viewed by researchers and clinicians alike as a time of *'Sturm und Drang'* (Hechinger & Hechinger, 1963) it is clear that, within the general population of adolescents, a significant proportion (80% or so) do not experience turmoil. They relate well to their family and peers, and are comfortable with their social and cultural values (Douvan & Adelson, 1986; Offer & Offer, 1975; Rutter *et al.*, 1976).

Of importance to the monitoring of their own health status is the fact that adolescence is a time when new mental capacities develop which allow the choice of a greater range of possibilities and alternatives than formerly (Keating, 1990). According to the influential psychologist Jean Piaget, adolescence is a time when 'formal operations' emerge, permitting the adolescent mentally to generate hypotheses and to seek alternative solutions to problems (Inhelder & Piaget, 1958). A refined ability to think in more abstract terms is known as 'meta-cognition' (Maccoby, 1983). Meta-cognition also implies an awareness of one's image as perceived by others. The capacity to use recursive thinking; to make statements such as 'he thinks that I think that she wants . . . ', is also a form of meta-cognition and emerges during adolescence (Santrock, 1990).

With adolescence comes the capacity to reflect, and to make deductions through the process of hypothetical reasoning. These abilities were not previously available. Adolescence is a time when young people begin to take a different view of handicaps and other personal disabilities which distinguish them from their peers. Adolescents with disabilities begin to reconstruct their childhoods. They begin to see that period of development from a very different perspective to that in which they perceived their childhood when they themselves were children (Elkind, 1985).

There is an emergent capacity to reflect on 'what might have been, if this hadn't happened to me. If only . . .'.

Adolescence is also a time when gender differences really begin to be important, with respect to a whole range of abilities related to the ability to cope with stressors. Girls tend to score more highly than boys on measures relating to social cognitive abilities such as empathy (Hoffman, 1977), and altruism (Krebs, 1975) as well as the interpretation of visual and auditory information (Kimura, 1992). Girls tend to have greater concerns than boys about health problems such as nervousness, fatigue and headaches (Dubow *et al.*, 1990). They perceive themselves as more vulnerable to illness, and they more readily express concerns about their health and about becoming sick (Radius *et al.*, 1980). Interestingly enough, adolescent boys, (especially those 16 years or older) describe themselves more frequently than do girls of an equivalent age as doing things they know are not good for their health, such as smoking cigarettes, drinking alcohol and taking drugs.

Girls are more likely than boys to associate emotional problems with poor physical health. They express more concerns about their personal appearance, especially the fear of growing overweight (Alexander, 1989; Garrick *et al.*, 1988; Feldman *et al.*, 1986; Dubow *et al.*, 1990).

The degree to which adolescents in general really do suffer emotional disturbance may be hard to gauge, because of their well-known reluctance to share personal information with adults. As children go through adolescence there is a marked change in whom they choose to confide, with a burgeoning preference for peers as confidantes rather than parents (Furman & Buhrmester, 1992). Changes in cognitive capacities allow adolescents to hide their true feelings, which may not be acceptable to those around them, and they tend to put on a misleading facade (Broughton, 1981). Failure accurately to 'read' an adolescent's state of mind is especially likely in the area of emotional adjustment, making it hard for an informant or observer to judge the presence of symptoms such as depression and anxiety (Pierce & Klein, 1982; Rutter *et al.*, 1976). Parents of adolescents have been shown to be less likely to report symptoms of depression in their children than the adolescents recognized in themselves when questioned directly (Fleming & Offord, 1990).

Little is known in general about the coping behaviors by which adolescents attempt to deal with their emotional problems, or about the individual variations in coping behavior that they employ (Hauser & Bowlds, 1990). Frequently they will try to handle stressful situations themselves, but they also engage in 'help seeking' behavior (DePaulo *et al.*, 1983). Why some young people seek help relatively readily, whereas others do not, is a relatively unresearched area. There are few data available and those studies which have looked at this issue have used hypothetical questions with healthy adolescents. Obviously, it would have been more helpful if adolescents in need of help had been studied and their actual behaviors observed (Whittaker *et al.*, 1990; Windle *et al.*, 1991).

For those professionals who are managing adolescents with a chronic illness, understanding how they cope, and the extent to which they are willing to seek help if they find it difficult to cope, is of the utmost importance. From the research findings to date it seems that adolescents prefer to counsel their families and friends, and possibly physicians, than to seek assistance for emotional difficulties from a mental health professional (Offer *et al.*, 1991). Reviewing the literature on this subject Offer and Schonert-Reichl (1992) emphasize the difficulties one faces as a clinician when attempting to intervene with children at this developmental stage; indeed there is some evidence that the severity of the problems being experienced by them is not linked to the propensity to seek help. Seiffge-Krenke (1989) found that as problems increased in severity, the propensity to seek therapeutic help actually decreased!

ACKNOWLEDGEMENTS

I am grateful for assistance in the preparation of this manuscript to Deborah Flynn, Linda Dowdney and Jennifer Smith.

REFERENCES

Abramson, L., Seligman, M.E and Teasdale, J.D. (1978) Learned helplessness in humans: critique and reformulation. *J. Abnormal Psychology*, **87**, 49–74.

Achenbach, T.M. (1991a) *Manual for the Child Behavior Checklist/4–18 and 1991 Profile*. University of Vermont, Department of Psychiatry, Burlington, VT.

Achenbach, T.M. (1991b) *Manual for the Teacher's Report Form and 1991 Profile*. University of Vermont, Department of Psychiatry, Burlington, VT.

Achenbach, T.M. (1991c) *Manual for the Youth Self-Report and 1991 Profile*. University of Vermont, Department of Psychiatry, Burlington, VT.

Ainsworth, M.D.S., Blehar, M.C., Waters, E. *et al.* (1978) *Patterns of Attachment*. Erlbaum, Hillsdale, NJ.

Alexander, C.S. (1989) Gender differences in adolescent health concerns and self assessed health. *J. Early Adolescence*, **9**, 467–79.

Altshuler, J.L. and Ruble, D.N. (1989) Developmental changes in children's awareness of strategies for coping with uncontrollable stress. *Child Devel.*, **60**, 1337–49.

Amiel, S.A., Sherwin, R.S., Simonson, D.C. *et al.* (1986) Impaired insulin action in puberty: a contributing factor to poor glycemic control in adolescents with diabetes. *N. Eng. J. Med.*, **315**, 215–19.

Antaki, A. and Bruen, C.R. (1982) *Attributions and Psychological Change*. Academic Press, London.

Band, E.B. and Weisz, J.R. (1988) How to feel better when it feels bad: children's perspectives on coping with everyday stress. *Developm. Psychol.*, **24**, 247–53.

Bates, J.E. (1989a) ' Concepts and measures of temperament', in G.A. Kohnstamm, J.E. Bates and M.K. Rothbart (eds). *Temperament in Childhood*, pp. 3–26, in Wiley, Chichester.

Bates, J.E. (1989b) 'Applications of temperament concepts'. G.A. Kohnstamm, J.E. Bates and M.K. Rothbart (eds). *Temperament in Childhood*, pp. 321–56. Wiley, Chichester.

Bates, J.E. and Bailes, K. (1984) Objective and subjective components in mothers' perceptions of their children from age 6 months to 3 years. *Merrill-Palmer Quarterly*, **30**, 111–30

Belsky, J. (1984) The determinants of parenting: a process model. *Child Devel.*, **55**, 83–96.

Blanchard-Fields, F. and Irion, J.C. (1988) The relation between locus of control and coping in two contexts: age as a moderator variable. *Psychology and Ageing*, **3**, 197–203.

Block, J., Block, J.H. and Jerde, P.F. (1988) Parental functioning and home environment in families of divorce: prospective and concurrent analyses. *J. Am. Acad. Child and Adoles. Psychiat.*, **27**, 207–213.

Bretherton, I. (1985) Attachment theory: retrospect and prospect. *Monographs of the Society for Research in Child Development*, **50**, 3–35.

Broughton, J.M. (1981) The divided self and adolescence. *Human Devel.*, **24**, 13–32.

Brouwen, C.R. and Shapiro, D.A. (1984) Beyond locus of control: attributions for responsibility for positive and negative outcomes. *Brit. J. Psychology*, **75**, 43–49.

Brown, J.M., O'Keefe, J., Sanders, S.H. *et al.* (1986) Developmental changes in children's cognition, distressful and painful situations. *J. Pediatr. Psychology*, **11**, 343–56.

Brown, R.T., Kaslow, N.J., Sansbury, L. *et al.* (1991) Internalising and externalising symptoms and attributional style in youth with diabetes. *J. Am. Acad. Child and Adoles. Psychiat.*, **30**, 921–25.

Buchanan, C.M., Eccles, J.S. and Becker, J.B. (1992) Are adolescents the victims of raging hormones: evidence for activational effects of hormones on moods and behaviour at adolescence. *Psychological Bull.*, **111**, 62–107.

Buss, A.H. and Plomin, R. (1984) *Temperament: early developing personality traits*. Erlbaum, Hillsdale, NJ.

Campos, J.J., Barratt, K., Lamb, M.E. *et al.* (1983) 'Socioemotional development', in M.M. Haith and J.J. Campos (eds). *Handbook of Child Psychology* (4th edition), Vol. IV, pp. 783–915. Wiley, New York.

Carey, W.B. and McDevitt, S.C. (1989) *Clinical and Educational Applications of Temperament Research*. Swets and Zeitlinger, Amsterdam-Lisse.

Cassidy, J. (1988) Child-mother attachment and the self in six year olds. *Child Devel.*, **59**, 121–34.

Compas, B.E., Malcarne, V.L. and Fondacaro, K.M. (1988) Coping with stressful events in older children and young adolescents. *J. Consult. Clin. Psychol.*, **56**, 405–411.

Crittenden, P.M. and Ainsworth, M.D.S. (1989) 'Child maltreatment and attachment theory', in D. Cicchetti and V. Carlson (eds). *Child Maltreatment*, pp. 432–63. Cambridge University Press, Cambridge.

Crnic, K.A. and Greenberg, M.T. (1990) Minor parenting stresses with young children. *Child Devel.*, **61**, 1628–37.

Curry, S.L. and Russ, S.W. (1985) Identifying coping strategies in children. *J. Consul. Clin. Psychol.*, **14**, 61–69.

De la Bruyere, J. (1991) The illusion of intelligence. *Lancet*, 7133769, 208–209.

DePaulo, B.M., Nadler, A. and Fischer, J.D. (1983) *New Directions in Helping*, Vol. 2. Academic Press, New York.

Ditesheim, J.A. and Templeton, J.M. (1987) Short term vs. long term quality of life in children following repair of high imperforate anus. *J. Pediatr. Surg.*, **22**, 581–87.

Douvan, E. and Adelson, J. (1986) *The Adolescent Experience*. Wiley, New York.

Downey, G. and Coyne, J.C. (1990) Children of depressed parents: an integrative review. *Psychol. Med.*, **108**, 50–76.

Drotar, D. (1981) Psychological perspectives in childhood chronic illness. *J. Pediatr. Psychol.*, **6**, 211–28.

Dubow, E.F., Lovko, K.R. Jr. and Kausch, D.F. (1990) Demographic differences in adolescents' health concerns and perceptions of helping agents. *J. Clin. Child Psychol.*, **19**, 44–54.

Earls, F. and Jung, K.G. (1987) Temperament and home environment characteristics as causal factors in the early development of child psychopathology. *J. Am. Acad. Child and Adoles. Psychiat.*, **26**, 491–98.

Elkind, D. (1985) Cognitive development and adolescent disabilities. *J. Adolescent Health Care*, **6**, 84–89.

Feldman, W., Hodgson, C., Corber, S. *et al.* (1986) Health concerns and health related behaviors of adolescents. *Can. Med. Assoc. J.*, **134**, 489–93.

Fleming, J.E. and Offord, D.R. (1990) Epidemiology of childhood depressive disorders: a critical review. *J. Am. Acad. Child and Adoles. Psychiat.*, **29**, 571–80.

Folkman, S. and Lazarus, R.S. (1988) The relationship between coping and emotion: implications for theory and research. *Social Science and Medicine*, **26**, 309–317.

Furman, W. and Buhrmester, D. (1992) Age and sex differences and perceptions of networks of personal relationships. *Child Devel.*, **63**, 103–115.

Garber, J. and Seligman, M.E.P. (1980) *Human Helplessness: Theory and Application*. Academic Press, New York.

Garmezy, N. (1985) 'Stress resistant children: the search for protective factors', in J.E. Stevenson (ed.). *Recent Research in Developmental Psychopathology*, pp. 213–33. Pergamon Press, Oxford.

Garrick, T., Ostrov, E. and Offer, D, (1988) Physical symptoms and self image in a group of normal adolescents. *J. Am. Med. Assoc.*, **29**, 73–80

Garrison, W.T., Biggs, D. and Williams, K. (1991) Temperament characteristics and clinical outcomes in young children with diabetes mellitus. *J. Child Psychol. Psychiat.*, **31**, 1079–88.

Goldsmith, H.H., Buss, A.H., Plomin, R. *et al.* (1987) Round table: what is temperament? Four approaches. *Child Devel.*, **58**, 505–529.

Goodyer, I. (1990) 'Social events, experiences and development', in I. Goodyer (ed.). *Life Experiences, Development and Childhood Psychopathology*, pp. 3–22. John Wiley & Sons, Chichester.

Graham, P., Rutter, M. and George, S. (1973) Temperamental characteristics as predictors of behaviour disorders in children. *Am. J. Orthopsychiatry*, **43**, 328–39.

Greenberg, M.T. and Crnic, K.A. (1988) Longitudinal predictors of a developmental status and social interaction in premature and full-term infants at age 2. *Child Devel.*, **59**, 554–70.

Harter, S. (1982) The perceived competence scale

for children. *Child Devel.*, **53**, 87–97.

Hauser, S.T. and Bowlds, M.K. (1990) 'Stress, coping and adaptation', in S. Feldman and G.R. Elliott (eds). *At the Threshold: The developing adolescent*, pp. 388–413. Harvard University Press, Cambridge, MA.

Hechinger, F. and Hechinger, G. (1963) *Teenage Tyranny*. William Morrow and Co., New York.

Hinde, R.A., Stevenson-Hinde, J. and Tamplin, A. (1985) Characteristics of 3–4 year olds assessed at home and their interaction in preschool. *Devel. Psychol.*, **21**, 130–40.

Hoffman, L.W. (1977) Changes in family roles, socialisation and sex differences. *Am. Psychologist*, **84**, 644–57.

Illingworth, R.S. and Holt, K.S. (1955) Children in hospital: some observations on their reactions with special reference to daily visiting. *Lancet*, **ii**, 1257–62.

Inhelder, B. and Piaget, J. (1958) *The Growth of Logical Thinking from Childhood to Adolescence*. Basic Books, New York.

Jenkins, J.M. and Smith, M.A. (1990) Factors protecting children living in dysharmonious homes: maternal reports. *J. Am. Acad. Child and Adoles. Psychiat.*, **29**, 60–69.

Johnson, J.H. (1986) *Life Events as Stressors in Childhood and Adolescence*. Sage, Beverly Hills, CA.

Johnson, S.B. (1980) Psychosocial factors in juvenile diabetes: a review. *J. Behav. Med.*, **3**, 95–115.

Johnson, S.B. (1988) Psychological aspects of childhood diabetes. *J. Child Psychol. Psychiat.*, **29**, 729–38.

Kager, V.A. and Holden, E.W. (1992) Preliminary investigation of the direct and moderating effects of family and individual variables on the adjustment of children and adolescents with diabetes. *J. Pediatr. Psychol.*, **17**, 491–502.

Keating, D. (1990) 'Adolescent thinking', in S.S. Feldman and G.R. Elliot (eds). *At the Threshold: The developing adolescent*, pp. 54–89. Harvard University Press, Cambridge, MA.

Kimura, D. (1992) Sex differences in brain. *Scien. Am.*, **267**, 81–87.

Klagsburn, M. and Bowlby, J. (1976) Responses to separation from parents: a clinical test for young children. *Projective Psychol.*, **21**, 7–26.

Kliewe, R. (1991) Coping in middle childhood: relations to competence, type A behaviour, monitoring, blunting, and locus of control. *Devel. Psychol.*, **27**, 689–97.

Krebs, D. (1975) Empathy and altruism. *J. Personality and Social Psychology*, **32**, 1124–46.

Kuttner, N.J., de la Mater, A.M. and Santiago, J.V. (1990) Learned helplessness in diabetic youths. *J. Pediatr. Psychol.*, **15**, 581–94.

LaMontagna, E.L.L. (1984) Children's locus of control beliefs as predictors of preoperative coping behaviour. *Nursing Research*, **33**, 76–85.

Lancaster, S., Prior, M. and Adler, R. (1989) Child behavior ratings: the influence of maternal characteristics and child temperament. *J. Child Psychol. Psychiat.*, **30**, 137–49.

Larson, R. and Lampman-Petraitis, C. (1989) Daily emotional states as reported by children and adolescents. *Child Devel.*, **60**, 1250–60.

Lazarus, R.S. (1984) Puzzles in the study of daily hassles. *J. Behav. Med.*, **7**, 375–89.

Lazarus, R.S., DeLongis, A., Folkman, S. *et al.* (1985) Stress and adaptational outcomes: the problem of confounded measures. *Am. Psychologist*, **40**, 770–79.

Lazarus, R.S. and Folkman, S. (1984) *Stress, Appraisal and Coping*. Springer, New York.

Lerner, R.M., Palermo, M., Spiro, A. *et al.* (1982) Assessing the dimensions of temperamental individuality across the lifespan: the Dimensions of Temperament Survery (DOTS). *Child Devel.*, **53**, 149–60.

Maccoby, E. (1983) 'Social-emotional development and response to stressors', in N. Garmezy and M. Rutter (eds). *Stress, Coping and Development in Children*, pp. 217–34. McGraw-Hill, New York.

Main, M. and Cassidy, J. (1988) Categories of response to reunion with a parent at age 6: predictive and infant attachment classifications and stable over a one month period. *Devel. Psychol.*, **24**, 415–26.

Marks, I. (1987) The development of normal fear: a review. *J. Child Psychol. Psychiat.*, **28**, 667–98.

Masten, A.S. (1989) 'Resilience in development: implications of the study of successful adaptation for developmental psychopathology', in D. Cicchetti (ed.). *The Emergence of a Discipline: Rochester Symposium on Developmental Psychopathology*. Erlbaum, Hillsdale, NJ.

Masten, A.M. and Garmezy, N. (1985) 'Risk, vulnerability, and protective factors in developmental psychopathology', in B.B. Lahey and A.E. Kazdin (eds). *Advances in Clinical Child Psy-*

chology, Vol. 8, pp. 1–52. Plenum, New York.

Matheny, A. (1989) 'Temperament and cognition: relations between temperament and mental test scores', in G.A. Kohnstamm, J.E. Bates and M.K. Rothbart (eds). *Temperament in Childhood*, pp. 283–98. Wiley, Chichester.

Matheny, A.P., Wilson, R.S. and Thoben, A.S. (1987) Home and mother: relations with infant temperament. *Devel. Psychol.*, **23**, 323–31.

Maziade, M., Caperaa, P., Laplante, B. *et al.* (1985) The value of difficult temperament amongst 7 year olds in the general population for predicting psychiatric diagnosis at age 12. *Am. J. Psychiat.*, **142**, 943–46.

Miller, S.N. and Green, M.L. (1985) 'Coping with stress and frustration: origins, nature and development', in M. Lewis and C. Saarni (eds). *The Socialisation of Emotions*, pp. 263–314. Plenum, New York.

Newcomb, A.F., Bukowski, W.M. and Pattee, L. (1993) Children's peer relations: a meta-analytic review of populat, rejected, neglected, controversial and average sociometric status. *Psychological Bull.*, **113**, 99–128.

Nowicki, S. and Strickland, B.R. (1973) A locus of control scale for children. *J. Consulting and Clinical Psychology*, **40**, 148–54.

Offer, D., Howard, K.I., Schonert, K.A. *et al.* (1991) To whom do adolescents turn for help? Differences between disturbed and non-disturbed adolescents. *J. Am. Acad. Child and Adolescent Psychiatry*, **30**, 623–30.

Offer, D. and Offer, J.B. (1975) *From Teenage to Young Manhood: a psychological study*. Basic, New York.

Offer, D. and Schonert-Reichl, K.A. (1992) Debunking the myths of adolescence: findings from recent research. *J. Am. Acad. Child and Adol. Psych.*, **31**, 1003–1014.

Orbach, I., Gross, Y., Gavbman, H. *et al.* (1985) Children's perception of death in humans and animals as a function of age, anxiety and cognitive ability. *J. Child Psychol. Psychiat.*, **26**:3, 453–63.

Pellegrini, D., Kosisky, S., Nackman, D. *et al.* (1986) Personal and social resources in children of patients with bipolar affective disorder and children of normal control subjects. *Am. J. Psychiatry*, **143**, 856–61.

Perrin, E.C., Ramsey, B.K. and Sandler, H.M. (1987) Competent kids: children and adolescents with a chronic illness. *Child Care, Health and Development*, **13**, 13–32.

Perrin, E.C., Stein, R.E.K. and Drotar, D. (1992) Cautions in using the Child Behavior Checklist: observations based on research about children with a chronic illness. *J. Pediatr. Psychol.*, **16**, 11–21.

Peterson, L. and Toler, S.M. (1986) An information-seeking disposition in child surgery patients. *Health Psychol.*, **5**, 343–58.

Phares, V. and Compas, B.E. (1992) The role of fathers in child and adolescent psychopathology: make room for Daddy. *Psychological Bull.*, **113**, 387–412.

Pierce, L. and Klein, H. (1982) A comparison of parent and child perception of the child's behavior. *Behav. Disorders*, **7**, 69–74.

Plomin, R. and DeFries, J.C. (1985) *Origins of Individual Differences in Infancy: the Colorado Adoption Project*. Academic Press, New York.

Prior, M. (1992) Childhood temperament. *J. Child Psychol. Psychiat.*, **33**, 249–80.

Radius, S.M., Dillman, T.E., Becker, M.H.*et al.* (1980) Adolescent perspectives on health and illness. *Adolescence*, **15**, 375–84.

Rae-Gant, N., Thomas, B.H., Offord, D.R. *et al.* (1989) Risk, protective factors, and the prevalence of behavioural and emotional disorders in children and adolescents. *J. Am. Acad. Child and Adolescent Psychiatry*, **28**, 262–68.

Rotter, J.B. (1966) Generalised expectancies for internal versus external control of reinforcement. *Psychological Monographs*, **80**:1.

Rovet, J.F. and Ehrlich, R.M. (1988) Effects of temperament on metabolic control in children with diabetes mellitus. *Diabetes Care*, **11**, 77–82.

Rutter, M. (1987) Psychosocial resilience and protective mechanisms. *Am. J. Orthopsychiatry*, **57**, 316–31.

Rutter, M., Graham, P., Chadwick, D.F. *et al.* (1976) Adolescent turmoil: fact or fiction? *J. Child Psychol. Psychiat.*, **17**, 35–56.

Sanson, A., Prior, M. and Kyrios, M. (1990) Further explorations of the link between temperament and behaviour problems: a reply to Bates. *Merrill-Palmer Quarterly*, **36**, 573–76.

Santrock, W. (1990) *Adolescence*. William C Brown, Dubuque, IA.

Schaffer, H.R. and Callender, W.M. (1959) Psychological effects of hospitalisation in infancy. *Pediatrics*, **24**, 528–39.

Seifer, R., Sameroff, A.J., Baldwin, C.P. *et al.* (1992) Child and family factors that ameliorate risk between 4 and 13 years of age. *J. Am Acad. Child and Adol. Psychiat.*, **31**, 893–903.

Seiffge-Krenke, I. (1989) 'Problem intensity and the disposition of adolescents to take therapeutic advice', in M. Brambring, F. Losel and H. Skowronek (eds). *Children at Risk: Assessment, Longitudinal Research and Intervention*, pp. 457–77. Walter De Gruyter, New York.

Seligman, M.E. (1975) *Helplessness: On Depression, Development and Death.* W. H. Freeman, San Francisco.

Seligman, M.E., Kaslow, N.J., Alloy, L.B. *et al.* (1984) Attributional style and depressive symptoms among children. *J. Abnormal Psychol.*, **93**, 235–38.

Shouldice, A. and Stevenson-Hinde, J. (1992) Coping with security distress: separation anxiety test and attachment classification at 4.5 years. *J. Child Psychol. Psychiat.*, **33**, 331–48.

Stevenson-Hinde, J. and Simpson, A.E. (1982) 'Temperament and relationships', in R. Porter, and G.M. Collins, (eds). *Temperamental Differences in Infants and Young Children*, pp. 51–61. Pitman/CIBA Foundation, London.

Stratton, P., Heard, D., Hanks, H.G.I. *et al.* (1986) Coding causal beliefs in natural discourse. *Brit. J. Soc. Psych.*, **25**, 299–313.

Tattersall, R.B. and Lowe, J. (1981) Diabetes in adolescence, *Diabetologia.*, **20**, 517–23

Thomas, A. and Chess, S. (1977) *Temperament and Development*. Brunner/Mazel, New York.

Thomas, A. and Chess, S. (1989) 'Temperament and personality', in G.A. Kohnstamm, J.E. Bates and M.K. Rothbart (eds). *Temperament in Childhood*, pp. 249–62. Wiley, Chichester.

Thomas, A., Chess, S. and Birch, H.G. (1968) *Temperament and Behavior Disorders in Children.* University Press, New York.

Thomas, A., Chess, S. and Korn, S. (1982) The reality of difficult temperament. *Merrill-Palmer Quarterly*, **28**, 1–20.

Van Eerdewegh, M.M., Bieri, M., Parilla, R., Clayton, P. (1982) The bereaved child. *Brit. J. Psychiatry*. **140**, 23–29.

Wahler, R. and Zigler, E. (1991) A review of resilience in childhood. *Am. J. Orthopsychiatry*, **61**, 6–22.

Walker, S.R. and Rosser, R. (1988) *Quality of Life: Assessment and Application.* MTP Press, Lancaster.

Wallander, J.L., Virani, J.W., Ballani, L., *et al.* (1988) Children with chronic physical disorders: maternal reports of their psychological adjustment. *J. Pediatr. Psychology*, **13**, 197–212.

Wallerstein, J.S. (1991) The long-term effects of divorce on children: a review. *J. Am. Acad. Child and Adol. Psychiat.*, **30**, 349–60.

Weinraub, M. and Wolf, E. (1983) Effects of stress and social supports on mother-child interaction in single and two parent families. *Child Devel.*, **54**, 1297–311.

Werner, E.E. and Smith, R.S. (1982) *Vulnerable but Invincible: A longitudinal study of resilient children and youth.* McGraw-Hill, New York.

Whittaker, A., Johnson, J., Schaffer, D. *et al.* (1990) Uncommon troubles in young people. *Arch. Gen. Psychiatry*, **47**, 487–96.

Windle, M., Miller-Tutzauer, C., Barnes, G.M. *et al.* (1991) Adolescent perceptions of help-seeking resources for substance abuse. *Child Devel.*, **62**, 179–89.

7

Childhood and adolescent psychological development in relation to diabetes

B.J. ANDERSON

7.1 INTRODUCTION

Successful treatment of insulin-dependent diabetes mellitus (IDDM) in children requires implementation of a complex therapeutic regimen involving multiple daily insulin injections, a complex meal plan, regular exercise, and frequent monitoring of blood glucose levels which must be closely coordinated in time with injections. IDDM is frequently singled out from among the spectrum of chronic childhood diseases for its demands for self-care and family responsibility for complex disease management (Anderson & Auslander, 1980). When a child is diagnosed with IDDM, the critical tasks of decision-making concerning the child's survival and daily treatment are transferred from health care providers to families and children soon after diagnosis (Drash & Becker, 1978). In the psychosocial literature on pediatric diabetes, it is well-documented that the tasks involved in the complex daily treatment regimen required of children with diabetes mellitus impact on every aspect of their development (Anderson *et al.*, 1991; Johnson, 1980). With respect to psychological development, at every period of development, 'good emotional adjustment' is strongly linked to 'good metabolic control' (Johnson, 1980). Sufficient studies have been conducted using standardized, objective measures, comparing groups of children with diabetes to nondiabetic comparison samples that we can conclude with confidence that children with diabetes are not a psychologically 'deviant' group. However, these global studies of groups of children with diabetes assessed by standardized psychological instruments shed little light on what it is about diabetes per se that affects the developing child and family. What is critical for future discussions and research on the psychological development of children with diabetes is to understand and identify the specific stresses of this disease which the child and/or parent must confront at each stage of development, and the coping responses with respect to disease-specific stressors, especially the treatment regimen, that lead to healthy psychological and physical outcomes in these children.

Childhood and Adolescent Diabetes
Published in 1994 by Chapman & Hall, London
ISBN 0 412 48610 5

Therefore, the focus of this chapter is how the normal tasks of each developmental period affect and are affected by the responsibilities required to manage diabetes. In this chapter, we will divide the discussion into: 1) Early-onset diabetes: the infant, toddler, and preschool years; 2) diabetes in school-aged children; and 3) diabetes in adolescence. For each developmental period, we will first briefly review the central milestones of normal psychological development and secondly, we will examine how the requirements of managing diabetes impact on the specific psychological tasks at each period. Throughout we will pay special attention to research on the development of self-esteem in children and adolescents with diabetes in relation to diabetes management requirements and responsibilities. This chapter will discuss only studies which include specifics of the disease and its treatment in assessing the psychological development of children with diabetes. Moreover, because there has been a revolution both in the technology as well as in the philosophy of diabetes management for pediatric populations during the last decade, this discussion will give priority to more recent investigations. For example, 15 years ago, we did not have the evidence that we now have concerning hypoglycemia as a risk factor to the cognitive development of toddlers with diabetes. Similarly, 15 years ago, children of 10–12 years of age with diabetes were expected by health care professionals, and therefore by parents, to achieve independence in disease management. As expectations for parents and for children have changed in response to new information about optimum diabetes management at different stages of development, the impact of this disease on the tasks of psychological development has necessarily changed as well. Finally, for each developmental period, we will conclude with brief recommendations for health care providers to assist in designing services to accommodate to the psychological needs of their pediatric patients with IDDM.

7.2 PSYCHOLOGICAL DEVELOPMENT AND EARLY-ONSET DIABETES: THE INFANT, TODDLER, AND PRESCHOOL YEARS

7.2.1 PSYCHOLOGICAL DEVELOPMENT DURING INFANCY (0–2 YEARS) IN RELATION TO DIABETES MELLITUS

Diabetes diagnosed during the first two years of life has a profound effect on the parent–infant relationship. The establishment of a mutually strong, emotional attachment between the infant and one or more primary caregivers is the central psychological task of the first two years of life (Erikson, 1950). The infant's psychological development is entirely dependent on the predictable presence of another human being, who meets the infant's survival needs and responds sensitively and reciprocally to the infant's early social signals. Therefore, psychological development in infancy involves the assessment of the infant-in-relationship, typically measures of infant–parent attachment and separation (Ainsworth *et al.*, 1971).

From the beginning of this discussion of psychological functioning during infancy in relation to diabetes, it is important to point out that there are, to date, no empirical studies focused specifically on this patient population. Most often when children under 24 months of age with diabetes are included in research studies, they are grouped with children under 6 years of age, and studied as a 'preschool sample'. When a child is diagnosed with IDDM during the first two years of life, the parent(s) or caregiver(s) become the real 'patient'. The grief experienced by parents of infants after diagnosis is often stronger and more disruptive emotionally to the parent than when a child is diagnosed at an older age because parents of young infants have more recently celebrated the birth of a 'healthy, perfect' child. Moreover, the diagnosis of IDDM during infancy is difficult to make by medical professionals as well as by parents because the classic signs and symptoms of increased thirst, increased hunger, weight loss, and more frequent urination are harder to identify when infants urinate on their own schedule into diapers and when appetites normally fluctuate. This means that many infants with diabetes go undiagnosed or are misdiagnosed, resulting in a child who is more critically ill at diagnosis, and may require an emergency hospital admission or intensive care unit. This heightens the trauma already experienced by the parents, and emphasizes the vulnerability of their child as well as the seriousness of diabetes. Finally, the parents of a very small infant may find it extremely difficult, both psychologically and physically, to inject insulin into or to take a drop of blood from their infant's tiny body. For these reasons, the diagnosis of IDDM during infancy is emotionally devastating to most parents.

On this foundation of grief, the day-to-day management of diabetes in an infant causes layers of stress for parents. Parents are given the clinical tools – insulin, syringes, glucagon, blood monitoring machine, finger-pricker, and food – and asked to make life-threatening and life-saving decisions. Around-the-clock vigilance is required in monitoring the baby for symptoms of hypoglycemia, which are difficult to differentiate from normal behavioral fluctuations in the baby during the day and night. For these reasons, many parents of diabetic babies are unable to find any 'relief' caregivers. It is well-documented that training a babysitter or a grandparent to be competent and comfortable caring for an infant with diabetes is a very difficult and often impossible task for many families (Anderson *et al.*, 1991). Therefore, the potential is high for parents of infants with diabetes to become very weary and fatigued, 'burned out', with constant monitoring, and no breaks. This is especially true for single parents or for families in which one parent carries all of the burden of responsibility for diabetes management. Parents are at risk of becoming isolated from other families with young children. Moreover, there are few resources (educational literature, parenting guidebooks, support groups, etc.) specific for families with infants with diabetes.

As detailed above, the diagnosis of diabetes and the day-to-day management of this disease create an often overwhelming stress for parents of infants. Parents easily become too exhausted and too isolated to leave their infant, creating a situation in which the infant with diabetes has fewer of the separation and reunion experiences which occur normally and naturally between infant and parent during the first year of life. This may put both baby and parent at risk for an over-dependent relationship. Again, we stress that this is a clinical conclusion, and that there are to date no empirical studies of the psychological functioning of the infant with diabetes nor of the infant–parent relationship. This is an important area for future empirical research by pediatric psychologists. The tasks of diabetes management exaggerate the normal bonding process of the infancy period, with parents constantly vigilant and fearing to separate from their baby. And for the baby with diabetes, this type of parental vigilance may interfere with learning that he or she can be safe and content without the parent. In summary, especially when parents do not have support resources and relief caregivers, diabetes may put the infant–parent relationship at risk for an over-closeness and may restrict positive separation experiences necessary during the infancy period. It is essential that health care providers in pediatric diabetes clinics begin to appreciate and address the stresses confronting parents of infants with diabetes by promoting the development of clinical services, childcare referral sources, educational materials, and support groups for families living with diabetes at this earliest developmental period.

7.2.2 PSYCHOLOGICAL DEVELOPMENT DURING THE TODDLER YEARS (2–4 YEARS) IN RELATION TO DIABETES MELLITUS

Diabetes during the second, third, and fourth years of life continues to have a profound effect on the parent–child relationship. At this developmental period, the toddler's two central psychological tasks are: to separate from the parent or primary caregiver and to establish him or herself as a separate person, by developing a sense of autonomy, with more clearly defined boundaries between the child and the parent; and to develop a sense of mastery over the environment and the confidence that they can act upon and produce results in the environment, including the people making up their social environment.

As is also true of infants with diabetes, when a two-, three-, or four-year-old child has IDDM, the parent(s) or caregiver(s) is the real 'patient'. Parents continue to be responsible for making complex, clinical decisions, and for vigilantly monitoring the child for symptoms of hypoglycemia. Parents with toddlers who have diabetes also have difficulty locating child caregivers who are competent to care for the toddler and in educating members of the extended family to provide childcare. Parents with toddlers also may have the additional stress of having a child who may actively resist and refuse insulin injections, blood monitoring, or needed meals and snacks. Parents often struggle to maintain the child's blood sugar within a safe and acceptable range due to the physiologic interference from the toddler's physical growth spurts, the child's inability to understand the importance of the regimen or to consistently cooperate with the diabetes treatment, and the toddler's inability to verbalize symptoms of high or low blood glucose.

Given the toddler's normal developmental task of establishing independence from the parent, diabetes only fuels the parent-child conflicts so typical of this age. Unfortunately, as with infants, toddlers with diabetes have been grouped with children under 6 years of age, and studied as a 'preschool sample'. One recent empirical research study by Wysocki *et al.* (1989) studied the psychological adjustment of 20 children, 24–72 months of age (2–6 years), with a mean age of 49 months (4 years), and their mothers. This study is the closest in the literature to an investigation of the psychological development of the toddler in relation to diabetes, although the sample did include older, preschool-aged children as well. Wysocki *et al.* (1989) indicated that mothers reported that their children showed significantly more 'internalizing' behavior problems on the standardized Child Behavior Checklist (Achenbach & Edelbrock, 1983): for example, symptoms of depression, anxiety, sleep problems, somatic complaints, or withdrawal; however, the authors emphasize that mothers did not rate their toddler and preschool children with diabetes in the clinically deviant range as measured on this standardized instrument. There were no assessments made of the toddler's behavior independent of maternal report. This is important to note in light of the other major finding by Wysocki and colleagues: that mothers with very young children with diabetes reported more overall stress in their families when contrasted with a nondiabetic standardization sample, with the child seen as the source of that stress. Children's psychological adjustment on the standardized child behavior assessment was not predictive of diabetes-specific behavior problems. With respect to diabetes management findings, Wysocki *et al.* (1989) reported that mothers perceived their children as more stigmatized by diabetes as compared with findings from a large sample of older children and adolescents with diabetes. Mothers reported more concerns about identifying hypoglycemia, and they perceived family disruption to be greater than that for the older diabetic sample. In discussing their findings, Wysocki and colleagues raise an issue of critical concern in the present chapter: '... If adjustment difficulties begin in the preschool years, are these problems predictive of poor adjustment in later childhood and adolescence?' (Wysocki *et al.*, 1989, p. 529). Unfortunately, there are to date no longitudinal studies following infants and toddlers with diabetes with follow-up psychological assessments made prospectively into childhood and adolescence.

The challenges of managing a chronic illness in a toddler are eloquently described by Garrison and McQuiston (1989):

> Behavioral and temperamental characteristics of toddlers, their wariness of strangers, reliance upon routines and rituals, poor impulse control, and limited ability to verbally communicate thoughts and feelings, together make it particularly difficult for this age group to cope with the stresses of chronic illness. Physical restraint or restriction of movement necessitated by medical procedures, and parental worry and overprotection, frustrate the child's motive to explore and master the environment ... If the illness impairs the child's developmental competencies resulting in regression or qualitative changes in behavior, the parents must adjust their expectations and alter caregiving patterns. From a transactional viewpoint, the changed child alters parental attitudes and behaviors which, in turn, affect the child's development and the nature of the parent-child relationship. (pp. 65–6)

In summary, clinically we can see that the restrictions of diabetes management stress the very normal drives of toddlers for autonomy and mastery. The research of Wysocki *et al.* (1989) emphasizes that mothers are reporting increased 'internalizing' symptoms in their children at this age, symptoms such as anxiety, depression, sleep problems, and appetite problems. The important question is not are these toddlers different from their peers living in families withort diabetes, but rather, what impact does this stressful beginning have on the developing psychological functioning of the child with diabetes? Again, there are no longitudinal studies following very young children with diabetes into childhood and adolescence. As we recommended for the infancy period, it is essential that health care providers in pediatric diabetes clinics begin to appreciate and address the stresses confronting parents of toddlers with diabetes by promoting the development of clinical services, educational materials, and parenting support programs for families living with diabetes at this period of development.

7.2.3 PSYCHOLOGICAL DEVELOPMENT DURING THE PRESCHOOL YEARS (4–6 YEARS) IN RELATION TO DIABETES MELLITUS

The central developmental task of the preschool-aged child is to put their newly-established sense of autonomy to work actively investigating the environment outside the home. The child is involved in gaining a sense of gender-identity, in developing new cognitive abilities which allow more cause-effect thinking, and in separating successfully from the parents for the first 'school' experience which, for many preschool-aged children, may be a day care experience. Nonetheless, at this developmental period the child must learn to adapt to the expectations of teachers or day care providers, to trust these adults to provide for his or her needs, and to begin to form relationships with peers and adults outside the family. The child takes increasing initiative and masters new skills in environments outside of the home.

For preschool-aged children with diabetes, entry into school may be their first awareness that they are 'different' from age-mates, in terms of eating at snack or lunch times, checking blood glucose levels, or wearing medical identification jewelry. Moreover, the preschool child must learn to trust adults other than parents to manage diabetes safely. Leaverton (1979) suggested that 'separation anxiety' is common for parents with 4–7-year-old children with diabetes and that there are some valid reasons for parental concerns as the child enters school. For both child and parent, entry into preschool may be the first public context within which the parent and child must cope with the social repercussions of diabetes, including the challenge of trusting and educating others about the disease.

With respect to recent empirical studies of 4–7-year-old children with diabetes, retrospective, cross-sectional neuropsychological reports have recently suggested that children diagnosed with diabetes before the age of 5 years have subtle cognitive deficits later in childhood or adolescence (Anderson *et al.*, 1984; Hale *et al.*, 1985; Holmes & Richman, 1985; Rovet *et al.*, 1987; Ryan *et al.*, 1985). To date, only one group of researchers, Rovet *et al.* (1990), has followed 4–7-year-old children with diabetes prospectively using neuropsychological assessments. The preliminary findings from this 3-year follow-up of newly-diagnosed children under 5 years of age indicated that there was no evidence of any neurocognitive impairment in these children at the onset of disease or one year after diagnosis (Rovet *et al.*, 1990). Rovet and colleagues report that they may not have yet followed their subjects long enough to observe any cognitive impairment or that subjects in the retrospective studies in which cognitive impairments were reported did not have the availability of blood glucose monitoring equipment, making metabolic control less adequate in contrast to the patients in their current study.

Only one published report, the previously discussed work of Wysocki *et al.* (1989) has investigated the preschool child's psychological adjustment (by maternal report). Mothers reported more sleep problems, social withdrawal, anxiety, and depression, as well as more family stress attributed to the target child than did mothers reporting in a standardization sample of healthy preschool children. Despite the cautious interpretation given to their findings by Wysocki and colleagues, it is unclear if such a 'standardization sample' is the appropriate comparison group for preschoolers with diabetes and their families. Both Eiser (1990) and Garrison and McQuiston (1989) have suggested that these types of behavioral changes in the very young child and changes in parental expectations are to be expected when any type of chronic illness occurs during the preschool years. Therefore, it is important not to conclude from the findings of Wysocki *et al.* (1989) that in all these preschool children it is diabetes that causes behavioral adjustment problems, or that all mothers with preschool children with IDDM see their families as severely stressed. Clearly, more research is needed with assessments of preschool children's adjustment other than solely by maternal report. However it is clear that families of preschool children with IDDM, similar to families with infants and toddlers, require additional supports within the health care system, specific to needs at this developmental period, resources such as parenting support programs and assistance in preparing the family and the school for the child's transition to school.

7.3 PSYCHOLOGICAL DEVELOPMENT IN SCHOOL-AGED CHILDREN (6–11 YEARS) WITH DIABETES

The primary developmental tasks of the child during the elementary school years include: forming close friendships with children of the same sex, gaining the approval from this peer group, developing new intellectual, athletic, and artistic skills, and evaluating themselves by comparing their abilities to those of the peer group.

Psychological development in school-aged children is assessed primarily with respect to the child's sense of self-esteem and the development of peer relationships. In a careful review of the early empirical psychosocial literature on children with diabetes, Johnson (1980) concluded

> most youngsters with diabetes do not have psychological problems, but among those who do, peer relationship difficulties are quite common . . . Among all of the personality traits assessed, the evidence for peer or social relationship problems seems the strongest. (p. 101)

Studies of self-esteem in children with diabetes have consistently linked low self-esteem and poor social-emotional adjustment to poorly-controlled diabetes (Johnson, 1980). Studies comparing groups of children with and without diabetes do not help us understand the origin of problems with peer relationships. However some of the older interview studies do suggest how diabetes interferes with peer solidarity in childhood. Bregani *et al.* (1979) emphasized that during this developmental period, children with diabetes often begin to feel a heightened sense of frustration and social stigma because of their diet restrictions. The authors point out that the child's emerging self-awareness and ability to reflect on diabetes and to compare him or herself with peers made the child very vulnerable to feelings of inadequacy. Similarly, Zuppinger *et al.* (1979) in interviews with 23 diabetic children at this age found that half of the sample identified teasing from peers and difficulty in accommodating meal schedules to school activities as the major difficulties in following the diabetic diet. Leaverton (1979) also suggested that the most common resentment of the child with diabetes during the elementary school years is following a planned diet because it gives an obvious sign to peers that the child is different.

These older studies make it clear that participation, positive self-image, and regimen flexibility (especially nutritional flexibility) are critical and interrelated goals for the school-aged child with diabetes. The implications for health care providers and parents are clear: avoid unrealistic demands for adhering to a meal, insulin, or monitoring schedule that restricts the elementary-school child from active participation in school and peer activities, and promote problem-solving skills for learning to be flexible concerning diabetes treatment. A second area of importance for health care providers with respect to elementary school children concerns the transference of diabetes care responsibilities from the parent to the child. While the expanding skills of the elementary school child make it seem reasonable to transfer more and more daily diabetes care responsibilities, and while research has shown that there is a naturally-occurring, gradual increase in the transfer of responsibility for diabetes management tasks during childhood (Anderson *et al.*, 1990), outcome research increasingly suggests that it is inappropriate for children at this age to assume complete independence or autonomy in diabetes care. Parental involvement in diabetes management is required throughout the early elementary school developmental period (Follansbee, 1989).

7.4 PSYCHOLOGICAL DEVELOPMENT IN ADOLESCENTS WITH DIABETES

7.4.1 NEW PERSPECTIVES ON THE DEVELOPMENTAL TASKS OF ADOLESCENCE

Early in this century, adolescence was characterized as the most stressful period of human development (Simmons, 1987). Pioneering American psychologist Hall, in 1904, originally described the adolescent years as one of '*sturm und drang*' (storm and stress). Later, Erikson called adolescence a time of 'identity crisis' (Erikson, 1968), and theorists such as Blos (1962 & 1979) suggested that puberty triggers a resurgence of psychosexual conflicts. The thrust of these major theories of adolescence was an emphasis on discontinuity and turmoil, and research was stimulated which focused on autonomy or separation, defined as freedom from parental influence (Irwin, 1987).

In contrast, during the last decade, several theorists have argued that issues of attachment and the transformation of significant interpersonal relationships during adolescence have been largely overlooked (Hill, 1987; Gilligan, 1987). There is a new theoretical focus on interdependence and the development of healthy interpersonal relationships. New conceptualizations of adolescent autonomy are emerging based on models of self-regulation as opposed to freedom from parents (Hill, 1987). Out of these new theoretical models of adolescent development, which place primary emphasis on the development of interdependency between adolescent and parent, has come the realization that the adolescent transition is also a time of family transition and reorganization. Including the family as a more central force in theories of adolescent development has resulted in a focus on defining and measuring those parenting styles which help to promote healthy adolescent development. Across a full range of families, 'authoritative' parenting (Baumrind, 1971) has been associated with increased competence in the adolescent, less susceptibility to antisocial influences and a variety of other desirable outcomes. This parenting style reflects open communication, give-and-take between parent and adolescent, and consistent support but also firm enforcement of clear rules (Baumrind, 1971). A consensus appears to be developing among investigators concerned with adolescent development that engagement with, rather than separation from, parents during early adolescence enhances adolescents' ego development (Hauser, 1991) and individuation by reducing their vulnerability to peer pressure.

Traditional theories emphasizing parent–adolescent conflict and adolescent independence led to the perspective during the 1960s that less supervision and earlier independence would better foster healthy adolescent development. According to Irwin (1987), however, current research indicates that 'early separation or emotional autonomy from the family can have a negative effect on the adolescent. This negative effect can be manifested by an increased risk of alienation or susceptibility to negative peer influence' (p. 3). In summary, early distancing from parents puts the young adolescent at risk for health-compromising behaviors. Indeed, researchers investigating school performance in adolescents have documented the benefits of a prolonged supportive environment and the importance of an 'arena of comfort' (Simmons, 1987) for adolescents coping with multiple transitions. Grolnick and Wellborn (1988) have developed a theory of parental support for adolescent autonomy and parental involvement as two critical components of adolescent academic success and lack of psychiatric symptomatology. Their theory is in sharp contrast to the traditional theories that have emphasized adolescent autonomy exclusively in opposition to an overdependence on parents. Research by Grolnick and Wellborn (1988) has suggested that adolescent development is fostered by closeness and attachment to parents in a climate of support for autonomy.

A pivotal summary of current theories of adolescent development was provided at the seminal National Invitational Conference on the Health Futures of Adolescents in 1986 (Irwin, 1987). Three of the five major knowledge outcomes of this critical meeting have direct relevance to adolescents with IDDM and are summarized below:

- Healthy adolescent development is fostered by providing a prolonged supportive environment during early adolescence, with graded steps toward autonomy.
- Adolescence is not inherently turbulent. Understanding positive growth, the acquisition of new skills and health-promoting behaviors, and the changing nature of interpersonal relationships deserve increased attention.
- Healthy development is encouraged by a process of mutual, positive engagement between the adolescent and various adults and peers. This process should occur through family and other significant adults and take place in schools, health institutions, and the community.

In summary, current developmental theories conceptualize the major task of the adolescent period as movement away from dependence on the family, not toward independence, but rather toward interdependence, and that this interdependence does not require adolescents to distance themselves emotionally from parents but rather, requires a reorganization in which family members renegotiate and redistribute responsibilities and obligations (Baumrind, 1987).

7.4.2 PSYCHOSOCIAL RESEARCH ON ADOLESCENTS WITH DIABETES

The vulnerability of adolescents with IDDM to medical and psychosocial problems has been consistently documented (Orr *et al.*, 1983). There is a consensus among empirical studies that adolescents as a group display the worst metabolic control, i.e., the highest blood glucose readings, as compared to other age groups (Report of the National Commission on Diabetes, 1976; Daneman *et al.*, 1981). Within this developmental period, the early adolescent years are consistently identified as a period of deteriorating blood glucose control (Blethen *et al.*, 1981; Cerreto & Travis, 1984; Daneman *et al.*, 1981). Recent studies indicate a network of influences disrupts metabolic stability during early adolescence (see Chapter 5). Despite increased insulin dosages during puberty, the hormonal upheaval and rapid physical growth of this period frequently continue to interfere with stable and acceptable blood glucose levels (Peterson *et al.*, 1978). Recently, several investigators have documented that the physiological changes of puberty, indeed, cause insulin resistance in both nondiabetic and diabetic adolescents and that this reduction in insulin sensitivity contributes to high blood glucose levels in young diabetic adolescents and may undermine self-care efforts (Amiel *et al.*, 1986; Bloch *et al.*, 1987).

While not all adolescent patients display a disrupted medical and psychological course, there are identifiable adolescents who experience a cycle of dysfunction, with medical and interpersonal crises closely intertwined. These adolescents experience repeated hospitalizations, symptoms of chronic poor control, with concomitant school problems and family conflicts over compliance with treatment responsibilities. Even if all families with adolescents do not experience these extreme disruptions, it is well-documented that family conflict over diabetes and diabetes management is higher during the adolescent years than at younger ages (Anderson, 1984; Johnson, 1980).

Prior to this new evidence documenting 'insulin resistance' during the pubertal period, investigators often focused exclusively on psychological factors and poor self-care behavior to explain the high and erratic blood glucose levels of adolescent patients (Orr *et al.*, 1983). Clearly, fundamental conflicts exist between the tasks of managing diabetes and the young adolescent's striving to be comfortable with a rapidly maturing body, to define an identity and to be positively accepted by peers (Greydanus & Hofmann, 1979). Moreover, these struggles occur within the broader context of increased expectations by parents and health care providers for the young adolescent to assume more independence in self-care responsibilities (Anderson *et al.*, 1989; Follansbee, 1989), as well as increased expectations by parents and physicians for good metabolic control. In summary, there is evidence that physiologic and psychological factors contribute to the vulnerability of adolescents with IDDM to both medical and psychosocial problems.

The unfortunate legacy from early studies of adolescents and diabetes management has been a bias in clinical recommendations for adolescent 'independence' with diabetes care tasks, despite no supporting empirical data. In fact, there is a growing consensus among recent empirical studies that children and adolescents given greater responsibility for their diabetes management have more mistakes in their self-care, are less adherent, and are in poorer metabolic control than those whose parents are more involved (Anderson *et al.*, 1990; Burns *et al.*, 1986; Ingersoll *et al.*, 1986). Studies using diabetes-specific instruments have consistently found that older children assume greater responsibility for the tasks of the treatment regimen (Anderson et al., 1990; Allen *et al.*, 1983; Rubin *et al.*, 1989). According to studies by LaGreca (1988), Allen *et al.* (1983), and Anderson *et al.* (1990), adolescents who assumed greater responsibility for regimen-specific tasks were in poorer metabolic control than those who assumed less responsibility.

In her important review of the empirical literature on family responsibility-sharing in diabetes, Follansbee (1989) concluded

> Cumulatively, these studies yield important information about the role of parent-child interaction in influencing youngsters' assumption of diabetes management. It seems that interdependence, rather than independence, is a worthwhile goal . . . A consistent finding is that for youths over age 12, parental supervision of diet, injections and charting is associated with better adherence and metabolic control. (p. 350)

There is convincing evidence that current patterns of medical care and educational approaches for adolescents with IDDM and their families are not effective in improving metabolic control and preventing the metabolic deterioration that predictably occurs during the adolescent years. Moreover, increasingly it is reported that improved metabolic control during adolescence has the potential to remediate or reverse some early physiologic complications, i.e., neuropathic and gastrointestinal complications (White *et al.*, 1981). Research evidence has also suggested that improved metabolic control may aid in prevention of two devastating later-onset complications of IDDM – diabetic nephropathy and diabetic retinopathy (*Clinical Practice Recommendations ADA 1991–1992,* 1992) (see also Chapters 39 and 40).

Innovative intervention strategies involving the families of adolescent patients have generally not been undertaken, probably due to the influence of outdated developmental theories which emphasize separation and detachment of the adolescent from the parents and focus exclusively on adolescent independence. It has been assumed that adolescent patients, because they have the eye-hand coordination skills to draw up and inject insulin or to test their blood using a monitor, are necessarily equipped cognitively and emotionally to carry out these tasks on a regular, day-to-day basis, motivated by concern about preventing long-term complications. Yet there is clear evidence in developmental psychology that adolescents are normally not capable of sustaining a long-term perspective (Baumrind, 1987), and therefore it is unrealistic to expect that their behavior will be motivated by long-term concerns. Moreover, creative research by Ingersoll and colleagues at the Diabetes Research and Training Center at the University of Indiana (Ingersoll *et al.*, 1986) has already demonstrated that many older teenagers with IDDM lack the cognitive skill to carry out the insulin adjustment or 'sliding scale' guidelines provided by their diabetes clinicians. This distinction between the mastery of a self-care skill and the expectation that the skill will be accurately and consistently executed on a routine basis is a critical distinction and one that has only recently been acknowledged in the psychosocial pediatric diabetes literature (e.g., Wysocki *et al.*, 1992). If pediatric diabetes health care providers and investigators were to be guided by the newer developmental theorists that emphasize the importance of interdependence between adolescent and parent, pediatric diabetes clinics, educational programs, and intervention studies would provide a much more active and powerful role for the parent–adolescent relationship. In pediatric diabetes care in the 1990s and the next century, new approaches are needed, targeted to parents and adolescents, concerning a family partnership with respect to sharing in the responsibilities of diabetes management.

7.5 CONCLUSION

Over the next decade, clinical and education approaches for youngsters with IDDM and their families will be transformed into delivery systems that are designed with a sense of the specific responsibilities and requirements of diabetes management which stress children and families at each developmental period. As this happens, new studies must be carried out of the psychological development of these children within this new health care context. As we anticipate a transformation in pediatric diabetes care into the twenty-first century, clinicians and researchers concerned with IDDM in the young and their families must pay close attention to the recommendations of Eiser (1990) concerning all children with chronic illnesses:

> For all parents, raising their children can be highly demanding and sometimes tedious . . . Parents of chronically sick children face the same dilemmas, with the added burden of reconciling the family activities within limits imposed by the disease. To this end they are families coping with very special circumstances, rather than pathological or deviant ones. (p. 126)

Similarly, the psychological development of children with IDDM must be seen as that of children coping with special stresses and responsibilities and not that of children with pathological or deviant personalities.

REFERENCES

Achenbach, T.M. and Edelbrock, D.S. (1983) *Manual for the Child Behavior Checklist and Revised Child Behavior Profile*. University of Vermont Press, Burlington, VT.

Ainsworth, M.D.S., Bell, S.M.V. and Stayton, D.J. (1971) 'Individual differences in strange-situational behavior of one-year-olds', in H.A. Schaffer (ed.). *The Origins of Human Social Relations*, pp. 17–52. Academic Press, London.

Allen, D.A., Tennen, H., McGrade, B.J. *et al.* (1983) Parent and child perceptions of the management of juvenile diabetes. *J. Pediatr. Psychol.*, **8**, 129–41.

Amiel, S.A., Sherwin, R.S., Simonson, D.C. *et al.* (1986) Impaired insulin action in puberty: A contributing factor to poor glycemic control in adolescents with diabetes. *N. Engl. J. Med.*, **315**, 215–19.

Anderson, B.J. (1984) 'The impact of diabetes on the developmental tasks of childhood and adolescence: a research perspective', in N. Nattras and J. Santiago (eds). *Recent Advances in Diabetes*, pp. 165–71. Churchill Livingstone, New York.

Anderson, B.J., Hagen, J., Barclay, C. *et al.* (1984) Cognitive and school performance in diabetic children. *Diabetes*, **23** (suppl. 1), 21.

Anderson, B.J. and Auslander, W.F. (1980) Research on diabetes management and the family: A critique. *Diabetes Care*, **3**, 696–702.

Anderson, B.J., Wolf, F.M., Burkhart, M.T. *et al.* (1989) Metabolic effects of a peer group intervention with adolescents with insulin-dependent diabetes mellitus: A randomized controlled study in an outpatient setting. *Diabetes Care*, **12**, 179–83.

Anderson, B.J., Auslander, W.F., Jung, K.C. *et al.* (1990) Assessing family sharing of diabetes responsibilities. *J. Pediatr. Psychol.*, **15**, 477–92.

Anderson, B.J., Wolfsdorf, J.I. and Jacobson, A.M. (1991) 'Psychosocial adjustment in children with Type I diabetes', in H. Libovitz (ed.). *Therapy for Diabetes Mellitus and Related Disorders*, pp. 51–58. American Diabetes Association, Alexandria, VA.

Baumrind, D. (1987) 'A developmental perspective on adolescent risk taking in contemporary America', in C.E. Irwin (ed.). *Adolescent Social Behavior and Health*, pp. 93–126. Jossey-Bass, San Francisco.

Baumrind, D. (1971) Current patterns of parental authority. *Developmental Psychology Monogragh*, **4** (1, part 2), 1–103.

Blethen, S.L., Sargeant, D.T., Whitlow, M.G. *et al.* (1981) Effect of pubertal stage and recent blood glucose control on plasma somatomedin C in children with insulin-dependent diabetes mellitus. *Diabetes*, **30**, 868–72.

Bloch, C.A., Clemons, P.S. and Sperling, M.A. (1987) Puberty decreases insulin sensitivity. *J. Pediatr.*, **110**, 481–87.

Blos, P. (1962) *On Adolescence: A Psychoanalytic Interpretation*. Free Press, New York.

Blos, P. (1979) *The Adolescent Passage*. International Universities Press, New York.

Bregani, P., Della Porta, V., Carbone, A. *et al.* (1979) Attitude of juvenile diabetics and their families towards dietetic regimen. *Pediatr. Adolesc. Endocrinol.*, **7**, 159–63.

Burns, K.L., Green, P. and Chase, H.P. (1986) Psychosocial correlates of glycemic control as a function of age in youth with IDDM. *J. Adolesc. Health Care*, **7**, 311–19.

Cerreto, M.C. and Travis, L.B. (1984) Implications of psychological and family factors in the treatment of diabetes. *Pediatric Clinics of North America*, **31**, 689–710.

Clinical Practice Recommendations, ADA 1991–1992. (1992) Screening for Diabetic Retinopathy. *Diabetes Care*, **15** (suppl. 2), 16–18.

Daneman, D., Wolfson, D.H., Becker, D.J. *et al.* (1981) Factors affecting glycosylated hemoglobin values in children with insulin-dependent diabetes. *J. Pediatrics*, **99**, 847–53.

Drash, A.L. and Becker, D. (1978) 'Diabetes mellitus in the child: Course, special problems, and related disorder', in H. Katzen and R. Mahler (eds). *Diabetes, Obesity, and Vascular Disease. Advances in Modern Nutrition*, Vol. 2, pp. 615–43. Wiley, New York.

Eiser, C. (1990) *Chronic Childhood Disease: An Introduction to Psychological Theory and Research.* Cambridge University Press, New York.

Erikson, E.H. (1950) *Childhood and Society*. Norton, New York.

Erikson, E.H. (1968) *Identity: Youth and Crisis.* Norton, New York.

Follansbee, D.S. (1989) Assuming responsibility for diabetes management: What age? What price? *Diabetes Educator*, **15**, 347–52.

Garrison, W.T. and McQuiston, S. (1989) *Chronic Illness During Childhood and Adolescence*. Sage Publications, Newbury Park, CA.

Gilligan, C. (1987) 'Adolescent development reconsidered', in C.E. Irwin (ed.). *Adolescent Social Behavior and Health*, pp. 63–92. Jossey-Bass, San Francisco.

Greydanus, D.E. and Hofmann, A.D. (1979) A perspective on the brittle teenage diabetic. *J. Family Practice*, **9**, 1007–12.

Grolnick, W.S. and Wellborn, J.G. (1988) 'Parent influences on children's school-related self-system process'. Paper presented at the meeting of the American Educational Research Association, New Orleans, LA.

Hale, D.B., Berenbaum, S.A., Traisman, H.S. *et al.*

(1985). Neuropsychological consequences of insulin-dependent diabetes in school-age children. *J. Clinical and Experimental Neuropsychology*, **7**, 606.

Hall, G.S. (1904) *Adolescence: Its Psychology and Its Relations to Physiology, Anthropology, Sociology, Sex, Crime, Religion, and Education*. Appleton, New York.

Hauser, S.T. (1991) *Adolescents and their Families: Paths of Ego Development*. Free Press, New York.

Hill, J.P. (1987) 'Research on adolescents and their families: Past and prospect', in C.E. Irwin (ed.). *Adolescent Social Behavior and Health*, pp. 13–32. Jossey-Bass, San Francisco.

Holmes, C.S. and Richman, L. (1985) Cognitive profiles of children with insulin-dependent diabetes. *Developmental and Behavioral Pediatrics*, **6**, 323–81.

Ingersoll, G.M., Orr, D.P., Herrold, A.J. *et al.* (1986) Cognitive maturity and self-management among adolescents with insulin-dependent diabetes mellitus. *J. Pediatrics*, **108**, 620–23.

Irwin, C.E. (ed.) (1987) *Adolescent Social Behavior and Health*. Jossey-Bass, San Francisco.

Johnson, S.B. (1980) Psychological factors in juvenile diabetes: A review. *Journal of Behavioral Medicine*, **3**, 95–116.

La Greca, A.M. (1988) 'Children with diabetes and their families: Coping and disease management', in T. Field, P. McCabe and N. Schneiderman (eds). *Stress and coping across development*, pp. 139–59. Erlbaum, Hillsdale, N.J.

Leaverton, D.R. (1979) 'The child with diabetes mellitus', in J.D. Noshpitz *et al.* (eds). *Basic Handbook of Child Psychiatry*, Vol. 1, p. 452. Basic Books, New York.

Orr, D.P., Golden, M.P., Myers, G. *et al.* (1983) Characteristics of adolescents with poorly controlled diabetes referred to a tertiary care center. *Diabetes Care*, **6**, 170–75.

Petersen, H., Korsgaard, B., Deckert, T. *et al.* (1978) Growth, body weight and insulin requirements in diabetic children. *Acta Paed. Scand.*, **67**, 453–57.

Report of the National Commission on Diabetes, Vol. III. (1976) US Department of Health, Education and Welfare, DHEW Publication No. (NIH), 76–1022.

Rovet, J.F., Ehrlich, R.M. and Hoppe, M. (1987) Intellectual deficits associated with early onset of insulin-dependent diabetes mellitus in children. *Diabetes Care*, **10**, 510–15.

Rovet, J.F., Ehrlich, R.M. and Czuchta, D. (1990) Intellectual characteristics of diabetic children at diagnosis and one years later. *J. Pediatric Psychology*, **15**, 775–88.

Rubin, R., Young-Hyman, D. and Peyrot, M. (1989) Parent-child responsibility and conflict in diabetes care (abstract). *Diabetes*, **38** (suppl. 2), 28.

Ryan, C., Vega, A. and Drash, A. (1985) Cognitive defects in adolescents who developed diabetes early in life. *Pediatrics*, **75**, 921–27.

Simmons, R.G. (1987) 'Social transition and adolescent development', in C.E. Irwin (ed.). *Adolescent Social Behavior and Health*, pp. 33–62. Jossey-Bass, San Francisco.

White, N.H., Waltman, S.R., Krupin, E. *et al.* (1981) Reversal of neuropathic and gastrointestinal complications related to diabetes mellitus in adolescents with improved metabolic control. *Pediatrics*, **99**, 41–45.

Wysocki, T., Huxtable, D., Linscheid, T. *et al.* (1989) Adjustment to diabetes mellitus in preschoolers and their mothers. *Diabetes Care*, **12**, 524–29.

Wysocki, T., Meinhold, P.A., Abrams, K.C. *et al.* (1992) Parental and professional estimates of self-care independence of children and adolescents with IDDM. *Diabetes Care*, **15**, 43–52.

Zuppinger, K., Schmid, E. and Schutz, B. (1979) Attitude of the juvenile diabetic, his family and peers toward a restricted dietetic regimen. *Pediatric and Adolescent Endocrinology*, **7**, 153–58.

PART TWO

8

The historical background

C.J.H. KELNAR

What follows is a partial list of some of the historical landmarks in the history of diabetes mellitus. Further information can be found in the papers and books cited in the bibliography which is itself highly selective.

BC

Diabetes known clinically since ancient times and claimed to have been first described in China, Egypt and India.

The Ebers papyrus (Egypt, 1550 BC) – found in a grave in Thebes in 1862 and now in the University of Leipzig – was named for the Egyptologist Prof Georg Ebers (1837–1898). It describes polyuria in a diabetes-like condition and contains dietary remedies – bones, wheat, grain, grit, green lead and earth – for those passing abundant urine.

'Diabetes' – Ionian Greek for 'a siphon' or to 'run through' – first used by **Aretæus of Cappodocia** (81–138 AD): 'a mysterious affection . . . melting down of flesh and limbs into urine . . . life is short, disgusting and painful, thirst unquenchable, death inevitable. . . .'. (Did not distinguish other polyuric diseases from diabetes mellitus.)

Childhood and Adolescent Diabetes
Published in 1994 by Chapman & Hall, London
ISBN 0 412 48610 5

AD

0–800

Roman Physician **Galen** (Claudius Galenus, 131–201 AD) thinks diabetes mellitus rare, employs the graphic term of 'diarrhoea urinosa' and thinks the disease is caused by the kidney's inability to retain water.

'Honeyed urine' (madhumea) in ancient Sanskrit (Indian Vedic) literature (5th–6th Cs AD). **Susruta** and **Charuka** (Indian physicians) noted the association of polyuria with sweet-tasting urine: like honey, sticky and attracting ants. Older, fatter and thin poor survivors distinguished. Contemporaneous Chinese and Japanese accounts include descriptions of boils.

800–1600

Avicenna (Ibn Sina 980–1037 AD) describes accurately the clinical features of diabetes including gangrene and impotence.

Maimonides (1135–1204 CE) is the name by which English-speaking scholars generally know the Jewish physician philosopher called 'Abu Imran Musa Ben Mai mum Ibn Abd Allah' (when he became physician to Saladin in Cairo) or 'Rabbi Moshe ben Maimon'. He is still thought of as the greatest of all Jewish physicians. Born in Cordova and familiar with the works of Hippocrates and Galen, he was a keen follower of Aristotle's teaching on the importance of observing nature and natural phenomena carefully. He realized that understanding comes and is advanced by 'performing the duty', that is, by being absorbed in the actual event rather than by meditation. Taking thought in itself is not enough.

In the 24th of 83 treatises consisting of some 1500 aphorisms, he discusses diabetes noting that it (the strong thirst) was rare in his native Spain but common in his adopted home of Egypt.

He was well aware of the interplay of psychic and somatic factors in disease (which was little thought about by his contemporaries) and which otherwise has been only a relatively recent concept in medical history.

During the Middle Ages, diabetes is known as the 'pissing evil'.

Theophrastus Bombastus von Hohenheim ('Paracelsus', 1493–1541) observes that diabetic urine contains an abnormal substance which remained as a white powder cake residue after evaporation and that this was salt which made the kidneys thirsty. (It is a pity he did not taste it!)

1600–1800

Thomas Willis (1621–1675, Guy's Hospital) notes the sweet taste of diabetic urine in 1674 but attributes it to salts and acids rather than sugar. He says it was rare in classical times but 'in our age, given to good fellowship and gusling down chiefly of unallayed wine, we meet with examples and instances enough, I may say daily, of this disease . . . wherefore the urine of the sick is so wonderfully sweet, or hath an honied taste . . . As to what belongs the cure, it seems a most hard thing in this disease to draw propositions for curing, for that its cause lies so deeply hid, and hath its origin so deep and remote.'

Thomas Sydenham (1624–1689) speculates that diabetes was a systemic disease due to incompletely digested chyle.

Johann Conrad Brunner in *Experimenta Nova Circa Pancreas* (Leyden, 1709) describes the excision of a dog pancreas which resulted in extreme thirst and polyuria.

Matthew Dobson (Liverpool physician, 1735–1784) graduates from Edinburgh in 1756 with a dissertation on menstruation. He publishes in the 'Medical Observations and Inquiries by a Society of Physicians in London, Volume 5' (Cadell, 1776) his 'Experiments and Obsevations on the urine in a diabetes' (*sic*) which was communicated by a friend Dr John Fothergill. He describes his own experience of sweet-tasting urine in diabetic patients and detailed observations in one Peter Dickonson who was admitted under his care in Liverpool on 22/10/1772 aged 33 years passing '28 pints of urine every 24 hours'. Crucially he also finds that Dickonson's blood tastes sweet and concluded, with foresight, that sugar in diabetic urine is not formed in the kidney but 'existed in the serum of the blood' and that emaciation is due to 'so large a proportion of the alimentary matter being drawn off by the kidney before it is perfectly assimilated and applied to the purpose of nutrition'. (Mellitus is derived from the Greek 'mell' – honey.)

At about the same time **William Cullen**, delivering the first lectures at the Royal Infirmary of Edinburgh pronounces diabetes to be a disease of the central nervous system, perhaps because he is impressed by its neuropathies.

Thomas Cawley (*London Medical Journal*, 1788) describes a case of diabetes which at autopsy showed marked pancreatic damage and the presence of pancreatic calculi. In the same year, **John Rollo** (d. 1809) locates the disease to the gastrointestinal tract attributing the abnormally high sugar production to stomach dysfunction. In 1798, Rollo makes the first controlled study of diabetes treatment, using a protein-rich, low-CHO diet to relieve the glycosuria of a 34-year-old man. He also describes diabetic cataracts and the odour of acetone (which he likened to decaying apples) on the breath of some diabetics.

1800–1900

1828 – The earliest mention of diabetes in pregnancy by **H.G. Bennewitz** in the Edinburgh Medical Journal (abstracted from a German publication).

1833 – A polarimetric assay for glucose is introduced by **Jean Baptiste Riot** (1774–1862).

1848–1850 – Metabolism of glucose formation in the liver and other aspects of carbohydrate metabolism are brilliantly described by **Claude Bernard** (1813–1878). By the mid-19th century, the existence of glucose is known – a carbohydrate (CHO) which could not be decomposed in water, circulated in the blood and which was utilized by living tissues to produce heat. (Lavoisier and Laplace thought glucose 'combustion' occurred in the lungs.) Bernard measures the glucose content of blood entering the liver (none) and compares it with that leaving. He concludes that the liver manufactures organic CHO, i.e., produces a substance which is transformed into sugar: glycogen ('which produces sugar'). He isolates it 7 years later in 1857. This was the first known example of 'internal secretions' – a concept that disturbance of blood glucose levels may cause diabetes and that there is normally consistency of the internal environment whose disequilibrium leads to illness.

1857 – Acetone in urine is first demonstrated by **Wilhelm Petters**.

1862 – **F.W. Pavy**, an English disciple of Claude Bernard, suggests a quantitative relationship between hyperglycemia and glycosuria and that, following a strict diet, patients could temporarily recover their health.

1869 – **Paul Langerhans** (1847–1888) who died of TB, was a student of and assistant to Rudolf Virchow (1821–1902). Whilst still a 22-year-old medical student, he wrote a treatise on the pancreas which describes for the first time two cell types in the pancreas: acinus glands producing digestive enzymes and islet cells of unknown function.

1870 – **Appolinaire Bouchardat** (1806–1886) observes that *rationing and forced exercise* caused by the siege of Paris led to the disappearence of glycosuria in some patients.

1874 – **Adolph Kussmaul** (1822–1902) describes three cases with the characteristic respiratory pattern without respiratory obstruction which bears his name.

1889 – In Strasbourg the relationship of pancreas to diabetes is first shown by **Joseph Freiherr von Mering** (1849–1908) and **Oscar Minkowski** (1859–1931) (who is also the first to describe pituitary hypertrophy in acromegaly). Experiments are initially on birds but then a pancreatectomized dog who develops polyuria and glycosuria (its urine attracted flies). When they ligate the pancreatic duct of another dog this causes malabsorption of food but not diabetes. **Hedon** repeats the experiment transplanting the pancreas under the animal's skin; no diabetes resultes but it develops when the organ was removed.

1893 – 'Islet cells of unknown function' called 'ilôts de Langerhans' (islets of Langerhans) are discovered by **Gustave Laguesse** (1861–1927) who suggests that they might produce an endocrine secretion.

Bernhard Naunyn (1839–1925) was the head of the Strasbourg institute where von Mering and Minkowski carried out their pancreatectomy. He was a great authority on the treatment of diabetes and made many studies and observations on ketosis. His famous diet was fat-rich, protein-poor and almost CHO-free.

1900–1950

1900 – **Leonid Szoboley** (1876–1919) in papers published around 1900 describes reduced numbers of islets and microscopic islet changes in some diabetics.

1900 – **E.L. Opie** (Johns Hopkins, 1873–1971) finds that destruction of islets causes diabetes.

Early 1900s – **Dr John Rennie** (1865–1929), in Aberdeen, Scotland, studies the occurrence of islets in bony fishes finding, in some species, the constant occurrence in a definite position of a particular islet, the 'principal islet'. With **Dr Thomas Fraser** (1872–1951) a local general practitioner and physician, tests the effects of an extract of 'principal islets' in 5 patients with diabetes; no convincing benefit is seen.

1902 – The first observation of cellular infiltration of the islets is probably made in Strasbourg by **M.B. Schmidt**.

1904 – The concept of hormones introduced by **Ernest Starling** (1866–1927).

1906 – **Bauer** first describes the glucose tolerance test.

1906 – **Dr (later Professor) J.J.R. Macleod** (1876–1935), in a contribution on 'The metabolism of the carbohydrates' in L. Hill (ed.), *Recent Advances in Physiology and Biochemistry*, devotes 74 pages to a review of current knowledge of carbohydrate metabolism and on the various forms of experimental diabetes. Subsequently, Macleod embarks on a major series of studies aimed at confirming and extending the work of Claude Bernard on the role of the nervous system in controlling blood glucose levels. *Studies in experimental glycosuria I–XII* are published in the American Journal of Physiology over the next 10 years.

1906 – **Georg Ludwig Zuelzer** (1870–1949, Berlin) extracts animal pancreas with alcohol and saline. After rabbit experiments, he gives injections of the extract to a dying diabetic. There seems to be improvement (no biochemical measurements are made) but within a few days the extract is used up and the patient relapses and dies. He carries out further experiments and publishes results in 1908. No significant progress is made and work ceases with the outbreak of the First World War in 1914. At around the same time **Ernest L. Scott** (Chicago) and **Israel S. Kleiner** (New York) were carrying out similar work searching for an effective pancreatic extract.

1908/9 – Fasting management introduced in the US by **R.T. Woodyat** at the Presbyterian Hospital, New York.

1909 – An internal secretion is named by **J. De Meyer** as produced by the islets but attempted extraction from pancreatic tissue fails.

1910 – **Elliott P. Joslin** (1870–1963), who contributed greatly to the practical management of the diabetic patient, founds the famous

Boston clinic which bears his name. During the dietary and insulin eras of diabetic treatment he adopted many of the calorific and dietary restrictions of his predecessor **Frederick M. Allen** (Rockefeller Institute, New York) who had published a large book *Studies Concerning Glycosuria and Diabetes* in 1913 and an important clinical study *Total dietary regulation in the treatment of diabetes* in 1917. This consisted of ruthless starvation until glycosuria disappeared followed by the very gradual reintroduction of food until the limits of tolerance were reached. Prolongation of life was at the expense of great suffering by the malnourished patients. (Banting attended Allen's lectures as a medical student.)

1912 – **Knowlton and E.H. Starling** (1866–1927) working at University College, London suggest that a hormone produced by the pancreas acts to increase the uptake and utilization of sugar in peripheral tissues and heart muscle.

1914 – The Harvey Lecture (Harvey Society of New York) is **J.J.R. Macleod**'s *Recent work on the physiological pathology of glycosuria*.

During the First world war (1914–18) **N.C. Paulesco** (Romania) carries out experiments with a preparation of pancreatic extracts ('pancreine') with hypoglycemic effect on dogs but publication is delayed by the war until 1921 when it appears as a sequence of short reports in an obscure French journal.

1920 – An important original method for *determination of blood glucose* is published by **Folin and Wu** and improved by **Folin** (1926 & 1929).

1920 – In separate physiology textbooks, **J.J.R. Macleod** and **E.H. Starling** both still state that there is no evidence for the existence of an internal secretion of the pancreas.

30.10.1920 – To pass a sleepless night and in preparation for a lecture on the pancreas, **F.G. Banting** (b. 14.11.1891, killed on active military service in an airplane crash in Newfoundland on 21.2.41), junior orthopedic doctor at Western University of London, Ontario reads an autopsy report by **Moses Barron** (Minneapolis). 'The relation of the islets of Langerhans to diabetes with special relationship to cases of pancreatic lithiasis', Surgery, Gynaecology and Obstetrics, Nov. 1920, Vol. XXXI describes a rare case of pancreatic stones which had blocked the pancreatic duct while the islets were unaffected. (Banting had been pall-bearer at the funeral of one of his schoolmates Jane who had died in diabetic coma at age 14.) At about 2 a.m., Banting has the inspiration that if the pancreatic duct was ligated, and the acini allowed to degenerate over several weeks, undamaged islets could be obtained from which the 'internal secretion' could be extracted. He writes in his notebook:

> Diabetus (*sic*)
> Ligate pancreatic ducts of dogs. Keep dogs alive until acini degenerate leaving islets. Try to isolate the internal secretion of these to relieve glycosurea (*sic*).

November, 1920 – Banting submits his idea to the leading Toronto physiologist **Professor J.J.R. Macleod** (1876–1935) who finds the idea interesting. The experiments have to be carried out in Toronto and Banting leaves his Ontario post. He arrives in Toronto 15.5.21.

Macleod selects **Charles Herbert Best** (1899–1978) – then still a medical student working for his Master's thesis in physiology–to be Banting's collaborator. Best also knew someone close who had died in diabetic coma – his paternal aunt after treatment at the Joslin Clinic, Boston in 1918. Work commences 17.5.21. Macleod goes on holiday in Scotland from mid-June to late-September.

June and July 1921 – Degenerated pancreas with undamaged islets is ground in Ringer's solution and injected into animals rendered diabetic by pancreatectomy – 1 hour later blood glucose levels had decreased by 40%. Late November 1921 – A further collaborator is assigned – **J.B. Collip**. Professor and Head of the Department of Biochemistry, Alberta, Edmonton. Collip had arrived to study for 6 months with Macleod on a Rockefeller Traveling Fellowship in April 1921. With his help, fractional precipitation using different concentrations of alcohol and other procedures, abstracts of islets are obtained which can be safely injected into humans. (This potent, effective and non-toxic material is used in the first effective clinical studies. The ability to extract insulin from beef pancreas thus laid the foundation of insulin production by the pharmaceutical industry. Insulin is available for clinical care throughout the world within 2 years.)

14 November 1921 – First presentation of findings by Banting and Best concerning the preparation of *insulin* is made to the Physiological Journal Club, University of Toronto.

December 1921 – Banting presents the work in the presence of Best and Collip before the American Physiological Society in a session chaired by Macleod.

11 January 1922 – Leonard Thomson, a 14-year-old boy in Toronto General Hospital is treated with pancreatic extract prepared by Banting and Best without evident clinical benefit.

23 January 1922 – Treatment is restarted using an extract prepared by Collip with immediate and dramatic success.

February 1922 – The first paper is published by Banting and Best on 'The Internal Secretion of the Pancreas' demonstrating that insulin could abolish ketosis and stimulate glycogen formation in the liver of diabetic dogs.

March, 1992 – The publication of the early clinical results in the Journal of the Canadian Medical Association (**2**, 141): *Banting, F.G., Best, C.H., Collip, J.B., Campbell, W.R., Fletcher, A.A.*: 'Pancreatic extracts in the treatment of diabetes mellitus', demonstrates that insulin reduced the blood sugar to normal values, abolished glycosuria, caused acetone bodies to disappear from the urine, and produced general clinical improvement in human patients with severe diabetes.

May, 1922 – Macleod makes the first public declaration that the effective abstract would be called 'insulin'. Macleod preferred the Latin root to the term 'isletin' used earlier by Banting and Best. He was unaware at that time that the name 'insulin' had already been suggested by **Sir Edward Sharpey-Shafer**, when Professor of Physiology in Edinburgh, who had advanced the hypothesis that the islets secreted a substance controlling the metabolism of CHO and had already suggested the name 'insulin' for the hypothetical hormone.

1922 – The Diabetic and Dietetic Department opens in the Edinburgh Royal Infirmary, Scotland – the first of its kind to be established in the UK. **Jonathan Campbell Meakins**, a Scottish Canadian, who had been appointed Professor of Therapeutics in Edinburgh in 1919, shows interest in the prospect of insulin for diabetic patients. With a group of Edinburgh workers and under the direction of Toronto, the first 'home-made' UK insulin is produced in Edinburgh and is used until commercial supplies (produced under a UK patent granted on Macleod's advice by the Toronto authorities through Sir Henry Dale to the Medical Research Council) become available in 1923.

The first vials of insulin were brought from Toronto to Prof. Meakins' ward in Edinburgh's Royal Infirmary by **Dr Lambie** (who later became the first Professor of Medicine in Australia). A diabetic doctor in Edinburgh was almost certainly the first patient in the UK to receive insulin in August 1922. **Sir Derrick Dunlop**, former Professor of Therapeutics and Clinical Medicine in Edinburgh who graduated in medicine at that time, has described how he had 'never seen anything in medicine more heart-warming or rewarding than to watch those diabetic patients raise themselves step by step out of the valley of the shadow'. As he remarked, insulin therapy was also unique in that it gave maximum relief with minimum toxicity. The diet recommended for some time was high in fat and contained less than 100 g CHO (ensuring only enough CHO for the proper combustion of fat) – resulting in the need for patients to eat great quantities of green vegetables drenched in margarine! Large portions of butter were smeared on small squares of oatcake or buns made of soya-bean meal. Good control was obtained on small amounts of insulin which was in short supply and expensive. So-called 'step-ladder' diets were used: 1) low calorie diet (40–50 g CHO) to render sugar-free (no glycosuria) 2) gradual build-up of calories and CHO to theoretical requirements – insulin was only administered if glycosuria appeared. These diets were used in children in whom they were particularly inappropriate – many failed to grow and their sexual development was often delayed. (Subsequently the pendulum of fashion for dietary management has swung from high fat/low CHO to low fat/high CHO, to (disastrous) *laissez-faire* where each meal should be 'an elegant satisfaction of the appetite rather than a problem in mental arithmetic and a trial in self-abnegation', to a good well-balanced food intake kept relatively constant from day to day so as to balance the insulin dose and avoiding an excess of concentrated sugars.)

1922 – **Macleod** and his research team embark on a series of studies on the physiologic actions of insulin. During a working holiday at the Atlantic Biological Station, New Brunswick, Canada, they prove that insulin is produced by the islets of Langerhans. The team prepares potent insulin preparations from the principal islets of bony fishes with much greater yield and more cheaply than from ox pancreases. **Dr W.R. Campbell** in Toronto shows these preparations to be satisfactory for clinical use in humans.

Early insulin preparations were in powder or tablet form and had to be dissolved in boiled water by the patients themselves, producing sterile abscesses. Early commercial insulin production (developed by the Eli Lilly company, Indianapolis), encountered problems with inadequate supplies and costly production. Problems were gradually solved: by August, 1922 supplies are available for Joslin (Boston) and Allen (New York) and, by 1924, sterile acid bovine insulin solutions in ampoules are available; the commercial production of fish insulin is not pursued.

25 October 1923 – It is announced that the award of the Nobel Prize for Medicine and Physiology is to be given jointly to **Banting** and **Macleod**. Banting shares his prize with **Best** and Macleod his with **Collip** (who subsequently goes on to discover parathyroid hormone). It is extremely unusual for a medical discovery to be honored in this way so soon. Protests soon follow: **Georg Zuelzer** (Berlin) claims priority, and **Nicholas Paulesco** (Romania) claims that he has been unjustly robbed of credit by the Toronto team.

1923 – **John Murlin** identifies a substance as an insulin contaminant which raised blood glucose and calls it **glucagon**.

1925 – Nobel lectures: **Macleod** – 'The physiology of insulin and its source in the animal body', 26 April 25; **Banting** – 'Diabetes and Insulin', 15 September 25.

1926 – **John J. Abel** (1857–1936) identifies *insulin as a protein* and first obtains it in crystalline form (the first protein for which this was achieved) which leads to much purer preparations uncontaminated by other proteins.

Blood glucose methods are developed by **H.C. Hagedorn** (1888–1971) and **B.N. Jensen** (1889–1946) [1923] and **Somogyi** [1930].

1930 – Effects of *other hormones on diabetes* are recorded. **B.A. Houssay** (1887–1971) and **Biasotti** note that the anterior pituitary gland contains a substance antagonistic to insulin, which if injected, might cause diabetes. Diabetic action of adrenal cortex is noted.

1931 – Modified *Glucose tolerance test* is described by **H. Shay** and coworkers. **T. Svedberg** determines the *molecular weight of insulin*.

1936 – **H.C. Hagedorn** (1888–1971) discovers that the addition of *protamine* to insulin results in a slowing of insulin absorption and thus produces a long-acting insulin. (See 1946 entry.)

1936 – *Microangiopathic complications*: **Poul Kimmelstiel** notes *nodular lesions in the glomeruli* of diabetics at autopsy. His findings are published with the help of **Charles Wilson**. Other renal vascular complications noted within a few years.

1944 – *Diabetic retinopathy* first described by **A.J. Ballantyne** and **Loewenstein**.

1946 – Crystalline protamine insulin is miscible with soluble insulin without loss of the two characteristic time courses – NPH = Neutral Protamine Hagedorn. Later it is found that the addition of *zinc* to the protamine further extended the insulin effect – lente series: semilente (amorphous precipitate), ultralente (crystalline suspension).

1947 – A review of the world literature by **W.E. Henley** shows a *fetal mortality* in diabetic mothers of 37.6% of 1269 cases. (The study of the prediabetic obstetric history of diabetic women first suggests that the clinical manifestations of diabetes reflect a metabolic abnormality which had gone on for a long time. Awareness of the 'prediabetic state' sows the seed for the research into prevention of the disease.)

1950–PRESENT

1953 – glucagon crystallized by **Staub, Sinn and Behrens** and found, by immunofluorescence techniques, to be produced in the pancreatic 'α' cells.

1954 – The concept of a specific and widespread diabetic small blood vessel disease affecting especially kidneys and retina is postulated by **Knud Lundbaek**. For the diabetic, the price of survival bought with insulin, is crippling degenerative vascular disease.

1955 – **Frederick Sanger** (b. 1918, Cambridge) describes the complete amino acid *sequence of bovine insulin*; he is awarded the Nobel Chemistry Prize in 1958. Species differences are described – the human insulin molecule differs from porcine by only 1 amino acid (C-B 30 threonine for alanine). Subsequently, **Dorothy Hodgkin** (1910–94) (Nobel Prize, 1964) elucidates the 3-D structure using X-ray crystallography.

1956–1962 – Understanding of the blood levels of insulin and other hormones is greatly advanced by the development of *immunoassay* techniques by **Solomon Berson** (1918–1972) and **Rosalyn Yalow** (Nobel Prize, 1978).

1964 – Insulin is synthesized by **Panavotis** and **Katsoyannis** (Pittsburgh), also by **Zahn** 1965, **Kung *et al.***, 1965.

1967 – The first step towards production of highly purified insulin preparations with fewer local side effects followed the work of **Donald Steiner** and coworkers who also discovered the structures of prepro-insulin, pro-insulin and its C-peptide.

1970s – *HLA (human leucocyte locus A)* antigenic system is found to be controlled by genes on short arm of chromosome 6 by **Baruj Benacerraf** (Nobel Prize, 1980). The discovery of the HLA system allowed the understanding of the autoimmune basis for many diseases.

1974 – **Jorn Nerup** (b. 1938) finds HLA B8 B15 B18 is significantly associated with IDDM but even closer associations are later found with Dw3 and Dw4 and a very low frequency of Dw2. Is autoimmunity a cause or an epiphenomenon? *Genetically engineered* insulin manufactured.

1972 – Twin studies (**Tattersall** and **Pyke**) show concordance for identical twins for IDDM was only around 50%. IDDM is not due entirely to genetic causes; attention is focused on environmental factors such as viral infections – mumps, coxsackie B, etc.

Further progress is made in the 1970s:

- Modern treatment of diabetic ketoacidotic coma heralded by low dose I/V insulin infusion regimes (**Alberti, Hockaday, Turner**, 1973).
- **Pfeiffer *et al.***, 1974: The *closed loop artificial beta cell* – a complex apparatus infusing insulin or glucose depending on the glucose level as determined by frequent analyses.
- **Deckert and Lorup**, 1976: Programmable *open loop* infusion devices for continuous subcutaneous infusion.
- Hyperglycemia related to the course and onset of complications (**Spiro**, 1976; **Job *et al.***, 1976).

Early 1980s – Knowledge of the basic amino acid *structure of insulin* and species differences leads eventually to the ability to chemically substitute C-B 30 threonine for alanine and produce 'human insulin'. A second method is developed altering genetic information by recombinant DNA technology and genetic engineering. The gene for human insulin (discovered by **Owerbach *et al.*** to be on the short arm of chromosome 11) is spliced into the DNA of a vector (e.g., plasmid from a bacterial cell) and inserted into the host cell (e.g., a bacterium such as *E. coli*). When the reprogrammed host cell is propagated, it expresses the 'foreign' gene and produces the product (insulin).

1980s – There is increasing understanding (often at descriptive level) of the epidemiology (genetic and environmental) of diabetes and its complications (physical and psychological).

1990s – The search continues for the fundamental causes of diabetes and its complications.

1993 – Evidence from American 10-year prospective *Diabetes Control and Complications Trial* (a large randomized prospective trial in diabetics over the age of 13 years) suggests that 'intensive' treatment which reduces hyperglycemia will unequivocally delay the onset and/or reduce the progression of microvascular complications.

The relative importance of 'tight' control in childhood and in adolescence remains to be determined as does the morbidity of 'tight' control (even if achievable) and hypoglycemia in childhood in terms of cognitive functioning. The achievement of euglycemia must be in the context of a child's normal physical and emotional growth and 'normal' family life style.

Prevention of complications and prevention of diabetes move from being inconceivable to realistically attainable future goals.

BIBLIOGRAPHY

Alberti, K.G.M.M., Hockaday, T.D.R. and Tumer, R.C. (1973) Small doses of intramuscular insulin in the treatment of diabetic 'coma'. *Lancet*, **ii**, 515–22.

Allen, F.M. (1913) *Studies concerning glycosuria and diabetes*. W.M. Leonard, Boston.

Aretaeus (1856) *The Extant Works*, edited and translated by Francis Adams. Sydenham Society, London. (*Reprint*: 1990 Classics of Medicine Library, Alabama.)

Banting, F.G. (1929) The history of insulin. *Edin. Med. J.*, **36**, 1–18.

Banting, F.G. and Best, C.H. (1922) The internal secretion of the pancreas. *J. Lab. Clin. Med.*, **7**, 251–66.

Banting, F.G., Best, C.H. and Macleod, J.J.R. (1922) The internal secretion of the pancreas. *Am. J. Physio.*, **59**, 479.

Banting, F.G., Best, C.H., Collip, J.B. *et al.* (1922) Pancreatic extracts in the treatment of diabetes mellitus. *Can. Med. Assoc. J.*, **12**, 141–46.

Banting, F.G., Best, C.H., Collip, J.B. *et al.* (1922) The effect produced on diabetes by extracts of pancreas. *Trans. Assoc. Am. Physicians*, **37**, 337–47.

Barron, M. (1920) The relation of the islets of Langerhans to diabetes with special reference to cases of pancreatic lithiasis. *Surgery, Gynecology and Obstetrics*, **31**, 437–48.

Bennewitz, H.G. (1828) Symptomatic diabetes mellitus. *Edin. Med. J.*, **30**, 217–18. (Abstracted from *Ossans Jahresbericht des Polyklinischen Institues zu Berlin*.)

Bernard, C. (1855) *Leçon de physiologie expérimentale*. Baillière, Paris.

Bernard, C. (1856) *Memoire sur le Pancreas* Baillière, Paris.

Bliss, M. (1982) Banting's, Best's and Collip's accounts of the discovery of insulin. *Bull. Hist. Med.*, **56**, 554–68.

Bliss, M. (1982) *The Discovery of Insulin*. McLelland and Stewart Ltd, Toronto.

Bliss, M. (1984) *Banting: a biography*. McLelland and Stewart Ltd, Toronto.

Bliss, M. (1989) J.J.R. Macleod and the discovery of insulin. *Quart. J. Exper. Physio.*, **74**, 87–96.

Brunner, J.C. (1709) *Experimenta Nova Circa Pancreas*. Theodore Haak, Leyden.

Cawley, T. (1788) A singular case of diabetes, consisting entirely in the quality of the urine; with an inquiry into the different theories of that disease. *London Med. J.*, **9**, 286–308.

Cullen, W. (1783) *First Lines of the Practice of Physic*. Creech, Edinburgh.

The DCCT Research Group. (1993) The effects of intensive treatment of diabetes in the development and progression of long-term complications in insulin-dependent diabetes mellitus. *N. Eng. J. Med.*, **329**, 977–86.

Dobson, M. (1776) *Experiments and Observations on the urine in Diabetes*. Medical Observations and Inquiries, **5**, 298–1784.

Dunlop, D.D. (1966) Opening address for 'Diabetes Mellitus' (Symposium of the University of Edinburgh Pfizer Foundation for Post-graduate Medical Research 1965), in L.P.J. Duncan (ed.). *Diabetes Mellitis*, pp. 1–6. University of Edinburgh Pfizer Medical Monographs, **1**, 1–6.

von Engelhardt, D. (ed.) (1989) *Diabetes: its medical and cultural history*. Springer Verlag, New York.

Joslin, E.P. (1917) *Treatment of Diabetes Mellitus*. Lea and Febiger, Philadelphia.

Joslin, E.P. (1918) *A Diabetic Manual*. Lea and Febiger, Philadelphia.

Joslin, E.P. (1956) Reminiscences of the discovery of insulin – a personal impression. *Diabetes*, **5**, 67–68.

Kleiner, I.S. (1919) The action of intravenous injection of pancreas emulsions in experimental diabetes. *J. Biol. Chem.*, **40**, 153–70.

Krogh, A. (1924) *Insulin – en opdagelse og dens betydning*. Københavns Universitets Festskrift, København.

Langerhans, P. (1869) 'Beiträge zur mikroscopischen Anatomie der Bauchspeicheldrüse', Inaugural-dissertation zur Erlangung der Doctorwürde. Berlin.

Lyon, P.L. (1990) The early days of insulin use in

Edinburgh. *Brit. Med. J.*, **2**, 1452–54.

MacFarlane, I.A. (1990) Matthew Dobson of Liverpool (1735–1784) and the history of diabetes. *Practical Diabetes*, **7**, 246–48.

Macleod, J.J.R. (1906) 'The metabolism of the carbohydrates', in L. Hill (ed.). *Recent advances in physiology and biochemistry*, pp. 312–86. Edward Arnold, London.

Macleod, J.J.R. (1913) *Diabetes: its pathological physiology*. Edward Arnold, London.

Martin E. (1989) 'Problems of priority in the discovery of insulin', in D. von Engelhardt (ed.). *Diabetes: its medical and cultural history*, pp. 420–26. Springer Verlag, New York.

Medvel, V.C. (1982) *A history of endocrinology*. MTP Press, Lancaster.

von Mering, F. and Minkowski, O. (1890) Archive für Pathologie und Pharmacologie, **26**, 371–87.

Murray, I. (1969) The search for insulin. *Scot. Med. J.*, **14**, 286–93.

Murray, I. (1971) Paulesco and the isolation of insulin. *J. Hist. Med.*, **26**, 150–57.

Naunyn, B. (1906) *Der diabetes mellitus* (2nd edn). Vienna.

Opie, E. (1900/1) The relation of diabetes mellitus to lesions of the pancreas. Hyaline degeneration of the islands of Langerhans. *J. Exper. Med.*, **5**, 527–40.

Papaspyros, N.S. (1964) *The history of diabetes mellitus* (2nd edn). Georg Thiemo Verlag, Stuttgart.

Pavy, F.W. (1862) *Researches on the Nature and Treatment of Diabetes*. John Churchill, London.

Poulsen, J.E. (1982) *Features of the history of diabetology*. Munksgaard, Copenhagen.

Pratt, J.H. (1954) A reappraisal of researches leading to the discovery of insulin. *J. Hist. Med. Allied Sciences*, **9**, 281–89.

Rollo, J. (1797) *Diabetes Mellitus: an account of two cases of the diabetes mellitus: with remarks as they arose during the progress of the cure*. Dilly, London.

Schadewalt, H. (1989) 'The history of diabetes', in D. von Engelhardt (ed.). *Diabetes: its medical and cultural history*, pp. 43–100. Springer Verlag, New York.

Scott, E.L. (1912) On the influence of intravenous injections of an extract of the pancreas on experimental pancreatic diabetes. *Am. J. Physiol.*, 306–310.

Tattersall, R.B. and Pyke, D.A. (1972) Diabetes in identical twins. *Lancet*, **ii**, 1120–25.

Williams, M.J. (1993) J.J.R. Macleod: the codiscoverer of insulin. *Proc. Royal Coll. Physicians of Edinburgh*, **23** (suppl. 1), 1–125.

Williams, M.J. (1993) Aberdonians, insulin and marine biology. *Proc. Royal Coll. Physicians of Edinburgh*, **23**, 186–92.

Willis, T. (1678) *Pharmaceutice Rationalis or an Exercitation of the Operations of Medicines in Humane Bodies*. Dring, Harper and Leigh, London.

Zuelzer, G.L. (1908) Über versuche einer specifischen fermenttherapie des diabetes. *Zeitschrift für Experimentalische Pathologie und Therapie*, **5**, 307–318.

9

Diabetes: definitions and classifications

D.I. JOHNSTON

9.1 DIABETES: DEFINITIONS

Childhood diabetes seldom presents as a problem in recognition (but see Brink in this volume) or classification. A child presenting with a combination of characteristic symptoms, obviously elevated blood glucose, and ketonuria clearly needs prompt insulin therapy and it is unlikely that the label 'insulin-dependent diabetes' will be disputed. Diagnostic problems do arise when an apparently healthy child is checked routinely, or because of a positive family history, and is found to have borderline hyperglycemia. What criteria should be used to confirm diabetes, and how do we justify starting insulin therapy with all that it implies? Current research into the natural history of early diabetes, and the promise of therapeutic maneuvers by which insulin dependence may be delayed or avoided, further emphasize the need for accepted definitions of diabetes and other categories of glucose intolerance. Measurement of glucose intolerance is also relevant to a range of genetic and acquired disorders which may be complicated by diabetes (Rimoin & Rotter, 1982) (see also Chapters 28 and 29). Glucose intolerance may have adverse effects on the prognosis of cystic fibrosis, and there needs to be an agreed strategy for investigation as the length of survival increases (Lanng *et al.*, 1991).

WHO Working Parties have provided clear criteria for diagnosing diabetes based on fasting and random plasma glucose levels, and on the interpretation of oral glucose tolerance tests (Table 9.1). Plasma glucose levels must, of course, be interpreted in the light of the child's general health, diet and coexistent drug treatment. It is unnecessary to perform confirmatory glucose tolerance testing in the face of unequivocally elevated fasting or random glucose levels. Plasma glucose measurements are convenient for clinical practice as well as being suitable for epidemiological studies. Other more sophisticated investigations, such as HLA typing, islet cell antibody titers and insulin secretory capacity, belong to the growing inventory of research tools applied to the classification of diabetes. However, they are not sufficiently robust to earn a place in widely-used definitions of the disease syndrome that makes up the spectrum of diabetes.

In addition to issues raised by persistent or deteriorating hyperglycemia, there are children who present with temporary glucose intolerance. It is well-recognized that plasma

Childhood and Adolescent Diabetes
Published in 1994 by Chapman & Hall, London
ISBN 0 412 48610 5

Table 9.1 Definitions of diabetes and impaired glucose tolerance (WHO, 1980).

	Glucose concentration mmol/l			
	whole blood		plasma	
	venous	capillary	venous	capillary
Diabetes				
fasting	⩾6.7	⩾6.7	⩾7.8	⩾7.8
random or 2 h after glucose load	⩾10.0	>11.1	>11.1	>12.2
Impaired glucose tolerance				
fasting	<6.7	<6.7	<7.8	<7.8
2 h after glucose load	6.7–10.0	7.8–11.1	7.8–11.1	8.9–12.2

Glucose load in oral GTT.
WHO recommendation: 1.75 g/kg body weight up to a maximum of 75 g (WHO, 1980).
ISGD recommendation: 45 g/m^2 body surface area (Weber, 1978).

glucose levels may be abnormally elevated during acute illness, particularly in association with convulsions or intracranial disease. This is unlikely to produce diagnostic confusion if the hyperglycemia is of short duration and there are no associated symptoms such as polydipsia, polyuria or prolonged weight loss. Ketonuria if present is transient and promptly corrected by restoration of an adequate fluid and food intake. Although it has been claimed that children presenting with illness, or stress-induced hyperglycemia are more at risk of subsequent diabetes, terminology such as prediabetes or potential diabetes should be avoided unless there is additional evidence derived from family studies or from raised islet-cell antibody titers. Not uncommonly, a coincidental illness or a surgical procedure brings to light persistent or fluctuating hyperglycemia in a child who may be in the pre-symptomatic phase of diabetes. This picture is usually clarified by serial home blood glucose monitoring, and by performing HbA_1 and islet-cell antibody measurements. An HbA_1 value exceeding three standard deviations above the normal mean is over 99% specific for diabetes. Unfortunately, HbA_1 measurement is too insensitive to be used as a sole screening test. An oral glucose tolerance test is occasionally needed to confirm diabetes in such children.

9.2 DIABETES: CLASSIFICATIONS

A disease classification that meets the requirements of clinicians, research scientists and epidemiologists has to be based on simple clinical and biochemical criteria. The categories need to be clearly defined, but capable of development to accommodate new patterns of the disease and greater understanding of causation. The long-established divisions into juvenile-onset or maturity-onset, or into insulin-dependent (IDDM) or non insulin-dependent (NIDDM) categories have stood the test of time. However, problems arise when young patients remain free of ketosis without insulin therapy, and when elderly patients develop ketosis and insulin dependence. These areas of overlap remind us that, although diabetes is conveniently defined by the presence of chronic hyperglycemia, it is the metabolic end-result of several very different etiological processes.

The traditional classification has had to be re-examined as our understanding of genetic and immune mechanisms responsible for diabetes has increased. Type 1 and Type 2 diabetes were originally introduced to describe clinical patterns largely equivalent to IDDM and NIDDM respectively. Cudworth (1976) subsequently recommended that Type 1 diabetes should have etiological meaning, and should be reserved for patients with HLA-associated diabetes linked to the occurrence of islet-cell antibodies. Type 1 diabetics are not necessarily insulin-dependent at the time of first diagnosis although they usually become so. Type 2 diabetes remains an imprecise category encompassing those who do not have Type 1 diabetes nor any of the other recognized causes.

Several authoritative bodies met during the 1970s and early 1980s in order to formulate an internationally acceptable classification. The scheme developed by the National Diabetes Data Group of the US National Institute of Health (NDDG, 1979), and adopted by the World Health Organization (WHO, 1980, 1985) remains in use (Table 9.2).

Table 9.2 Classification of diabetes (WHO, 1980 & 1985).

Diabetes mellitus

Clinical	Etiological
IDDM	Type 1
NIDDM	Type 2
a) non-obese	
b) obese	
c) young (MODY or NIDDMY)	
Malnutrition related diabetes, MRDM	
Other types	Pancreatic e.g., cystic fibrosis
	Hormonal e.g., Cushing syndrome
	Drug induced e.g., glucocorticoids
	Genetic e.g., DIDMOAD syndrome
	Receptor abnormalities
Gestational diabetes, GDM	
Impaired glucose tolerance	
a) non-obese	
b) obese	
c) secondary	

For explanation of abbreviations see text.

The WHO system is a clinical rather than an etiological classification. Although it equates IDDM with Type 1, and NIDDM with Type 2 diabetes respectively, it must be remembered that a single clinical type may arise from different etiologies, and a common etiological mechanism may produce a range of clinical types.

In the pediatric age-range, this is exemplified by the potential for incorrect classification of a young person presenting with mild hyperglycemia without ketosis. NIDDM of the young (NIDDMY), better known by the acronym for maturity onset diabetes of the young (MODY), is liable to be regarded as IDDM unless the clinician is alerted to a positive family history that suggests dominant inheritance with high penetrance (Table 9.3). The correct diagnosis may only emerge after some years when it is appreciated that the patient has never had ketosis even with provocation, and has remained free from microvascular disease. The situation is further complicated by the heterogeneity of MODY. Tattersall and Mansell (1991) have proposed a working definition of MODY: 'Diabetes diagnosed before age 25 years and treatable without insulin for more than 5 years in

Table 9.3 Differentiation of IDDM and MODY.

Feature	IDDM (Type 1)	MODY
Ketosis	prone	not prone
Onset	acute	insidious
Insulin treatment	essential	optional
HLA linkage	DR3, DR4 (DQA1, DQB1)	none
Islet cell antibodies	present	absent
Family history	10%	over 50%
Inheritance	polygenic control of disease susceptibility	autosomal dominant with high penetrance

patients who do not have islet-cell antibodies and are not HLA DR3/DR4 heterozygotes'.

MODY is rare in Caucasian children; a population-based survey in the former German Democratic Republic reported it as having been present in only 0.15% of 41 000 registered diabetics with onset before age 25 years (Panzram & Adolph, 1983). In spite of its rarity, large MODY kindreds with carefully documented phenotypes are attractive populations in which to search for the genetic basis of NIDDM (see also Chapters 11 and 29). In some pedigrees, the chronic hyperglycemia is caused by nonsense mutations in the gene encoding pancreatic β-cell and liver glucokinase (GCK). GCK has a key role at the beginning of the glycolytic pathway, regulating pancreatic insulin secretion in response to glucose and the uptake of glucose in the liver (Vionnet *et al.*, 1992). Undoubtably, separate mutations and enzyme defects will be defined in other kindreds and will reinforce the case for adjustments to the classification of diabetes.

REFERENCES

Cudworth, A. (1976) The aetiology of diabetes mellitus. *Brit. J. Hospital Med.*, **16**, 207–16.

Lanng, S., Thorsteinsson, B., Erichsen, G. *et al.* (1991) Glucose tolerance in cystic fibrosis. *Arch. Dis. Child.*, **66**, 612–16.

NDDG (1979) Classification and diagnosis of diabetes mellitus and other categories of glucose intolerance. *Diabetes*, **28**, 1039–57.

Panzram, G. and Adolph, W. (1983) Ergebnisse einer Populationsstudie uber den nichtinsulinabhangigen Diabetes Mellitus in Kindes-und Jugenalter. *Schweiz Med. Wochenschr.*, **113**, 779–84.

Rimoin, D. and Rotter, J. (1982) 'Genetic syndromes associated with diabetes mellitus and glucose intolerance', in J. Kobberling and R. Tattersall (eds). Serono Symposium No 47. *The genetics of diabetes mellitus.* Academic Press, London.

Tattersall, R. and Mansell, P. (1991) Maturity onset-type diabetes of the young (MODY): One condition or many? *Diabetic Med.*, **8**, 402–10.

Vionnet, N., Stoffel, M., Takeda, J. *et al.* (1992) Nonsense mutation in the glucose kinase gene causes early-onset noninsulin-dependent diabetes mellitus. *Nature*, **356**, 721–2.

Weber, B. (1978) Standardisation of the oral glucose test. *International Study Group of Diabetes in Children and Adolescents. Bulletin*, **2**, 23–7.

WHO (1980). *Expert Committee on Diabetes Mellitus.* No 646, WHO Technical report series, Geneva.

WHO (1985). *Expert Committee on Diabetes Mellitus.* No 727, WHO Technical report series, Geneva.

10

Epidemiology of childhood diabetes

J.S. DORMAN, L.A. O'LEARY and A.N. KOEHLER

10.1 INTRODUCTION

Insulin-dependent diabetes mellitus (IDDM) is one of the most common chronic childhood disorders, surpassing other conditions such as multiple sclerosis, leukemia, and muscular dystrophy (LaPorte & Cruickshanks, 1984). In the United States, the prevalence of IDDM in school-aged children is approximately 2 per 1000, with more than 120 000 children currently affected with the disease (LaPorte & Tajima, 1985). IDDM is associated with many severe long-term complications, including renal and cardiovascular diseases, amputations and blindness (Krolewski *et al.*, 1987; Orchard *et al.*, 1990). In addition, the mortality rates among young adults with IDDM are markedly increased compared to those for the general population of the same age (Dorman *et al.*, 1984). Although IDDM represents a major public health problem in many countries, the etiology of the disease remains unknown.

Due to recent major advancements in the field of diabetes epidemiology, descriptive studies of IDDM are currently being conducted in populations around the world. Moreover, in many areas, standardized research designs are being employed, permitting comparisons between and across countries. These investigations have led to new and exciting hypotheses which are now being tested by analytical studies through the use of molecular biology. The advantages of an interface between the laboratory sciences and epidemiology was recognized by Dr Kelly West, the founder of diabetes epidemiology, more than a decade ago (West, 1987). Since that time, the enormous advances in our understanding of the disease process, particularly in terms of the genetic determinants of the disease, as well as the dramatic improvements in molecular technology, have given epidemiologists the tools they require to study potential risk factors with the utmost sensitivity and specificity using traditional research designs. This is causing a paradigm shift in diabetes epidemiology, with the ultimate goal being disease prevention. The evolution of the field of diabetes epidemiology will be the focus of this chapter.

10.2 DESCRIPTIVE EPIDEMIOLOGY OF IDDM

10.2.1 INCIDENCE

During the past decade, our knowledge regarding the epidemiological patterns of IDDM worldwide has increased dramatically, due primarily to the establishment of standardized population-based incidence re-

Childhood and Adolescent Diabetes
Published in 1994 by Chapman & Hall, London
ISBN 0 412 48610 5

gistries across the world (LaPorte *et al.*, 1985). This has led to comparative studies of the descriptive epidemiology of the disease, which are now being facilitated by the WHO Multinational Project for Childhood Diabetes, known as DIAbetes MONDiale or the DIAMOND Project. DIAMOND has three specific aims: 1) the collection of standardized international information on incidence, risk factors and mortality associated with childhood diabetes, 2) an evaluation of the efficiency and effectiveness of health care and economics of diabetes and 3) the establishment of an international training program to strengthen national and international programs for diabetes (WHO DIAMOND Project Group, 1990). More than 70 countries around the world are currently participating in the DIAMOND Project through the establishment of standardized IDDM registries. In Europe, the EURODIAB ACE Study, which is also based on incidence registries, aims to determine the incidence of IDDM in Europe, test the hypothesis of a north-south gradient, and accumulate information regarding the etiology of IDDM (Green *et al.*, 1992).

As a result of these recently established multinational studies, there is clear evidence that the incidence of IDDM is highest in the Scandinavian countries, Finland (Tuomilehto *et al.*, 1991), Sweden (Dahlquist *et al.*, 1985), Norway (Joner & Sovik, 1989) and Sardinia, Italy (>20/100 000 per year) (Karvonen *et al.*, 1993), intermediate in countries such as the United States, New Zealand (Mason *et al.*, 1987), the Netherlands (Drykoningen *et al.*, 1992), and Spain (Serrano Rios *et al.*, 1990) (7–19/100 000 per year), and low in countries such as Poland (Rewers *et al.*, 1987), Italy (excluding Sardinia) and Israel (<7/100 000 per year) (Laron *et al.*, 1985). Countries in Asia (Diabetes Epidemiology Research International Group, 1988) and Latin America, such as Chile (Carrasco *et al.*, 1991) and Mexico (Robles Valdes *et al.*, 1987) are among the lowest risk populations in the world, with incidence rates of <3/100 000 per year. Thus, there is a 60-fold difference in incidence between Finland, the country with the highest IDDM incidence (42.9/100 000 per year) and China, with one of the lowest IDDM incidence rates (0.7/100 000 per year) (Bao *et al.*, 1989).

In addition to the variation in incidence across populations, differences within countries have also been observed. For example, there is more than a 6-fold difference in IDDM incidence within Italy (Diabetes Epidemiology Research International Group, 1990a), ranging from approximately 6–7/100 000 per year in the northern and central parts of the country (Bruno *et al.*, 1990; Calori *et al.*, 1990) to 30/100 000 per year in Sardinia (Muntoni *et al.*, 1992). Rates in the British Isles vary from 6.8/100 000 per year in the Republic of Ireland to 19.8/100 000 per year in Scotland (Metcalfe & Baum, 1991). In Norway, there also appears to be a gradient in IDDM incidence, with lower rates in the north compared to the south (Joner & Sovik, 1989).

Ethnic differences in the incidence of IDDM also exist. Studies within the United States have focused on Caucasians, African Americans, and Hispanics. In Allegheny County, Pennsylvania, the incidence of IDDM was higher among Caucasians (16/100 000 per year) compared to African Americans (10/100 000 per year) in the same geographic area (LaPorte *et al.*, 1986). Similar results were also observed from Jefferson County, Alabama (Wagenknecht *et al.*, 1989). Among Hispanics in the United States, the incidence of IDDM appears to be lower compared to that observed for non-Hispanics (9.5/100 000 per year and 15.3/100 000 per year, respectively) (Gay *et al.*, 1989). In Montreal, Canada, an area with a diverse ethnic background, IDDM incidence was highest among children of Jewish descent (17.2/100 000 per year), followed by those of British (15.3/100 000 per year), and Italian (10.7/100 000 per year) origin, while children of French descent had the lowest IDDM incidence (8.2/100 000 per year) (Siemiatycki *et al.*, 1988). These differences suggest that genetic factors contribute to the incidence of IDDM.

10.2.2 TEMPORAL TRENDS AND EPIDEMICS

The incidence of IDDM appears to be increasing in countries around the world. Data from standardized population-based registries show a linear increase in IDDM incidence during the past two decades for most of the European countries and those in the Western Pacific (Diabetes Epidemiology Research International Group, 1990b). On average, the annual increase in IDDM incidence ranged from 3–5% in the Scandinavian, Central European and Asian populations. No significant trends were observed in North America. However, recent data from Allegheny County, PA indicate a major increase in IDDM incidence after 1985, from an average of 14.4/100 000 per year during 1980–1984 to 18.1/100 000 per year during 1985–1989 (Dokheel, 1992).

Epidemics of IDDM have also been reported in several countries (WHO DIAMOND Project Group, 1992). The first recognized epidemic of IDDM occurred in midwest Poland (1982–1984) (Rewers *et al.*, 1987). During these three years, the incidence of IDDM nearly doubled (3.6/100 000–6.6/100 000 per year). An epidemic of childhood diabetes in the US Virgin Islands was also observed in 1984, where the incidence of IDDM increased from 5.3/100 000 per year in 1983, to 28.4/100 000 per year in 1984 (Tull *et al.*, 1991). In contrast to midwest Poland where the incidence remained elevated, the rates in the US Virgin Islands returned to those observed during the pre-epidemic time period (5.0/100 000 per year). Epidemics of IDDM have also been reported in countries such as Estonia (Podar *et al.*, 1992), Jefferson County, Alabama (Wagenknecht *et al.*, 1991), New Zealand (Scott *et al.*, 1991), and Asian immigrants to the United Kingdom (Burden *et al.*, 1991). Interestingly, these epidemics occurred during the early-to-mid 1980s, thus representing a global pandemic. Such marked increases over relatively short periods of time emphasize the role of environmental factors in the pathogenesis of IDDM.

10.2.3 MIGRANT STUDIES

Migrant studies represent an excellent approach for determining the contribution of genetic and environmental factors to a disease. If a disease is completely genetically determined, then individuals migrating to another country should maintain the risk of their native land. Conversely, if environmental factors are the sole contributor to a disease, then the migrant population would assume the risk of their new surroundings (Diabetes Epidemiology Research International Group, 1987).

Most migrant studies of IDDM indicate that the migrant population acquires the risk of their new homeland. Data from Montreal, Canada showed that the incidence of IDDM in Montreal French is twice the incidence reported in France, and among Jews in Montreal the incidence of IDDM is double that of Ashkenazi Jews in Israel (Siemiatycki *et al.*, 1988). Moreover, a recent study by Bodansky *et al.* (1992), which examined the incidence of IDDM in the offspring of transmigratory Asian families and non-Asian children in the Bradford District Metropolitan Council area of the United Kingdom found that the incidence of IDDM in the Asian children increased from 3.1/100 000 per year in 1978–1981 to 11.7/100 000 per year in 1988–1990, whereas there was no change in the incidence during that time for non-Asian children (10.5/100 000 per year). Similar results were described by Burden *et al.* (1990). Although these studies provide strong support for the contribution of environmental factors to the etiology of IDDM, a recent study by Podar *et al.* (1992) suggests that migrants do not always acquire the same risk of IDDM as the native population. In this study, native Estonians had an average annual IDDM incidence of 11.8/100 000 per year; whereas among the immigrant population (non-Estonians) the average annual incidence of IDDM was 7.6/100 000 per year.

10.2.4 AGE AND SEX DISTRIBUTION

IDDM during the first few months of life is rare; the risk increases after the age of 9 months until puberty and then declines in adulthood (Gamble, 1980). This pattern is similar to that for infectious diseases, which are rare during the first 6 months of life due to protection of the infant by maternal antibodies and limited exposure to infectious agents. The age of onset distribution for IDDM has been generally described as being bimodal, with some countries demonstrating a small peak occurring around age 5 in males, and a larger peak, seen in almost all populations and for both sexes, occurring near puberty (Gamble, 1980; Fleegler *et al.*, 1979; Joner & Sovik, 1981). Although this pattern is relatively consistent across the world, reasons for these apparent peaks are not clear. Several hypotheses have been proposed. The first peak, occurring around age 5, corresponds to the age at which most children begin school and thus have increased exposure to infectious agents (Gamble, 1980). The second peak, which occurs around age 11 in females and 1–2 years later in males, may be related to growth (Blom *et al.*, 1992) or hormonal changes that occur near puberty (see Chapters 4 and 5).

Overall the risk of developing IDDM appears to be similar for males and females. However, in countries with a high IDDM incidence, such as Finland, Sardinia, and Norway, a slight male excess is apparent. Among countries with low IDDM incidence rates, such as Israel, Poland, Romania and Japan, an excess of females has been observed (Diabetes Epidemiology Research International Group, 1990b; Green *et al.*, 1992).

10.2.5 SEASONAL VARIATION

Seasonal variation in the onset of IDDM has been observed worldwide. Most studies have been consistent, with a reduction in cases during the warm summer months (Fishbein *et al.*, 1982; Joner & Sovik, 1981; Elamin *et al.*, 1992). Data from Melbourne and Chile indicate that the seasonal variation in the Southern Hemisphere was similar to that of the Northern Hemisphere, but six months out of phase (Fleegler *et al.*, 1979). Slight variations have been seen within different age groups. Of interest is that the seasonal pattern appears to change during epidemic periods (Rewers *et al.*, 1987). Moreover, when examining the seasonal variation with respect to sex, some studies have shown a greater variation among males than females, reasons for which are unknown (Fishbein *et al.*, 1982; Siemiatycki *et al.*, 1986). These epidemiologic patterns indicate that environmental factors, such as viruses and infant nutrition, may be important risk factors. However, epidemiologic data also clearly provide evidence for a major contribution of genetic factors to the etiology of the disease.

10.3 GENETIC FACTORS AND IDDM

10.3.1 FAMILIAL AGGREGATION

IDDM is a disease which aggregates in families (Chern *et al.*, 1982; WHO DIAMOND Project Group, 1991). Cumulative risk estimates for first-degree relatives range from 3% to 10% by age 30 (Degnbol & Green, 1978; Wagener *et al.*, 1982; Tillil & Kobberling, 1987), as compared to rates of less than 1%

for the general population (LaPorte *et al.*, 1986; Diabetes Epidemiology Research International Group, 1988). Most of the available data on IDDM risk are from Caucasian populations in areas with similar incidence rates. There is a paucity of information for other racial groups and from populations with a very high or very low disease incidence (WHO DIAMOND Project Group, 1991).

One of the most intriguing patterns of familial aggregation is the sex difference in prevalence of parental diabetes. Diabetic children from families with an IDDM parent are significantly more likely to have an affected father than mother (Wagener *et al.*, 1982; Dahlquist *et al.*, 1989). There findings were corroborated by studies able to estimate directly IDDM recurrence risks among offspring of diabetic parents, which are approximately 6% and 2% for children of IDDM fathers and mothers, respectively (Warram *et al.*, 1984; Tillil *et al.*, 1987; Podar *et al.*, 1994). Several possible explanations have been proposed, including an increase in spontaneous abortions of susceptible fetuses by IDDM mothers (Warram *et al.*, 1984), maternal immunological tolerance of fetuses to autoantigens of the beta cells (Warram *et al.*, 1988), an increase in the paternal transmission of HLA susceptibility genes (Vadheim *et al.*, 1986), and genomic imprinting (McCarthy *et al.*, 1991). Although a specific mode of inheritance has not been identified (Spielman *et al.*, 1980; Thomson *et al.*, 1988; Field, 1988; Rotter & Rimoin, 1990), association (Wolf *et al.*, 1983; Bertram & Baur, 1984) and family studies (Barbosa *et al.*, 1980; Green *et al.*, 1985) confirm that IDDM susceptibility genes are located within the HLA region of chromosome 6 (also Chapter 11).

10.3.2 HLA AND IDDM

The HLA region of chromosome 6 contains genes that encode class I (HLA-A, B, C), class II (HLA-DR, DQ, DP), and class III antigens, as well as numerous other genes known to be involved in immune response (Trucco & Dorman, 1989). Class I molecules, which are expressed on the surface of most nucleated cells, present processed antigens to cytotoxic T lymphocytes. They consist of a polymorphic α chain non-covalently associated with β_2-micro-globulin, which is encoded by a gene located on chromosome 15 (Grey *et al.*, 1987). Crystallography studies of class I molecules have revealed that the outer domain of the molecule forms a cleft in which polypeptides from processed antigens bind (Bjorkman *et al.*, 1987). Class II molecules present antigens to helper T-lymphocytes, and they are expressed primarily on B lymphocytes, macrophages and activated T-cells. They also consist of two chains, α and β, which are both encoded by genes within the HLA complex. The structure of class II molecules is similar to that of class I molecules, with the shape of the antigen binding site being determined by hypervariable regions of the α and β chains. The HLA cleft-polypeptide complex is important in T-cell recognition and in determining an individual's T-cell repertoire (Marrack & Kappler, 1987).

There are several unique features of the HLA system which make these antigens excellent markers of host susceptibility: 1) the high degree of polymorphism at each locus, particularly with the B and D regions, 2) linkage disequilibrium between alleles at various loci, and 3) geographic and racial variation in the frequencies of specific HLA antigens (Dorman *et al.*, 1991). The polymorphic nature of HLA antigens, typically assessed at the protein level by HLA serological typing, permits the identification of genetic variation between individuals (Tiwari & Terasaki, 1985). However, the recognition of critical hypervariable sequences, which distinguish serologically-defined antigens at the DNA level, provides a far more accurate evaluation of the presence or absence of susceptibility alleles to autoimmune diseases, such as IDDM (Trucco, 1992). Linkage disequilibrium, another important feature of the HLA system, refers to the fact that particular haplotypes are much more common in a given population than expected, based upon the respective gene frequencies in the same population (Tiwari & Terasaki, 1985). This phenomenon has been suggested as one potential explanation for HLA-disease associations, which may be the result of linkage disequilibrium between HLA antigens and the 'true' disease susceptibility genes. Finally, there are major geographical and racial variations in the frequency of particular HLA antigens across populations (Tiwari & Terasaki, 1985). Population variation in the distribution of HLA antigens has been suggested to have a major influence on the strength of disease associations within populations, and affect the geographic distribution of autoimmune diseases such as IDDM (Tiwari & Terasaki, 1985). This has provided a rationale for international studies of IDDM.

Associations between HLA and IDDM began to be documented in the mid-1970s when it was observed that individuals with the disease were significantly more likely to be positive for the class I molecules HLA-B8 and B15 than nondiabetic controls (Nerup *et al.*, 1974; Cudworth & Woodrow, 1976). With the discovery of class II molecules, associations between DR locus antigens and IDDM became apparent. These studies revealed stronger relationships between IDDM and DR3 and/or DR4 than with the B locus antigens, which are in linkage disequilibrium with DR3 and DR4, respectively (Wolf *et al.*, 1983; Bertram & Baur, 1984). Approximately 95% of IDDM cases from most populations studied had either DR3 and/or DR4, and individuals with both DR3 and DR4 were particularly susceptible to developing the disease. However, racial differences were also observed. For example, associations to DR7 among African Americans (Reitnauer *et al.*, 1981) and/or DR9 among the Chinese (Hawkins *et al.*, 1987) and Japanese (Bertram & Baur, 1984) were reported. With advances in molecular biology, studies of the associations between HLA and IDDM are now being conducted at the DNA level in populations from across the world.

10.3.3 INTERNATIONAL MOLECULAR STUDIES OF IDDM

International comparative molecular studies of IDDM can be viewed from two perspectives (Table 10.1) (Dorman, 1992). One is that of the immunogeneticist, who investigates racial and ethnic differences in HLA susceptibility genes to study the etiology of the disease. Recent molecular immunogenetic studies in a variety of racial and ethnic groups have revealed that DNA sequences coding for the presence of an amino acid other than aspartic acid in the 57th position of the DQB1 gene (non-Asp-57) is highly associated with IDDM susceptibility (Todd *et al.*, 1985; Morel *et al.*, 1988; Dorman *et al.*, 1990; Mijovic *et al.*, 1991; Conti *et al.*, 1991; Ronningen *et al.*, 1991; Khalil *et al.*, 1992; Gutierrez-Lopez *et al.*, 1992). These associations were much stronger than those observed for HLA-DR3 and DR4. Moreover, non-DR3 and non-DR4 diabetic haplotypes typically carried non-Asp-57 alleles, suggesting that the DR associations were due to linkage disequilibrium with non-Asp-57 genes (Morel *et al.*, 1988). The consistency of these findings in most populations studied confirm their importance as IDDM susceptibility genes.

However, an interesting exception was found among the Japanese. The DR4-DQw4 haplotype which confers IDDM susceptibility in the Japanese contains DQA1*0301 and DQB1*0401. The latter is Asp-57 positive, but the DQA1 gene contained sequences coding for arginine in position 52 of the α chain (Todd *et al.*, 1990; Ronningen *et al.*, 1991; Awata *et al.*, 1992). DQA1*0301 was also found on African American, but not

Table 10.1 Importance of international comparative molecular studies of IDDM. (From Dorman, 1992.)

Immunogenetic perspective	Epidemiologic perspective
1. Evaluate racial/ethnic differences in linkage disequilibrium and their association with IDDM	1. Examine population differences in incidence and potential risk factors
2. Identify critical DNA sequences common to susceptibility genes	2. Evaluate contribution of genetic and environmental risk factors to patterns of disease
3. Examine interaction between IDDM susceptibility genes	3. Apply results to public health

Caucasian DR7 haplotypes, both of which encode DQB1*0201 (non-Asp-57). Caucasian DR7 haplotypes contain the DQA1*0201 allele and appear to be less diabetogenic. The Arg-52 α chain polymorphism has now been observed in other racial and ethnic groups and appears to contribute independently to IDDM risk (Todd *et al.*, 1990; Mijovic *et al.*, 1991; Awata *et al.*, 1992; Khalil *et al.*, 1992; Gutierrez-Lopez *et al.*, 1992). The heterodimer formed in trans between the DQA1*0501 (Arg-52) of the DQA1*0501-DQB1*0201 haplotype and the DQB1*0302 (non-Asp-57) of the DQA1*0301-DQB1*0302 haplotype, which are associated with DR3-DQw2 and DR4-DQw8, respectively, appears to be very 'diabetogenic' and may explain the high risk typically observed for DR3/DR4 heterozygotes. Moreover, there is a biological basis for these associations. Aspartic acid in position 57 of the DQ β chain, rather than a non-charged amino acid (i.e., alanine, valine, serine), and arginine in position 52 of the DQ α chain, alters the peptide-binding ability of the molecule which influences the recognition of the HLA-peptide complex by particular T-cell clones (Trucco, 1992). A structural modification of this type may explain the importance of specific amino acid sequences in determining susceptibility or resistance to autoimmune diseases, such as IDDM.

The second perspective illustrated in Table 10.1 is that of the epidemiologist, who conducts international comparative studies with a primary concern for public health (Dorman, 1992). These investigations, which focus on the genetic determinants of the disease, are now being conducted to examine population differences in the prevalence of IDDM susceptibility genes. Such studies also have the potential for assessing the contribution of genetic and environmental risk factors to the worldwide patterns of disease. Moreover, knowledge of the proportion of exposed or susceptible individuals in various populations, and the magnitude of their respective risks, will provide information necessary for the implementation of prevention strategies and health planning initiatives. Thus, each perspective, that of the immunogeneticist and the epidemiologist, will independently contribute to our knowledge concerning the etiology and prevention of IDDM. However, a combination of these approaches, representing an interface between molecular biology and epidemiology, will test unique hypotheses and achieve more in terms of scientific advancement and public health than either perspective alone.

10.3.4 MOLECULAR IDDM EPIDEMIOLOGY AND THE DIAMOND PROJECT

Molecular epidemiology has recently been defined as 'a science that focuses on the contribution of potential genetic and environmental risk factors, identified at the molecular level, to the etiology, distribution and prevention of disease within families and across populations' (Dorman, 1992). The objectives of molecular epidemiology are quite broad and include descriptive and analytical studies to evaluate host/environmental interactions in disease, and the development of prevention strategies, such as genetic screening to identify high-risk individuals, the use of recombinant vaccines, and the detection of bacteria, parasites and viruses at the molecular level.

At the present time, the Human Genome Project is the major stimulus for the evolution of molecular epidemiology (Dorman, 1992). During the next decade, information regarding the underlying susceptibility to most acute and chronic diseases will become available (Watson & Cook-Deegan, 1990). It will, therefore, be possible to evaluate host characteristics with extreme precision at the molecular level, and identify individuals with a genetic predisposition to virtually any disease. These DNA markers will be employed in clinical practices, as well as in descriptive and analytic epidemiologic research to replace more traditional measures of host susceptibility such as age, race, sex or a positive family history of the disease. An excellent example of the integration of DNA technology into epidemiology has been the evolution of international case-control molecular studies of IDDM through the WHO DIAMOND Project.

The identification of the HLA molecular polymorphisms which were strongly associated with IDDM susceptibility provided the rationale for the development of the DIAMOND Case-Control Molecular Epidemiology Sub-Project, which is based on a funded NIH grant (R01-DK42316) (Dorman, 1992). The objectives of this sub-project are: 1) to determine the degree to which the distribution of HLA class II genes, which are associated with IDDM, vary across racial groups and countries, and 2) to evaluate the contribution of differences in the frequency of HLA class II genes to the geographic and racial variation in IDDM incidence. The epidemiologic and laboratory standards required for this DIAMOND Sub-Project were developed during the NATO Advanced Research Work-shop 'Standardization of Epidemiologic Studies of Host Susceptibility' for the DIAMOND Project, held at the University of Pittsburgh in June, 1992 (Dorman *et al.*, 1994).

Our initial evaluation for this study focused on the DQB1 gene, and the association between non-Asp-57 and IDDM incidence across five populations: China (Bao *et al.*, 1989), African Americans and Caucasians from Allegheny County, Norway (Ronningen *et al.*, 1989) and Sardinia. The HLA-DQB1 genotype distributions varied significantly among IDDM cases ($p < 0.001$) and non-diabetic controls ($p < 0.001$), with an increase in non-Asp-57 homozygosity in high incidence areas (Dorman *et al.*, 1990). Moreover, in each of the five populations tested, relative risks for non-Asp-57 homozygotes compared to Asp-57 homozygotes were highly significant, ranging from 14 to 111, confirming that within all populations tested, non-Asp-57 was a strong marker of IDDM susceptibility. For Allegheny County Caucasians, the absolute risk was highest for non-Asp-57 homozygotes (47.6/100 000 per year), intermediate for heterozygous individuals (13.0/100 000 per year) and lowest for Asp-57 homozygotes (0.45/100 000 per year). Such estimates, which are only possible from population-based molecular studies, were suggestive of a dose-response relationship to IDDM susceptibility and further indicated that this genetic marker appears to play a critical role in the etiology of the disease.

If the geographic differences in disease incidence are due to variation in host susceptibility, then one would predict that the genotype-specific incidence rates would be similar across populations (Dorman *et al.*, 1990). Because the statistical properties of the

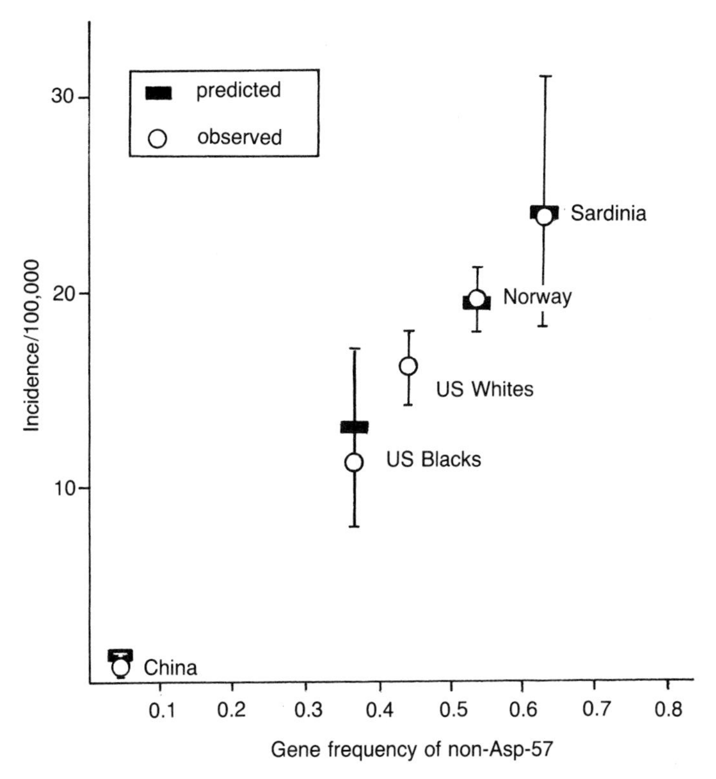

Figure 10.1 Association between actual and predicted age-adjusted annual IDDM incidence rates. The 95% confidence intervals are indicated by the bars associated with each observed incidence value (from Dorman *et al.*, 1990).

genotype-specific rates are currently under investigation, this issue was addressed indirectly by applying the point estimates for Allegheny County Caucasians to the other four populations to predict the overall IDDM incidence rate for each area. As shown in Figure 10.1, each of the predicted rates fell within the 95% confidence intervals for the rate established through IDDM registries. It will be possible in the future to evaluate directly the geographic variation in IDDM incidence among genetically homogeneous subgroups, and to quantify accurately the contribution of IDDM susceptibility genes to the global patterns of IDDM incidence.

A recent study from Madrid, using the standardized DIAMOND Protocol, illustrates the importance of arginine in position 52 of the DQα chain, particularly in the presence of non-Asp-57, from an epidemiologic perspective (Gutierrez-Lopez *et al.*, 1992). The absolute risk of developing IDDM was markedly increased (101.7/100 000 per year) among those who were homozygous for both non-Asp-57 and Arg-52, revealing a synergistic interaction between these two markers. Moreover, the attributable risk was estimated as 62%, indicating that approximately two-thirds of the incidence of IDDM in Madrid could be explained by these two high-risk alleles. In contrast, individuals who were heterozygous at one of the two loci had a risk similar to that for the general population (12.8/100 000 per year). This study provided evidence of a quantitative effect on IDDM susceptibility, since the absolute IDDM risk varied by the possibility of generating 4, 2, or 1 'diabetogenic' heterodimer, and emphasized the importance of the complete molecule rather than a single chain alone in the etiology of the disease. These associations with IDDM are currently being investigated as part of the DIAMOND Case-Control Molecular Epidemiology Sub-Project.

10.3.5 ISLET CELL ANTIBODIES AND IDDM

Organ-specific antibodies have long been recognized as one of the hallmarks of autoimmune disease. Antibodies against islet cell cytoplasmic antigens (ICAs) (Bottazzo *et al.*, 1974), as well as antibodies to insulin (Palmer *et al.*, 1983), the 64 kD islet cell antigen (Baekkeskov *et al.*, 1982), and most recently the enzyme glutamic acid decarboxylase (GAD) (Baekkeskov *et al.*, 1990) have been reported in IDDM. However, it is unclear whether they play a direct role in the disease process or serve as a marker of tissue damage initiated by other etiologic agents (Bottazzo, 1986). Despite immunological heterogeneity among ICAs and variation in laboratory methodology, most studies have reported a very high prevalence of ICAs (65–100%) among patients with newly diagnosed IDDM (Lipton & LaPorte, 1989). After disease onset, however, ICAs rarely persist. This contrasts with prevalence rates of 2–5% among first-degree relatives of IDDM patients and 0.5% or less among control subjects. ICAs are potent risk factors for IDDM, with relative risks ranging from 50–500 for first-degree relatives (Lipton & LaPorte, 1989). However, recent studies have shown that anti-GAD antibodies are much more sensitive and specific markers of IDDM than ICAs (Palmer & McCulloch, 1991; Baekkeskov *et al.*, 1987; Atkinson *et al.*, 1990; Christie *et al.*, 1992).

Since fewer than 50% of ICA positive individuals eventually develop the disease (Bruining *et al.*, 1989; Riley *et al.*, 1990; Bonifacio *et al.*, 1990), and approximately 20–30% of IDDM cases do not exhibit anti-GAD antibodies (Rowley *et al.*, 1992; Zimmet *et al.*, 1994), it is likely that genetic and/or other environmental factors further contribute to the risk of developing the disease. Data from studies which have evaluated both host susceptibility and immune markers have provided support for this hypothesis. For example, non-Asp-57 homozygosity was increased among ICA positive school children compared with local healthy controls (64.5% vs. 33.4%, $p < 0.01$) (Boehm *et al.*, 1991). Moreover, it was recently shown that the prevalence of anti-GAD antibodies among IDDMs who possessed DR3 and/or DR4 was significantly higher than that for diabetics who do not carry these high-risk alleles (76.9% vs. 47.8%, $p < 0.05$) (Serjeantson *et al.*, 1992). Interestingly, a study of French schoolchildren found a similar distribution of DQB1 non-Asp-57 alleles among ICA positive and negative individuals (Levy-Marchal *et al.*, 1992). These findings are consistent with our molecular studies of ICA positive and negative first-degree relatives from Allegheny County, PA (Lipton *et al.*, 1992). Although the proportions of first-degree relatives who were homozygous for both non-Asp-57 and Arg-52 were similar among the ICA positives (19%) and negatives (15%), the subsequent development of IDDM was restricted to individuals who were both ICA positive and genetically susceptible. By evaluating the presence or absence of high-risk IDDM susceptibility genes, organ-specific autoantibodies, and exposure to environmental risk factors in future family and case-control studies, one will be able to assess both the relative and absolute risks associated with these potential determinants of the disease.

10.4 ENVIRONMENTAL COMPONENTS OF IDDM ETIOLOGY

Monozygotic twin studies have provided important evidence for the role of environmental factors in the etiology of IDDM, revealing an IDDM concordance rate of approximately 36% (Olmos *et al.*, 1988). If the etiology of IDDM were entirely due to genetic factors, the concordance rate would be expected to be near 100%. Supporting evidence from migrant studies and the reported epidemics suggest that IDDM is a multifactorial disorder, and that genetic susceptibility is necessary, but not sufficient, for the development of the disease. Viruses, toxins, psychosocial factors and nutritional intake have all been implicated as potential environmental triggers.

10.4.1 VIRUSES

Strong arguments have been made for the role of the Coxsackie B virus in IDDM etiology. Coxsackie viruses B2, B3, B4 and B5 have all been isolated from the sera of persons with newly-diagnosed IDDM; however, the Coxsackie B4 virus has been the most commonly found. The most convincing evidence linking the Coxsackie B4 virus to the development of IDDM comes from a case report whereby a variant of the Coxsackie B4 virus was isolated from the pancreas of a 10-year-old boy who died seven days after the abrupt onset of IDDM following a flu-like illness (Yoon *et al.*, 1979). Lymphocytic infiltration of the islets of Langerhans and beta cell necrosis, as well as increased serum antibody titer to the virus was found at autopsy. Genetically susceptible mice were subsequently injected with the virus and developed IDDM. Higher mean Coxsackie B virus antibody titers have also been observed in persons with recent onset IDDM (Gamble, 1980). A study by King *et al.* (1983) also found a positive relationship between Coxsackie B virus infection and recent onset of IDDM.

On the other hand, Palmer *et al.* (1982) did not find more Coxsackie B antibody in persons with IDDM (46%) versus age-matched controls (52%). It is hypothesized that variants of the Coxsackie B virus have different diabetogenic potential, although it is unknown whether the virus initiates or accelerates beta cell destruction. Since estimates have shown that only 30% of IDDM cases are associated with Coxsackie B viruses, the search for other environmental etiological factors remains (Yoon & Rayfield, 1986).

Attention has recently focused on persistent viral infections as possible triggers of autoimmune disease (Yoon, 1990). The incorporation of human cytomegalovirus (CMV) gene segments into genomic DNA has been significantly associated with IDDM among newly-diagnosed patients (Pak *et al.*, 1988) and a relationship between CMV genome positive and islet cell antibodies has also been reported (Pak *et al.*, 1988; Nicoletti *et al.*, 1990). Persistent CMV infection may lead to the expression of viral or host antigens on the beta cells of the pancreas, resulting in the production of ICA. Alternatively, molecular mimicry may contribute to the production of antibodies that recognize both viral and host antigens. Aberrant beta cell expression of HLA class II molecules may also contribute to the beginning of an autoimmune response, particularly if non-Asp-57 is present. These issues need to be further explored in etiologic research.

Congenital rubella syndrome (CRS) has been associated with the development of IDDM due to the high prevalence of IDDM in persons with CRS (approximately 20% in the United States) compared to the general population (Menser *et al.*, 1978). Studies by Ginsberg-Fellner *et al.* (1984 & 1985) found a high frequency of IDDM-associated HLA antigens (DR3/DR4) in persons with CRS. In addition, islet cell surface antibodies were discovered in 20% of individuals with CRS which is consistent with that of the IDDM population. It has therefore been hypothesized that exposure to rubella infection *in utero* triggers an autoimmune mechanism in genetically susceptible individuals subsequently resulting in IDDM.

Several case reports have described a temporal relationship between mumps virus infection and the development of IDDM (King, 1962; Messaritikas *et al.*, 1971). Epidemiological studies validating this observation have met with limited success. The incidence data for IDDM was found to parallel the incidence data for mumps after allowing for a 4-year lag period in Erie County, New York. Also noted was that approximately 50% of children with IDDM in this population also had mumps or exposure to mumps approximately 4 years prior to IDDM onset (Sultz *et al.*, 1975). Methodologic problems, including the fact that only one-third of the IDDM population of Erie County was evaluated, limit the validity of this study. A study by West *et al.* (1981) found no evidence of antecedent mumps infection and subsequent onset of IDDM in residents of Montreal. As with Coxsackie B virus, it has been suggested that a particular variant of the mumps virus in combination with genetic susceptibility is necessary for development of IDDM. If mumps is a cause of IDDM it is likely to be so in only a small proportion of cases.

10.4.2 TOXINS AND CHEMICALS

Several case reports have related the ingestion of the rodenticide, Vacor, which contains the active chemical N-3-pyridylmethyl n^1-p-nitrophenylurea with the occurrence of IDDM (Pont *et al.*, 1979). It is unlikely, however that toxic chemicals are a predominant cause of IDDM. Arner *et al.* (1983) described steroid-induced diabetes in 46% of renal transplant recipients receiving corticosteroids. As this type of diabetes is dose-dependent, and in some cases reversible once the drug dosage is lowered, it shows a higher resemblance to non-insulin dependent diabetes mellitus.

10.4.3 STRESS

Stressful events have also been suggested to be triggering factors involved in the etiology of IDDM, perhaps by lowering the resistance to infection in genetically susceptible individuals through direct or indirect mechanisms (Craighead, 1978; Williams *et al.*, 1981). Early studies on stress and IDDM showed conflicting results and suffered from methodological problems, such as inadequate control groups, poor data collection instruments for measuring psychological stress, recall bias, and small sample sizes (Hauser & Pollets, 1979). However, a relatively recent 3-year retrospective study by Robinson and Fuller (1985) found that persons with IDDM had a higher frequency of one or more severe life events and severe difficulties prior to diagnosis than did matched siblings and neighbors. More research needs to be done to clarify the role of stress in the etiology of IDDM.

10.4.4 NUTRITION

Various nutrients and nutritional practices have been associated with the development of IDDM. Helgason and Jonasson (1981) implicated the ingestion of smoked/cured mutton by Icelandish women near the time of conception as a potential cause of IDDM in male offspring; however, a study from Scotland by Symon *et al.* (1984) failed to find a relationship between smoked food intake by mothers and subsequent development of IDDM in their children. Dahlquist *et al.* (1990) found a positive linear relationship between the intake of solid foods containing high amounts of protein and nitrosamines and the risk of IDDM. A significant but non-linear relationship between carbohydrate intake and IDDM was also found. Theories include the possibilities that proteins and certain amino acids may trigger an autoimmune response, that long-term exposure to nitrosamines or gliadin proteins in carbohydrates may have toxic effects on β-cells or increase their susceptibility to other agents. These effects may also be potentiated by the occurrence of frequent infections (Dahlquist *et al.*, 1991).

Coffee consumption, in particular caffeine and other metabolites by women during pregnancy, has also been hypothesized to be toxic to the intrauterine development of pancreatic cells in genetically susceptible fetuses. This hypothesis arose from a recent study by Tuomilehto *et al.* (1990) that found a correlation between coffee consumption of various countries and the incidence of IDDM in persons <15 year ($r = 0.74$). Pozzilli and Bottazzo (1991) noted that many countries with a high coffee consumption also have a high sugar intake and that the correlation between sugar consumption and IDDM ($r = 0.55$) closely matches that of coffee, which may be more relevant to the pathogenesis of the disease.

Nicotinamide is a water-soluble vitamin that functions in the body as a component of two coenzymes, nicotinamide adenine dinucleotide (NAD) and nicotinamide adenine dinucleotide phosphate (NADP) (National Research Council, 1989). Animal studies have shown that treatment with high doses of nicotinamide prevents the induction of diabetes by streptozotocin in rats by increasing the NAD content, and subsequently proinsulin synthesis, in the β cells (Uchigata, 1983). Nicotinamide has also been shown to favor the regeneration of β cells in partially pancreatectomized rats (Yonemura *et al.*, 1984). Vague *et al.* (1989) provided nicotinamide at 3 g/day for 9 months to adults with IDDM who had received insulin for 1–5 years and found that residual insulin secretion could be protected post-honeymoon period in those receiving nicotinamide versus placebo. However, Chase *et al.* (1990) did not observe a preservation of residual insulin secretion in children with newly-diagnosed IDDM who received a nicotinamide dose of 1.5 g/day or less for 1 year. Finally, Elliott and Chase (1991) examined the effect of a maximum 3 g/day nicotinamide administration to children considered to be at a high IDDM risk (first-degree relatives of persons with IDDM, islet cell antibody levels of 80 IUs or more and first phase insulin release <5th percentile). Remarkably, only one child in 14 who received nicotinamide has developed IDDM, whereas all eight children who did not receive treatment have since been diagnosed. Further research certainly needs to be conducted to determine the length of the delay that nicotinamide may permit and the dosage required (see also Chapter 46).

By far the most widely studied nutritional factor with regard to IDDM etiology is cow milk protein. An increased incidence of diabetes has been shown in BB rats with early exposure to dairy proteins (Daneman *et al.*, 1987). A Scandinavian study by Borch-Johnsen *et al.* (1984) found that children with IDDM were completely or partially breast-fed for a significantly shorter period of time ($p < 0.02$) compared to non-IDDM siblings. Evidence supporting this finding includes a Colorado study by Mayer *et al.* (1988) which discovered a decreased risk of IDDM among persons who had been breast-fed to an older age (OR = 0.54 for a duration of breast-feeding of over 12 months) and the ecologic analyses of Scott (1990), who reported a negative relationship between breast-feeding at age 3 months and IDDM risk ($r = -0.53$). A recent Finnish study also found a decreased risk of IDDM among children breast-fed for at least 7 months (OR = 0.45) and those exclusively breast-fed for at least 3 months (OR = 0.33). Children over 4 months of age at the time of supplementary cow's milk feeding also had a lower risk of IDDM (OR = 0.48) (Virtanen *et al.*, 1991).

In a matched case-control study Kostraba *et al.* (1992) found that in whites, persons with IDDM were less likely than those without IDDM to have been breast-fed (OR = 0.5). Duration of breast-feeding did not differ by diabetes status for whites or blacks. Blacks with IDDM were more likely to have received breast milk substitutes and cow's milk-based substitutes earlier than blacks without IDDM. This association, however, was not found in whites which the authors felt may have indicated a larger genetic influence in whites, or that other environmental factors were playing a role.

The whey protein bovine serum albumin (BSA) is the suggested milk protein trigger molecule which results in an autoimmune response in genetically susceptible individuals. Antibodies to a 17-amino-acid section of the BSA molecule (ABBOS) have been found in children with IDDM which have been shown to react with p69, a β cell surface protein (Karjalainen *et al.*, 1992). Infants have immature digestive systems which allow large protein chains, such as BSA, to pass directly into the bloodstream. It has been proposed that genetically susceptible children who have been exposed to cow's milk at an early age and prior to 'gut closure', which occurs between 3 and 12 months of age, build up an immunity to ABBOS. The sensitized immune system then mistakes the p69 β cell protein for ABBOS and ultimately destroys the β cell resulting in IDDM (Karjalainen *et al.*, 1992). However, genetically susceptible individuals do not always develop IDDM. The p69 protein is known to be displayed on the surface of the β cell during periods of stress, such as a viral infections. If during development an infant's immune system has had the opportunity to recognize p69 as self, the β cells do not risk attack. It has been theorized that multiple viral attacks are required, after a sensitivity to ABBOS has been developed, for enough β cell destruction to result in IDDM. This may partially explain the variation in age of IDDM onset that is observed (Karjalainen *et al.*, 1992). Without reference to IDDM, breast-feeding or iron-fortified infant formula is encouraged by the American Academy of Pediatrics to assure good nutrition for the first 6–12 months of life (McCarren, 1992).

10.5 SUMMARY

In his landmark book, Dr Kelly West, the founder of diabetes epidemiology, said

> It has become evident that many factors contribute in an important way in increasing or decreasing susceptibility to diabetes, and that systematic epidemiologic study has great potential for elucidating mechanisms by which both diabetes and its specific manifestations are caused or prevented. (West, 1978, p. 3)

Since that time, much has been learned about the epidemiologic patterns of IDDM in racial and ethnic groups around the world. This is primarily the result of collaborative international projects, such as the WHO DIAMOND Project, which has stimulated IDDM epidemiologic research worldwide. On almost every continent in the world, new data are beginning to emerge regarding the incidence of IDDM and its potential risk factors, particularly the genetic determinants, which vary in prevalence across populations. These efforts, as well as advances in DNA technology, have led to the development of a molecular epidemiologic research approach, which is being applied by the WHO Multinational Project for Childhood Diabetes to investigate the contribution of specific genetic markers, identified at the molecular level, to the overall incidence of IDDM within and across populations. These studies will provide critically important information regarding IDDM etiology during the next decade, and represent a new paradigm in the field of diabetes epidemiology.

In the future, issues such as morbidity and mortality, health care delivery and the economics of IDDM will also be addressed through the DIAMOND Project. Moreover, young epidemiologists are being trained in diabetes epidemiology, so that they will be able to monitor the patterns of disease in their communities and ultimately eliminate its occurrence, perhaps through modification of potential risk factors. These endeavors are expanding in all corners of the world and have resulted in an incredible network of scientists and clinicians who are directing their efforts towards a common goal: the prevention of insulin-dependent diabetes mellitus through epidemiologic approaches. With their continued efforts and the rapid progression of the field of diabetes epidemiology, Dr Kelly West's vision will be achieved.

ACKNOWLEDGEMENTS

This research was supported by NIH grants R01 DK42316 and R01 DK24021. The authors would like to acknowledge the collaboration and technology developments for the HLA class II molecular analyses by Dr Massimo Trucco at the University of Pittsburgh, and the support of the WHO Diamond Project Group, and in particular, Dr Ronald E. LaPorte, Dr Jaakko Tuomilehto (Principal Investigators) and Dr Hilary King (WHO Representative).

REFERENCES

Arner, P., Gunnarsson, R., Blomdahl, S. *et al.* (1983) Some characteristics of steroid diabetes: a study in renal-transplant recipients receiving high-dose corticosteroid therapy. *Diabetes Care*, **6**, 23–25.

Atkinson, M.A., Maclaren, N.K., Scharp, D.W. *et al.* (1990) 64 000 M^1 autoantibodies as predictors of insulin-dependent diabetes. *Lancet*, **335**, 1357.

Awata, T., Kuzuya, T., Matsuda, A. *et al.* (1992) Genetic analysis of HLA class II alleles and susceptibility to Type 1 (insulin-dependent) diabetes mellitus in Japanese subjects. *Diabetologia*, **35**, 419–24.

Baekkeskov, S., Nielsen, J.H., Marner, B. *et al.* (1982) Autoantibodies in newly diagnosed diabetic children immunoprecipitate human pancreatic islet cell proteins. *Nature*, **298**, 167.

Baekkeskov, S., Kristensen, J.K., Srikanta, S. *et al.* (1987) Antibodies to a M 64 000 human islet cell antigen precede the clinical onset of insulin-dependent diabetes. *J. Clin. Invest.*, **479**, 926.

Baekkeskov, S., Aanstoot, H.-K., Christgau, S. *et al.* (1990) Identification of the 64K autoantigen in insulin-dependent diabetes as the GABA-synthesizing enzyme glutamic acid decarboxylase. *Nature*, **347**, 151–56.

Bao, M.Z., Wang, J.X., Dorman, J.S. *et al.* (1989) HLA-DQ beta non-Asp-57 allele and incidence of diabetes in China and the USA. *Lancet*, **ii**, 497–98.

Barbosa, J., Chern, M.M., Anderson, V.E. *et al.* (1980) Linkage analysis between the major histocompatibility system and insulin-dependent diabetes in families with patients in two consecutive generations. *J. Clin. Invest.*, **65**, 592–601.

Bertram, J. and Baur, M. (1984) Insulin-dependent diabetes mellitus, in *Histocompatibility Testing*, pp. 348–68. Springer-Verlag, Heidelberg.

Bjorkman, P., Saper, M., Samraoui, W. *et al.* (1987) Structure of the human class I histocompatibility antigen, HLA-A2. *Nature*, **329**, 512–17.

Blom, L., Persson, L.A. and Dahlquist, G. (1992) A high linear growth is associated with an increased risk of childhood diabetes mellitus. *Diabetologia*, **35**, 528–33.

Bodansky, H.J., Staines, A., Stephenson, C. *et al.* (1992) Evidence for an environmental effect in the aetiology of insulin dependent diabetes in a transmigratory population. *Br. Med. J.*, **304**, 1020–22.

Boehm, B.B., Manfras, B., Seibler, J. *et al.* (1991) Epidemiology and immunogenetic background of islet cell antibody-positive nondiabetic schoolchildren. *Diabetes*, **40**, 1435–39.

Bonifacio, E., Bingley, P.J., Shattock, M. *et al.* (1990) Quantification of islet cell antibodies and prediction of insulin-dependent diabetes mellitus. *Lancet*, **335**, 147–49.

Borch-Johnsen, K., Mandrup-Poulsen, T., Zachau-Christiansen, B. *et al.* (1984) Relation between breast-feeding and incidence rates of insulin-dependent diabetes mellitus. *Lancet*, **ii**, 1083–86.

Bottazzo, G.F. (1986) Death of a β-cell. Homicide or suicide? *Diabetic Med.*, **3**, 119–30.

Bottazzo, G.F., Florin-Christensen, A. and Doniach, D. (1974) Islet cell antibodies in diabetes mellitus with autoimmune polyendocrine deficiencies. *Lancet*, **ii**, 1279.

Bruining, G.J., Molenaar, J.L., Grobbee, D.E. *et al.* (1989) Ten-year follow-up study of islet cell antibodies and childhood diabetes mellitus. *Lancet*, **i**, 1100–13.

Bruno, G., Merletti, F., Pisu, E. *et al.* (1990) Incidence of IDDM during 1984–1986 in population aged <30 yr. residents of Turin, Italy. *Diabetes Care*, **13** (10), 1051–56.

Burden, A.C., Samanta, A. and Chaudhuri, K.R. (1990) The prevalence and incidence of insulin-dependent diabetes in White (W) and Indian (I) children in Leicester City (UK). *Intnl. J. Diab. Dev. Countries*, **10**, 8–10.

Burden, A.C., Burden, M.L., Williams, E.R. *et al.* (1991) Evidence of frequent epidemics of childhood diabetes. *Diabetes*, **40**, 373A.

Calori, G., Gallus, G., Garancini, P. *et al.* (1990) Identification of the cohort of type 1 diabetes presenting in Lombardy in 1983–84: A validated assessment. *Diabetic Med.*, **7**, 595–99.

Carrasco, E., Lopez, G., Garcia de los Rios, M. *et al.* (1991) Incidencia de diabetes mellitus insulinodependiente en la region metropolitana. *Rev. Med. Chile*, **119**, 709–14.

Chase, H.P., Butler-Simon, N., Garg, S. *et al.* (1990) A trial of nicotinamide in newly diagnosed patients with type 1 (insulin-dependent) diabetes mellitus. *Diabetologia*, **33**, 444–46.

Chern, M.M., Anderson, V.E. and Barbosa, J. (1982) Empirical risk for insulin-dependent diabetes (IDD) in sibs: Further definition of genetic heterogeneity. *Diabetes*, **31**, 1115–18.

Christie, M.R., Tunry, R., Lo, S.S. *et al.* (1992) Antibodies to GAD and tryptic fragments of islet 64K antigens as distinct markers in the development of IDDM. Studies with identical twins. *Diabetes*, **41**, 782–87.

Contu, L., Carcassi, C. and Trucco, M. (1991) Diabetes susceptibility in Sardinia. *Lancet*, **338**, 65.

Craighead, J.E. (1978) Current views on the etiology of insulin dependent diabetes mellitus. *New Engl. J. Med.*, **299**, 1439–45.

Cudworth, A.G. and Woodrow, J.D. (1976) Genetic susceptibility in diabetes mellitus: analyses of the HLA association. *Br. Med. J.*, **2**, 846–68.

Dahlquist, G., Blom, L., Holmgren, G. *et al.* (1985) The epidemiology of diabetes in Swedish children 0–14 years – a six year prospective study. *Diabetologia*, **28**, 802–808.

Dahlquist, G., Blom, L., Tuvemo, T. *et al.* (1989) The Swedish childhood diabetes study. Results from a nine year case registry and a one year case-referent study indicating that Type I (insulin-dependent) diabetes mellitus is associated with both Type II (non-insulin-dependent) diabetes mellitus and autoimmune disorders. *Diabetologia*, **32**, 2–6.

Dahlquist, G.G., Blom, L.G., Persson, L. *et al.* (1990) Dietary factors and the risk of developing insulin dependent diabetes in childhood. *Br. Med. J.*, **300**, 1302–1306.

Dahlquist, G., Blom, L. and Lonnberg, G. (1991) The Swedish childhood diabetes study – A multivariate analysis of risk determinants for diabetes in different age groups. *Diabetologia*, **34**, 757–62.

Daneman, D., Fishman, L., Clarson, C. *et al.* (1987) Dietary triggers of insulin-dependent diabetes in the BB rat. *Diabetes Res.*, **5**, 93–97.

Degnbol, B. and Green, A. (1978) Diabetes mellitus among first and second degree relatives of early onset diabetics. *Ann. Hum. Genet.*, **42**, 25–47.

Diabetes Epidemiology Research International Group (1987) Preventing insulin dependent diabetes mellitus: The environmental challenge. *Br. Med. J.*, **295**, 479–81.

Diabetes Epidemiology Research International Group (1988) Geographic patterns of childhood insulin-dependent diabetes mellitus. *Diabetes*, **37**, 1113–19.

Diabetes Epidemiology Research International Group (1990a) The epidemiology and immunogenetics of IDDM in Italian-heritage populations. *Diab. Metab. Rev.*, **6**, 63–69.

Diabetes Epidemiology Research International Group (1990b) Secular trends in incidence of childhood IDDM in 10 countries. *Diabetes*, **39**, 858–64.

Dokheel, T. (1992) Personal Communication.

Dorman, J.S. (1992) Genetic epidemiology of insulin-dependent diabetes mellitus: international comparisons using molecular genetics. *Ann. Med.*, **24**, 393–99.

Dorman, J.S., LaPorte, R.E., Kuller, L.H. *et al.* (1984). The Pittsburgh insulin-dependent diabetes mellitus (IDDM) morbidity and mortality study. Mortality results. *Diabetes*, **33**, 271–76.

Dorman, J.S., LaPorte, R.E., Stone, R.A. *et al.* (1990) Worldwide differences in the incidence of type I diabetes are associated with amino acid variation at position 57 of the HLA-DQ β chain. *Proc. Natl. Acad. Sci.*, **87**, 7370–74.

Dorman, J.S., LaPorte, R.E., and Trucco, M. (1991) 'Genes and environment', in B. Tait and L. Harrison (eds). *The Genetics of Diabetes Mellitus*, pp. 229–45. Bailliere Tindall, London.

Dorman, J.S., Kocova, M., O'Leary, L.A. *et al.* (1994) 'Case-control molecular epidemiology studies: standards for the WHO DIAMOND Project', in J. Dorman (ed.). *Standardization of epidemiologic studies of host susceptibility, NATO ASI Series*, Plenum Publishing Corp., New York.

Drykoningen, C.E.M., Mulder, A.L.M., Vaandrager, G.J. *et al.* (1992) The incidence of male childhood Type 1 (insulin-dependent) diabetes mellitus is rising rapidly in The Netherlands. *Diabetologia*, **35**, 139–42.

Elamin, A., Omer, M.I.A., Zein, K. *et al.* (1992) Epidemiology of childhood type I diabetes in Sudan, 1987–1990. *Diabetes Care*, **15**, 1556–59.

Elliott, R.B. and Chase, H.P. (1991) Prevention or delay of type 1 (insulin-dependent) diabetes mellitus in children using nicotinamide. *Diabetologia*, **34**, 362–65.

Field, L.L. (1988) Insulin-dependent diabetes mellitus: A model for the study of multifactorial disorders. *Am. J. Hum. Genet.*, **43**, 793–98.

Fishbein, H.A., LaPorte, R.E., Orchard, T.J. *et al.* (1982) The Pittsburgh insulin-dependent diabetes mellitus registry: Seasonal incidence. *Diabetologia*, **23**, 83–85.

Fleegler, F.M., Rogers, K.D., Drash, A. *et al.* (1979) Age, sex and season of onset of juvenile diabetes in different geographic areas. *Pediatrics*, **63**, 374–79.

Gamble, D.R. (1980) The epidemiology of insulin-dependent diabetes, with particular reference to the relationship of virus infection to its etiology. *Epidemiologic Rev.*, **2**, 49–70.

Gay, E.C., Hamman, R.F. and Carosone-Link, P.J. (1989) Colorado IDDM Registry: Lower incidence of IDDM in hispanics – Comparisons of disease characteristics and care patterns in biethnic population. *Diabetes Care*, **12**, 701–708.

Ginsberg-Fellner, F., Witt, M.E., Yagihashi, S. *et al.* (1984) Congenital rubella syndrome as a model for type I (insulin-dependent) diabetes mellitus: increased prevalence of islet cell surface antibodies. *Diabetologia*, **27**, 87–89.

Ginsberg-Fellner, F., Witt, M.E., Fedun, B. *et al.* (1985) Diabetes mellitus and autoimmunity in patients with the congenital rubella syndrome. *Rev. Inf. Dis.*, **7** (suppl. 1), S170–74.

Green, A., Svejgaard, A., Platz, P. *et al.* (1985) The genetic susceptibility to insulin-dependent diabetes mellitus: Combined segregation and linkage analyses. *Genet. Epidemiol.*, **2**, 1–15.

Green, A., Gale, E.A.M. and Patterson, C.C. (1992) Incidence of childhood-onset insulin-dependent diabetes mellitus: the EURODIAB ACE study. *Lancet*, **339**, 905–909.

Grey, A., Kubo, R., Colon, S. *et al.* (1987) The small subunit of HLA antigens is beta 2 microglobulin. *J. Exp. Med.*, **138**, 1608–1616.

Gutierrez-Lopez, M.D., Bertera, S., Chantres, M.T. *et al.* (1992) Susceptibility to Type 1 (insulin-dependent) diabetes mellitus in Spanish patients correlates quantitatively with expression of HLA-DQα Arg 52 and HLA-DQβ non-Asp 57 alleles. *Diabetologia*, **35**, 583–88.

Hauser, S.T. and Pollets, D. (1979) Psychological aspects of diabetes mellitus: A critical review. *Diabetes Care*, **2**, 227–32.

Hawkins, B.R., Lam, K.S., Ma, J.T. *et al.* (1987) Strong associations of HLA-DR3/DRw9 heterozygosity with early onset insulin-dependent diabetes mellitus in Chinese. *Diabetes*, **36**, 1297–1300.

Helgason, T. and Jonasson, M.R. (1981) Evidence for a food additive as a cause of ketosis-prone diabetes. *Lancet*, **ii**, 716–20.

Joner, G. and Sovik, O. (1981) Incidence, age at onset and seasonal variation of diabetes mellitus in Norwegian children. *Acta Paed. Scand.*, **70**, 329–35.

Joner, G. and Sovik, O. (1989) Increasing incidence of diabetes mellitus in Norwegian children 0–14 years of age 1973–1982. *Diabetologia*, **32**, 79–83.

Karjalainen, J., Martin, J.M., Knip, M. *et al.* (1992) A bovine albumin peptide as a possible trigger of insulin-dependent diabetes mellitus. *New*

Engl. J. Med., **327**, 302–307.

Karvonen, M., Tuomilehto, J., Libman, I. *et al.* (1993) A review of the recent epidemiological data on the worldwide incidence of Type I (insulin-dependent) diabetes mellitus. *Diabetologia*, **36**, 883–92.

Khalil, I., Deschamps, I., Lepage, V. *et al.* (1992) Dose effect of cis- and trans-encoded HLA-DQαβ heterodimers in IDDM susceptibility. *Diabetes*, **41**, 378–84.

King, M.L., Bidwell, D., Shaikh, A. *et al.* (1983) Coxsackie-B-virus-specific IgM responses in children with insulin-dependent (juvenile-onset; Type I) diabetes mellitus. *Lancet*, **i**, 1397–99.

King, R.C. (1962) Mumps followed by diabetes. *Lancet*, **ii**, 1055.

Kostraba, J.N., Dorman, J.S., LaPorte, R.E. *et al.* (1992) Early infant diet and risk of IDDM in blacks and whites. *Diabetes Care*, **15**, 626–31.

Krolewski, A.S., Warram, J.H., Rand, L.I. *et al.* (1987) Epidemiologic approach to the etiology of type I diabetes mellitus and its complications. *New Engl. J. Med.*, **317**, 1390–98.

LaPorte, R.E. and Cruickshanks, K.J. (1984) 'Incidence and risk factors for insulin-dependent diabetes mellitus', in *Diabetes In America, Data Compiled 1984*. National Diabetes Group, Washington, DC, United States Department of Health and Human Services 1985:V-1-8 (NIH Publication No. 85-1468).

LaPorte, R.E. and Tajima, N. (1985) 'Prevalence of insulin-dependent diabetes', in *Diabetes In America, Data Compiled 1984*. National Diabetes Group, Washington, DC, United States Department of Health and Human Services 1985:V-1-8 (NIH Publication No. 85-1468).

LaPorte, R.E., Tajima, N., Akerblom, H.K. *et al.* (1985) Geographic differences in the risk of insulin-dependent diabetes mellitus: The importance of registries. *Diabetes Care*, **8** (suppl. 1), 101–107.

LaPorte, R.E., Tajima, N., Dorman, J.S. *et al.* (1986) Differences between blacks and whites in the epidemiology of insulin-dependent diabetes mellitus in Allegheny County, Pennsylvania. *Am. J. Epidemiol.*, **123**, 592–602.

Laron, Z., Karp, M., Modan, M. (1985) The incidence of insulin-dependent diabetes mellitus in Israeli children and adolescents 0–20 years of age: a retrospective study, 1975–1980. *Diabetes Care*, **6** (suppl. 1), 24–28.

Levy-Marchal, C., Tichet, J., Fajardy, I. *et al.* (1992) Islet cell antibodies in normal French schoolchildren. *Diabetologia*, **35** (6), 577–82.

Lipton, R.B. and LaPorte, R.E. (1989) Epidemiology of islet cell antibodies. *Epidemiol. Rev.*, **11**, 182–203.

Lipton, R.B., Kocova, M., LaPorte, R.E. *et al.* (1992) Autoimmunity and genetics contribute to the risk of insulin-dependent diabetes mellitus in families: islet cell antibodies and HLA DQ heterodimers. *Am. J. Epidemiol.*, **136**, 503–512.

Marrack, P. and Kappler, J. (1987) The T cell receptor. *Science*, **238**, 1073–79.

Mason, D.R., Scott, R.S. and Darlow, B.A. (1987) Epidemiology of insulin-dependent diabetes mellitus in Canterbury, New Zealand. *Diab. Res. Clin. Pract.*, **3**, 21–29.

Mayer, E.J., Hamman, R.F., Gay, E.C. *et al.* (1988) Reduced risk of IDDM among breast-fed children. *Diabetes*, **37**, 1625–32.

McCarren, M. (1992) A case of mistaken identity. *Diabetes Forecast*, December.

McCarthy, B.J., Dorman, J.S., Aston, C.E. *et al.* (1991) Investigating genomic imprinting and susceptibility to insulin-dependent diabetes mellitus (IDDM): An epidemiologic approach. *Genetic Epidemiol.*, **8**, 177–86.

Menser, M.A., Forrest, J.M. and Bransky, R.O. (1978) Rubella infection and diabetes mellitus. *Lancet*, **i**, 57–60.

Messaritikas, J., Karabula, C., Kattamis, C. *et al.* (1971) Diabetes following mumps in sibs. *Arch. Dis. Child.*, **46**, 561–62.

Metcalfe, M.A. and Baum, J.D. (1991) Incidence of insulin-dependent diabetes in children aged under 15 years in the British Isles during 1988. *Brit. Med. J.*, **302**, 443–47.

Mijovic, C.H., Jenkins, D., Jacobs, K.H. *et al.* (1991) HLA-DQA1 and -DQB1 alleles associated with genetic susceptibility to IDDM in a black population. *Diabetes*, **40**, 748–53.

Morel, P.A., Dorman, J.S., Todd, J.A. *et al.* (1988) Aspartic acid at position 57 of the HLA-DQ beta chain protects against Type 1 diabetes. *Proc. Natl. Acad. Sci.*, **85**, 8111–16.

Muntoni, S., Songini, M. *et al.* (1992) High incidence rate of IDDM in Sardinia. *Diabetes Care*, **15**, 1317–22.

National Research Council (1989) *Recommended Dietary Allowances*, 10th edn. National Academy Press, Washington, DC.

Nerup, J., Platz, P., Anderson, O. *et al.* (1974) HLA antigens and diabetes mellitus. *Lancet*, **ii**, 864–67.

Nicoletti, F., Scalia, G., Lunetta, M. *et al.* (1990) Correlation between islet cell antibodies and anti-cytomegalovirus IgM and IgG antibodies in healthy first-degree relatives of type 1 (insulin-dependent) diabetic patients. *Clin. Immun. Immunopath.*, **55**, 139–47.

Olmos, P., A'Hern, R., Heaton, D.A. *et al.* (1988) The significance of concordance rate for type 1 (insulin-dependent) diabetes in identical twins. *Diabetologia*, **31**, 747–50.

Orchard, T.J., Dorman, J.S., Maser, R.E. *et al.* (1990) The prevalence of complications in insulin-dependent diabetes mellitus by sex and duration: Pittsburgh epidemiology of diabetes complications study – I. *Diabetes*, **39**, 1116–24.

Pak, C.Y., Eun, H.M., McArthur, R.G. *et al.* (1988) Association of cytomegalovirus infection with autoimmune type 1 diabetes. *Lancet*, **ii**, 1–4.

Palmer, J.P., Cooney, M.K., Ward, R.H. *et al.* (1982) Reduced Coxsackie antibody titers in type I (insulin-dependent) diabetic patients presenting during an outbreak of Coxsackie B3 and B4 infection. *Diabetologia*, **22**, 426–29.

Palmer, J.P., Asplin, C.M., Clemons, P. *et al.* (1983) Insulin antibodies in insulin-dependent diabetes before insulin treatment. *Science*, **222**, 1337.

Palmer, J.P. and McCulloch, D.K. (1991) Prediction and prevention of IDDM – 1991. *Diabetes*, **40**, 943.

Podar, T., Tuomilehto-Wolf, E., Tuomilehto, J. *et al.* (1992) Insulin-dependent diabetes mellitus in native Estonians and immigrants to Estonia. *Am. J. Epidemiol.*, **135** (11), 1231–36.

Podar, T., Tuomilehto, J., Tuomilehto-Wolf, E. *et al.* (1994) 'The risk of insulin-dependent diabetes in offspring of parents with insulin-dependent diabetes, a review', in J. Dorman (ed.). *Standardization of epidemiologic studies of host susceptibility, NATO ASI Series*, Plenum Publishing Corp., New York.

Pont, A., Rubino, J.M., Bishop, D. *et al.* (1979) Diabetes mellitus and neuropathy following vacor ingestion in man. *Arch. Inter. Med.*, **139**, 185–87.

Pozzilli, P. and Bottazzo, G.F. (1991) Coffee or sugar: which is to blame in IDDM? *Diabetes Care*, **14**, 144–45.

Reitnauer, P.J., Roseman, J.M., Barger, B.O. *et al.* (1981) HLA associations with insulin-dependent diabetes mellitus in a sample of the American black population. *Tissue Antigens*, **17**, 286–93.

Rewers, M., LaPorte, R.E., Walczak, M. *et al.* (1987) Apparent epidemic of insulin-dependent diabetes mellitus in midwestern Poland. *Diabetes*, **36**, 106–13.

Riley, W.J., Maclaren, N.K., Krischer, J. *et al.* (1990) A prospective study of the development of diabetes in relatives of patients with insulin-dependent diabetes. *New Eng. J. Med.*, **323**, 1167–72.

Robinson, N. and Fuller, J.H. (1985) Role of life events and difficulties in the onset of diabetes mellitus. *J. Psych. Res.*, **29**, 583–91.

Robles Valdes, C., Cornejo, B.J., Dorantes, A.L. *et al.* (1987) Incidencia de la diabetes mellitus tipo I, 1984–1986, en el D.F. y area metropolitana (A.M.). *Proc. Soc. Mex. Nutr. Endocrinol.*, Merida.

Ronningen, K.S., Gjertsen, H.A., Iwe, T. *et al.* (1991) Particular HLA-DQ αβ heterodimer associated with IDDM susceptibility in both DR4-DQw4 Japanese and DR4-DQw8/DRw8-DQw4 whites. *Diabetes*, **40**, 759–63.

Ronningen, L.S., Halstensen, T.S., Spurkland, A. *et al.* (1989) The amino acid at position 57 of the HLA-DQ beta chain and susceptibility to develop insulin-dependent diabetes mellitus. *Human. Immunol.*, **26**, 215–25.

Rotter, J.I. and Rimoin, D. (1990) 'Genetics of diabetes mellitus', in H. Rifkin and D. Porte (eds). *Diabetes Mellitus: Theory and Practice*, pp. 378–413. Elsevier, New York.

Rowley, M.J., Mackay, I.R., Chen, Q.-Y. *et al.* (1992) Antibodies to glutamic acid decarboxylase discriminate major types of diabetes mellitus. *Diabetes*, **41**, 548.

Scott, F. (1990) Cow milk and insulin-dependent diabetes mellitus: Is there a relationship? *Am. J. Clin. Nutr.*, **51**, 489–91.

Scott, R.S., Brown, L.J. and Moir, C.L. (1991) The Canterbury (NZ) diabetes registry – 30 years survival data for IDDM. *Diabetes* (Abstract No. 1485), **40** (suppl. 1), 372A.

Serjeantson, S.W., Kohonen-Corish, M.J.,

Rowley, M.J. *et al.* (1992) Antibodies to glutamic acid decarboxylase are associated with HLA-DR genotypes in both Australians and Asians with insulin-dependent diabetes mellitus. *Diabetologia*, **35** (10), 996–1001.
Serrano Rios, M., Moy, C.S., Martin Serrano, R. *et al.* (1990) Incidence of Type 1 (insulin-dependent) diabetes mellitus in subjects 0–14 years of age in the Comunidad of Madrid, Spain. *Diabetologia*, **33**, 422–24.
Siemiatycki, J., Colle, E., Aubert, D. *et al.* (1986) The distribution of type I (insulin-dependent) diabetes mellitus by age, sex, secular trend, seasonality, time clusters and space-time clusters: Evidence from Montreal, 1971–1983. *Am. J. Epidemiol.*, **124** (4), 545–60.
Siemiatycki, J., Colle, E., Campbell, S. *et al.* (1988) Incidence of IDDM in Montreal by ethnic group and by social class and comparisons with ethnic groups elsewhere. *Diabetes*, **37**, 1096–102.
Spielman, R.S., Baker L. and Zmijewski, C.M. (1980) Gene dosage and susceptibility to insulin-dependent diabetes. *Ann. Hum. Genet.*, **43**, 399–414.
Sultz, H.A., Hart, B.A., Zielezny, M. *et al.* (1975) Is mumps virus an etiologic factor in juvenile diabetes mellitus? *J. Pediatr.*, **86** (4), 654–56.
Symon, D.N., Hennessy, E.R. and Small, P.J. (1984) Smoked foods in the diets of mothers of diabetic children. *Lancet*, **ii**, 514.
Thomson, G., Robinson, W.P., Kuhner, M.K. *et al.* (1988) Genetic heterogeneity, modes of inheritance and risk estimates for a joint study of Caucasians with insulin-dependent diabetes mellitus. *Am. J. Hum. Genet.*, **43**, 799–816.
Tillil, H. and Kobberling, J. (1987) Age-corrected empirical genetic risk estimates for first degree relatives of IDDM patients. *Diabetes*, **36**, 93–99.
Tiwari, J.L. and Terasaki, P.I. (1985) *HLA and Disease Associations*, pp. 4–18. Springer-Verlag, New York.
Todd, J.A., Bell, J.L. and McDevitt, H.L. (1985) HLA-DQ beta gene contributes to susceptibility and resistance to insulin-dependent diabetes mellitus. *Nature*, **329**, 559–604.
Todd, J.A., Fukul, Y., Kitagawa, T. *et al.* (1990) The A3 allele of the HLA-DQA1 locus is associated with susceptibility to Type 1 diabetes in Japanese. *Proc. Natl. Acad. Sci.*, **87**, 1094–99.
Trucco, M. (1992) To be or not to be ASP 57, that is the question. *Diabetes Care*, **15**, 705–715.
Trucco, M. and Dorman, J.S. (1989) Immunogenetics of insulin-dependent diabetes mellitus in humans. *CRC Reviews*, **9** (3), 201–45.
Tull, E.S., Roseman, J.M. and Christian, C.L.E. (1991) Epidemiology of childhood IDDM in US Virgin Islands from 1979 to 1988. Evidence of an epidemic in early 1980s and variation by degree of racial admixture. *Diabetes Care*, **14** (7), 558–64.
Tuomilehto, J., Tuomilehto-Wolf, E., Virtala, E. *et al.* (1990) Coffee consumption as trigger for insulin dependent diabetes mellitus in childhood. *Br. Med. J.*, **300**, 642–43.
Tuomilehto, J., Lounamaa, R., Tuomilehto-Wolf, E. *et al.* (1991) Epidemiology of childhood diabetes in Finland – background of a nationwide study of type 1 (insulin-dependent) diabetes mellitus. *Diabetologia*, **35**, 70–76.
Uchigata, Y., Yamamoto, H., Nagai, H. *et al.* (1983) Effect of poly (ADP-ribose) synthetase inhibitor administration to rats before and after injection of alloxan and streptozotocin on islet proinsulin synthesis. *Diabetes*, **32**, 316–18.
Vadheim, C.M., Rotter, J.I., Maclaren, N.K. *et al.* (1986) Preferential transmission of diabetic alleles within the HLA gene complex. *New Eng. J. Med.*, **315**, 1314–18.
Vague, P., Picq, R., Bernal, M. *et al.* (1989) Effect of nicotinamide treatment on the residual insulin secretion in type 1 (insulin-dependent) diabetic patients. *Diabetologia*, **32**, 316–21.
Virtanen, S.M., Rasanen, L., Aro, A. *et al.* (1991) Infant feeding in Finnish children <7 yr of age with newly diagnosed IDDM. *Diabetes Care*, **14**, 415–17.
Wagener, D.K., Sacks, J.M., LaPorte, R.E. *et al.* (1982) The Pittsburgh study of insulin-dependent diabetes mellitus: Risk for diabetes among relatives of IDDM. *Diabetes*, **31**, 136–44.
Wagenknecht, L.E., Roseman, J.M. and Alexander, W.J. (1989) Epidemiology of IDDM in black and white children in Jefferson County, Alabama, 1979–1985. *Diabetes*, **38**, 629–33.
Wagenknecht, L.E., Roseman, J.M. and Herman, W.H. (1991) Increase incidence of insulin-dependent diabetes mellitus following an epidemic of Coxsackie virus B5. *Am. J. Epidemiol.*, **133**, 1024–31.
Warram, J.H., Krolewski, A.S., Gottlieb, M.S. *et al.* (1984) Differences in risk of insulin-

dependent diabetes in offspring of diabetic mothers and diabetic fathers. *New Eng. J. Med.*, **311**, 149–52.

Warram, J.H., Krolewski, A.S. and Kahn, C.R. (1988) Determinants of IDDM and perinatal mortality in children of diabetic mothers. *Diabetes*, **37**, 1328–34.

Watson, J.D. and Cook-Deegan, R.M. (1990) Human genome project and international health. *J. Am. Med. Assoc.*, **364**, 3322–24.

West, K. (1978) *Epidemiology of Diabetes and Its Vascular Lesions*, Elsevier, New York.

West, R., Colle, E., Belmonte, M.M. *et al.* (1981) Prospective study of insulin-dependent diabetes mellitus. *Diabetes*, **30**, 584–29.

WHO DIAMOND Project Group (1990) WHO multinational project for childhood diabetes. *Diabetes Care*, **13**, 1062–68.

WHO DIAMOND Project Group (1991) Familial IDDM epidemiology: Standardization of data for the DIAMOND Project. *Bull. WHO*, **69**, 767–77.

WHO DIAMOND Project Group (1992) Childhood diabetes, epidemics, and epidemiology: an approach for controlling diabetes. *Am. J. Epidemiol.*, **135**, 803–16.

Williams, J.M., Peterson, R.G., Shea, P.A. *et al.* (1981) Sympathetic innovation of murine rhymus and spleen: evidence for a functional link between the nervous and immune systems. *Brain Res. Bull.*, **6**, 83–94.

Wolf, E., Spencer, K.M. and Cudworth, A.G. (1983) The genetic susceptibility to Type I (insulin-dependent) diabetes: analyses of the HLA-DR associations. *Diabetologia*, **23**, 224–49.

Yonemura, Y., Takashima, T., Miwa, K. *et al.* (1984) Amelioration of diabetes mellitus in partially depancreatized rats by poly (ADP-ribose) synthetase inhibitors. Evidence of islet B-cell regeneration. *Diabetes*, **33**, 401–404.

Yoon, J.W. (1990) 'Role of viruses and environmental factors in induction of diabetes', in S. Baekkeskov and B. Hansen (eds). *Current topics in Microbiology and Immunology*, pp. 164, 95–123. Springer-Verlag, Heidelberg.

Yoon, J.W., Austin, M., Onodera, T. *et al.* (1979) Virus-induced diabetes mellitus. Isolation of a virus from the pancreas of a child with diabetic ketoacidosis. *New Eng. J. Med.*, **300**, 1173–79.

Yoon, J.W. and Rayfield, E.J. (1986) 'Two possible pathogenic mechanisms for virus-induced diabetes', in G.D. Molinar and M.A. Jaworski (eds). *The Immunology of Diabetes Mellitus*, pp. 287–98. Elsevier Science Publisher, New York.

Zimmet, P., Mackay, I.R., Rowley, M. *et al.* (1994) 'Geographic differences in antibodies to glutamic acid decarboxylase in insulin-dependent diabetes mellitis', in J. Dorman (ed.). *Standardization of epidemiologic studies of host susceptibility, NATO ASI Series*, Plenum Publishing Corp., New York.

11

Inheritance/genetics of childhood diabetes

J.M. CONNOR

Genetic analysis in childhood diabetes seeks to determine whether and which genes are involved in the predisposition to the occurrence, the prognosis and response to various forms of therapy. Broadly these analyses are divided into complementary 'old' and 'new' approaches.

11.1 BACKGROUND TO 'OLD' GENETIC ANALYSES

Genetic conditions may be subdivided, in order of frequency, into multifactorial, somatic cell genetic, single gene, chromosomal and mitochondrial disorders (Table 11.1). Multiple subtypes are apparent with a collective frequency of 33% of all births. This large number of subtypes (>5600) and the limited repertoire of disease presentation means that most diseases have a variety of different genetic origins (genetic heterogeneity). Within a family, however, a single origin is likely and classification is aided by pedigree analysis, twin studies and family correlation studies. Single gene disorders and mitochondrial disorders have diagnostic patterns of inheritance within a family whereas for the remaining disorders the distribution of patients within a family is not characteristic and a familial component may not be evident without twin or family studies. Identical twins have the same genetic makeup whereas non-identical twins have 50% of their genes in common (as do brothers and sisters). For single gene, chromosomal and mitochondrial disorders, identical twins are always either both affected or both unaffected (100% concordance). For somatic cell genetic disorders such as cancer where one or more independent mutations occur after birth, the concordance rates are similar in identical and non-identical twins whereas in multifactorial traits the concordance rate in identical twins exceeds that in non-identical twins but is less than 100% due to the involvement of environmental factors. Multifactorial inheritance with the interaction of one or more genetic loci with one or more environmental factors is suspected for many common disorders on the basis of this characteristic pattern of twin concordance. Family correlation studies are a direct extension of twin studies and seek to compare the frequency of a condition among groups of relatives who share the same proportions of their genes. For multifactorial conditions the frequency falls rapidly with each step further away in the pedigree whereas for single gene

Childhood and Adolescent Diabetes
Published in 1994 by Chapman & Hall, London
ISBN 0 412 48610 5

Table 11.1 Types of genetic disease (after Connor and Ferguson-Smith, 1993).

Type	Frequency/1000 births	No. of subtypes	Pedigree analysis	Twin concordance
Multi-factorial disorders	60	>100	non-diagnostic	diagnostic
Somatic cell genetic disorders	250	>100	non-diagnostic	non-diagnostic
Single gene disorders	14	>5000	diagnostic	non-diagnostic
Chromosomal disorders	6	>400	non-diagnostic	non-diagnostic
Mitochondrial disorders	rare	>10	diagnostic	non-diagnostic

disorders the risk remains high in affected branches of the family. These observed frequencies in different relatives of patients with a multifactorial condition are called empiric risks and are useful for genetic counselling.

11.2 CHILDHOOD DIABETES AND 'OLD' GENETIC ANALYSES

Twin studies have consistently shown an increased frequency of childhood diabetes in identical twins (ranging from 10–55%, average 30–40%) as compared with 6% in non-identical twins (reviewed by Vadheim *et al.*, 1990). Family studies also support multifactorial inheritance in most families with early onset diabetes.

Thus, although the majority of evidence from these analyses supports multifactorial inheritance, there are exceptional families where alternative mechanisms are involved. For example, pedigree analysis indicates autosomal dominant single gene inheritance in some but not all families with maturity onset diabetes of youth (MODY) (Panzram & Adolph, 1981) and mitochondrial inheritance in an exceptional family with variable combinations of diabetes, deafness and cardiomyopathy (Reardon *et al.*, 1992). Childhood diabetes may also be a secondary feature in several chromosomal disorders and over 60 rare genetic syndromes (Vadheim *et al.*, 1990) (see also Chapter 29).

Thus genetic heterogeneity is apparent for childhood diabetes with rare variants secondary to chromosomal, single gene and mitochondrial defects but in the majority of families multifactorial inheritance appears to be involved. This implies that one or more genetic loci are contributing to the predisposition to diabetes with an important interaction with one or more environmental factors.

11.3 BACKGROUND TO 'NEW' GENETIC ANALYSES

The approaches outlined under 'old' genetic analyses provide evidence for a genetic contribution to the occurrence of childhood diabetes but do not help to identify the nature of this contribution. Other approaches are required to identify which genes are involved and these are considered under linkage analysis, association analysis, sib-pair analysis and mutational analysis of candidate genes.

Linkage analysis is particularly helpful in

single gene disorders and seeks to find cosegregation of the disease trait with a genetic marker within families. These studies have been greatly assisted in recent years by the development of polymorphic DNA markers. Prior to 1978 only polymorphic proteins (blood groups, enzymes, etc.) could be used as genetic markers and this approach was restricted by their limited number and uneven distribution throughout the chromosomes. DNA polymorphisms (restriction fragment length polymorphisms (RFLPs); variable number of tandem repeats (VNTRs); and cytosine and adenine (CA) repeats), in contrast, are numerous (over 2000 identified to date) and are available for all chromosomal regions. DNA from a single blood sample can be analyzed for multiple markers and it has been estimated that if 150–200 are analyzed then this will screen all chromosomes and allow identification of cosegregation of a particular chromosomal region with the disease (Botstein *et al.*, 1980). In this type of linkage study the statistical significance of observed cosegregation is measured by the **lod score**. The lod score is the logarithm to the base 10 of the odds of the observed cosegregation versus that expected by chance alone and is estimated for a range of potential distances (called recombination fractions of 0–50%) between the disease and the marker (Conneally & Rivas, 1980). A lod score of 3 (odds of 1000 to 1) is accepted as evidence of linkage and allows assignment of the disease to the chromosomal region of origin of the DNA marker. Lod scores have the advantage that information from different families can be combined in this type of study. Conversely, failure of a DNA marker from within a particular gene to be co-inherited with a disease effectively excludes that gene as the cause of the disease.

Association analysis (or population association) compares the frequency of a particular genetic marker between patients and matched controls. A significant association with disease suggests either a causative role for the polymorphism or linkage between the polymorphism and a disease susceptibility allele. To date, most association analyses have been published in respect of the major histocompatibility complex (MHC) on the short arm of chromosome 6. The MHC consists of a tightly-linked cluster of genes, and the DNA polymorphisms within such a tightly-linked cluster show the phenomenon of linkage disequilibrium. Crossing over within the cluster is infrequent and hence DNA markers in the group tend to be inherited en bloc as a haplotype. New markers or disease-causing mutations arising within the cluster are associated, therefore, with the haplotype of origin and only slowly lose this association over many generations. In the meantime, linkage disequilibrium or marker association exists and an association study would reveal an excess of a particular haplotype amongst the patients as compared with the general population. It is important in these studies that the patients and controls are precisely matched for ethnic background since different patterns of linkage disequilibrium have resulted in haplotype differences between racial groups. Assuming genetic susceptibility to the disease to be identical in all races, any allele consistently associated with disease in all races studied is likely to be a primary disease determinant and not secondary to linkage disequilibrium. Transracial analysis thus helps to distinguish primary from secondary disease associations.

Association analysis is hampered if a condition can be caused by different mutations in the same gene in different families (mutational heterogeneity) and in this respect the **affected relative pair method** has an advantage (Suarez & Hodge, 1979; Weeks & Lange, 1988). In this analysis the frequency with which relatives with the disease share 0, 1 or 2 marker loci/haplotypes identical by descent is compared with the frequencies expected if the marker and the disease were unrelated.

Thus, for example, 25% of sibs (brothers and sisters) have identical HLA haplotypes, 50% share one HLA haplotype and 25% have different genotypes at this locus. Demonstration of genotypic concordance among affected relatives in excess of what would be expected is taken as evidence for existence of a disease susceptibility locus linked to the marker. This approach has the advantage that it needs no a priori information about the mode of inheritance or penetrance for a single gene disorder (both required for linkage analysis).

These approaches can identify particular chromosomal regions of interest and candidate genes from these regions can then be studied by **mutational analysis**. Selection of candidate genes has been greatly assisted by the growth in knowledge about the human genome (Human Gene Mapping 11, 1992) and a variety of laboratory strategies have been developed for screening for mutations in these candidate genes (Cotton, 1989).

11.4 CHILDHOOD DIABETES AND 'NEW' GENETIC ANALYSES

Linkage analysis has been utilized in many families with maturity-onset diabetes of youth (MODY) and shows evidence of linkage to the short arm of chromosome 7 (Froguel *et al.*, 1992). This linkage finding led to the identification of mutations in the candidate gene, glucokinase (Vionnet *et al.*, 1992). The structures of human pedigrees with the commoner multifactorial type of diabetes are less suited to linkage analysis but this approach has been successfully used to identify genetic determinants in the non-obese diabetic (NOD) mouse. The NOD mouse is an inbred strain which spontaneously develops diabetes which is similar to the human disorder. These animals have been used in outcross and backcross experiments to search for cosegregation between DNA polymorphic markers and the disease (Todd *et al.*, 1991; Cornall *et al.*, 1991). Using this strategy, three new regions in the NOD mouse which are associated with diabetes susceptibility, namely idd 3, 4 and 5, have been identified which, from comparative mapping studies, correspond to areas of human chromosomes 1, 2, 4 and 17. This information can now be used to identify polymorphic markers for human studies and for identification of potential candidate genes. For example, the region on chromosome 2 (homologous to idd 5 on mouse chromosome 1) contains two potential candidate genes, interleukin-1 receptor gene and a gene which influences macrophage activation.

The original MHC associations were described with HLA B8 or B15 (Singal & Blajchman, 1973; Nerup *et al.*, 1974) (which were found in about 60% of patients) and these were clues to stronger associations with DR3 and DR4 respectively which are in linkage disequilibrium. Of patients with childhood diabetes, 95% have HLA DR3 or DR4 as compared with the combined frequency of these antigens of 50% in the general population (Wolf *et al.*, 1983). The association and relative risk increased still further when restriction fragment length polymorphisms at the neighbouring DQ beta-1 (DQB1) locus were studied (Nepom *et al.*, 1986). Ninety per cent of Caucasian DR4 positive diabetics possessed the DQB1*0302 allele and only 10% the DQB1*0301 allele whereas both alleles were equally represented in a DR4 positive control population. This association was not, however, confirmed in southern Chinese or Japanese populations and thus DQB1*0302 is unlikely to be a primary disease susceptibility determinant (Cavan *et al.*, 1992). Similarly the DQB1*0201 allele (which is associated with the DR3 haplotype in Caucasians) and the DQA1*0301 allele (which is associated with the DR4 haplotype) show associations with diabetes in some but not all ethnic groups suggesting that each is in linkage disequilibrium with susceptibility alleles.

One strong candidate for a susceptibility allele was revealed by DNA sequencing of DQB1 genes. This revealed consistent changes at amino acid position 57 which is part of the putative antigen binding cleft. If alanine, valine or serine was present at this site then individuals were susceptible whereas aspartate conferred resistance (Todd *et al.*, 1987). Overall, 90% of Caucasian insulin dependent diabetics are aspartate negative homozygotes and the remainder are heterozygous as compared with the general population frequency of aspartate negative homozygotes of 19.5%. Data from other races, however, do not support this candidate: only 27% of Chinese diabetics are aspartate negative homozygotes and in Japanese diabetics the frequency of this allele does not differ from controls (Cavan *et al.*, 1992).

Conversely, certain HLA haplotypes appear to be at reduced risk for childhood diabetes. DR2 and DRw6 appear to have a protective effect in many ethnic groups and two DQB1 alleles, DQB1*0602 and DQB1*0603, which occur on DR2 and DRw6 haplotypes respectively, are negatively associated with disease in all races studied and may thus represent primary protective genes (Cavan *et al.*, 1992).

Sib-pair analysis has also been used to support the involvement of the HLA complex. In sib-pairs with insulin-dependent diabetes mellitus, 57% have the same genes from the major histocompatibility complex (25% expected), 38% have one gene in common (50% expected) and only 5% have no gene in common for this complex (25% expected) (Field, 1988). This approach should be of value in identifying other chromosomal regions of interest; the assembly of the British Diabetic Association-Warren Repository of EBV-transformed cell lines from 100 diabetic multiplex families (affected sibs plus both parents) will facilitate this task (Bain *et al.*, 1990).

Overall, the HLA complex is believed to contribute 60–70% of the genetic suceptibility to insulin-dependent diabetes. Several other loci have been implicated but, with the exception of the insulin gene region on the short arm of chromosome 11, the results of different studies have been in conflict. The major polymorphism in the insulin gene region is located 5′ to the start of transcription of the insulin gene and, in Caucasians, two main classes of alleles are observed: small alleles of approximately 40 repeats (class I alleles) and large alleles of approximately 170 repeats (class III alleles). Almost all population studies have shown an increase in the frequency of the class I alleles in patients with insulin-dependent diabetes compared with controls (Todd, 1990). Linkage analyses in multiplex families, however, have failed to confirm this finding (Tuomilehto-Wolf *et al.*, 1989). This conflict between association and linkage analysis is believed to reflect the high frequency of disease-associated alleles in the general population and perhaps genomic imprinting of this region of chromosome 11 whereby the parental origin of the insulin gene influences disease susceptibility (Julier *et al.*, 1991).

Thus, to date, the genetic basis is unclear, although the HLA-DQ loci are strongly implicated. The DQA1 and DQB1 gene products form a single molecule whose function is likely to be determined by its overall structure. If DQ polymorphism is important in disease predisposition, specific combinations of DQA1 and DQB1 allele products will result in molecular structures which may present antigens critical to beta cell destruction either to promote or damp down that process. Alternatively, since class II molecules restrict T cell repertoire, DQ polymorphisms may delete clones of T cells so that β-cell antigens are not recognized, thus protecting against disease (Cavan *et al.*, 1992). Non-HLA genes are also involved although their identity is, as yet, undetermined.

11.5 GENETIC COUNSELLING IN CHILDHOOD DIABETES

As always, when giving genetic counselling, it is first necessary to confirm the diagnosis and to construct a family tree. Confirmation of the diagnosis needs to exclude the unusual causes of diabetes as discussed in Chapter 29 and the pedigree will also help to identify exceptional patients who have a single gene or mitochondrial disorder. Most patients will have a negative family history and non-syndromic diabetes and in this situation the overall risk to brothers and sisters is 6% (Table 11.2) (Chern *et al.*, 1982; Tillil & Kobberling, 1987).

These risks can be modified by HLA studies. Sibs of an affected patient have a 12% risk if HLA identical, a 5% risk if only one haplotype is in common and a 1% risk if neither haplotype is shared (Eisenbarth, 1987). There is an unexplained preferential transmission of both high risk (DR3 or DR4) haplotypes from fathers and of the DR3 (but not the DR4) haplotype from mothers (Vadheim *et al.*, 1986). This reduced rate of transmission of the DR4 haplotype from mothers presumably influences the observed lower risk to a child (2%) when the mother is affected as compared with the father (5% risk to offspring) (Warram *et al.*, 1984).

In practice, most families will be reassured by the low empiric recurrence risk for siblings (6%), and HLA typing (by immunological or DNA analysis) is mainly used for research purposes.

Table 11.2 Genetic counseling risks for childhood diabetes mellitus in Caucasians.

Situation	Risk
General population	1 in 500
No family history but HLA DR3/DR3 or DR4/DR4	1 in 150
No family history but HLA DR3/DR4	1 in 40
No family history but DQ beta-1 aspartate negative homozygote	1 in 50
Sib with diabetes	1 in 16
Sib with diabetes and	
• 0 HLA haplotypes in common	1 in 100
• 1 HLA haplotype in common	1 in 20
• 2 HLA haplotypes in common	1 in 8
Identical twin with diabetes	1 in 3
Offspring of affected mother	1 in 50
Offspring of affected father	1 in 20

REFERENCES

Bain, S.C., Todd, J.A. and Barnett, A.H. (1990) The British Diabetic Association-Warren Repository. *Autoimmunity*, **7**, 83–85.

Botstein, D., White, R.L., Skolnick, M. *et al.* (1980) Construction of a genetic linkage map using restriction fragment length polymorphisms. *Am. J. Hum. Gen.*, **32**, 314–31.

Cavan, D., Bain, S. and Barnett, A. (1992) The genetics of type I (insulin dependent) diabetes mellitus. *J. Med. Gen.*, **29**, 441–46.

Chern, M.M., Anderson, V.E. and Barbosa, J. (1982) Empirical risk for insulin-dependent diabetes (IDD) in sibs. Further definition of genetic heterogeneity. *Diabetes*, **31**, 1115–18.

Conneally, P.M. and Rivas, M.C. (1980) Linkage analysis in man. *Adv. Hum. Gen.*, **10**, 209–266.

Connor, J.M. and Ferguson-Smith, M.A. (1993) *Essential Medical Genetics*, 4th edn. Blackwell Scientific Publications, Oxford.

Cornall, R.J., Prins, J.-B., Todd, J.A. *et al.* (1991) Type 1 diabetes in mice is linked to the interleukin-1 receptor and Lsh/Ity/Bcg genes on chromosome 1. *Nature*, **353**, 262–65.

Cotton, R.G.H. (1989) Detection of single base changes in nucleic acid. *Biochem. J.*, **263**, 1–10.

Eisenbarth, G.S. (1987) Genes, generator of diversity, glycoconjugates, and autoimmune beta cell insufficiency in type 1 diabetes. *Diabetes*, **36**, 355–64.

Field, L.L. (1988) Insulin dependent diabetes mellitus: a model for the study of multifuctioned disorders. *Am. J. Hum. Gen.*, **43**, 753–58.

Froguel, Ph., Vaxillaire, M., Jun, F. *et al.* (1992)

The glucokinase locus on chromosome 7p is closely linked to early onset non-insulin dependent diabetes mellitus. *Nature*, **356**, 162–64.

Human Gene Mapping 11. (1992) Eleventh international workshop on human gene mapping. *Cytogen. Cell Gen.*, **58**, 1–2180.

Julier, C., Hyer, R.N., Davies, J. *et al.* (1991) Insulin-IGF2 region on chromosome 11p encodes a gene implicated in HLA-DR4 dependent diabetes susceptibility. *Nature*, **354**, 155–59.

Nepom, B.S., Palmer, J., Kim, S.J. *et al.* (1986) Specific genomic markers for the HLA-DQ subregion discriminate between DR4+ insulin-dependent diabetes mellitus and DR4+ seropositive juvenile rheumatoid arthritis. *J. Exper. Med.*, **164**, 345–50.

Nerup, J., Platz, P., Andersen, O.O. *et al.* (1974) HL-A antigens in diabetes mellitus. *Lancet*, **ii**, 864–66.

Panzram, G. and Adolph, W. (1981) Heterogeneity of maturity-onset diabetes at young age (MODY). *Lancet*, **ii**, 986.

Reardon, W., Ross, R.J.M., Sweeney, M.G. *et al.* (1992) Diabetes mellitus associated with a pathogenic point mutation in mitochondrial DNA. *Lancet*, **340**, 1376–79.

Singal, D.P. and Blajchman, M.A. (1973) Histocompatibility (HL-A) antigens, lymphocytotoxic antibodies and tissue-specific antibodies in patients with diabetes mellitus. *Diabetes*, **22**, 429–32.

Suarez, B.K., Hodge, S.E. (1979) A simple method to detect linkage for rare recessive diseases: an application to juvenile diabetes. *Clin. Gen.*, **15**, 126–36.

Tillil, H. and Kobberling, J. (1987) Age-corrected empirical genetic risk estimates for first-degree relatives of IDDM patients. *Diabetes*, **36**, 93–99.

Todd, J.A. (1990) Genetic control of autoimmunity in type 1 diabetes. *Immunology Today*, **11**, 122–29.

Todd, J.A., Aitman, T.J., Cornall, R.J. *et al.* (1991) Genetic analysis of an autoimmune disease, murine type 1 (insulin dependent) diabetes mellitus. *Nature*, **351**, 542–47.

Todd, J.A., Bell, J.I. and McDevitt, H.O. (1987) HLA-DQB gene contributes to susceptibility and resistance to insulin-dependent diabetes mellitus. *Nature*, **329**, 599–604.

Tuomilehto-Wolf, E., Tuomilehto, J., Cepaitis, Z. *et al.* (1989) New susceptibility haplotype for type 1 diabetes. *Lancet*, **ii**, 299–302.

Vadheim, C.M., Rimoin, D.L. and Rotter, J.I. (1990) 'Diabetes mellitus', in A.E.H. Emery and D.L. Rimoin (eds). *Principles and Practice of Medical Genetics*, 2nd edn, pp. 1521–58. Churchill-Livingston, Edinburgh.

Vadheim, C.M., Rotter, J.I., Maclaren, N.K. *et al.* (1986) Preferential transmission of diabetic alleles within the HLA gene complex. *New Eng. J. Med.*, **315**, 1314–18.

Vionnet, N., Stoffel, M., Takeda, J. *et al.* (1992) Nonsense mutation in the glucokinase gene causes early onset non-insulin dependent diabetes mellitus. *Nature*, **356**, 721–22.

Warram, J.H., Krolewski, A.A., Gottlieb, M.S. *et al.* (1984) Differences in risk of insulin-dependent diabetes in offspring of diabetic mothers and diabetic fathers. *New Eng. J. Med.*, **311**, 149–52.

Weeks, D.E. and Lange, K. (1988) The affected-pedigree member method of linkage analysis. *Am. J. Hum. Gen.*, **42**, 315–26.

Wolf, E., Spencer, K.M. and Cudworth, A.G. (1983) The genetic susceptibility to type 1 (insulin-dependent) diabetes: analysis of the HLA-DR association. *Diabetologica*, **24**, 224–30.

12

Pancreatic morphology/islet cellular morphology

A.K. FOULIS

12.1 INTRODUCTION

Childhood diabetes is fundamentally a pancreatic disease. However, children rarely die of diabetes and biopsy of the pancreas is potentially dangerous and not necessary to make a diagnosis of diabetes. Thus studies of the histopathology of the pancreas in juvenile diabetes are rare. The only circumstance where such an examination is generally possible is in the tragic event of an autopsy on a child who has died of diabetic ketoacidosis. The findings described in this chapter are essentially drawn from such material. Before discussing the abnormal, it is first necessary to describe normal pancreatic microanatomy.

12.2 PANCREATIC HISTOLOGY

The pancreas develops from two separate buds of the primitive foregut. The dorsal bud eventually forms 90% of the volume of the pancreas and constitutes the tail, body and anterior part of the pancreatic head. The ventral bud forms the posterior part of the pancreatic head.

Endocrine cells are largely aggregated into groups known as 'islets'. These occupy approximately 2–5% of the total pancreatic mass in adults and are randomly distributed in the exocrine pancreas with a slightly increased density in the head of the organ (Clark *et al.*, 1988). However endocrine cells are not solely confined to islets. They can be grouped in such small numbers as to be unrecognizable as islets and they can even occur singly within exocrine acinar tissue or ducts.

Four endocrine cell types are found in the pancreas: the insulin-secreting β cell, glucagon-secreting α cell, somatostatin-secreting D cell and pancreatic polypeptide-secreting PP cell. Malaisse-Lagae *et al.* (1979) were the first to recognize that PP cells were not distributed evenly within the pancreas. They showed that the vast majority of these cells were found in the posterior part of the pancreatic head, in an area that corresponded to that part of the pancreas derived from the ventral bud. This area has become known as the 'PP rich lobe', while the remainder of the gland is known as the 'PP poor lobe'. In the PP poor lobe of an adult, 82% of endocrine cells are β cells, 13% α cells, 4% D cells and 1% PP cells. By contrast, in the PP rich lobe, 18% are β cells, less than 1% α cells, 1% D cells and 80% are PP cells (Stefan *et al.*, 1982).

Childhood and Adolescent Diabetes
Published in 1994 by Chapman & Hall, London
ISBN 0 412 48610 5

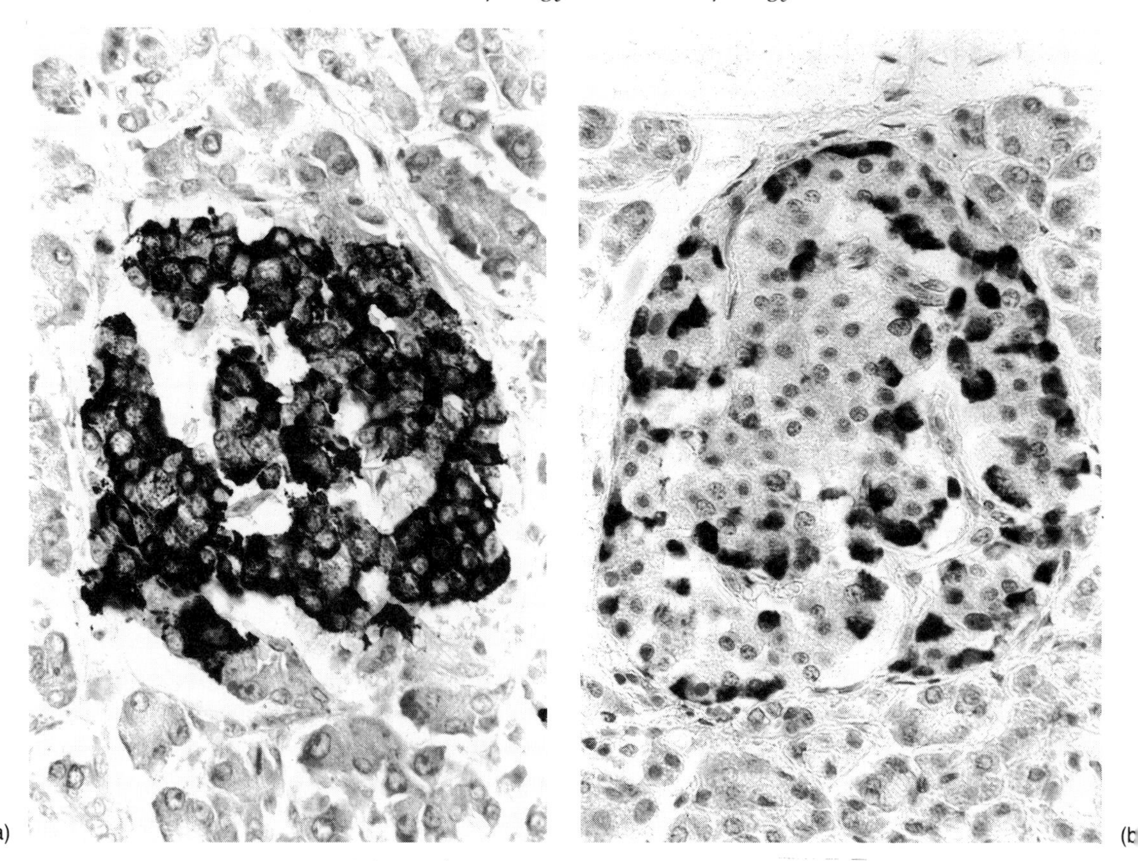

Figure 12.1 Normal islets from the PP-poor lobe immunostained to show (a) insulin-containing β cells, (b) glucagon-containing A cells and (c) somatostatin-containing D cells (×500).

Islets in the PP poor lobe are generally well-defined, and spherical. The α cells appear to line the vascular sinusoids and the β cells lie in small groups separated from the sinusoids by the other endocrine cells (Figure 12.1). By contrast, islets in the PP rich lobe are much more numerous relative to the exocrine tissue, are ill-defined and appear to merge into the surrounding exocrine tissue. They are not spherical but are totally irregular in outline (Figure 12.2).

The exocrine pancreas is divided into lobules (approximately 1–3 mm in diameter) by connective tissue septa. Within the lobule, the secretory unit is the acinus, and pancreatic enzymes from these cells drain into intralobular and interlobular ducts. The blood supply of the pancreas is of interest. Most islets are supplied by an arteriole which splits up into intra-islet sinusoids. The islet is not drained by a vein but rather the sinusoids branch into capillaries which ramify among the peri-islet acini (Plate 1) (Yaginuma *et al.*, 1986). This arrangement means that acini near to islets are bathed in capillary blood which has very high levels of islet hormones compared to other tissues in the body (Henderson, 1969).

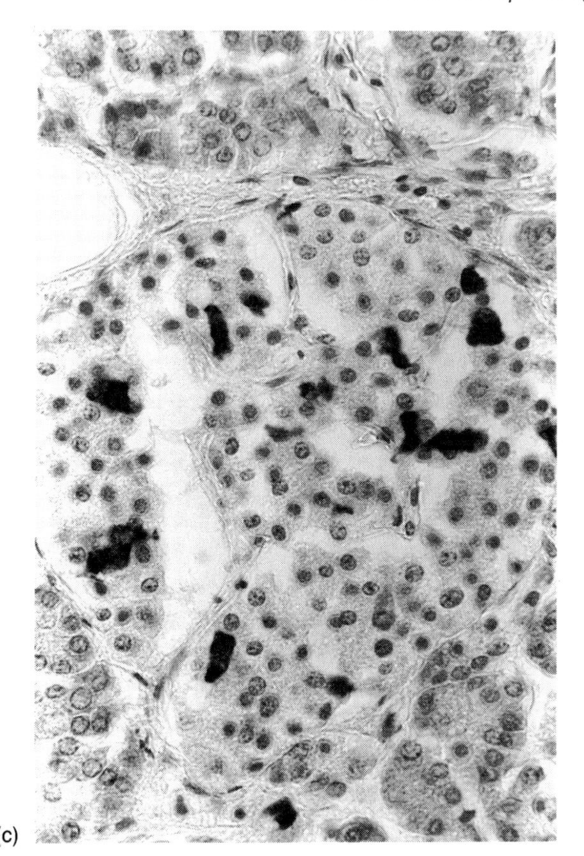

Figure 12.1 *Continued*

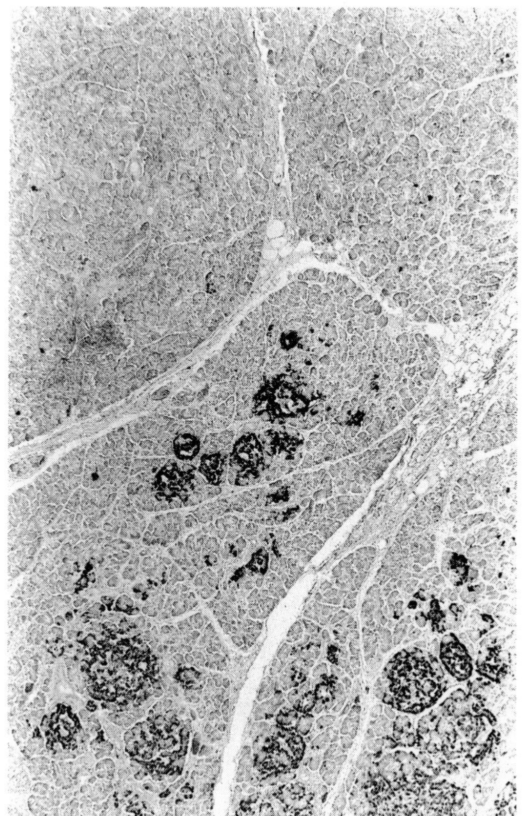

Figure 12.2 This photograph is taken through the junction of the PP-poor lobe (top) and PP-rich lobe (bottom) of a normal child's pancreas. It has been immunostained to show PP cells. Note the density and irregular outline of the PP islets (×50).

12.3 PANCREATIC HISTOPATHOLOGY IN TYPE 1 DIABETES

Type 1 (insulin-dependent, juvenile) diabetes occurs usually in young people. The vast majority of children with insulin-dependent diabetes in Western countries have this disease.

In the pancreas, the disease is characterized by selective destruction of β cells within islets. This appears to be the result of an autoimmune response in which the β cell is the target (Bottazzo, 1984). At the same time, there seems to be relatively little alteration in the numbers of α, D and PP cells. Thus, if the pancreas of a patient with type 1 diabetes of many years duration is examined, very few residual β cells, if any, will be found (Gepts, 1965; Gepts & De Mey, 1978). In the PP poor lobe these 'insulin deficient islets' consist almost entirely of α and D cells (Figure 12.3). Similarly, islets in the PP rich lobe will have lost their B cells and consist virtually exclusively of PP cells.

Although patients with this disease may present clinically with a relatively acute illness, there is evidence that the destruction of β cells proceeds very slowly and may well have been present for years before diagnosis

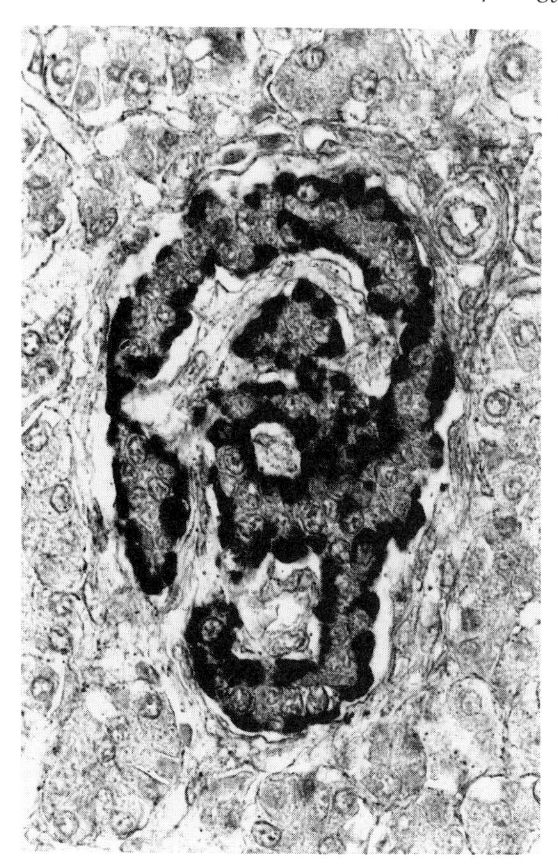

Figure 12.3 This is an insulin-deficient islet from the PP-poor lobe. The section has been immunostained to show α, D and PP cells. All the endocrine cells in the islet have been stained. There has thus been destruction of β cells, cf. Figure 12.1 (×600).

(Tarn *et al.*, 1987). There is considerable reserve within the endocrine pancreas and it has been estimated that it is not until the patient has lost approximately 80% of their β cell mass that they decompensate and present with clinical diabetes (Klöppel *et al.*, 1984).

If the pancreas is examined at clinical presentation of the disease it can be seen that there are essentially three morphological types of islet. First, the great majority of the islets are insulin deficient. Second, there are islets which contain residual β cells but which are also infiltrated by chronic inflammatory cells ('insulitis'). Finally, islets are present which appear histologically normal and which have a normal complement of β cells. These different islet types probably represent different stages of the autoimmune disease process. Thus, in the insulin deficient islets the β cells have been destroyed, in the islets affected by insulitis they are being destroyed and in the normal islets they are yet to be destroyed (Foulis *et al.*, 1986). The remarkable thing is that representatives of the three islet types can be found in a single pancreatic section taken at autopsy. An unexplained phenomenon is that within a given pancreatic exocrine lobule all the islets tend to be at the same stage of the disease process. Thus a lobule in which all the islets are insulin deficient can lie alongside one in which they are all affected by insulitis or one in which they all appear normal (Foulis *et al.*, 1986).

12.3.1 INSULITIS

Insulitis was a recognized feature of some diabetic pancreases for many years but it was not until Gepts published his account of the pathology of the pancreas in recent onset juvenile diabetes (Gepts, 1965) that it came to be recognized as the pathognomonic lesion.

Gepts described the appearances of islets in autopsy pancreases derived from 22 patients who had died within six months of first experiencing diabetic symptoms. In 15 of these cases, he noted that a proportion of the islets were inflamed. The inflammation consisted primarily of lymphocytes with very few polymorphs and no plasma cells (Figure 12.4). There is controversy in the literature concerning the frequency of insulitis in autoimmune type 1 diabetes (Foulis *et al.*, 1986; Maclean & Ogilvie, 1959; Junker *et al.*, 1977) with one study denying its very existence (Doniach & Morgan, 1973).

However, it now seems likely that insulitis is present in virtually every case of type 1

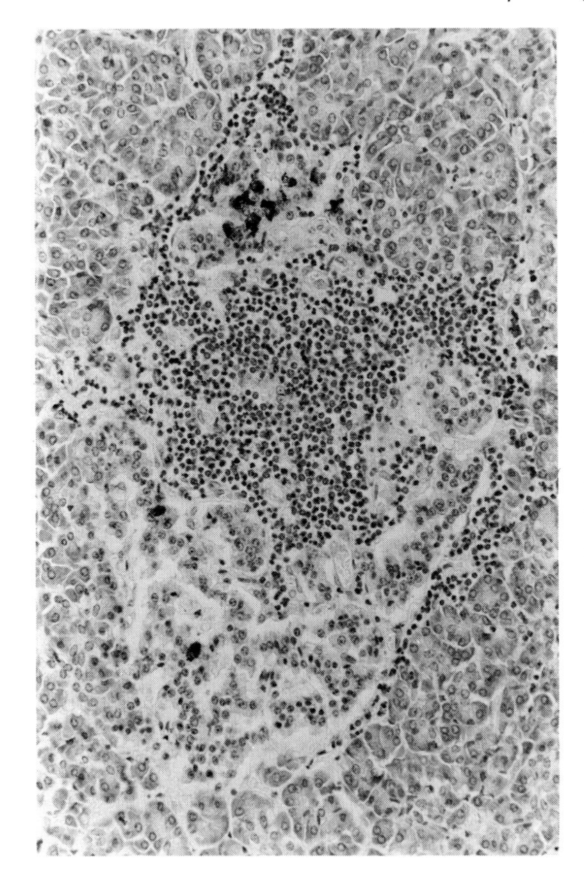

Figure 12.4 Insulitis. There is a marked lymphocytic infiltrate centered on the islet. The section has been immunostained to show the presence of β cells. Note how few are left, cf. Figure 12.1 (×250).

diabetes. It was probably previously missed because of sampling error at autopsy and a lack of appreciation of how minimal the islet infiltrate may be (Foulis *et al.*, 1986).

If insulitis is the pathognomonic lesion of autoimmune diabetes, what process does it represent? In a study of a single case, in which frozen material was available, the majority of lymphocytes in the islets were T cells with a predominance of those belonging to the CD8 phenotype (cytotoxic/suppressor cells). While helper T lymphocytes and natural killer cells were also present in small numbers, macrophages were inconspicuous (Bottazzo *et al.*, 1985). These findings, taken in conjunction with the fact that insulitis preferentially affects islets which contain residual β cells (Foulis *et al.*, 1986), makes it seem very likely that insulitis represents the immunologically-mediated, selective destruction of β cells (Gepts, 1965; Foulis *et al.*, 1986).

Given the fact that the loss of B cells seems to be a very slow process one would expect to find insulitis before and after clinical presentation. This is indeed the case. It has been seen in patients who were thought to be prediabetic (Foulis *et al.*, 1988, 1991) and it was also found affecting insulin-containing islets in the pancreas of a child who had had clinical diabetes for six years (Foulis *et al.*, 1986).

12.3.2 B CELL REGENERATION

Since the destructive process affecting β cells is a chronic one, it is not surprising that there may be evidence of regeneration of residual β cells at clinical presentation. In many cases, some insulin-containing islets are enlarged and contain an increased number of β cells, some of which have polyploid nuclei (Gepts, 1965; Foulis *et al.*, 1986). However, there is little convincing evidence of neoformation of islets from ductal elements and the fact that diabetes actually occurs following such a slow disease process implies that the regenerative capacity of β cells is very limited.

12.3.3 CHANGES IN THE EXOCRINE PANCREAS

The pancreas in patients who have had type 1 diabetes for many years is often reduced in weight (Gepts, 1965). There is a moderate degree of acinar atrophy associated with periacinar and perilobular fibrosis. In recent onset diabetes, acini around insulin-deficient islets are atrophic while acini around insulin-containing islets appear normal (Foulis & Stewart, 1984). These findings in the acini are probably the direct consequence of the loss of β cells from islets and the associated loss of locally-produced insulin. As has been described earlier, acini around islets are bathed in blood in which pancreatic hormone levels are very high. Insulin is a trophic hormone to the exocrine pancreas while glucagon and somatostatin are inhibitory. Acini around insulin-deficient islets will thus be supplied by blood having very high levels of only inhibitory hormones – thus causing atrophy, while acini around insulin-containing islets will have a balance of trophic and non-trophic hormones. Not surprisingly, patients with long-standing type 1 diabetes have measurable evidence of exocrine pancreatic malfunction (Frier *et al.*, 1976, 1978) although this is not sufficient to manifest as steatorrhea. These findings point to the importance of the islets of Langerhans in normal exocrine pancreatic function (Henderson, 1969; Foulis & Frier, 1984).

12.4 IMMUNOLOGICAL EVENTS IN ISLETS IN TYPE 1 DIABETES

With the advent of immunohistochemistry has come the possibility of not only documenting differences in morphology between normal and diseased tissues but also differences in the expression of individual proteins and other chemicals. The pioneering work in applying these techniques to the study of the diabetic pancreas was done by Bottazzo *et al.* (1985). These authors studied a single pancreas of a child who had died of recent onset diabetes. They had obtained fresh frozen pancreas from the autopsy and were able to study the expression of major histocompatibility complex (MHC) molecules in the pancreas as well as the nature of the inflammatory cell infiltrate in insulitis. Subsequently, these observations were expanded and extended by Foulis who used immunohistochemical techniques capable of detecting relevant proteins in formalin-fixed diabetic pancreases (Foulis & Farquharson, 1986; Foulis *et al.*, 1987a, 1987b).

12.4.1.1 Aberrant expression of class II MHC by β cells

There is a marked genetic component to the development of type 1 diabetes. While several different genes are likely to be involved, the closest linkage so far defined is to the class II MHC genes, HLA-DR, DP & DQ (Wolf *et al.*, 1983) (see also Chapters 10 and 11). These genes code for proteins which are expressed on the surface of certain cells and whose function seems to be involvement in antigen presentation.

Normally T helper lymphocytes, the cells which initiate the immune response, only recognize the antigen to which they are directed if the antigen is presented to them by cells which express class II MHC molecules. Many cells in the body, including pancreatic β cells, do not normally express class II MHC molecules (Natali *et al.*, 1981; Alejandro *et al.*, 1982). Thus, even if there were potentially autoreactive T lymphocytes present which could recognize antigens on these cells, they would not react because the antigens would not be 'presented' to them in the context of class II MHC. Bottazzo *et al.* (1983) proposed that one event which may provoke organ specific autoimmunity would be aberrant expression of class II MHC molecules by target cells, such as pancreatic β cells. This could theoretically convert them into antigen-presenting cells, capable of presenting their own surface antigens to potentially autoreactive T lymphocytes. Support for this hypothesis would be forthcoming if β cells but not α, D or PP cells expressed class II MHC in the disease, since only the β cells are destroyed. This is exactly what has been observed. In 22 out of 24 cases of recent onset diabetes, aberrant expression of class II MHC has been found, confined to β cells (Bottazzo *et al.*, 1985; Foulis & Farquharson, 1986; Foulis *et al.*, 1987) (Plate 2). Such expression has not been found in normal or chronically inflamed pancreases or pancreases affected by graft versus host disease, type 2 diabetes or viral infection. Like the presence of insulitis, it is a unique finding to type 1 diabetes.

12.4.1.2 Hyperexpression of class I MHC

Whilst helper T-lymphocytes can only recognize the antigen to which they are directed in the context of class II MHC molecules, cytotoxic T lymphocytes, which are the cells most likely to be responsible for destroying islet B cells (Bottazzo *et al.*, 1985), recognize the antigen only in the presence of class I MHC (HLA-A, B and C in humans). Islet β cells, in common with most nucleated cells in the body, normally express these molecules. However, hyperexpression of class I MHC molecules may make them more susceptible to the action of cytotoxic T lymphocytes. In their preliminary report, Bottazzo *et al.* (1985) found that some islets in their diabetic pancreas hyperexpressed class I MHC. Further analysis of this phenomenon in a large number of cases showed that in pancreases from recent onset diabetic patients, 92% of insulin-containing islets hyperexpressed class I MHC but only 1% of insulin-deficient islets displayed this phenomenon (Foulis *et al.*, 1987a) (Figure 12.5). Within affected islets, α, D and PP cells as well as β cells hyperexpressed class I MHC. Hyperexpression of this product by endocrine cells in islets also appeared to be a finding characteristic of type 1 diabetes – being absent in over 90 control pancreases from nondiabetic subjects or patients with type 2 diabetes.

12.4.1.3 Interferon-alpha expression by B cells

As has been described above, α and D cells hyperexpressed class I MHC when they were adjacent to β cells in insulin-containing islets. However, when they were physically divorced from β cells, in insulin-deficient islets, they ceased to hyperexpress this product. This, in conjunction with the fact that many islets which hyperexpressed class I MHC did not appear to be inflamed, suggested that the β cells may be secreting some factor which caused adjacent endocrine cells to hyperexpress class I MHC. Substances which are known to be able to do this to cultured islet endocrine cells *in vitro* include interferons-alpha, -beta and -gamma (Pujol-Borrell *et al.*, 1986). Interferon-gamma is produced only by T lymphocytes and the presence of interferon-beta cannot yet be reliably studied in autopsy-fixed tissues. In an immunohistochemical study of 37 diabetic pancreases, immunoreactive interferon-alpha, confined to β cells, was found in 93% of islets which hyperexpressed class I MHC but only in 0.4% of those showing no hyperexpression (Figure 12.5). Among 80 normal and diseased pancreases from nondiabetic patients and patients with type 2 diabetes, significant numbers of β cells containing interferon-alpha were present only in 4 cases of acute infantile Coxsackie viral pancreatitis (Foulis *et al.*, 1987b).

Histopathology is more than a mere description of morbid anatomical changes. An attempt is usually made to try to interpret the underlying disease process causing the observed histological changes. Thus Gepts (1965) suggested that autoimmunity may play a part in the destruction of β cells after highlighting the presence of insulitis in juvenile diabetes. This suggestion came nine years before the discovery of islet cell autoantibodies. What interpretations can be put on the immunological abnormalities seen in the pancreas in recent onset diabetes?

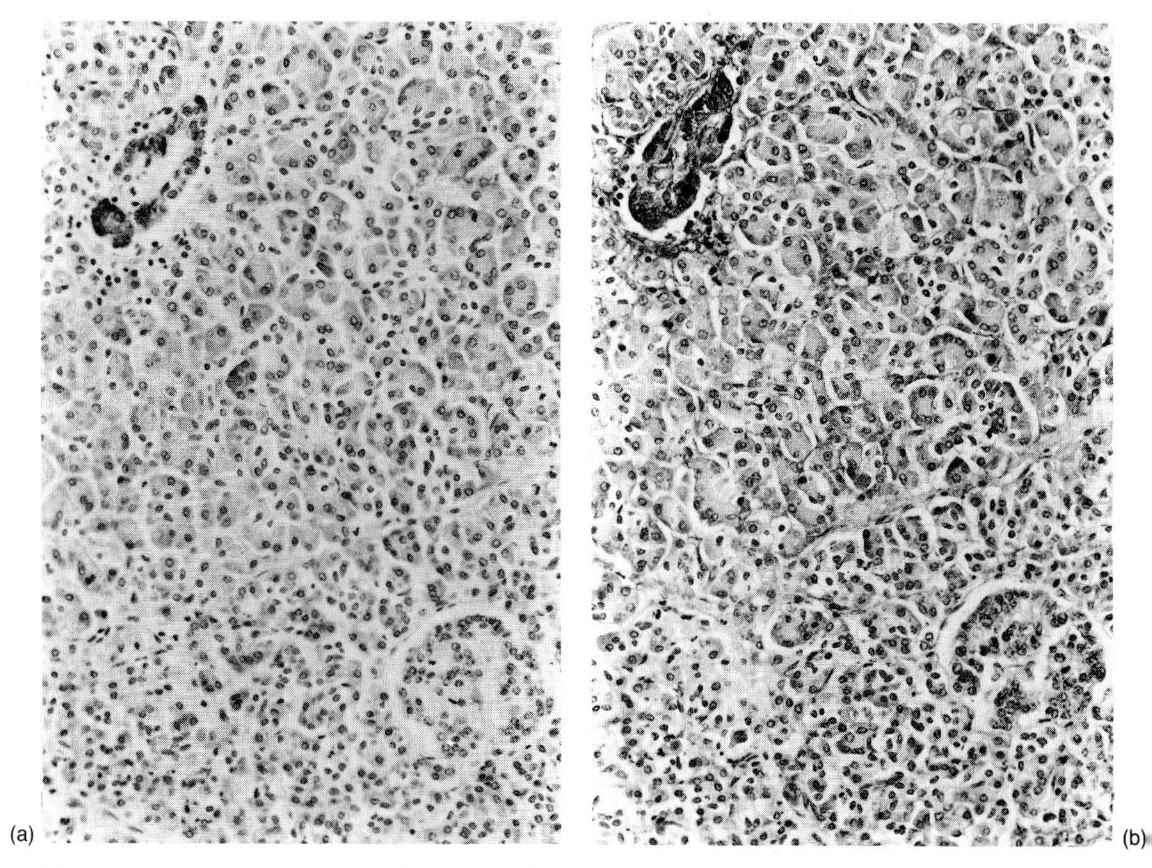

Figure 12.5 Hyperexpression of class I MHC by insulin-containing islets and the correlation with the presence of interferon-alpha. Section (a) has been immunostained for insulin, (b) for class I MHC and (c) (p. 177) for interferon-alpha. There is an insulin-containing islet in the top left of the photograph and an insulin-deficient islet in the bottom right. Endocrine cells in the former hyperexpress class I MHC and contain interferon-alpha (×250).

12.4.2 SEQUENCE OF IMMUNOLOGICAL EVENTS

If it is correct that the three populations of islet observed in the pancreas at clinical presentation of diabetes – normal, inflamed and insulin deficient – represent three different stages of the disease process as it affects individual islets, i.e., the stages before, during and after β cell destruction, then it should be possible to assign the observed immunological abnormalities to these various stages (Figure 12.6).

In the pancreas at clinical presentation of type 1 diabetes, many histologically normal islets, which show no loss of β cells or evidence of insulitis, hyperexpress class I MHC (Foulis *et al.*, 1987a). At least one reason for the hyperexpression of class I MHC by islet endocrine cells is liable to be interferon-alpha secretion by β cells and so both these phenomena are likely to precede insulitis and destruction of β cells. They both probably also occur before aberrant expression of class II MHC by β cells within the islet. This is deduced from the fact that all islets in which

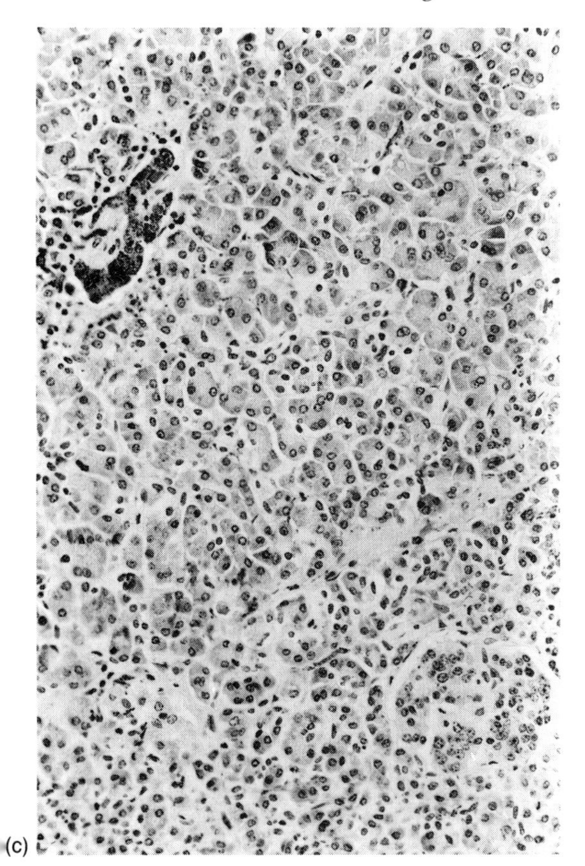

Figure 12.5 *Continued*

β cell expression of class II MHC was observed also hyperexpressed class I MHC. By contrast, islets could be found which hyperexpressed class I MHC but in which β cells did not display class II MHC molecules (Foulis *et al.*, 1987a). Whether aberrant expression of class II MHC is a consequence of insulitis or precedes it remains uncertain.

12.4.3 HYPOTHESIS

Type 1 diabetes is liable to be the result of an interplay between genetic predisposition and environmental agents. If the disease were entirely genetic in its pathogenesis, the concordance rate in monozygotic twins would approach 100%. In fact the observed rate is less than 50% (Tattersall & Pyke, 1972). While there has been recent interest in the possible role of diet as a relevant environmental agent, the principal suspects studied to date have been viruses. Chief among these have been Coxsackie, mumps, rubella and cytomegalovirus (Banatvala *et al.*, 1985; Mueller-Eckhardt *et al.*, 1984; Forrest *et al.*, 1971; Pak *et al.*, 1988).

The finding that B cells in both diabetes and Coxsackie viral pancreatitis express interferon-alpha raises the possibility that β cells are chronically infected by a virus in diabetes. This infection is not likely to be cytopathic, given the long time required for destruction of β cells in the disease. However, if a 'slow' viral infection provoked the β cells to secrete interferon-alpha, this might cause hyperexpression of class I MHC by islet endocrine cells. In the absence of a genetic predisposition perhaps nothing further would happen. However, it is conceivable that either the virus alone, or the virus plus cytokines, such as interferon-gamma and tumor necrosis factor, released in an inflammatory infiltrate, may cause β cells to express class II MHC in persons carrying the genetic susceptibility for diabetes. Support for this idea comes from the fact that those patients with congenital rubella who develop diabetes carry the class II MHC alleles DR3 and/or DR4 (Rubinstein *et al.*, 1982). It is proposed that aberrant expression of class II MHC by β cells is a crucial pathogenic event in diabetes, causing induction of autoimmunity and eventually destruction of the insulin-secreting cells in a cell-mediated fashion. This hypothesis suggests that the development of diabetes is a 'multistep' process involving both environmental and genetic components (Foulis, 1989).

One published attempt has been made to test this hypothesis by looking for evidence of Coxsackie virus infection in diabetic pancreases. A technique was developed which could demonstrate the Coxsackie viral capsid

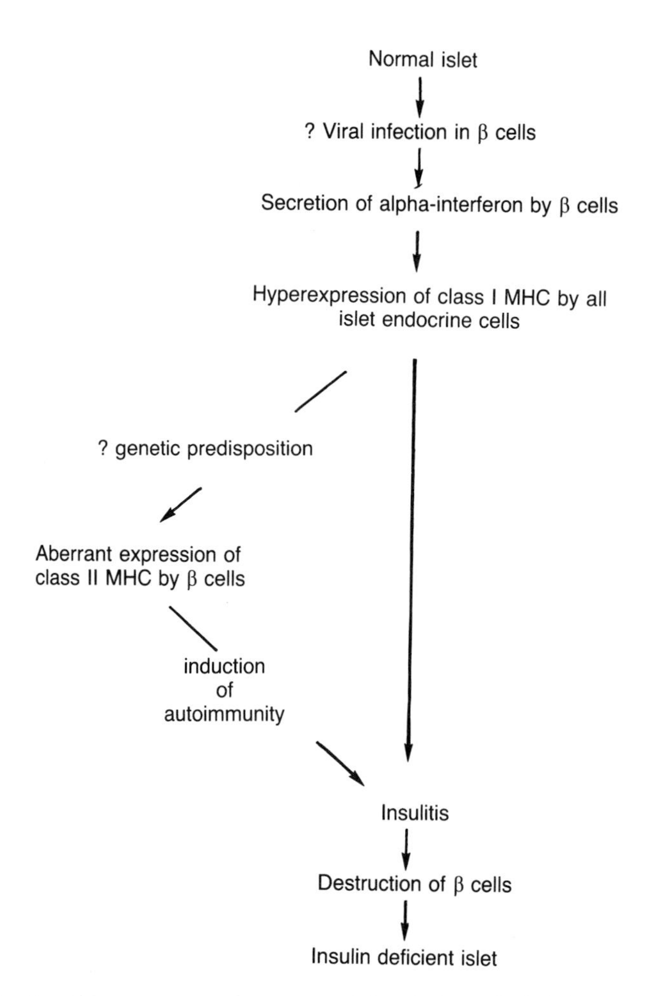

Figure 12.6 Possible sequence of events in islets in type 1 diabetes.

protein immunohistochemically in fixed tissue. Examination of pancreases of infants who had died of Coxsackie viral myocarditis showed that the virus exhibited very marked tropism to islets and appeared to infect β cells preferentially, causing widespread necrosis of these cells. However, examination of 88 autopsy diabetic pancreases with this technique failed to reveal any evidence of infection by this type of virus (Foulis *et al.*, 1990). This result certainly excluded a massive cytolytic Coxsackie viral infection of β cells as a significant cause of type 1 diabetes.

In acute systemic infections, Coxsackie viruses show tropism to myocardium as well as endocrine pancreas. Recent work has provided evidence of enteroviral RNA in heart tissue of patients suffering from congestive cardiomyopathy (Bowles *et al.*, 1986; Kandolf *et al.*, 1987), but in such patients viral capsid protein could not be detected in cardiac myocytes. This finding suggests that chronic low-grade enteroviral infection may cause disease in the absence of demonstrable capsid protein. Thus, until attempts have been made to detect enteroviral nucleic acid in diabetic pancreases, the possibility that chronic infection by such viruses predisposes to childhood diabetes cannot be excluded.

12.5 OTHER CAUSES OF DIABETES IN CHILDREN

12.5.1 CYSTIC FIBROSIS

In this disease ductal concretions cause duct obstruction which results in progressive loss of pancreatic exocrine tissue. This exocrine atrophy is initially associated with fibrosis, but in some patients the pancreas is progressively replaced by fat, so that macroscopically it comes to resemble a piece of adipose tissue. Pancreatic islets do not disappear as a result of the exocrine atrophy but become embedded in fibrous or adipose tissue (Figure 12.7) (Löhr *et al.*, 1989).

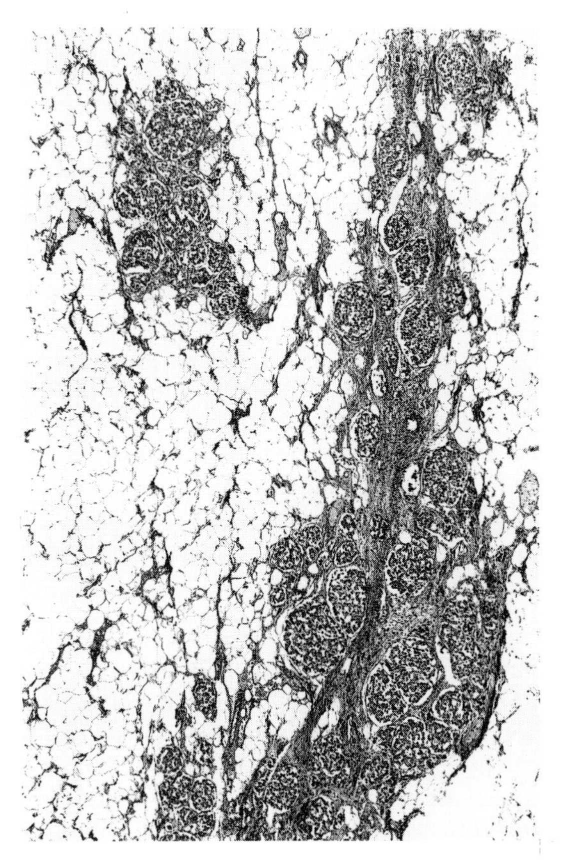

Figure 12.7 This pancreas is from a 14-year-old child with cystic fibrosis who had also developed diabetes. Note the complete exocrine atrophy. Some islets are present in adipose tissue and some are embedded in fibrous tissue. All islets are insulin-containing (Hematoxylin & Eosin ×30).

12.5.2 FIBROCALCULUS PANCREATIC DIABETES

Whilst types 1 and 2 diabetes do occur in the tropics a third cause of diabetes in this area, which can present in childhood, is a separate disease related to malnutrition. The histology of this disease is essentially the same as that seen in adults with chronic calcifying pancreatitis secondary to alcohol abuse in Western countries. Thus calcified ductal concretions are present which cause widespread exocrine atrophy and fibrosis. Just as cirrhosis can be the final outcome of many forms of chronic hepatitis, so this appearance in the pancreas is probably the end result of several different diseases which cause chronic damage to the epithelial lining of pancreatic ducts. Consumption of various toxins has been implicated in the development of fibrocalculus pancreatic diabetes, including the chronic consumption of cassava (Bajaj & Subba Rao, 1988).

The 'end stage' pancreases of cystic fibrosis and fibrocalculus pancreatic diabetes are in many respects very alike. There is almost total loss of exocrine pancreas, islets are preserved but may be embedded in fibrous tissue, and there may be a relative loss of β cells compared to α cells. Thus the mechanism of the development of clinical diabetes in these diseases is probably similar. At least two factors are liable to be involved. First, isolated islets surrounded by fibrous tissue may be relatively ischemic due to disruption of their normal vasculature during the preceding inflammatory damage. Second, endocrine failure (diabetes) usually occurs when there is also exocrine failure (steatorrhea). Intestinal malabsorption due to pancreatic failure may result in decreased secretion of 'incretins', such as glucose-dependent insulinotropic peptide (GIP) with resulting diminished insulin release from islets (Marks, 1978; Ebert & Creutzfeldt, 1980).

12.6 DIABETES WITH NO HISTOLOGICAL ABNORMALITY IN THE PANCREAS

In a study of British children who had died of ketoacidosis, four patients, all under the age of 18 months, were indentified in whom pancreatic histology was entirely normal (Foulis *et al.*, 1986). Subsequent studies of these four pancreases have failed to detect any abnormalities of MHC expression or insulitis. Exactly what syndrome these patients had is not known, but the histology would be compatible with the development of biochemical non-responsiveness to insulin. A personally observed pancreas from a youth with diabetes and *acanthosis nigricans* was also entirely normal histologically. This syndrome is associated with very marked insulin resistance.

REFERENCES

Alejandro, R., Shienvold, F.L., Hajek, S.V. *et al.* (1982) Immunocytochemical localization of HLA-DR in human islets of Langerhans. *Diabetes*, **31** (suppl. 4), 17–22.

Bajaj, J.S. and Subba Rao, G. (1988) 'Malnutrition-related diabetes mellitus', in L.P. Krall (ed.). *World Book of diabetes in practice 3*. Elsevier Science Publishing, New York.

Banatvala, J.E., Bryant, J., Schernthaner, G. *et al.* (1985) Coxsackie B, Mumps, Rubella and Cytomegalovirus specific IgM responses in patients with juvenile-onset insulin-dependent diabetes mellitus in Britain, Austria and Australia. *Lancet*, **i**, 1409–1412.

Bottazzo, G.F. (1984) Beta-Cell damage in diabetic insulitis: are we approaching a solution? *Diabetologia*, **26**, 241–49.

Bottazzo, G.F., Dean, B.M., McNally, J.M. *et al.* (1985) *In situ* characterization of autoimmune phenomena and expression of HLA molecules in the pancreas in diabetic insulitis. *N. Eng. J. Med.*, **313**, 353–60.

Bottazzo, G.F., Pujol-Borrell, R., Hanafusa, T. *et al.* (1983) Role of aberrant HLA-DR expression and antigen presentation in iduction of endocrine autoimmunity. *Lancet*, **ii**, 1115–18.

Bowles, N.E., Richardson, P.J., Olsen, E.G.J. *et al.* (1986) Detection of Coxsackie-B-virus-specific RNA sequences in myocardial biopsy samples from patients with myocarditis and dilated cardiomyopathy. *Lancet* **i**, 1120–22.

Clark, A., Wells, C.A., Buley, I.D. *et al.* (1988) Islet amyloid, increased A-cells, reduced B-cells and exocrine fibrosis: quantitative changes in the pancreas in type 2 diabetes. *Diabetes Res.*, **9**, 151–59.

Doniach, I. and Morgan, A.G. (1973) Islets of Langerhans in Juvenile Diabetes Mellitus. *Clin. Endocrin.*, **2**, 233–48.

Ebert, R. and Creutzfeldt, W. (1980) Reversal of impaired GIP and insulin secretion in patients with pancreatogenic steatorrhoea following enzyme substitution. *Diabetologia*, **19**, 198–204.

Forrest, J.M., Menser, M.A. and Burgess, J.A. (1971) High frequency of diabetes mellitus in young adults with congenital rubella. *Lancet*, **ii**, 332–34.

Foulis, A.K. (1989) Lawrence Lecture: 'In type 1 diabetes, does a non-cytopathic viral infection of insulin-secreting β-cells initiate the disease process leading to their autoimmune destruction?' *Diabetic Med.*, **6**, 666–74.

Foulis, A.K. and Farquharson, M.A. (1986) Aberrant expression of HLA-DR antigens by insulin containing beta cells in recent onset type 1 (insulin-dependent) diabetes mellitus. *Diabetes*, **35**, 1215–24.

Foulis, A.K., Farquharson, M.A., Cameron, S.O. *et al.* (1990) A search for the presence of the enteroviral capsid protein VP1 in pancreases of patients with type 1 (insulin-dependent) diabetes and pancreases and hearts of infants who died of Coxsackie-viral myocarditis. *Diabetologia*, **33**, 290–98.

Foulis, A.K., Farquharson, M.A. and Hardman, R. (1987a) Aberrant expression of Class II major histocompatibility complex molecules by β cells and hyperexpression of Class I major histocompatibility complex molecules by insulin containing islets in Type 1 (insulin-dependent) diabetes mellitus. *Diabetologia*, **30**, 333–43.

Foulis, A.K., Farquharson, M.A. and Meager, A. (1987b) Immunoreactive alpha-interferon in insulin-secreting beta cells in Type 1 diabetes mellitus. *Lancet*, **ii**, 1423–27.

Foulis, A.K. and Frier, B.M. (1984) Pancreatic endocrine-function in diabetes: an old alliance disturbed. *Diabetic Med.*, **1**, 263–66.

Foulis, A.K., Jackson, R. and Farquharson, M.A. (1988) The pancreas in idiopathic Addison's disease – a search for a prediabetic pancreas. *Histopathology*, **12**, 481–90.

Foulis, A.K., Liddle, C.N., Farquharson, M.A. *et al.* (1986) The histopathology of the pancreas in Type 1 (insulin-dependent) diabetes mellitus: a 25-year review of deaths in patients under 20 years of age in the United Kingdom. *Diabetologia*, **29**, 267–74.

Foulis, A.K., McGill, M. and Farquharson M.A. (1991) Insulitis in Type 1 (insulin-dependent) diabetes mellitus in man – macrophages, lymphocytes and interferon-gamma containing cells. *J. Patholo.*, **165**, 97–103.

Foulis, A.K. and Stewart, J.A. (1984) The pancreas in recent-onset type 1 (insulin-dependent) diabetes mellitus: insulin content of islets, insulitis and associated changes in the exocrine acinar tissue. *Diabetologia*, **26**, 456–61.

Frier, B.M., Saunders, J.H.B., Wormsley, K.G. *et al.* (1976) Exocrine pancreatic function in juvenile-onset diabetes mellitus. *Gut*, **17**, 685–91.

Frier, B.M., Faber, O.K., Binder, C. *et al.* (1978) The effect of residual insulin secretion on exocrine pancreatic function in juvenile-onset diabetes mellitus. *Diabetologia*, **14**, 301–304.

Gepts, W. (1965) Pathologic anatomy of the pancreas in juvenile diabetes mellitus. *Diabetes*, **14**, 619–33.

Gepts, W. and De Mey, J. (1978) Islet cell survival determined by morphology – an immunocytochemical study of the islets of Langerhans in juvenile diabetes mellitus. *Diabetes*, **27** (suppl. 1), 251–61.

Henderson, J.R. (1969) Why are the Islets of Langerhans? *Lancet*, **ii**, 466–70.

Junker, K., Egeberg, J., Kromann, H. *et al.* (1977) An autopsy study of the Islets of Langerhans in acute-onset juvenile diabetes mellitus. *Acta Pathol. Microbiol. Scand.*, Section A, **85**, 699–706.

Kandolf, R., Ameis, D., Kirschner, P. *et al.* (1987) In situ detection of enteroviral genomes in myocardial cells by nucleic acid hybridization: An approach to the diagnosis of viral heart disease. *Proc. Nat. Acad. Sci. USA*, **84**, 6272–76.

Klöppel, G., Drenck, C.R., Oberholzer, M. *et al.* (1984) Morphometric evidence for a striking B-cell reduction at the clinical onset of type 1 diabetes. *Virchows Archives (Pathological Anatomy)*, **403**, 441–52.

Löhr, M., Goertchen, P., Nizze, H. *et al.* (1989) Cystic fibrosis associated islet changes may provide a basis for diabetes. *Virchows Archives (Pathological Anatomy)*, **414**, 179–85.

Maclean, N. and Ogilvie, R.F. (1959) Observations on the pancreatic islet tissue of young diabetic subjects. *Diabetes*, **8**, 83–91.

Malaisse-Lagae, F., Stefan, Y., Cox, J. *et al.* (1979) Identification of a lobe in the adult human pancreas rich in pancreatic polypeptide. *Diabetologia*, **17**, 361–65.

Marks, V. (1978) The enteroinsular axis. *J. Clin. Pathol.*, **33** (supp. 8), 38–42.

Mueller-Eckhardt, G., Stief, T., Otten, A. *et al.* (1984) Complications of mumps infection, islet-cell antibodies, and HLA. *Immunobiology*, **167**, 338–44.

Natali, P.G., De Martino, C.D., Quaranta, V. *et al.* (1981) Expression of Ia-like antigens in normal human non-lymphoid tissues. *Transplantation*, **31**, 75–78.

Pak, C.Y., Eun, H.-M., McArthur, R.G. *et al.* (1988) Association of cytomegalovirus infection with autoimmune type 1 diabetes. *Lancet*, **ii**, 1–4.

Pujol-Borrell, R., Todd, I., Doshi, M. *et al.* (1986) Differential expression and regulation of MHC products in the endocrine and exorine cells of the human pancreas. *Clin. Exper. Immunol.*, **65**, 128–29.

Rubinstein, P., Walker, M.E., Fedun, B. *et al.*

(1982) The HLA system in congenital rubella patients with and without diabetes. *Diabetes*, **31**, 1088–91.
Stefan, Y., Orci, L., Malaisse-Lagae, F. *et al.* (1982) Quantitation of endocrine cell content in the pancreas of non-diabetic and diabetic humans. *Diabetes*, **31**, 694–700.
Tarn, A.C., Smith, C.P., Spencer, K.M. *et al.* (1987) Type 1 (insulin-dependent) diabetes: a disease of slow clinical onset? *Brit. Med. J.*, **294**, 342–45.
Tattersall, R.B. and Pyke, D.A. (1972) Diabetes in identical twins. *Lancet*, **ii**, 1120–25.
Wolf, E., Spencer, K.M. and Cudworth, A.G. (1983) The genetic susceptibility to Type 1 (insulin-dependent) diabetes: Analysis of the HLA-DR association. *Diabetologia*, **24**, 224–30.
Yaginuma, N., Takahashi, T., Saito, K. *et al.* (1986) The microvasculature of the human pancreas and its relation to Langerhans islets and lobules. *Pathological Research Practices*, **181**, 77–84.

13

Pathogenesis of childhood diabetes

T. MANDRUP-POULSEN and J. NERUP

13.1 INTRODUCTION

Insulin-dependent diabetes mellitus (IDDM) is caused by a selective destruction of the insulin-producing pancreatic β cells, leading to insulin deficiency. The evidence for the classification of human IDDM as an autoimmune disease (listed in Table 13.1) is indirect and circumstantial (for review, see DeFronzo, 1993). To fulfil the formal criteria of an autoimmune disease the autoantigen(s) should be identified and either serum or mononuclear cells must be able to tranfer the disease. However, the existing evidence is compelling, and the fact that immunosuppression can preserve β-cell function and induce clinical remission in recently diagnosed IDDM patients strongly supports the concept of IDDM as an immune-mediated disorder.

In the following we will deal with immune mechanisms supposed to cause β cell destruction in IDDM and how these mechanisms may be genetically controlled. Detailed descriptions of the genetics of IDDM, environmental determinants and the histopathology of IDDM are found elsewhere in this volume.

13.2 AUTOIMMUNITY AND AUTOIMMUNE DISEASE

Immune reactivity to endogeneous antigens (autoimmunity) is an integrated part of the normal immune system. A significant percentage of the normal population develops circulating autoantibodies with age without presenting clinical symptoms. Autoimmune disease occurs when an autoimmune reaction causes impairment of normal function or tissue destruction leading to symptoms and overt disease.

Proposed causes of immune reactivity to self-antigens (loss of immunological 'tolerance') include the lack of deletion of 'forbidden' autoreactive T-cell clones in the thymus or imbalance between stimulatory and mitogenic versus suppressive signals to the immune cells. Little is known about the factors that determine whether autoreactivity remains under control in health or develops into disease. There is no evidence that lack of tolerance to β cell antigen is an initial cause of IDDM in animal models of IDDM or in human IDDM. Rather, the coincidence of 1) environmental factors causing β cell antigen release and 2) an unfavorable combination of genes encoding for a) efficient presentation of β cell antigen, b) imbalanced cytokine response to antigen presentation, and c) a low level of β cell defense against immune attack,

Childhood and Adolescent Diabetes
Published in 1994 by Chapman & Hall, London
ISBN 0 412 48610 5

Table 13.1 Evidence for human IDDM as an autoimmune disease.

- Association with genes that control the immune response
- Association with other organ-specific autoimmune disorders
- β-cell destructive mononuclear cell infiltration in the islets
- Circulating autoantibodies reacting against islet cell components
- Cell-mediated immune reactivity against islet cell components
- Preservation of β cell function in immunosuppressed new-onset IDDM

may be the causes of immune-mediated β-cell destruction in IDDM.

13.3 AUTOANTIGENS IN IDDM

No single important autoantigen has been identified in IDDM. The heterogeneous pattern of the T-cell usage of certain parts of the T-cell receptor (the so-called V_{β}-chains) in early IDDM in animal models underlines that a variety of β cell antigenic epitopes is recognized by T-cells in IDDM.

Two major approaches have been taken to identify autoantigens in IDDM:

a) the use of sera from IDDM patients to detect binding of autoantibodies in the sera with islet components and other antigens,
b) the registration of proliferation of T-cells from IDDM patients to islet components and other antigens.

The relative role of these candidate antigens (Table 13.2) remains to be determined.

Table 13.2 Candidate antigens in IDDM.

Antigen	Humoral reactivity	T-cell reactivity
β-cell specific		
Insulin/proinsulin	x	
38 K insulin secretory granule membrane protein	x	x
Carboxypeptidase H proinsulin processing enzyme	x	
p52 rat insulinoma cell membrane protein	x	
155 kD rat insulinoma cell membrane protein	x	
β-cell non-specific		
Gangliosides	x	
Glutamic acid decarboxylase (GAD) 65 and 67 kD	x	x
37/40 kD tryptic fragment of a 64 kD non-GAD islet protein	x	
32, 55–72, 120–170 kD islet proteins		x
Glucose-transporter GLUT-2	x	
Peripherin (58 kD)	x	
Heat shock proteins 62 and 65	x	
Bovine serum albumin (BSA)	x	
ABBOS (linear BSA epitope)	x	x
p69 BSA homologous peptide	x	
Sulphatides	x	

13.4 AUTOANTIBODIES IN IDDM

Many circulating autoantibodies have been detected in the sera of recent-onset IDDM patients, recognizing many different β cell specific and non-specific antigens (Table 13.2). None of these antibodies are considered to have primary pathogenetic importance but rather to be consequences of a polymorphic and polyclonal activation of B-lymphocytes. They may, however, serve as valuable markers of β cell destruction.

13.4.1 ISLET CELL CYTOPLASMIC ANTIBODIES (ICA)

Of the autoantibodies in IDDM, islet cell cytoplasmic antibodies (ICA) have been studied most extensively. This family of IgG antibodies recognizes several different islet components, among others gangliosides which are also abundant in the nervous system and glutamic acid decarboxylase 65, a GABA-synthesizing enzyme also found in the brain and peripheral nerves. ICA can be demonstrated in 60–90% of new-onset IDDM patients depending on the sensitivity of the assay used. The ICA titer and prevalence decline with increasing disease duration, and high-titered ICA predict a rapid loss of β-cell function after diagnosis. Presence of ICA, in particular high-titered ICA, increases the risk of developing IDDM in family members of IDDM patients and also in the general population, albeit less significantly in the latter group. ICA is therefore an important and useful scientific tool in the prediction of IDDM.

13.4.2 ANTI-GLUTAMIC ACID DECARBOXYLASE (GAD) ANTIBODIES

Anti-GAD antibodies (GAD) may be the earliest autoantibodies detectable in people at risk of developing IDDM, found up to 10 years before development of clinical disease. The prevalence of GAD 65 antibodies at diagnosis is 65–80% and these antibodies are remarkably stable after diagnosis. Their independent predictive value in the prediabetic phase remains to be investigated, but they seem to confer an additional risk of IDDM development when combined with ICA.

13.4.3 ANTI-INSULIN AUTOANTIBODIES

Anti-insulin autoantibodies (IAA) can be found in people at risk for IDDM and in 30–40% of new-onset IDDM patients before the administration of insulin. Their prevalence is inversely correlated with age, at onset being most frequent in young IDDM children. When combined with ICA, presence of IAA seems to confer additional risk of IDDM development. The combination of three or more autoantibodies appears to increase the positive predictive value to approximately 90% in a 10-year follow-up period in family studies.

13.5 CELL-MEDIATED IMMUNITY IN IDDM

The mononuclear cell infiltrate in the islets in IDDM is suggestive of a delayed cell-mediated hypersensitivity (Type IV) reaction. Strong support for an important role of cell-mediated immunity in human IDDM (Table 13.3) stems from animal studies (for review, see Mandrup-Poulsen & Nerup, 1990; DeFronzo, 1993). Spleen cells from acutely diabetic animals can adoptively transfer IDDM, and measures that inhibit the cell-mediated immune system prevent disease in the rodent models of IDDM.

13.6 IMMUNOBIOLOGY OF THE ISLET-INFILTRATING MONONUCLEAR CELLS

At the time of diagnosis the islet inflammatory infiltrate is composed of most types of

Table 13.3 Evidence for cell-mediated anti-β-cell immunity in IDDM.

- Mononuclear cell (MNC) infiltration in islets
- Cutaneous hypersensitivity to islet mterial in new-onset IDDM
- New-onset IDDM MNC reactivity to islet material *in vitro*
- Homing of MNC from new-onset IDDM patients to islets in immunocompromised mice
- Isolation of islet reactive CD4+ (T helper) cell clones from new-onset IDDM patients
- Elevated activated (HLA-class II positive) T cells
- Defective IL-2 production from new-onset IDDM MNC

lymphocytic and monocytic cells. This infiltrate represents the end-stage of the destructive process. There are no human data concerning the types of cells infiltrating the islets in the earliest phases of the natural course of IDDM, but in animal models of IDDM dendritic cells, macrophages and T-helper (Th or CD4+) lymphocytes – in this order – are the first to be detected in the islets.

The relative role of monocytic cells and CD4+ Th and T cytotoxic/suppressor (Tc/s or CD8+) lymphocytes as effector-cells mediating directly the killing of the β-cells is controversial (reviews: Mandrup-Poulsen & Nerup, 1990; DeFronzo, 1993). IDDM can be prevented in animal models by eliminating either of these cells. There is evidence that CD8+ T-cells are not required for β-cell destruction, but they may accelerate an ongoing β-cell destructive process. Of the T-cells proliferative, non-cytotoxic CD4+ clones isolated from the infiltrate in the islets of rodent models can transfer IDDM, underlining the importance of the Th-cell in the early stages of IDDM pathogenesis.

13.7 EFFECTOR MECHANISMS

The cellular and biochemical mechanisms by which the immune cells destroy the β cells are not completely understood. Cell-to-cell contact between CD4+ T-cells and β cells does not seem to be required for β cell killing in animal models, suggesting that humoral factors may be involved in delivering the lethal hit. Early infiltrating monocytic cells express messenger RNA for several soluble proinflammatory mediators (cytokines), i.e., interleukin-1 (IL-1), interleukin-6 (IL-6) and tumor necrosis factor α (TNFα). There is good evidence that cytokines act as effector molecules in IDDM (Mandrup-Poulsen, 1989; Sandler, 1991) (Table 13.4).

Table 13.4 Evidence for cytokines as effector molecules in IDDM.

- Major IDDM predisposing gene located close to the IL-1 gene cluster in mice with IDDM
- IL-1 gene polymorphism associated with HLA non-DR 3 or 4 IDDM
- IDDM associated IL-1 gene polymorphism associated with elevated MNC IL-1 synthesis
- IL-1 receptor antagonist (IL-1Ra) gene polymorphism associated with familial IDDM
- IL-1 and TNFα messenger RNA abundant in early inflammatory infiltrate in islets of rodent IDDM models
- Islet β-cells express IL-1 receptors
- IL-1 selectively cytotoxic to rat β cells, synergy with TNFs and IFNy
- IL-1 plus TNFs or IFNy cytotoxic to human β cells
- IL-1 produces transient diabetes in normal rats
- IL-1ra delays IDDM onset in rat IDDM model

The biochemical mode of action of cytokines is not fully clarified, but involves induction of toxic nitric oxide and probably also superoxide radicals that damage DNA and inactivate mitochondrial respiratory enzymes, leading to defective energy generation (Sandler, 1991; Corbett, 1992). For unknown reasons, cytokines fail to induce the cytokine inducible nitric oxide-generating enzyme (iNOS) in non-β cells, providing an attractive explanation for the selectivity of β cell destruction in IDDM.

13.8 GENETIC CONTROL OF β-CELL DESTRUCTIVE AND PROTECTIVE EVENTS IN IDDM

Several normal genes have been associated with IDDM susceptibility (Table 13.5) (Nerup, 1989; DeFronzo, 1993). Major histocompatibility complex class II genes, in particular sequences of the HLA-DQ locus (A1*0301, B1*0302, B1*0201, A1*0501) have shown the strongest association with IDDM. However, no single gene locus has been found to be either necessary or sufficient

Table 13.5 Genes associated with IDDM susceptibility in humans.

Gene locus	Chromosomal location
• IL-1 gene polymorphism	2
• IL-1 receptor antagonist gene polymorphism	2
• Major histocompatibility complex class II genes (HLA-DQ)	6
• Tumor necrosis factor α (TNFα) gene promotor polymorphism	6
• Heat shock protein 70 gene polymorphism	6
• Mn superoxide dismutase gene polymorphism	6
• Insulin gene flanking polymorphism	11

for disease development. Sequencing of susceptibility genes have failed to identify sequences unique for IDDM. Hence, IDDM-specific genes or gene mutations may not exist. The inheritance of IDDM can only be explained by combinations of several genes with varying penetrance. Thus, IDDM is a polygenic disease, and most IDDM-associated gene loci have been suggested to confer susceptibility by controlling specific elements of the pathogenesis (Figure 13.1).

HLA-DQ heterodimers associated with IDDM presumably affect the shape of the antigen-binding groove on the class II MHC molecules expressed on antigen-presenting cells, thereby determining the efficacy of presentation of β cell autoantigens to autoreactive T-cells. It has been suggested that class II molecules associated with IDDM bind β-cell antigens more avidly than those other class II molecules, thereby increasing the probability of recognition of the antigen by β cell reactive Th-cells.

Thus, the HLA class II DQ locus may be a major IDDM susceptibility locus. However, in the HLA class III region polymorphic genes associated with IDDM can be found that may add to genetic susceptibility. A polymorphism in the TNFα gene promoter region controls TNFα secretion from peripheral blood monocytes and an IDDM-associated polymorphism encodes for hypersecretion of TNFα. In the HLA class III region are located two heat shock protein (HSP) genes. Both of these genes show a simple diallelic polymorphism and one of them, probably associated with low inducibility of heat shock proteins, is positively associated with IDDM on DR 3 haplotypes.

The IL-1 gene cluster on chromosome 2 contains several genes of interest in IDDM susceptibility. This gene cluster contains genes coding for IL-1 secretion, IL-1 type I and type II receptors and the IL-1 receptor antagonist. In the IL-1β gene there is a diallelic polymorphism of which the allele encoding for IL-1β hypersecretion is positively associated with IDDM. In the IL-1 receptor antagonist gene a penta-allelic polymorphism is identified. A particular IL-1 receptor antagonist genotype encoding for low levels of circulating IL-1 receptor antagonist peptide is positively associated with IDDM. Taken together the cytokine gene polymorphisms associated with IDDM seem to increase agonists with β cell cytotoxic properties and to reduce the production of antagonist with protective properties. Furthermore, the chromosome 2 IDDM-associated polymorphisms seem to be able to distinguish between familial and true sporadic cases of IDDM.

The manganese superoxide dismutase gene of the long arm of chromosome 6 as well as a polymorphism of the insulin gene (chromosome 11) also show association with IDDM. The functional implications of these genes in relation to IDDM pathogenesis are still to be elucidated.

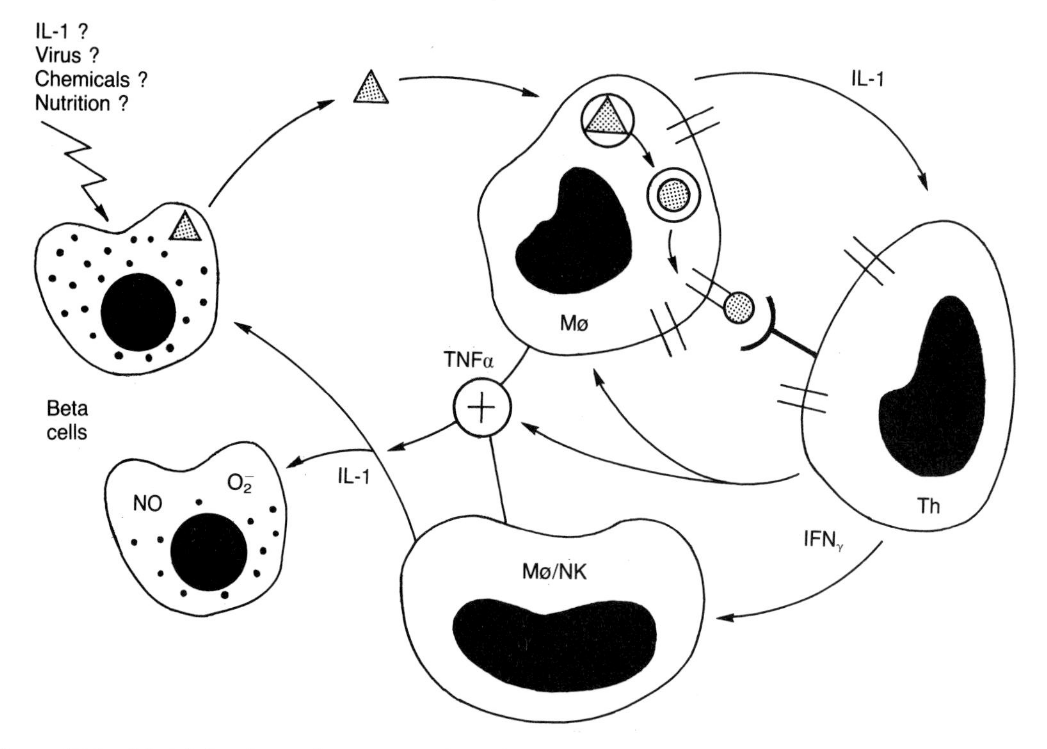

Figure 13.1 Model for the pathogenesis of insulin-dependent diabetes mellitus. Abbreviations: IL-1: interleukin-1; ▲: native β cell antigen; •: processed β cell antigen; ||: MHC class II molecule; Mø: macrophage; [Y]: T-cell receptor; Th: CD4+ T helper lymphocyte; TNFα: tumor necrosis factor α; IFN_{γ}: interferon γ; ⊕: synergy; NK: natural killer cell; NO: nitric oxide radical; O_2^-: free oxygen radical.

13.9 SUMMARY AND CONCLUSIONS

In summary, IDDM is caused by a Th-cell dependent, cytokine mediated destruction of the β cells in individuals genetically predisposed by an unfavorable combination of normal genes, most of which have known functional effects on the immune response to the β cells, and some of which may control β cell defense against immune attack. The etiological triggers and the autoantigens driving this process are unknown. Autoantibodies against β-cell components have little if any pathogenetic importance, but may serve as valuable markers of disease activity, allowing increasingly precise risk assessments.

We propose the following model for IDDM pathogenesis (Figure 13.1):

Any triggering event that causes focal, limited β cell damage and liberation of β cell components will allow processing and presentation of the β cell antigen to specifically reactive Th-cells. Recognition of the antigen-MHC class II molecule complex and a co-stimulatory signal provided by IL-1 will induce T-cell lymphokine gene expression and secretion. Lymphokines attract and activate lymphocytes and monocytes which secrete cytokines (IL-1, TNFα and IFN) in high local concentrations which are synergistically β cell toxic by inducing free oxygen- and nitrogen-derived radicals against which β cells have limited protective properties.

REFERENCES

Corbett, J.A. and McDaniel, M.L. (1992) Does nitric oxide mediate autoimmune destruction of β-cells? Possible therapeutic interventions in IDDM. *Diabetes*, **41**, 897–903.

DeFronzo, R.A. (ed.). (1993) Immunology and IDDM. *Diabetes Reviews*, **1**, 1–126.

Mandrup-Poulsen, T., Helqvist, S., Mølvig, J. *et al.* (1989) Cytokines as immune effector molecules in autoimmune endocrine diseases with special reference to insulin-dependent diabetes mellitus. *Autoimmunity*, **4**, 191–218.

Mandrup-Poulsen, T. and Nerup, J. (1990) 'The Autoimmune Hypothesis of Insulin-Dependent Diabetes: 1965 to the Present', in F. Ginsberg-Fellner and R.C. McEvoy (eds.). *Autoimmunity and the Pathogenesis of Diabetes*, pp. 1–28. Springer-Verlag, New York.

Nerup, J. Mandrup-Poulsen, T. and Hökfelt, B. (eds). (1989) *Genes and Gene Products in the Development of Diabetes Mellitus. Basic and Clinical Aspects*. Excerpta Medica, Amsterdam.

Sandler, S., Eizirik, D.L., Svensson, C. *et al.* (1991) Biochemical and molecular actions of interleukin-1 on pancreatic β-cells. *Autoimmunity*, **10**, 241–53.

14

Biochemistry and intermediate metabolism

J.W. GREGORY and R. TAYLOR

14.1 INTRODUCTION

The control mechanisms leading to glucose homeostasis in healthy infants and children have been previously described in Chapters 1–3. Childhood diabetes is recognized clinically as an inability to control blood glucose concentrations. The major feature of insulin-dependent diabetes mellitus (IDDM) in childhood is postprandial hyperglycemia which occurs because glucose appearance in the plasma exceeds glucose removal, primarily due to insulin deficiency. However, insulin deficiency is also associated with disturbances of the whole of intermediary metabolism (Madsbad *et al.*, 1981) and the metabolic abnormalities associated with this state are reviewed in this chapter (Figure 14.1). Many of the studies cited which have led to our understanding of the metabolic disturbance associated with IDDM necessarily relate to research work in young adults rather than children, because of the difficulty of undertaking invasive investigations in the pediatric age group.

Childhood and Adolescent Diabetes
Published in 1994 by Chapman & Hall, London
ISBN 0 412 48610 5

14.2 METABOLIC ABNORMALITIES IN INSULIN-DEPENDENT DIABETES MELLITUS

14.2.1 GLUCOSE PRODUCTION

The majority (over 75%) of glucose production originates from the liver with a small contribution from the kidneys. Hepatic glucose production results from glycogenolysis and gluconeogenesis. Precursors for the latter include alanine, glutamine, glycerol, lactate and pyruvate. In regulating both glycogenolysis and gluconeogenesis, insulin and glucagon have opposite effects as previously described in Chapters 1–3. In insulin-deficient states such as childhood diabetes, the insulin:glucagon ratio is decreased and as a consequence, hepatic glycogenolysis and gluconeogenesis are increased (Cherrington *et al.*, 1987). Furthermore, increased amino acid release from muscle and glycerol release from adipose tissue drives gluconeogenesis by increasing substrate supply. In addition, the elevated fatty acid oxidation rate further stimulates hepatic gluconeogenesis.

With more prolonged insulin deficiency, stress hormone secretion is increased and this may be exacerbated by intercurrent ill-

Tissue	Substrate	Normal uptake (←) output (→) of substrate	Insulin-deficient uptake (←) output (→) of substrate
Liver	Glucose	→	⇛
	Lactate	←	⇚
	NEFA	←	⇚
	Ketones	→	⇛
Muscle	Lactate	→	⇉
	NEFA	←	←
	Ketones	←	⇇ *
Adipocyte	NEFA	→	⇉
Brain	Glucose	←	⇇ *
Blood	Glucose	↔	↑↑↑
	Lactate	↔	↑
	NEFA	↔	↑↑
	Ketones	↔	↑↑↑

Figure 14.1 The effect of insulin deficiency on fasting metabolism. The increased tissue uptake of substrates labelled * is due to mass action effect of elevated plasma concentrations. ↑ refers to elevated substrate concentration in blood secondary to insulin deficiency.

ness which may be a predisposing factor to the development of diabetic ketoacidosis. Glucagon secretion may be increased, further depressing the insulin : glucagon ratio. Glucocorticoid hormones are released and promote the release of gluconeogenic precursors such as amino acids and glycerol from muscle and adipose tissue respectively. Growth hormone secretion is also increased in the stress response and this promotes lipolysis and the availability of glycerol for gluconeogenesis. Increased sympathetic activity and catecholamine release have a potent effect in stimulating lipolysis and also glycogenolysis and gluconeogenesis by direct hepatic action. The consequences of the metabolic effects described above are that glucose production rates are excessive for the elevated blood glucose concentrations present during development of diabetic ketoacidosis. It is of note that these glucose production rates are within the range of values in nondiabetic individuals with normal blood glucose concentrations. However, in nondiabetics, glucose production rates decrease by 80–85% for each 1 mmol rise in blood glucose concentrations (Sharp & Johnston, 1991).

14.2.2 GLUCOSE CONSUMPTION

Glucose uptake in cardiac and skeletal muscle is decreased in subjects with IDDM with inadequate insulin replacement. This is an

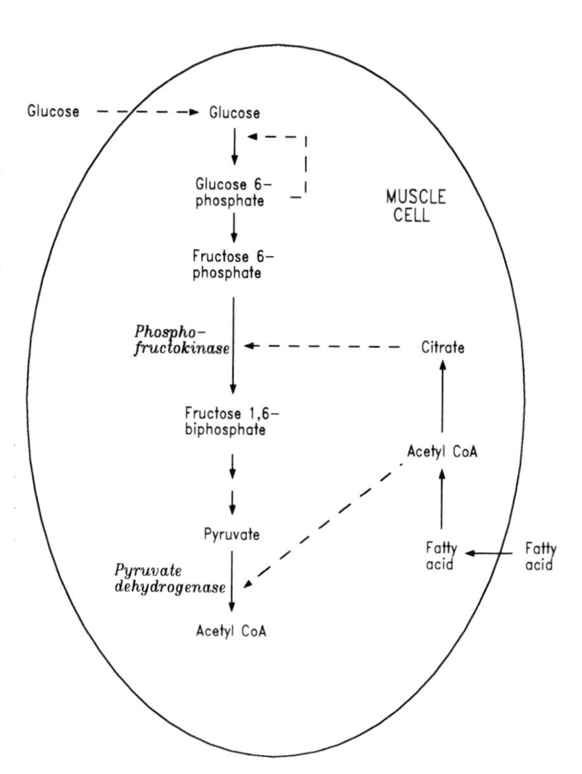

Figure 14.2 The glucose–fatty acid (Randle) cycle in muscle. The inhibitory effects of this cycle on glucose transport and metabolism are shown by interrupted arrows.

effect both of decreased insulin stimulation of glucose transport and decreased glucose utilization as a consequence of the glucose–fatty acid (Randle) cycle (Randle *et al.*, 1963) (Figure 14.2). Glucose metabolism is inhibited within muscle cells because insulin deficiency results in increased non-esterified fatty acid (NEFA) release from intracellular stores. Metabolism of NEFA produces citrate which is itself an inhibitor of 6-phosphofructo-1-kinase. Also, acetyl CoA production from NEFA metabolism inhibits activation of pyruvate dehydrogenase, thus reducing metabolism of pyruvate.

Insulin deficiency also results in an increased production of ketone bodies (3-hydroxybutyrate, acetoacetate and acetone) in the liver. Metabolism of ketone bodies by the brain, intestine and kidney tends to increase concentrations of citrate and acetyl CoA. Hence by a similar mechanism to that described above for NEFA metabolism, glucose uptake and metabolism is inhibited.

With progressive hyperglycemia, glucose is lost in the urine and over a period of hours, dehydration develops. As salt and water loss decreases renal perfusion, glucose clearance from the plasma is decreased, thus causing further elevation of plasma glucose concentration.

A further factor which predisposes to decreased tissue glucose consumption in patients with IDDM receiving conventional insulin replacement, relates to the relative portal hypoinsulinism which results from the injection of insulin into the systemic circulation. This imbalance of insulin action on peripheral tissues compared to the liver is also thought to predispose to the hyperlactatemia (Taylor & Agius, 1988) which has been observed in most studies of adults with IDDM (Nosadini *et al.*, 1982; Capaldo *et al.*, 1984). In addition there is some evidence that peripheral insulin resistance occurs (Proietto *et al.*, 1983; Yki-Jarvinen *et al.*, 1984b), decreasing glucose uptake by muscle. Delivery of insulin into the portal circulation to restore the porto-peripheral gradient produces normalization of these metabolic abnormalities (Stevenson *et al.*, 1983a & 1983b; Jimenez *et al.*, 1985).

In subjects with IDDM and inadequate insulin replacement, glucose metabolism is increased by the sorbitol pathway (Figure 14.3). Glucose is reduced to sorbitol by aldose reductase which requires NADPH and forms $NADP^+$ (section 14.5 below) and sorbitol is then oxidized to fructose by sorbitol dehydrogenase. The initial step is coupled to reduction of NAD^+ to NADH which competes with glycolysis at the glyceraldehyde dehydrogenase step for NAD^+ (Gonzalez *et al.*, 1986). An increased $NADH/NAD^+$ ratio favors increased conversion of dihydroxyacetone phosphate to glycerol 3-phosphate.

14.2.3 LIPID METABOLISM

Insulin is the major factor which inhibits lipolysis in humans, and in subjects with IDDM, lipolysis occurs as a result of both insulin lack and insulin resistance (Singh *et al.*, 1987; Jensen *et al.*, 1989). Lipolysis and fatty acid mobilization occur as a consequence of the unopposed stimulation of triacylglycerol lipase by catecholamine release associated with the β-adrenergic effects of sympathetic activity. In subjects who are ill, sympathetic activity is high and the elevated lipolysis contributes to the risk of developing ketoacidosis. Furthermore, this effect is exacerbated by elevated levels of growth hormone and cortisol which also have lipolytic effects (Johnston & Alberti, 1982) and decrease tissue sensitivity to insulin (MacGorman *et al.*, 1981; Bratusch-Marrain *et al.*, 1982).

Fatty acids are metabolized by conversion into their CoA esters and then esterification into glycerolipid or oxidation into acetyl CoA in the mitochondria. For the latter step, the rate of transfer into the mitochondria is reg-

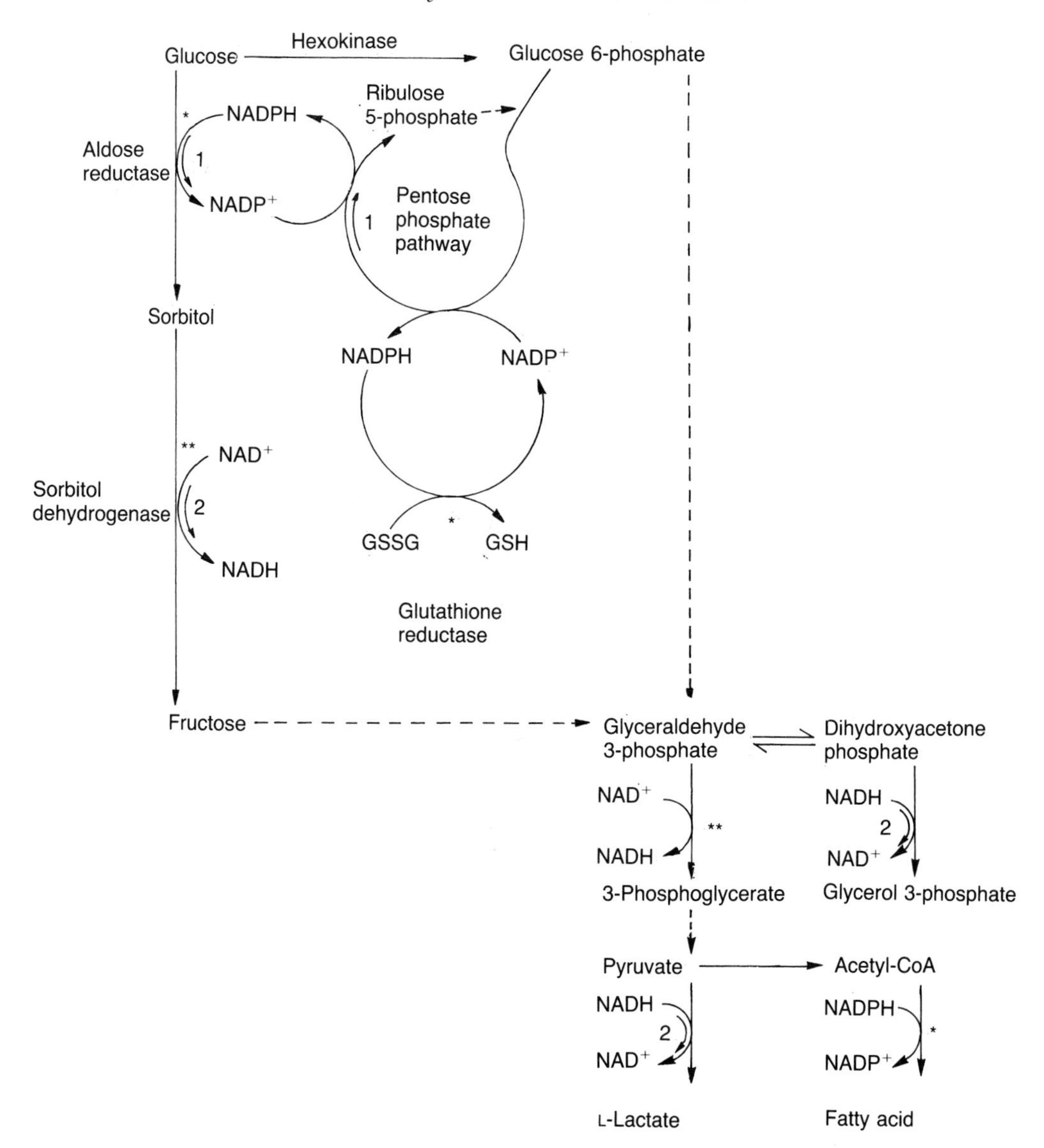

Figure 14.3 The sorbitol pathway and its links with the pentose phosphate pathway and glycolysis through the $NADP^+$ and NAD^+ redox couples (Gonzalez *et al.*, 1983 & 1986).

Reactions coupled to oxidation of NADPH are indicated by * and reactions coupled to reduction of NAD^+ are indicated by **. (Reproduced with permission from Taylor & Agius (1988).)

ulated by the activity of carnitine palmitoyltransferase 1 which itself is inhibited by malonyl CoA which is an intermediate in fatty acid synthesis. In insulin deficiency, fatty acid synthesis and malonyl CoA concentrations decrease, relieving the inhibition on carnitine palmitoyltransferase, thus favoring increased transfer of long chain fatty acids into the mitochondria. However, in ketoacidosis, ketone body synthesis increases to a point that saturation of the mechanisms utilizing ketone bodies as fuels occurs (Owen & Reichard, 1971) and their concentrations increase. In insulin-deficient states, the low insulin:glucagon ratio stimulates ketone body synthesis secondary to the increased production of NEFA from lipolysis. Furthermore, uptake of ketone bodies by extrahepatic tissues is reduced.

More recent work has suggested that in subjects with IDDM whose insulin replacement is deficient, acetone which is synthesized from acetoacetate may be a potential gluconeogenic substrate, via pyruvate and lactate or acetate (Reichard *et al.*, 1986).

Triacylglycerol is synthesized in the liver and either stored intracellularly or secreted with apoproteins in the form of VLDL. Triacylglycerol concentrations in plasma are elevated in individuals with IDDM due to decreased clearance (Bagdade *et al.*, 1968; Nikkila *et al.*, 1977; Taskinen & Nikkila, 1979). In insulin deficiency, plasma fatty acid concentration and turnover are increased but intensive insulin therapy results in a decrease in triacylglycerol secretion rate (Pietri *et al.*, 1983; Dunn *et al.*, 1987). Poorly-controlled IDDM is associated with histological changes of fatty liver, elevated serum transaminase and hepatomegaly.

14.3 HORMONE ACTIONS IN INSULIN-DEPENDENT DIABETES MELLITUS

14.3.1 INSULIN

Evidence is accumulating that the liver of patients with IDDM is relatively insensitive to the effects of insulin (Bell *et al.*, 1986). Adipocytes from patients with poorly-controlled IDDM demonstrate decreased insulin receptor binding with impaired sensitivity of some pathways (glucose transport and antilipolysis) but normal insulin sensitivity with respect to glucose oxidation and lipogenesis, implying a post-receptor modulation of some of the metabolic effects of insulin to counterbalance the decrease in insulin receptor binding (Pedersen & Hjollund, 1982; Lönnroth *et al.*, 1983). Impaired insulin action is thought to be a consequence of the metabolic sequelae of hyperglycemia. The role of the peripheral hyperinsulinism caused by conventional intermittent injections of insulin is uncertain. Despite the lower daily doses of insulin required by continuous subcutaneous insulin infusion (CSII) therapy compared to intermittent injections, glycemic control and patterns of intermediary metabolites and counter-regulatory hormones were similar in groups of adult patients treated with both regimens longterm. There was no evidence of increased peripheral insulin sensitivity on CSII, though insulin-stimulated rates of glucose uptake by adipocytes were increased with CSII (Marshall *et al.*, 1988).

14.3.2 GLUCAGON AND GUT HORMONES

Glucagon causes a transient increase in glycogenolysis, stimulates gluconeogenesis, fatty acid oxidation and ketogenesis (Gerich *et al.*, 1975) and exerts a weak effect on peripheral lipolysis (Honnor & Saggerson, 1980). In nondiabetics, the effects of glucagon are counterbalanced by insulin but in states of insulin deficiency with a decreased insulin: glucagon ratio, the metabolic effects of glucagon are increased. In patients with IDDM, the regulating effect of blood glucose concentrations on glucagon secretion are diminished and plasma glucagon levels are elevated in untreated patients and in those with ketoacidosis, whereas in response to hypoglycemia, glucagon secretion is diminished. The latter effect becomes more pronounced with time after diagnosis (Gerich *et al.*, 1973; Benson *et al.*, 1977; Bolli *et al.*, 1983).

Somatostatin is released from D cells of the pancreatic islets and gut, particularly the stomach. Secretion from the pancreatic D cells is stimulated by a variety of nutrients, peptides and neurotransmitters, including in particular glucose, free fatty acids and 3-hydroxybutyrate (Wasada *et al.*, 1981). Somatostatin release from the stomach is precipitated mainly by glucose, secretin and cholecystokinin and inhibited by somatostatin, insulin, acetylcholine and bicarbonate ions. The majority of plasma somatostatin derives from the stomach (Gutniak *et al.*, 1987). Of potential importance to subjects with IDDM is its inhibitory effect on release of glucagon, growth hormone and any residual insulin (Alberti *et al.*, 1973; Mortimer *et al.*, 1974). In patients with IDDM, particularly with ketoacidosis, plasma somatostatin concentrations are increased, presumably due to the relative deficiency of insulin (Skare *et al.*, 1985; Binimelis *et al.*, 1987). Despite the potential effects on glucose homeostasis, it is probable that the abnormal dynamics of somatostatin secretion in IDDM are a secondary effect rather than a primary etiological factor. It also has to be considered that the major effect of somatostatin on the pancreas is via a paracrine mechanism. Furthermore, somatostatin analogues have to date proved disappointing as potential therapeutic tools in the management of IDDM (Davies *et al.*, 1989).

A number of other gut hormones (e.g., gastric inhibitory peptide, GLP-1 7–36 amide, cholecystokinin and secretin) and pancreatic polypeptide are released in response to meals and some stimulate insulin release. However, most of these hormones do not appear to have a specific role in the metabolic abnormalities of IDDM (Kreymann & Bloom, 1991) though a blunted pancreatic polypeptide response to hypoglycemia may be a marker of defective glucose counter-regulation in IDDM, perhaps predictive of the development of sympathetic autonomic neuropathy (White *et al.*, 1985).

14.3.3 CATECHOLAMINES

Plasma catecholamine levels are increased in patients with IDDM and poor glycemic control or ketoacidosis (Christensen, 1974). They may have an important role in ketogenesis, by augmenting lipolysis (Keller *et al.*, 1984; Keller, 1986; Muller *et al.*, 1989) and as a result of α-adrenergic effects, inhibiting release of any remaining insulin in newly-presenting patients with IDDM. Catecholamines may also have an important role in glucose counter-regulation when glucagon secretion is impaired (Hansen *et al.*, 1986).

14.3.4 GROWTH HORMONE (SEE ALSO CHAPTER 5)

Plasma growth hormone concentrations are elevated in the patient with poorly controlled IDDM (Fineberg & Merimee, 1974; Gerich, 1984). In such patients, growth hormone clearance from the plasma is normal (Navalesi *et al.*, 1975) and so an increase in growth hormone secretion seems the most likely mechanism. Growth hormone secretion in response to a variety of physiologic and pharmacological stimuli including growth hormone-releasing hormone is increased (Holly *et al.*, 1988; Press *et al.*, 1984b). The mechanism for the hypersecretion of growth hormone is unknown but may result from altered hypothalamic-pituitary control or from a lack of feedback inhibition from low levels of insulin-like growth factor 1 (IGF-1), production of which may be decreased in insulin deficiency (Holly *et al.*, 1988). Indirect evidence for the latter comes from studies demonstrating that improvement of glycemic control is associated with increased IGF-1 and decreased growth hormone levels (Tamborlane *et al.*, 1981; Amiel *et al.*, 1984; Press *et al.*, 1984a). Suppression of IGF-1 production in IDDM has been speculated to be a mechanism for muting the growth-promoting properties of growth hormone, thus permitting utilization of mobilized substrates for fuel homeostasis rather than for cell growth and proliferation (Holly *et al.*, 1988).

Increases in growth hormone secretion are particularly apparent in adolescents with IDDM. Studies have shown that the increase in growth hormone secretion is primarily due to an increase in growth hormone pulse amplitude (Edge *et al.*, 1990a; Pal *et al.*, 1992). Growth hormone appears to have a role in the dawn phenomenon (Campbell *et al.*, 1984; Edge *et al.*, 1990b & 1990c) in which it augments the effect of a relative functional hypoinsulinism (Skor *et al.*, 1983 & 1984), producing hyperglycemia. This is discussed further in section 14.4.2.

At a biochemical level in nondiabetics, growth hormone has mainly anti-insulin effects, stimulating hepatic gluconeogenesis, impairment of tissue glucose utilization, and increasing lipolysis which produces glycerol as a substrate for gluconeogenesis and fatty acids which inhibit glucose oxidation and utilization (Randle *et al.*, 1963). Growth hormone also appears to induce insulin resistance through a site distal to the insulin receptor (Rosenfeld *et al.*, 1982). The above mechanisms operate in patients with IDDM but in response to insulin resistance, a compensatory increase in pancreatic insulin secretion which occurs in nondiabetics is not possible (Press *et al.*, 1984a). This predisposes to worse glycemic control and a vicious circle in which growth hormone secretion is stimulated further.

14.3.5 CORTISOL

Cortisol is of importance in patients with IDDM who are under-insulinized, producing increased hepatic glucose output and ketogenesis (Barnes *et al.*, 1978; Johnston & Alberti, 1982). Cortisol enhances amino acid production from muscle protein catabolism thus increasing the availability of substrates for gluconeogenesis though it appears to probably have a relatively minor role in the regulation of ketogenesis in such patients (Taylor & Agius, 1988).

14.4 THE EFFECT OF AGE ON THE METABOLIC DISTURBANCE CAUSED BY INSULIN-DEPENDENT DIABETES MELLITUS

14.4.1 INFANTS AND YOUNG CHILDREN

Neonatal IDDM which may be transient or permanent (Chapter 30) is very rare and there are few data on intermediary metabolism at this age. In transient neonatal IDDM, which is probably due to delayed β cell maturation (Milner *et al.*, 1971; Pagliara *et al.*, 1973; Cavallo *et al.*, 1987), hyperglycemia is often accompanied by minimal or absent ketonuria (Gentz & Cornblath, 1969). Similarly, in the presence of congenital absence of the β cells and other causes of permanent IDDM in infancy, hyperglycemia is associated with mild ketonuria (Blum *et al.*, 1993). Insulin levels tend to be low for the raised plasma glucose concentration (Milner *et al.*, 1971; Knip *et al.*, 1983) but insulin sensitivity appears to be normal (Ivarsson *et al.*, 1988). Counter-regulatory hormone secretion in both forms of neonatal diabetes does not appear to be increased (Cavallo *et al.*, 1987).

In children under the age of 5 years with IDDM, ketoacidosis is a relatively common finding at diagnosis (Golden *et al.*, 1985), perhaps because of delayed clinical recognition of the disease. However, after the initial presenting episode, ketonuria is either absent or mild (Goldman, 1979) and the frequency of ketoacidosis is relatively decreased compared to that in the older population (Ternand *et al.*, 1982; Golden *et al.*, 1985). This is likely to reflect the fact that intercurrent infection precipitates ketoacidosis when insulin secretory capacity is still present (Heinze *et al.*, 1978), having been decreased to around 20% of normal. After control of the initial episode, ketogenesis is easily suppressed as the very slow steady decline of β cell mass continues (Baker *et al.*, 1967; Hernandez *et al.*, 1968; Illig & Prader, 1968; Weber, 1972). The relative resistance to the development of ketoacidosis which has been suggested (Ternand *et al.*, 1982) may also be assisted by a decreased frequency of missed insulin injections because of greater parental supervision than occurs in older children (Golden *et al.*, 1985).

Overnight metabolic profiles in children aged under 6 years have shown, as in older children and young adults, the clear presence of a dawn phenomenon. The association of an increase in blood glucose at this time with changes in intermediary metabolite concentrations in blood, particularly an increase in 3-hydroxybutyrate and glycerol, suggest the presence of functional hypoinsulinism (de Beaufort *et al.*, 1986). In the same study, blood alanine levels remained relatively constant implying the absence of severe insulin deficiency. The presence of concurrent normal levels of insulin have been interpreted as evidence of a relative increase in insulin resistance (de Beaufort *et al.*, 1986), despite the previously recognized increased insulin sensitivity of young children (Rosenbloom *et al.*, 1975).

Young children with IDDM are also recognized to have an increased susceptibility to hypoglycemia (Ternand *et al.*, 1982). This phenomenon in addition to the decreased propensity to ketoacidosis might suggest a defect in the secretion of counter-regulatory hormones. However, metabolic studies in such children have shown the presence of insulin insufficiency only. No evidence of an abnormality of secretion of other pancreatic islet hormones or of gastric inhibitory peptide was found (Ternand *et al.*, 1982).

The effects of CSII on intermediary metabolism have been studied during attempts to improve metabolic control in older children with IDDM. Short-term CSII for 8–10 days in both newly-diagnosed and chronically-treated children with IDDM produced normoglycemia, associated with normalization of fasting plasma-free insulin, growth hormone, free fatty acid, triglyceride and total cholesterol levels (Soltesz *et al.*, 1988). However, normoglycemia was achieved at the expense of relatively large total doses of insulin which produced fasting hypoglucagonemia and hypoketonemia. Longer-term therapy for two years with CSII also resulted in improved glycemic control compared to a regimen of intermittent injections (de Beaufort *et al.*, 1989). Fasting intermediary metabolites were within the normal range with the exception of β-hydroxybutyrate which was minimally elevated, suggesting early morning insulin deficiency. However, the latter phenomenon was much more marked in patients treated with intermittent injections (de Beaufort *et al.*, 1989).

14.4.2 PUBERTY

Glycemic control frequently deteriorates in children at puberty (Blethen *et al.*, 1981; Mann & Johnston, 1982). Whereas many factors such as rebellion and emotional lability may contribute to this phenomenon (Tattersall & Lowe, 1981), there is clear evidence that a reversible decrease in insulin sensitivity occuring during puberty is partly responsible (see also Chapter 5) (Amiel *et al.*, 1986). Euglycemic insulin-clamp studies have demonstrated a decrease in insulin-stimulated glucose metabolism in children in puberty compared to prepubertal children and adults but occurring to an even greater degree in those with IDDM compared to non-diabetic children (Figure 14.4) (Amiel *et al.*, 1986). Increased physical fitness and improved glycemic control also appear to alter

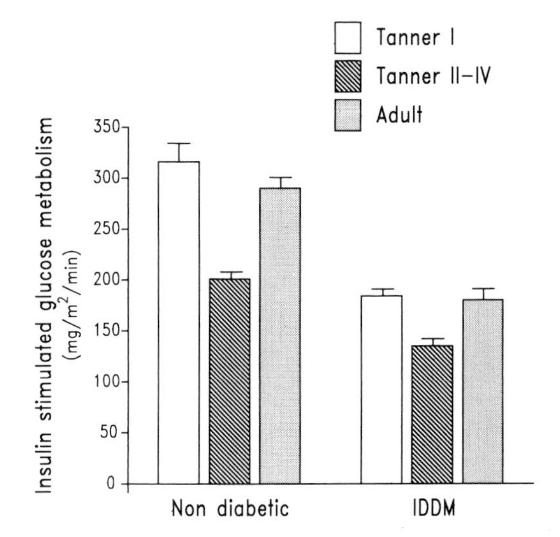

Figure 14.4 The effect of puberty on insulin-stimulated glucose metabolism (mean ± SE) in subjects with and without IDDM. (Reprinted by permission from Amiel *et al.*, 1986, Impaired insulin action in puberty: a contributing factor to poor glycemic control in adolescents with diabetes; *New England Journal of Medicine*, **35**, 215–19.)

insulin sensitivity in adolescents and young adults, producing increased insulin-mediated glucose metabolism (Yki-Jarvinen *et al.*, 1984a; Landt *et al.*, 1985; Arslanian *et al.*, 1990).

Biochemical studies in pubertal patients with IDDM have shown that the response to insulin appears to be inversely correlated with mean 24-hour levels of growth hormone but not with plasma levels of IGF-1, catecholamines or cortisol (Amiel *et al.*, 1986). Insulin resistance in puberty appears to reduce glucose uptake during euglycemic insulin-clamp studies but to have no effect on endogenous glucose production. Furthermore, basal plasma concentrations and response to insulin of total branched chain amino acids, free fatty acids and β-hydroxybutyrate are unaffected by puberty. These findings suggest that the insulin resistance of puberty is confined to glucose metabolism in muscle and has no effect on hepatic glucose production, lipolysis, ketogenesis and anabolism (Amiel *et al.*, 1991). As in normal subjects, insulin resistance in patients with IDDM is maximal in late puberty (Beaufrere *et al.*, 1988; Dunger, 1992).

In pubertal patients with IDDM, growth hormone pulse amplitude and baseline concentrations are elevated (Edge *et al.*, 1990a) and are uninfluenced by improvements in glycemic control (Miller *et al.*, 1992). Euglycemic clamp studies of the dawn phenomenon have shown that overnight growth hormone secretion is related to the dawn increase in insulin requirement (Beaufrere *et al.*, 1988; Edge *et al.*, 1990b), though there is debate as to whether this is the primary cause of the dawn phenomenon or whether increased insulin clearance is responsible (Arslanian *et al.*, 1992). Administration of pirenzepine to adolescents with IDDM suppresses growth hormone pulse amplitude, reduces the dawn rise in β-hydroxybutyrate and the insulin requirements to maintain normoglycemia as measured by a euglycemic clamp (Dunger *et al.*, 1991). This may not be beneficial overall and pirenzepine is not used therapeutically. However, a similar effect of recombinant IGF-1 on overnight growth hormone secretion and insulin requirements (Cheetham *et al*, 1993) may prove to be therapeutically useful (Usala *et al.*, 1992).

Despite elevated growth hormone levels in patients with IDDM, IGF-1 levels are decreased. Serum levels of growth hormone binding protein as a measure of the concentration of hepatic growth hormone receptors are reduced in children and adolescents with IDDM, though there is no association with circulating levels of IGF-1 (Massa *et al.*, 1993). This finding suggests that the reduced concentrations of IGF-1 seen in IDDM may be related to a post-growth hormone receptor defect or to changes in the insulin-like growth factor binding proteins. Circulating concentrations of insulin-like growth factor binding protein 1 (IGFBP-1) which inhibit IGF-1 bioavailability are inversely associated with insulin concentrations and in the presence of inadequate nocturnal insulin levels, IGFBP-1 levels may be increased, thus further reducing the bioactivity of IGF-1 (Holly *et al.*, 1990; Batch *et al.*, 1991).

14.5 BIOCHEMICAL ASPECTS OF COMPLICATIONS

14.5.1 DIABETIC KETOACIDOSIS

Diabetic ketoacidosis is the result of relative or absolute insulin deficiency in association with excessive counter-regulatory hormone (glucagon, cortisol, growth hormone and epinephrine) secretion. The actions of these individual hormones at a metabolic level have been described earlier in this chapter and they result in hyperglycemia, hyperlipidemia and ketonemia. With the accumulation of ketones, a rapid dissociation of β-hydroxybutyrate and acetoacetate occurs with the release of hydrogen ions that exceeds buffering capacity and produces a lowering of the plasma bicarbonate concentration. The actions of the counter-regulatory hormones are increased in the presence of insulin deficiency and, furthermore, the hyperglycemic effect of all these hormones together appears to be greater than the sum of the individual hormones (Shamoon *et al.*, 1981). Although the presence of insulin deficiency is a prerequisite, it appears that concurrently elevated concentrations of counter-regulatory hormones are essential to produce substantial metabolic decompensation (Gerich *et al.*, 1975; McGarry & Foster, 1977; Schade & Eaton, 1977a & 1977b; Schade *et al.*, 1977; Barnes *et al.*, 1978; McGarry, 1979; Schade & Eaton, 1980; MacGillivray *et al.*, 1981 & 1982).

Although the acidosis of diabetic ketoacidosis is predominantly due to the accumulation and dissociation of organic ketoacids, other contributory factors include lactic acidosis from hypoperfusion and hyperchloremic acidosis particularly after intravenous fluids and during recovery from ketoacidosis (Hammeke *et al.*, 1978; Oh *et al.*, 1978; Halperin *et al.*, 1981; Adrogué *et al.*, 1982).

Cerebral edema is a complication of diabetic ketoacidosis, seen most commonly in newly-presenting patients with IDDM or in children under 5 years of age (Rosenbloom, 1990). Subclinical brain swelling has been demonstrated by CT scanning to be a very common occurrence during the treatment of ketoacidosis in children (Krane *et al.*, 1985). The etiology of cerebral edema is, however, under much debate and three possible biochemical mechanisms may contribute to its development (Hammond & Wallis, 1992):

1) Treatment of ketoacidosis which produces a rapid decrease in blood glucose and plasma sodium concentrations and thus a precipitate fall in plasma osmolality might be expected to predispose to cerebral edema. However, studies have shown that approximately half the cases of cerebral edema have received inadequate fluid replacement and more than half have experienced a fall in blood glucose concentrations of less than 2.8 mmol/l/h (Rosenbloom, 1990). However, one-third of patients had plasma sodium concentrations of less than 130 mmol/l at the time of cerebral herniation (Duck & Wyatt, 1988) and 60% had a fall in plasma sodium concentration between admission and collapse of over 4 mmol/l (Rosenbloom, 1990).

2) The generation of osmoprotective molecules in brain cells during the development of ketoacidosis may be a causative factor in the development of cerebral edema. Animal studies have shown that glucose may be metabolized within brain cells by the polyol pathway (Figure 14.3), to produce osmotically active substances such as sorbitol (Clements *et al.*, 1968). However, other experimental work has not demonstrated excess concentrations of these substances in the brain

extracellular space and half of the increase in brain osmolality has been proposed to be secondary to unidentified idiogenic osmoles (Arieff & Kleeman, 1973).

3) An alternative mechanism for the development of cerebral edema may be secondary to impaired ion transport. Cerebral tissue hypoxia may occur during ketoacidosis (Young & Bradley, 1967), leading to an increase in glutamate concentration. This in turn may activate the *n*-methyl-D-aspartate (NMDA) receptor, producing excitotoxic cell swelling as a result of the subsequent ion influx and a toxic increase in intracellular calcium (Collins *et al.*, 1989).

14.5.2 HYPOGLYCEMIA

Hypoglycemia is the most frequent acute complication of IDDM in children. Clinical aspects of this problem are discussed elsewhere in this volume. The blood glucose concentration at which symptoms of hypoglycemia occur appears to vary, dependent on the previous glycemic control experienced by the child (Soltesz, 1993). However, a clear hierarchy of responses occur as plasma glucose concentrations decrease (Mitrakou *et al.*, 1991). The initial response is that of increased counter-regulatory hormone (glucagon, epinephrine, cortisol and growth hormone) secretion. Thereafter, at lower glucose concentrations still, autonomic nervous system activity produces symptoms and finally, neuroglycopenic symptoms occur.

In nondiabetic adult subjects insulin-induced hypoglycemia suppresses hepatic glucose production and increases glucose uptake. Hypoglycemia reverses when hepatic glucose output due to glycogenolysis and later gluconeogenesis (Lecavalier *et al.*, 1989) exceeds glucose consumption (Rizza *et al.*, 1979; Bolli *et al.*, 1984a). Later, as the effects of the insulin wear off, glucose utilization decreases, plasma glucose levels return to normal and counter-regulatory hormone secretion decreases (Gerich, 1993). Glucagon appears to be the major counter-regulatory hormone when plasma glucose concentrations decrease rapidly and epinephrine secretion is of major importance only in the absence of glucagon (Figure 14.5) (Rizza *et al.*, 1979; Cryer & Gerich, 1985).

In children with IDDM, growth hormone, cortisol and catecholamine responses to hypoglycemia appear normal (Brambilla *et al.*, 1987), but as in adults with IDDM, the glucagon response is lost shortly after the onset of the disease (Aman & Wranne, 1988; Singer-Granick *et al.*, 1988) and they are therefore at greater risk of an increase in frequency and severity of episodes of hypoglycemia. However, several studies in children with IDDM have demonstrated that they show a vigorous epinephrine response to mild hypoglycemia which is greater than that observed in studies in adults with IDDM (Amiel *et al.*, 1987; Hoffman *et al.*, 1991). In children with poor glycemic control, the epinephrine response occurs at higher plasma glucose values than in nondiabetic children (Jones *et al.*, 1991). With increasing duration of IDDM, studies in adults have shown that the catecholamine response is also lost and counter-regulation in the presence of acute hypoglycemia is severely compromised (Cryer, 1992).

Patients with IDDM also demonstrate an increased rebound of plasma glucose concentrations compared to nondiabetic subjects following hypoglycemia. This phenomenon is also known as the 'Somogyi effect' and may have a detrimental effect on overall glycemic control (Bolli *et al.*, 1984b; Perriello *et al.*, 1988). The rebound in plasma glucose concentration is likely to be caused by relative insulin deficiency, following the increased rate of release of insulin from the subcutaneous depot which led to the occurrence of hypoglycemia.

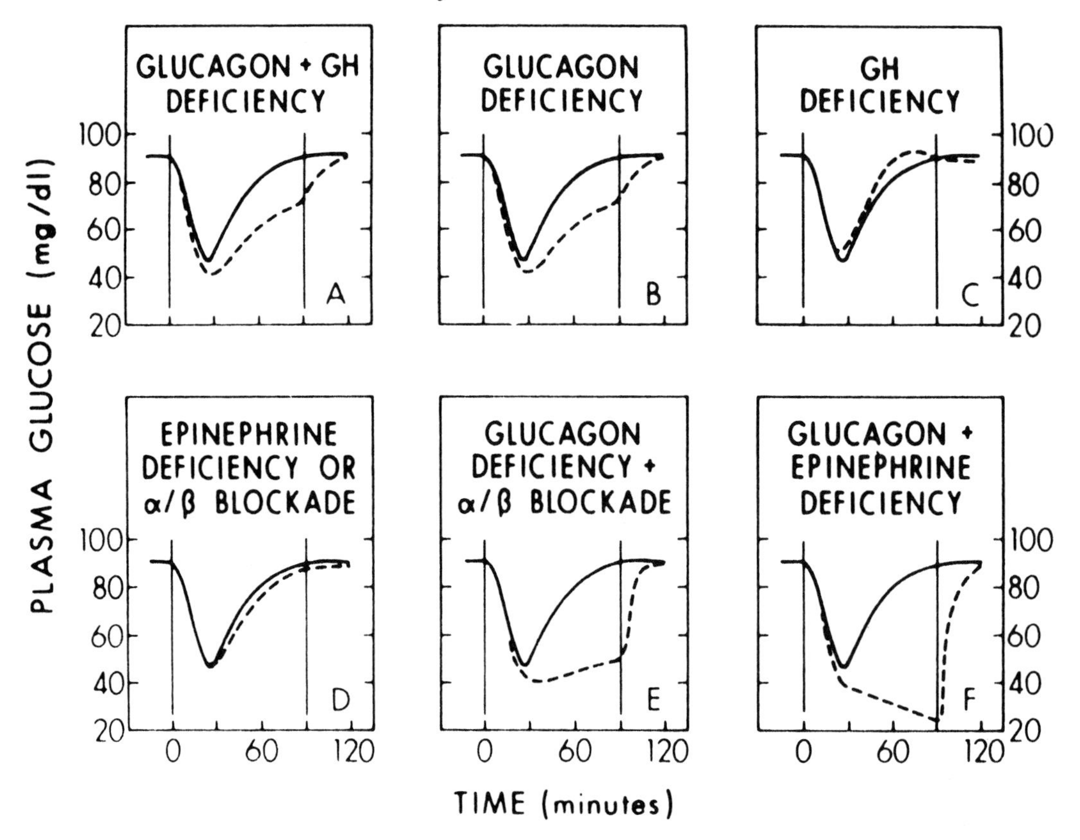

Figure 14.5 The effect of counter-regulatory hormone deficiency on plasma glucose curves during insulin-induced hypoglycemia in nondiabetic subjects. Control subjects are shown by solid lines and the effect of interventions by interrupted lines. Panels A–C demonstrate the primary role of glucagon, whereas panels D–F show the secondary importance of catecholamines in the presence of glucagon deficiency in recovery from hypoglycemia. These idealized curves were derived from Clarke *et al.* (1979), Gerich *et al.* (1979) and Rizza *et al.* (1979). (Reproduced with permission from Cryer, 1981.)

14.5.3 LONG-TERM COMPLICATIONS

The presence of clinically detectable chronic complications of IDDM are relatively unusual in children. Nevertheless, histological evidence of the onset of complications is seen in childhood. Basement membrane thickening develops within 5 years of diagnosis (Osterby, 1986) and though the role of collagen glycosylation in its development is unclear (Cohen *et al.*, 1980), this phenomenon does not develop prior to the onset of the biochemical disturbance of IDDM (Steffes *et al.*, 1985). Furthermore, the increment in glomerular basement membrane thickness in young adults with microalbuminuria has been shown to be correlated with glycemic control (Bangstad *et al.*, 1993). Basement membrane thickening has been observed in several tissues, including muscle (Kilo *et al.*, 1972; Sheikholislam *et al.*, 1976a & 1976b; Williamson & Kilo, 1978).

Non-enzymic glycosylation of proteins is promoted by chronic elevation of plasma glucose concentrations. Lysine and valine residues are affected and undergo aldimine and then ketoamine formation which may alter the stereochemical configuration and thus the functional properties of chemicals. It is hypothesized that these chemical effects may predispose to the development of many of the longer-term complications seen in patients with IDDM (Kirschenbaum, 1984). For example, glycosylated albumin inhibits hepatic uptake of glycoproteins (Summerfield *et al.*, 1982); glycosylated fibrin is more resistant to breakdown increasing the risk of thrombus formation (Brownlee *et al.*, 1983); glycosylated apoprotein B reduces the affinity for low density lipoprotein receptors thus decreasing low density lipoprotein cholesterol metabolism (Kesaniemi *et al.*, 1983), a change which may relate to the development of atherosclerosis; glycosylated collagen demonstrates increased crosslinkage (Kohn & Schnider, 1982) which may predispose to the small joint mobility problems seen in patients with longstanding IDDM.

The production and metabolism of polyols seems to have an important role in the development of the chronic complications of IDDM. Accumulation of osmotically active sorbitol within cells may predispose to cellular swelling and the development of cataracts and disordered nerve conduction (Gabbay, 1975). Myoinositol content of nerve tissue is decreased in patients with IDDM and this may predispose to the development of neuropathy (Finegold *et al.*, 1983). Maintenance of neural myoinositol content by supplementation or by the use of a specific aldose reductase inhibitor may provide a therapeutic option in the prevention of neuropathy (Salway *et al.*, 1978). The requirement for NADPH for the initial reduction of sorbitol competes with other reactions requiring NADPH e.g., the conversion of oxidized to reduced glutathione (Figure 14.3) which protects cellular components from oxidative damage due to its powerful antioxidant effect.

Growth hormone may have a role in the development of microangiopathy (Gerich, 1984). It is known that proliferative retinopathy in diabetics progresses more slowly in patients after hypophysectomy (Lundbaek *et al.*, 1970) and that such findings are rare in patients who also have isolated growth hormone deficiency (Merimee *et al.*, 1973). However, the precise role of growth hormone in the development of complications is not well understood.

REFERENCES

Adrogué, H.J., Wilson, H., Boyd, A.E. *et al.* (1982) Plasma acid-base patterns in diabetic ketoacidosis. *N. Eng. J. Med.*, **307**, 1603–160.

Alberti, K.G.M.M., Christensen, N.J., Christensen, S.E. *et al.* (1973) Inhibition of insulin secretion by somatostatin. *Lancet*, **ii**, 1299–1301.

Aman, J. and Wranne, L. (1988) Hypoglycaemia in childhood diabetes: 1. Clinical signs and hormonal counterregulation. *Acta Paed. Scand.*, **77**, 542–47.

Amiel, S.A., Caprio, S., Sherwin, R.S. *et al.* (1991) Insulin resistance of puberty: a defect restricted to peripheral glucose metabolism. *J. Clin. Endocrin. and Metab.*, **72**, 277–82.

Amiel, S.A., Sherwin, R.S., Hintz, R.L. *et al.* (1984) Effect of diabetes and its control on insulin-like growth factors in the young subject with type 1 diabetes. *Diabetes*, **33**, 1175–79.

Amiel, S.A., Sherwin, R.S., Simonson, D.C. *et al.* (1986) Impaired insulin action in puberty: a contributing factor to poor glycemic control in adolescents with diabetes. *N. Eng. J. Med.*, **315**, 215–19.

Amiel, S.A., Simonson, D.C., Sherwin, R.S. *et al.* (1987) Exaggerated epinephrine responses to hypoglycemia in normal and insulin-dependent diabetic children. *J. Pediatr.*, **110**, 832–37.

Arieff, A.I. and Kleeman, C.R. (1973) Studies on mechanisms of cerebral edema in diabetic comas: effects of hyperglycemia and rapid lowering of plasma glucose in normal rabbits. *J. Clin. Invest.*, **52**, 571–83.

Arslanian, S., Ohki, Y., Becker, O.D.J. *et al.* (1992) The dawn phenomenon: comparison between normal and insulin-dependent diabetic adolescents. *Pediatr. Res.*, **31**, 203–206.

Arslanian, S., Nixon, P.A., Becker, D. *et al.* (1990) Impact of physical fitness and glycemic control on *in vivo* insulin action in adolescents with IDDM. *Diabetes Care*, **13**, 9–15.

Bagdade, J.D., Porte, D. and Bierman, E.L. (1968) Acute insulin withdrawal and the regulation of plasma triglyceride removal in diabetic subjects. *Diabetes*, **17**, 127–32.

Baker, L., Kaye, R. and Root, A.W. (1967) The early partial remission of juvenile diabetes mellitus: the roles of insulin and growth hormone. *J. Pediatr.*, **71**, 825–31.

Bangstad, H-J., Osterby, R., Dahl-Jorgensen, K. *et al.* (1993) Early glomerulopathy is present in young, type 1 (insulin-dependent) diabetic patients with microalbuminuria. *Diabetologia*, **36**, 523–29.

Barnes, A.J., Kohner, E.M., Bloom, S.R. *et al.* (1978) Importance of pituitary hormones in aetiology of diabetic ketoacidosis. *Lancet*, **i**, 1171–74.

Batch, J.A., Baxter, R.C. and Werther, G. (1991) Abnormal regulation of insulin-like growth factor binding proteins in adolescents with insulin-dependent diabetes. *J. Clin. Endocrin. Metab.*, **73**, 964–68.

de Beaufort, C.E., Bruining, G.J., Home, P.D. *et al.* (1986) Overnight metabolic profiles in very young insulin-dependent diabetic children. *Eur. J. Pediatr.*, **145**, 73–76.

de Beaufort, C.E., Houtzagers, C.M.G.J., Bruining, G.J. *et al.* (1989) Continuous subcutaneous insulin infusion (CSII) versus conventional injection therapy in newly diagnosed diabetic children: two-year follow-up of a randomized, prospective trial. *Diabetic Med.*, **6**, 766–71.

Beaufrere, B., Beylot, M., Metz, C. *et al.* (1988) Dawn phenomenon in type 1 (insulin-dependent) diabetic adolescents: influence of nocturnal growth hormone secretion. *Diabetologia*, **31**, 607–611.

Bell, P.M., Firth, R.G. and Rizza, R.A. (1986) Assessment of insulin action in insulin-dependent diabetes mellitus using [6^{14}C]glucose, [3^{3}H]glucose, and [2^{3}H]glucose: differences in the apparent pattern of insulin resistance depending on the isotope used. *J. Clin. Invest.*, **78**, 1479–86.

Benson, J.W., Johnson, D.G., Palmer, J.P. *et al.* (1977) Glucagon and catecholamine secretion during hypoglycemia in normal and diabetic man. *J. Clin. Endocrin. and Metab.*, **44**, 459–64.

Binimelis, J., Webb, S.M., Serrano, J. *et al.* (1987) Plasma immunoreactive somatostatin is elevated in diabetic ketoacidosis and correlates with plasma non-esterified fatty acid concentration. *Diabetic Med.*, **4**, 221–24.

Blethen, S.L., Sargeant, D.T., Whitlow, M.G. *et al.* (1981) Effect of pubertal stage and recent blood glucose control on plasma somatomedin C in children with insulin-dependent diabetes mellitus. *Diabetes*, **30**, 868–72.

Blum, D., Dorchy, H., Mouraux, T. *et al.* (1993) Congenital absence of insulin cells in a neonate with diabetes mellitus and mutase-deficient methylmalonic acidaemia. *Diabetologia*, **36**, 352–57.

Bolli, G.B., Gottesman, I.S., Campbell, P.J. *et al.* (1984b) Glucose counterregulation and waning of insulin in the Somogyi phenomenon (posthypoglycemic hyperglycemia). *N. Eng. J. Med.*, **311**, 1214–19.

Bolli, G.B., Gottesman, I.S., Cryer, P.E. *et al.* (1984a) Glucose counterregulation during prolonged hypoglycemia in normal humans. *Am. J. Physiol.*, **247** (Endocrinol. Metab. 10), E206–214.

Bolli, G., de Feo, P., Compagnucci, P. *et al.* (1983) Abnormal glucose counterregulation in insulin-dependent diabetes mellitus: interaction of anti-insulin antibodies and impaired glucagon and epinephrine secretion. *Diabetes*, **32**, 134–41.

Brambilla, P., Bougneres, P.F., Santiago, J.V. *et al.* (1987) Glucose counterregulation in pre-school-age diabetic children with recurrent hypoglycemia during conventional treatment. *Diabetes*, **36**, 300–304.

Bratusch-Marrain, P.R., Smith, D. and DeFronzo, R.A. (1982) The effect of growth hormone on glucose metabolism and insulin secretion in man. *J. Clin. Endocrin. and Metab.*, **55**, 973–82.

Brownlee, M., Vlassara, H. and Cerami, A. (1983) Nonenzymatic glycosylation reduces the susceptibility of fibrin to degradation by plasmin. *Diabetes*, **32**, 680–84.

Campbell, P.J., Bolli, G.B., Cryer, P.E. *et al.* (1984) Nocturnal spikes in growth hormone secretion cause the dawn phenomenon. *Diabetologia*, **27**, 262A.

Capaldo, B., Home, P.D., Massi-Benedetti, M. *et al.* (1984) The response of blood intermediary metabolite levels to 24 hours treatment with a blood glucose-controlled insulin infusion system in type 1 diabetes. *Diabetes Res.*, **1**, 187–93.

Cavallo, L., Mautone, A., Laforgia, N. *et al.* (1987) Neonatal diabetes mellitus: evaluation of pancreatic β-cell function in two cases. *Helvet. Paed. Acta.*, **42**, 437–43.

Cheetham, T.D., Jones, J., Taylor, A.M. *et al.* (1993) The effects of recombinant insulin-like growth factor 1 administration on growth hormone levels and insulin requirements in adolescents with type 1 (insulin-dependent) diabetes mellitus. *Diabetologia*, **36**, 678–81.

Cherrington, A.D., Stevenson, R.W., Steiner, K.E. *et al.* (1987) Insulin, glucagon, and glucose as regulators of hepatic glucose uptake and production *in vivo*. *Diabetes/Metab. Rev.*, **3**, 307–332.

Christensen, N.J. (1974) Plasma norepinephrine and epinephrine in untreated diabetics, during fasting and after insulin administration. *Diabetes*, **23**, 1–8.

Clarke, W.L., Santiago, J.V., Thomas, L. *et al.* (1979) Adrenergic mechanisms in recovery from hypoglycemia in man: adrenergic blockade. *Am. J. Physiol.*, **236** (Endocrinol. Metab. Gastointest. Physiol. 5), E147–52.

Clements, R.S., Prockop, L.D. and Winegrad, A.I. (1968) Acute cerebral oedema during treatment of hyperglycaemia. *Lancet*, **ii**, 384–86.

Cohen, M.P., Urdanivia, E., Surma, M. *et al.* (1980) Increased glycosylation of glomerular basement membrane collagen in diabetes. *Biochem. and Biophys. Res. Comm.*, **95**, 765–69.

Collins, R.C., Dobkin, B.H., Choi, D.W. (1989) Selective vulnerability of the brain: new insights into the pathophysiology of stroke. *Ann. Int. Med.*, **110**, 992–1000.

Cryer, P.E. (1981) Glucose counterregulation in man. *Diabetes*, **30**, 261–64.

Cryer, P.E. (1992) Iatrogenic hypoglycemia as a cause of hypoglycemia-associated autonomic failure in IDDM: a vicious cycle. *Diabetes*, **41**, 255–60.

Cryer, P.E. and Gerich, J.E. (1985) Glucose counterregulation, hypoglycemia, and intensive insulin therapy in diabetes mellitus. *N. Eng. J. Med.*, **313**, 232–41.

Davies, R.R., Turner, S.J., Alberti, K.G.M.M. *et al.* (1989) Somatostatin analogues in diabetes mellitus. *Diabetic Med.*, **6**, 103–111.

Duck, S.C. and Wyatt, D.T. (1988) Factors associated with brain herniation in the treatment of diabetic ketoacidosis. *J. Pediatr.*, **113**, 10–14.

Dunger, D.B. (1992) Diabetes in puberty. *Arch. Dis. Child.*, **67**, 569–73.

Dunger, D.B., Edge, J.A., Pal, R. *et al.* (1991) Impact of increased growth hormone secretion on carbohydrate metabolism in adolescents with diabetes. *Acta Paed. Scand.*, **377** (Suppl.), 69–77.

Dunn, F.L., Carroll, P.B. and Beltz, W.F. (1987) Treatment with artificial β-cell decreases very-low-density lipoprotein triglyceride synthesis in type 1 diabetes. *Diabetes*, **36**, 661–66.

Edge, J.A., Dunger, D.B., Matthews, D.R. *et al.* (1990a) Increased overnight growth hormone concentrations in diabetic compared with normal adolescents. *J. Clin. Endocrin. Metab.*, **71**, 1356–62.

Edge, J.A., Matthews, D.R. and Dunger, D.B. (1990b) The dawn phenomenon is related to overnight growth hormone release in adolescent diabetics. *Clin. Endocrin.*, **33**, 729–37.

Edge, J.A., Matthews, D.R. and Dunger, D.B. (1990c) Failure of current insulin regimes to meet the overnight requirements of adolescents with insulin-dependent diabetes. *Diabetes Res.*, **15**, 109–112.

Fineberg, S.E. and Merimee, T.J. (1974) Acute metabolic effects of human growth hormone. *Diabetes*, **23**, 499–504.

Finegold, D., Lattimer, S.A., Nolle, S. *et al.* (1983) Polyol pathway activity and *myo*-inositol metabolism: a suggested relationship in the pathogenesis of diabetic neuropathy. *Diabetes*, **32**, 988–92.

Gabbay, K.H. (1975) Hyperglycemia, polyol metabolism, and complications of diabetes mellitus. *Ann. Rev. Med.*, **26**, 521–36.

Gentz, J.C.H. and Cornblath, M. (1969) Transient diabetes of the newborn. *Adv. in Pediatr.*, **16**, 345–63.

Gerich, J.E. (1984) Role of growth hormone in diabetes mellitus. *N. Eng. J. Med.*, **310**, 848–50.

Gerich, J.E. (1993) Control of glycaemia. *Balliere's Clin. Endocrin. and Metab.*, **7**, 551–86.

Gerich, J., Davis, J., Lorenzi, M. *et al.* (1979) Hormonal mechanisms of recovery from insulin-induced hypoglycemia in man. *Am. J. Physiol.*,

236 (Endocrinol. Metab. Gastrointest. Physiol. 5), E380–85.

Gerich, J.E., Langlois, M., Noacco, C. *et al.* (1973) Lack of glucagon response to hypoglycemia in diabetes: evidence for an intrinsic pancreatic alpha cell defect. *Science*, **182**, 171–73.

Gerich, J.E., Lorenzi, M., Bier, D.M. *et al.* (1975) Prevention of human diabetic ketoacidosis by somatostatin: evidence for an essential role of glucagon. *N. Eng. J. Med.*, **292**, 985–89.

Golden, M.P., Russell, B.P., Ingersoll, G.M. *et al.* (1985) Management of diabetes mellitus in children younger than 5 years of age. *Am. J. Dis. in Children*, **139**, 448–52.

Goldman, S.L. (1979) Hyperglycemic hyperosmolar coma in a 9-month-old child. *Am. J. Dis. in Children*, **133**, 181–83.

Gonzalez, A.-M., Sochor, M., Hothersall, J.S., McLean, P. (1986) Effect of aldose reductase inhibitor (Sorbinil) on integration of polyol pathway, pentose phosphate pathway, and glycolytic route in diabetic rat lens. *Diabetes*, **35**, 1200–1205.

Gonzalez, A.-M., Sochor, M. and McLean, P. (1983) The effect of an aldose reductase inhibitor (Sorbinil) on the level of metabolites in lenses of diabetic rats. *Diabetes*, **32**, 482–85.

Gutniak, M., Grill, V., Wiechel, K-L. *et al.* (1987) Basal and meal-induced somatostatin-like immunoreactivity in healthy subjects and in IDDM and toally pancreatectomized patients: effects of acute blood glucose normalization. *Diabetes*, **36**, 802–807.

Halperin, M.L., Bear, R.A., Hannaford, M.C. *et al.* (1981) Selected aspects of the pathophysiology of metabolic acidosis in diabetes mellitus. *Diabetes*, **30**, 781–87.

Hammeke, M., Bear, R., Lee, R. *et al.* (1978) Hyperchloremic metabolic acidosis in diabetes mellitus: a case report and discussion of the pathophysiologic mechanisms. *Diabetes*, **27**, 16–20.

Hammond, P. and Wallis, S. (1992) Cerebral oedema in diabetic ketoacidosis: still puzzling – and often fatal. *British Medical Journal*, **305**, 203–44.

Hansen I., Firth, R., Haymond, M. *et al.* (1986) The role of autoregulation of the hepatic glucose production in man: response to a physiologic decrement in plasma glucose. *Diabetes*, **35**, 186–91.

Heinze, E., Beischer, W., Keller, L. *et al.* (1978) C-peptide secretion during the remission phase of juvenile diabetes. *Diabetes*, **27**, 670–76.

Hernandez, A., Zorrilla, E. and Gershberg, H. (1968) Serum-insulin in remission of juvenile diabetes. *Lancet*, **ii**, 223.

Hoffman, R.P., Singer-Granick, C., Drash, A.L. *et al.* (1991) Plasma catecholamine responses to hypoglycemia in children and adolescents with IDDM. *Diabetes Care*, **14**, 81–88.

Holly, J.M.P., Amiel, S.A., Sandhu, R.R. *et al.* (1988) The role of growth hormone in diabetes mellitus. *J. Endocrin.*, **118**, 353–64.

Holly, J.M.P., Dunger, D.B., Edge, J.A. *et al.* (1990) Insulin-like growth factor binding protein-1 levels in diabetic adolescents and their relationship to metabolic control. *Diabetic Med.*, **7**, 618–23.

Honnor, R.C. and Saggerson, E.D. (1980) Altered lipolytic response to glucagon and adenosine deaminase in adipocytes from starved rats. *Biochem. J.*, **188**, 757–61.

Illig, R. and Prader, A. (1968) Remission of juvenile diabetes. *Lancet*, **ii**, 1190.

Ivarsson, S-A., Marner, B., Lernmark, A. *et al.* (1988) Nonislet pancreatic autoantibodies in sibship with permanent neonatal insulin-dependent diabetes mellitus. *Diabetes*, **37**, 347–50.

Jensen, M.D., Caruso, M., Heiling, V. *et al.* (1989) Insulin regulation of lipolysis in nondiabetic and IDDM subjects. *Diabetes*, **38**, 1595–1601.

Jimenez, J.T., Walford, S., Home, P.D. *et al.* (1985) Free insulin levels and metabolic effects of meal-time bolus and square-wave intraperitoneal insulin infusion in insulin-dependent diabetic patients. *Diabetologia*, **28**, 728–33.

Johnston, D.G. and Alberti, K.G.M.M. (1982) Hormonal control of ketone body metabolism in the normal and diabetic state. *Clin. Endocrin. and Metab.*, **11**, 329–61.

Jones, T.W., Boulware, S.D., Kraemer, D.T. *et al.* (1991) Independent effects of youth and poor diabetes control on responses to hypoglycemia in children. *Diabetes*, **40**, 358–63.

Keller, U. (1986) Diabetic ketoacidosis: current views on pathogenesis and treatment. *Diabetologia*, **29**, 71–77.

Keller, U., Gerber, P.P.G. and Stauffacher, W. (1984) Stimulatory effect of norepinephrine on ketogenesis in normal and insulin-deficient humans. *Am. J. Physiol.*, **247** (Endocrinol. Metab. 10), E732–39.

Kesaniemi, Y.A., Witztum, J.L. and Steinbrecher, U.P. (1983) Receptor-mediated catabolism of low density lipoprotein in man: quantitation using glucosylated low density lipoprotein. *J. Clin. Invest.*, **71**, 950–59.

Kilo, C., Vogler, N. and Williamson, J.R. (1972) Muscle capillary basement membrane changes related to aging and to diabetes mellitus. *Diabetes*, **21**, 881–905.

Kirschenbaum, D.M. (1984) Glycosylation of proteins: its implications in diabetic control and complications. *Pediatr. Clin. N. America*, **31**, 611–21.

Knip, M., Koivisto, M., Kaar, M-L. *et al.* (1983) Pancreatic islet cell function and metabolic control in an infant with permanent neonatal diabetes. *Acta Paed. Scand.*, **72**, 303–307.

Kohn, R.R. and Schnider, S.L. (1982) Glucosylation of human collagen. *Diabetes*, **31** (suppl. 3), 47–51.

Krane, E.J., Rockoff, M.A., Wallman, J.K. *et al.* (1985) Subclinical brain swelling in children during treatment of diabetic ketoacidosis. *N. Eng. J. Med.*, **312**, 1147–51.

Kreymann, B. and Bloom, S.R. (1991) 'Glucagon and the gut hormones in diabetes mellitus', in J. Pickup and G. Williams (eds). *Textbook of Diabetes*, 1st edn, pp. 313–24. Blackwell Scientific Publications, Oxford.

Landt, K.W., Campaigne, B.N., James, F.W. *et al.* (1985) Effects of exercise training on insulin sensitivity in adolescents with type 1 diabetes. *Diabetes Care*, **8**, 461–65.

Lecavalier, L., Bolli, G., Cryer, P., Gerich, J. (1989) Contributions of gluconeogenesis and glycogenolysis during glucose counterregulation in normal humans. *Am. J. Physiol.*, **256** (Endocrinol. Metab. 19), E844–51.

Lönnroth, P., Blohme, G., Lager, I. *et al.* (1983) Insulin resistance in fat cells from insulin-treated type 1 diabetic individuals. *Diabetes Care*, **6**, 586–90.

Lundbaek, K., Christensen, N.J., Jensen, V.A. *et al.* (1970) Diabetes, diabetic angiopathy, and growth hormone. *Lancet*, **ii**, 131–33.

McGarry, J.D. (1979) New perspectives in the regulation of ketogenesis. *Diabetes*, **28**, 517–23.

McGarry, J.D. and Foster, D.W. (1977) Hormonal control of ketogenesis. *Arch. Int. Med.*, **137**, 495–501.

MacGillivray, M.H., Bruck, E. and Voorhess, M.L. (1981) Acute diabetic ketoacidosis in children: role of the stress hormones. *Pediatr. Res.*, **15**, 99–106.

MacGillivray, M.H., Voorhess, M.L., Putnam, T.I. *et al.* (1982) Hormone and metabolic profiles in children and adolescents with type 1 diabetes mellitus. *Diabetes Care*, **5** (suppl. 1), 38–47.

MacGorman, L.R., Rizza, R.A. and Gerich, J.E. (1981) Physiological concentrations of growth hormone exert insulin-like and insulin antagonistic effects on both hepatic and extrahepatic tissues in man. *J. Clin. Endocrin. Metab.*, **53**, 556–59.

Madsbad, S., Faber, O.K., Binder, C. *et al.* (1981) Diurnal profiles of intermediary metabolites in insulin-dependent diabetes and their relationship to different degrees of residual B-cell function. *Acta Diabetologia Latina*, **18**, 115–21.

Mann, N.P. and Johnston, D.I. (1982) Total glycosylated haemoglobin (HbA_1) levels in diabetic children. *Arch. Dis. Child.*, **57**, 434–37.

Marshall, S.M., Taylor, R., Home, P.D. *et al.* (1988) Intermediary metabolism, insulin sensitivity and insulin receptor status under comparable long-term therapy with insulin injections and continuous subcutaneous insulin infusion. *Acta Endocrin. (Copenh.)*, **117**, 417–27.

Massa, G., Dooms, L., Bouillon, R. *et al.* (1993) Serum levels of growth hormone-binding protein and insulin-like growth factor 1 in children and adolescents with type 1 (insulin-dependent) diabetes mellitus. *Diabetologia*, **36**, 239–43.

Merimee, T.J., Fineberg, S.E. and Hollander, W. (1973) Vascular disease in the chronic HGH-deficient state. *Diabetes*, **22**, 813–19.

Miller, J.D., Wright, N.M., Lester, S.E. *et al.* (1992) Spontaneous and stimulated growth hormone release in adolescents with type 1 diabetes mellitus: effects of metabolic control. *J. Clin. Endocrin. and Metab.*, **75**, 1087–91.

Milner, R.D.G., Ferguson, A.W. and Naidu, S.H. (1971) Aetiology of transient neonatal diabetes. *Arch. Dis. in Child.*, **46**, 724–26.

Mitrakou, A., Ryan, C., Veneman, T. *et al.* (1991) Hierarchy of glycemic thresholds for counterregulatory hormone secretion, symptoms, and cerebral dysfunction. *Am. J. Physiol.*, **260** (Endocrinol. Metab. 23), E67–E74.

Mortimer, C.H., Tunbridge, W.M.G., Carr, D. *et al.* (1974) Effects of growth-hormone release-inhibiting hormone on circulating glucagon, insulin, and growth hormone in normal, diabetic, acromegalic, and hypo-pituitary patients. *Lancet*, **i**, 697–701.

Muller, M.J., von zur Muhlen, A., Lautz, H.U. *et al.* (1989) Energy expenditure in children with type 1 diabetes: evidence for increased thermogenesis. *Brit. Med. J.*, **299**, 487–91.

Navalesi, R., Pilo, A. and Vigneri, R. (1975) Growth hormone kinetics in diabetic patients. *Diabetes*, **24**, 317–27.

Nikkila, E.A., Huttunen, J.K. and Ehnholm, C. (1977) Postheparin plasma lipoprotein lipase and hepatic lipase in diabetes mellitus: relationship to plasma triglyceride metabolism. *Diabetes*, **26**, 11–21.

Nosadini, R., Noy, G.A., Nattrass, M. *et al.* (1982) The metabolic and hormonal responses to acute normoglycemia in type 1 (insulin-dependent) diabetes: studies with a glucose controlled insulin infusion system (artificial endocrine pancreas). *Diabetologia*, **23**, 220–28.

Oh, M.S., Carroll, H.J., Goldstein, D.A. *et al.* (1978) Hyperchloremic acidosis during recovery phase of diabetic ketosis. *Ann. Int. Med.*, **89**, 925–27.

Osterby, R. (1986) Structural changes in the diabetic kidney. *Clin. in Endocrin. and Metab.*, **15**, 733–51.

Owen, O.E. and Reichard, G.A. (1971) Human forearm metabolism during progressive starvation. *J. Clin. Invest.*, **50**, 1536–45.

Pagliara, A.S., Karl, I.E. and Kipnis, D.B. (1973) Transient neonatal diabetes: delayed maturation of the pancreatic beta cell. *J. Pediatr.*, **82**, 97–101.

Pal, B.R., Phillips, P.E., Matthews, D.R. *et al.* (1992) Contrasting metabolic effects of continuous and pulsatile growth hormone administration in young adults with type 1 (insulin-dependent) diabetes mellitus. *Diabetologia*, **35**, 542–49.

Pedersen, O. and Hjollund, E. (1982) Insulin receptor binding to fat and blood cells and insulin action in fat cells from insulin-dependent diabetics. *Diabetes*, **31**, 706–715.

Perriello, G., de Feo, P., Torlone, E. *et al.* (1988) The effect of asymptomatic nocturnal hypoglycemia on glycemic control in diabetes mellitus. *N. Eng. J. Med.*, **319**, 1233–39.

Pietri, A.O., Dunn, F.L., Grundy, S.M. *et al.* (1983) The effect of continuous subcutaneous insulin infusion on very-low-density lipoprotein triglyceride metabolism in type 1 diabetes mellitus. *Diabetes*, **32**, 75–81.

Press, M., Tamborlane, W.V. and Sherwin, R.S. (1984a) Importance of raised growth hormone levels in mediating the metabolic derangements of diabetes. *N. Eng. J. Med.*, **310**, 810–15.

Press, M., Tamborlane, W.V., Thorner, M.O. *et al.* (1984b) Pituitary response to growth hormone-releasing factor in diabetes: failure of glucose-mediated suppression. *Diabetes*, **33**, 804–806.

Proietto, J., Nankervis, A., Aitken, P. *et al.* (1983) Glucose utilization in type 1 (insulin-dependent) diabetes: evidence for a defect not reversible by acute elevations of insulin. *Diabetologia*, **25**, 331–35.

Randle, P.J., Garland, P.B., Hales, C.N. *et al.* (1963) The glucose fatty-acid cycle: its role in insulin sensitivity and the metabolic disturbances of diabetes mellitus. *Lancet*, **i**, 785–9.

Reichard, G.A., Skutches, C.L., Hoeldtke, R.D. *et al.* (1986) Acetone metabolism in humans during diabetic ketoacidosis. *Diabetes*, **35**, 668–74.

Rizza, R.A., Cryer, P.E. and Gerich, J.E. (1979) Role of glucagon, catecholamines, and growth hormone in human glucose counterregulation: effects of somatostatin and combined α- and β-adrenergic blockade on plasma glucose recovery and glucose flux rates after insulin-induced hypoglycemia. *J. Clin. Invest.*, **64**, 62–71.

Rosenbloom, A.L. (1990) Intracerebral crises during treatment of diabetic ketoacidosis. *Diabetes Care*, **13**, 22–33.

Rosenbloom, A.L., Wheeler, L., Bianchi, R. *et al.* (1975) Age-adjusted analysis of insulin responses during normal and abnormal glucose tolerance tests in children and adolescents. *Diabetes*, **24**, 820–28.

Rosenfeld, R.G., Wilson, D.M., Dollar, L.A. *et al.* (1982) Both human pituitary growth hormone and recombinant DNA-derived human growth hormone cause insulin resistance at a postreceptor site. *J. Clin. Endocrin. and Metab.*, **54**, 1033–38.

Salway, J.G., Whitehead, L., Finnegan, J.A. *et al.*

(1978) Effect of *myo*-inositol on peripheral-nerve function in diabetes. *Lancet*, **ii**, 1282–84.

Schade, D.S. and Eaton, R.P. (1977a) Dose response to insulin in man: differential effects on glucose and ketone body regulation. *J. Clin. Endocrin. and Metab.*, **44**, 1038–53.

Schade, D.S. and Eaton, R.P. (1977b) The controversy concerning counterregulatory hormone secretion: a hypothesis for the prevention of diabetic ketoacidosis? *Diabetes*, **26**, 596–601.

Schade, D.S., Eaton, R.P. and Standefer, J. (1977) Glucocorticoid regulation of plasma ketone body concentration in insulin deficient man. *J. Clin. Endocrin. and Metab.*, **44**, 1069–79.

Schade, D.S. and Eaton, R.P. (1980) The temporal relationship between endogenously secreted stress hormones and metabolic decompensation in diabetic man. *J. Clin. Endocrin. and Metab.*, **50**, 131–36.

Shamoon, H., Hendler, R. and Sherwin, R.S. (1981) Synergistic interactions among anti-insulin hormones in the pathogenesis of stress hyperglycemia in humans. *J. Clin. Endocrin. and Metab.*, **52**, 1235–41.

Sharp, P. and Johnston, D.G. (1991) 'Mechanisms of Hyperglycaemia and Disorders of Intermediary Metabolism', in J. Pickup and G. Williams (eds). *Textbook of Diabetes*, 1st edn, pp. 303–12. Blackwell Scientific Publications, Oxford.

Sheikholislam, B.M., Irias, J.J., Lin, H.-J. *et al.* (1976a) Carbohydrate metabolism and capillary basement-membrane thickness in children: I. Cross-sectional studies. *Diabetes*, **25**, 650–60.

Sheikholislam, B.M., Irias, J.J., Lowrey, G.H. *et al.* (1976b) Carbohydrate metabolism and capillary basement-membrane thickness in children: II. Longitudinal studies. *Diabetes*, **25**, 661–66.

Singer-Granick, C., Hoffman, R.P., Kerensky, K. *et al.* (1988) Glucagon responses to hypoglycemia in children and adolescents with IDDM. *Diabetes Care*, **11**, 643–49.

Singh, B.M., Palma, M.A. and Nattrass, M. (1987) Multiple aspects of insulin resistance: comparison of glucose and intermediary metabolite response to incremental insulin infusion in IDDM subjects of short and long duration. *Diabetes*, **36**, 740–48.

Skare, S., Dahl-Jorgensen, K., Hanssen, K.F. *et al.* (1985) Increased peripheral venous somatostatin concentration and decreased glucagon response to arginine in patients with insulin-dependent diabetes mellitus without residual B-cell function. *Acta Endocrin.*, **109**, 517–21.

Skor, D.A., White, N.H., Thomas, L. *et al.* (1983) Examination of the role of the pituitary-adrenocortical axis, counterregulatory hormones, and insulin clearance in variable nocturnal insulin requirements in insulin-dependent diabetes. *Diabetes*, **32**, 403–407.

Skor, D.A., White, N.H., Thomas, L. *et al.* (1984) Relative roles of insulin clearance and insulin sensitivity in the prebreakfast increase in insulin requirements in insulin-dependent diabetic patients. *Diabetes*, **33**, 60–63.

Soltesz, G. (1993) Hypoglycaemia in the diabetic child. *Ballière's Clin. Endocrin. and Metab.*, **7**, 741–55.

Soltesz, G., Molnar, D., Decsi, T. *et al.* (1988) The metabolic and hormonal effects of continuous subcutaneous insulin infusion therapy in diabetic children. *Diabetologia*, **31**, 30–34.

Steffes, M.W., Sutherland, D.E.R., Goetz, F.C. *et al.* (1985) Studies of kidney and muscle biopsy specimens from identical twins discordant for type 1 diabetes mellitus. *N. Eng. J. Med.*, **312**, 1282–87.

Stevenson, R.W., Orskov, H., Parsons, J.A. *et al.* (1983a) Metabolic responses to intraduodenal glucose loading in insulin-infused diabetic dogs. *Am. J. Physiol.*, **245** (Endocrinol. Metab. 8), E200–208.

Stevenson, R.W., Parsons, J.A. and Alberti, K.G.M.M. (1983b) Effect of intraportal and peripheral insulin on glucose turnover and recycling in diabetic dogs. *Am. J. Physiol.*, **244** (Endocrinol. Metab. 7), E190–95.

Summerfield, J.A., Vergalla, J. and Jones, E.A. (1982) Modulation of a glycoprotein recognition system on rat hepatic endothelial cells by glucose and diabetes mellitus. *J. Clin. Invest.*, **69**, 1337–47.

Tamborlane, W.V., Hintz, R.L., Bergman, M. *et al.* (1981) Insulin-infusion-pump treatment of diabetes: influence of improved metabolic control on plasma somatomedin levels. *N. Eng. J. Med.*, **305**, 303–307.

Taskinen, M.-R. and Nikkila, E.A. (1979) Lipoprotein lipase activity of adipose tissue and skeletal muscle in insulin-deficient human diabetes. *Diabetologia*, **17**, 351–56.

Tattersall, R.B. and Lowe, J. (1981) Diabetes in adolescence. *Diabetologia*, **20**, 517–23.

Taylor, R. and Agius, L. (1988) The biochemistry of diabetes. *Biochem. J.*, **250**, 625–40.

Ternand, C., Go, V.L.W., Gerich, J.E. *et al.* (1982) Endocrine pancreatic response of children with onset of insulin-requiring diabetes before age 3 and after age 5. *J. Pediatr.*, **101**, 36–39.

Usala, A.-L., Madigan, T., Burguera, B. *et al.* (1992) Brief report: treatment of insulin-resistant diabetic ketoacidosis with insulin-like growth factor 1 in an adolescent with insulin-dependent diabetes. *New Eng. J. Med.*, **327**, 853–57.

Wasada, T., Howard, B., McCorkle, K. *et al.* (1981) High plasma free fatty acid levels contribute to the hypersomatostatinemia of insulin deficiency. *Diabetes*, **30**, 358–61.

Weber, B. (1972) Glucose-stimulated insulin secretion during 'remission' of juvenile diabetes. *Diabetologia*, **8**, 189–95.

White, N.H., Gingerich, R.L., Levandoski, L.A. *et al.* (1985) Plasma pancreatic polypeptide response to insulin-induced hypoglycemia as a marker for defective glucose counterregulation in insulin-dependent diabetes mellitus. *Diabetes*, **34**, 870–75.

Williamson, J.R. and Kilo, C. (1978) The relationship between glomerular and skeletal muscle capillary basement membrane. *Diabetes*, 513 (abstract).

Yki-Jarvinen, H., DeFronzo, R.A. and Koivisto, V.A. (1984a) Normalization of insulin sensitvity in type 1 diabetic subjects by physical training during insulin pump therapy. *Diabetes Care*, **7**, 520–27.

Yki-Jarvinen, H., Taskinen, M.-R., Kiviluoto, T. *et al.* (1984b) Site of insulin resistance in type 1 diabetes: insulin-mediated glucose disposal *in vivo* in relation to insulin binding and action in adipocytes *in vitro*. *J. Clin. Endocrin. and Metab.*, **59**, 1183–92.

Young, E. and Bradley, R.F. (1967) Cerebral edema with irreversible coma in severe diabetic ketoacidosis. *N. Eng. J. Med.*, **276**, 665–69.

PART THREE

15

Presentation and ketoacidosis

S.J. BRINK

15.1 CLASSICAL PRESENTATION OF TYPE I IDDM

Youngsters with IDDM generally present (Brink, 1987; Drash, 1987; Travis *et al.*, 1987; Baum & Kinmoth, 1985; Jackson & Guthrie, 1986) with the classical symptoms of polyuria, polydipsia, nocturia and occasionally enuresis. This reflects absolute or relative insulin deficiency with resultant hyperglycemia and osmotic diuresis from varying degrees of glycosuria. Many lose weight rapidly over several days or weeks but occasionally IDDM presents with slower onset over weeks or months particularly in older teenagers and young adults. In such cases, weight loss occurs from not only fluid losses but also from catabolism of muscle protein and fat in combination with glycosuria. Insulin deficiency produces profound disturbances in not only carbohydrate but also protein and fat metabolism.

If family members, teachers or sometimes the children or teenagers themselves are observant, symptoms are noticeable and medical attention results in quick diagnosis. In-office urinalysis demonstrates glycosuria and/or ketonuria on random urinalysis and is confirmed with random hyperglycemia on blood testing. Glucose tolerance testing is usually not required to confirm the diagnosis when obvious signs and symptoms are coupled with abnormal urinalysis and elevated blood glucose levels. Most but not all such youngsters will have evidence of an active autoimmune process (positive islet cell and/or insulin antibodies and other biologic markers of an activated immune system). These autoantibodies as well as other markers are not important for clinical decision-making at diagnosis even though they have profound research implications (see Chapter 12). Occasionally, random urinalysis done at the time of camp, sports, school or regular physical exams is abnormal.

Insulin deficiency is also present but need not be documented for routine care. Clinical care decisions are based upon severity of signs and symptoms and degree of metabolic decompensation present: for example, is the patient vomiting or capable of taking oral fluids, how clinically dehydrated are they, what are the initial serum electrolyte and acid-base parameters, how ketotic is the patient, how elevated is the initial glucose level, what are the family economic and psychosocial circumstances?

Clinically, childhood and adolescent IDDM can present with severe dehydration and rapidly progress to coma and death, or youngsters can be totally asymptomatic.

Childhood and Adolescent Diabetes
Published in 1994 by Chapman & Hall, London
ISBN 0 412 48610 5

Sophisticated families usually recognize symptoms early enough to avoid automatic inpatient hospitalization where adequate primary care facilities exist. When medical care access is remote, when psychosocial circumstances interfere with prompt diagnosis and/or when there is very rapid onset or few recognizable warning symptoms, morbidity and even death can result so that the diagnosis of IDDM must remain a true medical emergency until electrolyte and fluid balance is restored and insulin begun.

The patient may be detected (Bingley *et al.*, 1993) through screening programs (especially if he or she has a first degree relative with known IDDM) or may present with mild, moderate or severe signs and symptoms related to insulin deficiency. Pathophysiologically, current research suggests that the following events are likely to take place as β-cell function decreases.

An autoimmune process, perhaps genetically predispositioned but precipitated by unknown factors (viruses, cross reactive exogenous antigens), begins. β cells are targeted by the immune system with activated T cells and a host of immune-related phenomena self-perpetuating destruction of β cells (Botazzo, 1992). The variability in the rapidity with which this process destroys insulin production and in producing clinical symptoms is unexplained. Islet cell antibodies and/or insulin autoantibodies are often but not always detected in the serum before frank insulin deficiency or abnormalities of intravenous or oral glucose tolerance testing occur. Youngsters with certain HLA haplotypes are more likely to have such autoimmune phenomena documented (see Chapters 10 and 11). Large generalized screening programs have been attempted but are extremely costly and cumbersome outside of a research setting (Bingley *et al.*, 1993). However, screening of targeted populations such as first degree relatives produces an approximately 2–5% positive antibody detection rate prior to clinical hyperglycemia (Bingley *et al.*, 1993).

The earliest abnormalities may be detected months or years before clinical hyperglycemia (Brink *et al.*, 1986; Vardi *et al.*, 1991). Asymptomatic patients who go on to clinical diabetes have abnormalities detected by low levels of first phase insulin secretion. This is tested following intravenous glucose challenge and measurement of the first and third minute insulin levels. Hypoinsulinemia or hyperglycemia on oral glucose tolerance tests is a very late phenomenon and is not thought to occur until significant and measurable β cell destruction and insulin deficiency has taken place. Discussion of what interventions might be attempted in the 'prediabetic' phase of IDDM are presented in Chapter 38 and can be summarized as (a) experiments involving ways to 'rest' the damaged β cells so that they might last longer, (b) attempts to 'protect' the β cells as targets for ongoing autoimmune processes and (c) mechanisms to 'interfere' with the immune system itself. At present, all these remain theoretical and experimental. None have shown sufficient benefit to be attempted outside of well-controlled scientific trials around the world because of risks involved.

15.1.1 DELAYED DIAGNOSIS

Rarely, signs and symptoms of IDDM are not detected either because the diagnosis is not so commonly entertained by parents and health care providers (infants, toddlers and preschool age children) when its incidence is relatively low or because the youngest children do not often communicate in detail. In adolescents, delay may occur because parents are no longer in a position to closely observe their teenager's behavior and must rely upon the relatively reticent teenagers questioning how their body is working (publicly!). In some economically disadvantaged parts of the world, IDDM is

Table 15.1 Delayed diagnosis of IDDM.

1. Nonverbal infants and toddlers
2. Symptoms not recognized in age groups where incidence is very low, i.e., preschool age children
3. Confused with concomitant viral or bacterial illnesses or other diagnosis (e.g., mononucleosis)
4. Medical care unavailable
5. Weight loss mistakenly thought to be positive result in obese child or adolescent rather than sign of disease
6. Symptoms not reported by 'independent' adolescent
7. Urinalysis not checked
8. Blood glucose not available or not requested

thought to be extremely rare because access to sophisticated medical care is not available and youngsters most likely present in florid ketoacidosis or with signs and symptoms of overwhelming infection which produces severe dehydration and metabolic disturbances in its own right (i.e., acute gastroenteritis) (Table 15.1).

If diagnosis is delayed, mild symptoms can quickly lead to severe fluid, electrolyte and acid-base disturbances followed by vomiting, dehydration, coma and death. This is particularly a problem in very young patients whose metabolic reserves are not as great as in older children or teenagers. Patients who present in frank diabetic ketoacidosis (DKA) will be discussed in detail below.

15.1.2 OUTPATIENT MANAGEMENT IN ASYMPTOMATIC OR MILDLY TO MODERATELY SYMPTOMATIC CHILD OR ADOLESCENT

Once hyperglycemia is confirmed by laboratory blood glucose testing, it is irrelevant whether or not that child or adolescent is symptomatic since treatment involves fluid, electrolyte replenishment and correction of insulin deficiency. The asymptomatic or mildly symptomatic youngster will not be significantly dehydrated. If symptoms are minimal, he or she will merely be compensating by polydipsia for the osmotic diuresis taking place. The longer the insulin deficiency and the more other fluid and electrolyte losses that have taken place (i.e., from diarrhea, vomiting or associated with fever), the more likely that symptoms will have been present for a long period of time. As long as such youngsters are able to take oral fluids – and as long as there is not significant nausea and vomiting – treatment can be instituted out of hospital. This can only take place, however, if the pediatric and adolescent diabetes specialty team is equipped to provide frequent telephone contact and daily outpatient visits to begin the initial survival training of patient and family. Certain interfering circumstances can exist which prevent outpatient management of IDDM and these are listed as what might be called 'energy diversions' in Table 15.2.

In certain parts of the world and in areas where outpatient management teams have

Table 15.2 Energy diversions (adapted from Brink, 1987).

A. Patient with already existing:
   1. Other chronic medical problem (e.g., celiac, epilepsy, asthma, cystic fibrosis)
   2. Learning problems (mild through frank retardation)
   3. Behavioral or psychiatric problems
B. Parent with already existing:
   1. Chronic medical problem including IDDM or NIDDM
   2. Substance abuse (nicotine, alcohol, drugs)
   3. Learning problems
   4. Behavioral or psychiatric problems
   5. Abnormal spousal relationship (separation, divorce)
   6. Low socioeconomic status

not been established, it will be mandatory to provide such initial teaching and support in inpatient facilities until the condition of the youngster stabilizes sufficiently that ambulatory follow-up can be arranged.

15.2 INITIAL TREATMENT ISSUES

Initial treatment issues are listed in Table 15.3.

15.2.1 CONFIRM DIAGNOSIS

With gentleness, confirmation of the diagnosis of IDDM must occur quickly and alternative differential diagnostic possibilities ruled out. This must be done so that the child or teenager and his or her family members understand the process. It is often extremely helpful to encourage verbalization of alternative diagnoses being considered by the youngster or family member. Allowing expression of the patient or family's own explanatory model for IDDM immediately sets the stage for having the patient and family members as an integral part of the treatment team and helps to establish rapport. Frequently health care providers will need to offer their own explanations for why this is not merely a bad case of 'the flu', gastroenteritis, bladder or urinary tract infection, 'mono' (mononucleosis) or a laboratory error, etc. It is often helpful if a detailed past medical and family history has been obtained since questions about 'which side of the family was responsible' can also be addressed and immediate issues of guilt or fear for other family members discussed. Knowledge about family members who have had problems with their heart, blood pressure, cholesterol or who have autoimmune disorders known to be associated with IDDM (thyroid, adrenal, celiac disease) help place some of the immediate treatment decisions into perspective and focus on lab tests needed.

Table 15.3 Initial treatment issues (Brink, 1987).

A. Confirm diagnosis. Answer questions. Debunk myths
B. Offer psychological support
   1. Guilt
   2. Anxiety and fears
   3. Establish team treatment, philosophy and relationships
C. Urine ketone testing
D. Capillary blood glucose testing and record keeping
E. Insulin technique, administration, protocols
F. Initial survival meal planning. Broad concepts
   1. Weigh and measure to promote portion learning
G. More detailed insulin dose decisions
   1. Slow, steady insulinization
   2. Aggressive insulinization to promote beta cell 'rest'
H. Emergency procedures for hypoglycemia
   1. Medic-alert tags, bracelets, wallet cards
   2. Rapid carbohydrate oral treatment options
   3. Glucagon
I. When and how to contact diabetes team
   1. Telephone numbers
   2. Emergency room and ambulance
   3. Review role of all team members
      a. Physician
      b. Nurse educator
      c. Dietician
      d. Social worker, psychologist, psychiatrist
      e. Exercise specialist
      f. Patient and family members
J. Establish need for and procedures for ongoing in-depth education, re-education and motivation
K. Provide for ongoing psychosocial support and involvement
   1. Patient
   2. Both mother and father
   3. Siblings
   4. Babysitters
   5. Grandparents
   6. Other relatives
   7. Neighbors, coaches, teachers
   8. Peers

15.2.2 SETTING THE STAGE FOR PSYCHOLOGICAL SUPPORT

IDDM is a chronic illness that requires an enormous amount of technical skill coupled with huge behavioral changes for many family members. No other chronic illness places such demands on the patient and his or her family in such an all-encompassing fashion and without respite. Those families who succeed often do so by working together as a team. If diabetes health care professionals are successful, they formulate such a working relationship and focus on transferring decision-making from them to the patient and the family as is appropriate for age, development and intellectual capability (see Chapter 7).

Special efforts should be made to involve not only the mother but also the father at the time of diagnosis and at all future educational and training sessions. This should take place whether or not outpatient or inpatient teaching is being used. Not all fathers will be willing and able to participate in such an egalitarian model; not all mothers will allow their spouses to become so involved; certain cultures may shun this as unmanly. But the child and even teenagers who have both parents directly participating seem to benefit from knowing that care is being provided and the situation taken seriously.

Having siblings come to teaching sessions and learn what is required to care for IDDM is also important as is having close relatives like grandparents learning initial survival skills together with other family members.

Introducing the concept of a health care team where numerous professionals will be involved is helpful as is identifying the patient as the focus of the team and identifying age-appropriate responsibilities. De-emphasizing who actually gives insulin injections and focusing on broad treatment concepts can help avoid future problems of lack of supervision and inappropriate self-care. Demonstrating the different roles of the various health care professionals, identifying the importance of the emotional component of IDDM by bringing examples immediately to the surface for discussion, and giving lots of praise for initial efforts will lay the groundwork for positive progression as skills are mastered and more independent self-care behaviors introduced.

Diabetes health care must be individualized based upon age, the emotional well-being of the family and the child or adolescent, ethnic and cultural issues, financial concerns and previous fears and myths about dealing with doctors, nurses and medical personnel. Knowledge about health care belief theory as well as psychological constructs for working through the first stages of diagnosis are critical. Positive role-modeling and a positive attitude about techniques and procedures that can be mastered are important tools for all diabetes educators to pass along to patients and family members. The 'imprinting' and sustained positive behavior that takes place following such organized team diabetes education – compared to the never-ending battles when such positive team approaches are not available or not utilized – is very impressive. Introducing the notion that others (peers, parents, siblings) have felt the same way and been able to overcome initial hesitancy allows validation of such fears and frustrations with scary, painful procedures either to oneself or to one's child. Appropriate assistance with initial techniques, even for some teenagers, is required if fears prevent them from learning to master initial diabetes self-care tasks. Avoiding feelings of failure by slow step-wise introduction of concepts and gentle support often produces desired results.

Local national and international diabetes associations should be mentioned and perhaps applications completed for patients and family members by health care professionals as a way of introducing and indicating the support networks available for youngsters as well as family members. Summer as well as winter, weekend and day camp experiences can provide much needed solace. Books in which characters have diabetes (Martin, 1986) and deal with its vicissitudes, including the emotions of learning to live with diabetes, are an excellent resource as are monthly magazines like the American Diabetes Association's *Diabetes Forecast*, especially its 'Kid's Corner' section, and *Balance* from the British Diabetic Association.

In sequence, the following technical skills are demonstrated and then actually done by patient and parent almost immediately after the diagnosis is confirmed in the office or outpatient setting. If hospitalization is required, these same steps are followed with delay produced only by how physically ill the patient is at the moment.

15.2.3 URINE KETONE TESTING

This is an easy first procedure to master since it involves no pain but only a bit of embarrassment at having to urinate into a cup! Light banter about 'yucky' urine can ease tensions. Simple ketone testing strips, chemically impregnated with pads or tablets that will change color if acetone or acetoacetate is present in a urine sample, are easy to demonstrate. Having one or several other family members also produce a urine sample and test their own specimen in similar fashion provides a quick reassurance that no other family members are 'incubating' diabetes at the moment and also demonstrates what a 'negative' result is like compared to the patient's specimen (if ketonuria is present). Some diabetologists prefer combination strips where urinary glucose and ketone testing can be done simultaneously.

15.2.4 CAPILLARY BLOOD GLUCOSE TESTING

Parents, other direct caretakers and often siblings should be shown how to obtain capillary blood for blood glucose sampling. One favorite technique involves demonstration of a visual blood glucose strip on a parent and then having each parent test the other while the patient and siblings observe the procedures. This is then followed immediately by having different partners test each other using a memory chip meter that will allow future downloading into office or home computers for statistical analysis. This author prefers memory meters for all patients and has set up his diabetes office follow-up visits so that all such patients have their meters automatically downloaded for analysis together with patient and family as a teaching technique. Ongoing computer analysis also allows identification of those not testing, those testing but not keeping written logbooks, and most importantly, those not able to do appropriate self-analysis of their own data. Within 15 minutes of beginning such teaching protocols, multiple family members have paired off to test each other until either the youngsters with IDDM test themselves or one of the parents – generally the most reluctant one is whom I choose for this task – is helped to obtain a blood glucose sample on the patient just diagnosed. At times, it is more appropriate for the slightly older patient to do their own testing after having practiced and observed testing on their parent(s). This serves as another confirmation of the elevated blood glucose and often also as an opportunity to discuss blood glucose variability from the original sample result.

Establishing a system of record keeping is another important early task to be mastered. Record books organized with insulin doses in a series of columns on one side of the page and sufficient space for longitudinal weekly assessment of patterns of blood glucose readings on the opposite seem to facilitate learning about insulin action as well as identifying opportunities to adjust food, activity or insulin. An example of a logbook offered at NEDEC is illustrated in Figure 15.1.

NEW ENGLAND DIABETES & ENDOCRINOLOGY CENTER (NEDEC)
25 BOYLSTON STREET, SUITE 211, CHESTNUT HILL, MA 02167

Date	Insulin					Test Results: Blood and Urine									Notes
	Type	Dose				Test	Breakfast		Lunch		Dinner		Bedtime	Night	
		Morn	Noon	Eve	Night		Before		Before		Before				
Mon ___						Blood glucose									
						Urine ketones									
	Time taken					Time of test									
Tue ___						Blood glucose									
						Urine ketones									
	Time taken					Time of test									
Wed ___						Blood glucose									
						Urine ketones									
	Time taken					Time of test									
Thu ___						Blood glucose									
						Urine ketones									
	Time taken					Time of test									
Fri ___						Blood glucose									
						Urine ketones									
	Time taken					Time of test									
Sat ___						Blood glucose									
						Urine ketones									
	Time taken					Time of test									
Sun ___						Blood glucose									
						Urine ketones									
	Time taken					Time of test									

Figure 15.1 New England Diabetes & Endocrinology Center (NEDEC) logbook.

Using color-coded pens to highlight ranges of blood glucose is a useful tool to teach children, teenagers and parents to use. For instance, red can represent 'potential danger' and used for blood glucose values ≤4 mmol/L (≤66 mg/100 ml) whereas green (green traffic light = safe to proceed) can represent values between 4 mmol/L (66 mg/100 ml) and 8 mmol/L (140 mg/100 ml). Black can represent values between 8 mmol/L (140 mg/100 ml) and 11 mmol/L (180 mg/100ml) and values ≥11 mmol/L (180 mg/100 ml) in blue ('sad'). Pattern control teaching is facilitated and the need to analyze the actual blood glucose data reinforced. At NEDEC, we demonstrate blood glucose analysis by first defining goals of our treatment (i.e., 75% of values between 4 mmol/L and 9 mmol/L for teenagers; 75% of values between 5 mmol/L and 11 mmol/L for toddlers) and then printing out bar charts, graphic displays of standard or modal days, pie charts or statistical summaries of different times of the day and night for the prior month. Exactly what degree of blood glucose control is achievable must be individualized and changes in the remission phase from what is possible once full clinical diabetes exists (i.e., 75% of values between 4 mmol/L and 8 mmol/L). Some families have access to personal computers and either enter their own data manually or use the same downloading systems that we use in the office to do this process every week at home. Others are taught to manually make graphs to identify patterns each week.

15.2.5 SYRINGE AND INSULIN TECHNIQUE AND ADMINISTRATION

After urine ketone testing and capillary blood glucose testing is practiced a few times, with the entire family present, sterile saline is used to demonstrate insulin administration. Generally, patients under the age of 10–12 years should not be shamed or forced to self-administer insulin. While each child and circumstance must be considered individually, it will usually be obvious whether or not the child or teenager is ready to self-administer an injection by direct observation and questioning. Too often in the past, health care providers have focused on this issue only to produce extreme non-compliance and outright rebellion weeks, months or years later. It is clearly preferable for parents to assume this responsibility and to work towards self-reliance in a non-crisis situation later rather than produce a situation which will have more negative consequences as a result of inappropriate early coercion. Here again, verbalizing the rationale for such decisions, indicating that reluctance to self-administer of insulin is not equivalent to being 'chicken', 'dumb' or 'a coward' will be beneficial.

Sterile saline can be used to teach how and why to remove syringe bubbles, how to determine the correct dose and to allow self-administration or 'partner'-administration in much the same way that urine and blood glucose testing was taught. In the process of having multiple family members practice on themselves and on each other, fears can be ascertained, learning disabilities identified (who can follow instructions, is learning best done concretely or in the abstract, can two numbers be added together correctly?), and decisions regarding insulin assistance devices (spring-loaded injection gadgets) can be considered earlier rather than later. Using multiple dose insulin programs with cartridge syringes is generally easier to learn than having to learn how to withdraw and/or mix different types of insulin in a syringe. The immediate medical emergency now comes to a close with insulin actually administered to the child or teenager as the final step in this process.

15.2.6 SURVIVAL FLUID AND MEAL PLANNING

At this point, the only immediate 'food' advice that is required involves survival skills for fluid, electrolyte replacement and food intake for the next few hours. Simply omitting juice, candy (sweets) and obvious concentrated sugars is readily accepted and not overly complicated. It's important to remember that almost all youngsters just diagnosed with IDDM will have some need for increased fluid requirements and salt replenishment. Giving them simple guidelines such as what kind of soup or broth they can have and why it is important to have large amounts the first few days will help them feel better and understand some of what has happened to their body metabolism. Instructions for the next few meals and/or snacks will also be helpful with encouragement to eat in simple fashion and, if possible, foods that they usually were eating before the diabetes was diagnosed. For instance, a hamburger or sandwich, small portion of French fries (chips) and a diet soda or glass of skimmed milk would be a very appropriate initial meal, simple to make for most families and providing proof that diabetes meal planning can be handled without major food deprivation. Listing which types of liquids are readily available and can be used to correct any subtle dehydration while the insulin begins to work will also be received favorably. A bedtime snack of popcorn and a glass of milk or a small sandwich with meat, peanut butter or cheese is also an easy recommendation. Exact and specific details of meal planning are not required in this initial visit but can await the next few days when emotions are less strained and ability to listen is improved. Learning will be easier as a consequence of being more calm, feeling better and having some control resumed.

15.2.7 SUMMATION

Usually all of the above are accomplished in the late afternoon or early evening. Generally it takes about 2–3 hours of physician and/or nurse educator time to meet a new patient and his/her family, obtain a detailed medical and family history, examine the patient and complete the above survival skill training for urine and blood glucose testing as well as insulin administration. The observant physician and health care providers involved in such an intensive training experience get to know a great deal about how the newly-diagnosed patient will function and how the family interacts. This will set the groundwork for future progress, based upon small hints in response to questions that arise and experience shared.

The final requirement is the exchanging of telephone numbers. This allows the patient and his/her family to return home, do a urine and blood glucose check a few hours later and report to the physician how things are progressing. This author provides his home telephone number in addition to a 24-hour 'beeper' number and often has the teenager, child or parent call in a few hours merely to provide reassurance. A follow-up appointment is then scheduled for early the next morning before breakfast and all procedures repeated together under supervision once again: urine testing, blood glucose testing, insulin administration and some initial breakfast meal planning that next day.

15.2.8 MORE DETAILED MEAL PLANNING

On this return visit major concepts of meal planning can be explained and some sample meals chosen. Use of the exchange concept for food choice or other similar approaches can be reviewed. This should be done in some detail, based upon knowledge of usual and customary ethnic and individual preferences for certain foods. Global concepts about sugar content of certain foods, fast and slow acting carbohydrate effects, decreasing protein and decreasing animal/saturated fat intake can be introduced (Brink, 1992). Involving the entire family with food decisions, times for meal and snacks to be eaten, compromises with school and work schedules, likes and dislikes is useful. The more the entire family adjusts their eating habits together at this stage, the better. Here again is an opportunity to allow expression for common myths faced by the newly-diagnosed patient: diabetes is not contagious and cannot be produced by eating sugary foods; special vitamin and mineral supplements are usually not required; special occasions and holiday food variability can be mentioned for a future session once treatment has stabilized. Type I and Type II diabetes can be discussed and similarities as well as differences mentioned in terms of food and medication, age of usual onset, etc.

15.2.9 INSULIN ADMINISTRATION/ TREATMENT PHILOSOPHY

Survival skills for insulin administration include the obvious ones of which syringe to use, how to measure exact doses and how to remove air bubbles. If mixed doses of rapid and slower-acting insulins are to be used, this too must be taught in a manner which minimizes contamination of regular insulin by the NPH or lente insulins. Many diabetologists prefer abdominal injections of insulin especially if multidose insulin protocols are to be used since this may decrease some day-to-day absorption differences and produce more predictable glucose response to insulin injections. It is generally believed that in the non-exercised state, abdominal insulin absorption is faster compared to arm or leg sites. However, following exercise, injections of insulin in the exercised arm or leg show much more dramatic increases in vascular perfusion and this is associated with increased absorption of insulin from arm and leg sites as a result. Some of the day-to-day 'brittility' of glucose levels may be related to burst activity which is unexpected and therefore interferes with smoother glucose control. Whether or not injection site choices is of significant clinical (as opposed to research) importance remains controversial.

Many diabetologists also prefer using specific sites at specific times of the day or night to promote reproducibility of absorption characteristics. For instance, on an insulin schedule prebreakfast, prelunch, predinner and prebedtime snack, I might suggest the 7 a.m. insulin dose be administered in the buttocks with rotations from right to left; the prelunch 12 noon insulin dose be given in arms with rotations from left to right arm; the predinner 6 p.m. insulin dose be given on both sides of the abdomen and prebedtime 9 p.m. insulin dose be given in both anterior thigh regions. The importance of making insulin injection in different parts of specific body sites to avoid insulin hypertrophy – and its attendant insulin malabsorption and leakage problems – should also be stated. As in many other aspects of IDDM care, setting up good initial principles will prevent having to 'unlearn' bad habits months and years later.

The philosophy of gradual or aggressive insulinization should be briefly explained to patient and family members to explain why a two or three injection dose schedule is chosen vs. a more aggressive four dose per day schedule. If 'tight' control is expected and accepted, more doses of smaller amounts may prove more beneficial coupled with frequent capillary blood glucose monitoring (Ludvigsson *et al.*, 1989 and DCCT Research Group, 1993). At the present time, there are many different insulin dosing schedules in use around the world (Chapter 17). None have been proven superior in any rigorous, prospective scientific study. Most diabetologists prefer human insulin since it is the least allergenic of the available insulin preparatios. Pure pork insulin is nearly in the same category and in certain patients may provide slightly slower and longer duration of effect. This may be particularly true for the very young patient. Availability of insulins in different parts of the world may be the most important factor in choice of insulin whereas cost of certain insulins may become the dominant factor rather than supply. No rules about insulin choice (or dose, for that matter), however, apply to all patients under all circumstances. There are many individual exceptions to any rule provided. In certain situations, using pure beef or beef/pork ultralente may be selected to provide lowered peak insulin effect while multiple bursts of regular insulin are given around meal times to mimic normal insulin release without using an insulin pump. The insulin pump has been

Table 15.4 Some insulin dosing schedules at NEDEC.

A. Four injections daily
 1. Premeal regular insulin with human NPH @ bedtime
 2. Same with human lente @ bedtime
 3. Same with human ultralente @ bedtime
 4. Same with animal source ultralente @ bedtime
 5. Premeal regular insulin with some other intermediate or long-acting insulins divided at different times of day or evening
  (a) R+N prebreakfast, R alone prelunch and predinner and R+N at bedtime
  (b) R+N prebreakfast, R alone prelunch and R+N predinner and R+N at bedtime
  (c) Animal ultralente breakfast and bedtime with premeal regular insulins
 6. Premeal regular insulin with different intermediate or long acting insulin given at breakfast and bedtime
  (a) R+ultralente prebreakfast, R alone prelunch, R alone predinner and R+NPH at bedtime
  (b) Same but with lente at bedtime
B. Three injections daily
 1. Premeal regular insulin with either NPH (or lente or ultralente), and source, as combination with regular predinner
 2. Premeal regular insulin with ultralente as combination prebreakfast
 3. Premeal regular insulin with ultralente at breakfast and dinner
 4. Breakfast split mix of regular + NPH (or lente or ultralente), nothing prelunch, regular alone predinner and NPH (or lente or ultralente) alone at bedtime
C. Two injections daily
 1. NPH or lente or ultralente alone prebreakfast and either predinner or bedtime
 2. Split mixes of regular plus NPH (or lente or ultralente)
 3. Regular plus NPH (or lente or ultralente) prebreakfast with NPH (or lente or ultralente) alone at bedtime or predinner

used successfully in several pediatric and adolescent settings with similar benefits and problems as in adult populations studied (De Beaufort, 1986; Brink & Stewart, 1986).

Table 15.4 presents some insulin protocols currently being used. The selection of exactly which insulin is chosen, whether human or pure pork, depends upon specific absorption characteristics of the individual patient, timing and amount of food usually eaten, timing and amount of snacks eaten, activity pattern and capillary blood glucose results to fine tune the choice. If an aggressive insulinization protocol is started at diagnosis, for example, Humulin™ or Novolin™ (also called Actrapid Human™) regular insulin alone might be used before breakfast, lunch and dinner with Humulin™ NPH alone at bedtime. However, if middle-of-the-night glucose monitoring suggests that the NPH was not lasting for sufficiently long duration to provide prebreakfast glycemic control, a switch to the slightly longer acting Humulin lente or even the longer duration Humulin ultralente might be given at bedtime.

Similarly, in some circumstances, Humulin or Novolin (human) insulins do not provide sufficient duration of action to last until the next meal and a change to a pork regular insulin may be helpful to improve glycemic control under such circumstances. Some diabetologists find that more complex combinations of ultralente at bedtime with NPH or lente in the morning work better than keeping both intermediate acting insulins the same type. The message for the 1990s is to match the insulin effect desired – and proven with capillary blood glucose monitoring data – with all the other variables in a given patient in an effort to provide optimal insulinization, minimize plasma hyperinsulinemia if possible and decrease the chances of severe or recurrent hypoglycemia. Whether and how this can be accomplished in clinical (as opposed to research settings) is not yet known. Alternative insulin delivery devices like pen devices can be used with cartridges designed to make multiple dose programs easier to accept. Some patients use standard syringes at home but choose cartridge insulin for simplicity of use at school away from parental supervision (Ludvigsson *et al.*, 1989).

Current commercial insulins exist in hexamer formation. As a result, insulins must be partially metabolized at subcutaneous injection sites before they produce their metabolic effects. By using monomers or other insulin analogs, speed of action and duration of action can be affected (see Chapter 42). Studies currently underway in various centers around the world show promise with improved immediate postprandial glycemic control because of speedier absorption of such monomeric insulins compared to current human or pork insulin. In addition, because duration of effect is also shorter, the late hypoglycemic effects that necessitate forced snacking several hours after insulin is given or produce excessive clinical hypoglycemic reactions, may be minimized or avoided. Efficacy studies with scientifically correct crossover design will answer such questions shortly. The final practical benefit of such monomeric insulins is that the suggested 30–45 minute wait from insulin injection to time of the meal may be unnecessary since absorption will be sufficiently rapid to have this accomplished simultaneously. Many patients have great difficulty being consistent with their insulin-to-food timing from day to day. In toddlers where food intake cannot be mandated and enforced, knowing how much a child has actually eaten and then dosing insulin accordingly will be a tremendous improvement compared to current practical limitations of insulin use in such very young children.

15.2.10 HYPOGLYCEMIA, EMERGENCY PROCEDURES, MEDIC-ALERT

Survival skills regarding hypoglycemia include defining at what level of blood glucose this is an issue and the fact that many instances of hypoglycemia can occur without warning signals. Teaching classical symptoms is nevertheless important (shakiness, confusion, headache, strange hunger cravings, dizziness, unconsciousness, coma and convulsions) but also must emphasize that symptoms sometimes change, do not always have to occur and often change in character over time. It is also important to try to distinguish early vs. late symptoms as well as qualitative symptomatology: mild hypoglycemic reactions that are self-treated or resolve spontaneously, moderate hypoglycemic reactions which require the assistance of another and severe hypoglycemic reactions which involve unconsciousness or seizures or both (Brink, 1987). Mild and moderate hypo-

Table 15.5 Hypoglycemia treatment options.

A. Mild to moderate reactions during daytime:
   1. 4–6 oz (120–180 cc) unsweetened orange juice
   2. 4–6 oz (120–180 cc) sweetened carbonated or noncarbonated drinks (e.g., Coca Cola, 7Up, Lucozade)
   3. 2–3 glucose tablets (various brands)
   4. 30 grams honey
   5. 1–2 teaspoons of granulated sugar
   6. 7–10 LifeSaver candies (or other hard candies)
B. Mild to moderate nocturnal reactions:
   1. same options as 1–6 above plus one bread exchange plus one meat exchange
C. Severe reactions:
   1. 1/4–1 ml glucagon given SC, IM or IV (exact dose according to approximate weight)
   2. 10–15 grams of intravenous glucose if medical personnel and venous access available

glycemic reactions can usually be treated with oral quick-acting carbohydrate as listed in Table 15.5 whereas severe hypoglycemic reactions often require glucagon subcutaneously, intramuscularly or intravenously (or intravenous glucose, if it is available).

Infants and toddlers, because they are often non-verbal, may have greater difficulty with hypoglycemia since they do not provide early warning signals for their caretakers' response. Close skilled observation, while ideal, is clearly not always practical (i.e., in the middle of the night or when others, not parents, provide intermittent care). In patients who have behavioral or intellectual compromise, detection of hypoglycemia may also be problematic. In adolescents, intake of alcohol, blocking the liver's ability to correct hypoglycemia, may turn mild to moderate hypoglycemic reactions into a severe hypoglycemic episode. A patient with diabetes who is drinking (and/or abusing drugs), may not have the ability or motivation to respond to what would otherwise be easily recognizable symptoms of hypoglycemia. All these issues must at least be discussed briefly as part of survival training regarding hypoglycemia recognition and treatment.

Hypoglycemia prevention education should include the importance of food and snacks at set times as well as insulin kinetics for the particular child or adolescent. Effect of exercise, whether burst exercise or prolonged aerobic exercise, and whether the hypoglycemic effect is immediate, shortly after exercise takes place or several hours later must all be discussed and action plans instituted to counterbalance predicted likelihood. Capillary blood glucose monitoring once again plays a pivotal role in defining and teaching about such events.

Medic-Alert identification cards or bracelets or necklaces must be introduced in a positive and reassuring fashion. Options for type and style of Medic-Alert 'jewelry' provides an opportunity to allow choice to the youngster or teenagers. A teaching opportunity can be created changing the focus from 'being tagged and therefore different from one's peers' to one of 'being unique, taking charge of one's needs and boosting self esteem'.

15.2.11 ONGOING EDUCATION, FREQUENCY OF CONTACTS AND AMBULATORY VISITS, ONGOING PSYCHOSOCIAL ASSESSMENT AND SUPPORT

Specific issues such as ongoing education needs and the importance of working with a team consisting of physician, diabetes educator and dietician should be specifically stated. An overview of how this will be accomplished should be outlined after initial survival education has concluded. Establishing the importance of maintaining newly-taught skills, reviewing issues periodically and updating for increasing responsibility as age and maturity dictate is an essential factor in the success of the multidisciplinary team involved with diabetes education. Stressing the role of psychosocial support staff (social workers, psychologist and/or psychiatrists, depending upon circumstances) and the possible role of exercise physiologists, camp counselors and voluntary diabetes organizations may facilitate future introduction. Reinforcing how and why to contact staff, how often follow-up visits are likely to be needed and circumstances under which such guidelines will change is also important. Deciding which teaching manuals will be used (if not already obtained) suggest that these too can be used as a future as well as current resource. Many insulin and diabetes supply companies provide specific pamphlets and coloring books that can be used for specific issue reinforcement. Children's books whose main characters get diagnosed with IDDM or have diabetes are also extremely useful adjuncts to supporting the daily trials and tribulations of learning to live with diabetes (Brink & Wilson, 1990) just as some lay publications and books provide such resources for parents and teachers as well as health care professionals.

15.3 DIABETIC KETOACIDOSIS: SEVERE METABOLIC DECOMPENSATION

If the diagnosis of IDDM is delayed for any reason or if it occurs in a very young child where it is usually unsuspected until severe decompensation occurs, diabetic ketoacidosis (DKA) can occur. This can also occur in the already diagnosed patient with IDDM as discussed below and the medical treatment remains the same. DKA is life-threatening yet with proper recognition and treatment virtually never fatal. Effective therapy demands sophisticated knowledge of the pathophysiology of the disorder and of the interrelationships of not only insulin deficiency but also fluid and electrolyte replacement as well as carbohydrate and fat energy utilization.

All stages of ketoacidosis from the earliest increases in blood glucose through increasing generation of ketone bodies to ketonemia, acidemia and eventually ketoacidosis may be steps in the process leading to coma and death if appropriate intervention does not occur. The patient with diabetes out of control is said to be in diabetic ketoacidosis (DKA) or 'diabetic coma' when the carbon dioxide level (or serum bicarbonate) is 10 mmol/l or less. The term 'diabetic coma' is often misleading since most patients with severe diabetic ketoacidosis are not unconscious. A clear goal for all diabetes health care professionals is proper early recognition and treatment by the patient and/or his or her family before hospitalization as a necessity.

15.4 INITIAL FLUID AND ELECTROLYTE MANAGEMENT

On the assumption that dehydration is mainly reflected by body weight loss, the weight of the patient can be used for initial calculation of replacement while surface area can be utilized to best reflect the differences in infancy, childhood and adulthood for maintenance needs. The severity of the signs and symptoms of dehydration reflect extracellular fluid loss; the minimal detectable evidence of dehydration is approximately 3–5% loss of body weight; the maximal acute body weight loss which is compatible with life is estimated to be approximately 20%. With 20% acute volume depletion the patient is, by definition, in profound shock and moribund. (Note that 20% acute plus chronic weight loss is not all water loss so that patients who are newly diagnosed and give a history of significant weight loss are not necessarily 20% dehydrated since they have lost muscle and fat as well as water weight.) Because extracellular fluid loss represents, for the most part, loss of sodium and water, immediate restitution of blood volume should be estimated at 10–20 ml/kg of body weight as normal (0.9%) saline given over the first 1–2 hours of treatment. This effectively removes the patient from the immediate consequences of potential or overt shock and does not cause any delay searching for special intravenous solutions (blood, plasma, Ringer's lactate, albumin, etc.).

Maintenance water, sodium and potassium can be estimated according to standard pediatric guidelines based on surface area estimations:

water: 2000 (1500–2500 range) ml/m^2/24 hours
sodium: 40 (30–60 range) mmol/m^2/24 hours
potassium: 40 (30–50 range) mmol/m^2/24 hours

Total body deficits can be enormous with changes not always reflected in initial laboratory measurements. The serum sodium may be high, normal or low but this is not an accurate measure of the sodium requirement especially if there has been technical artifact added to the measurement because of concomitant hyperlipidemia. Because of the acidotic state, potassium is usually driven out of the intracellular space but, at the same time, it is also being lost in the urine. Initially, serum potassium levels are usually normal or slightly elevated because of acid-base shifts. As tissue dehydration is corrected, lactic acid production decreases with increased body perfusion; simultaneously, insulin administration will begin to allow a decrease in ketoacid production so that the acidotic state begins to reverse. Serum potassium should be expected to decrease soon after therapy for ketoacidosis begins. The clinician should be alerted to the dangers of hypokalemia by monitoring serum potassium values as well as by obtaining sequential bedside EKG rhythm strips for evaluation of T and U wave changes. Occasionally, metabolic decompensation has progressed to the point that hypokalemia is present initially; this has a more ominous prognosis because of the cardiac arrhythmias that can coexist at that time or shortly after the acidotic state begins to change.

Most treatment centers suggest the use of normal saline (0.9%) intravenously for the first 1–4 hours with a switch to half-normal (0.45%) saline with added potassium in subsequent bottles; this takes into account the hypotonic nature of the losses relative to the extracellular space. More recent information concerning the possibility that cerebral edema is more common than appreciated (Harris *et al.*, 1992) has led some to recommend that normal saline be continued for a longer time period (for example until blood glucose ≤13 mmol/l) in order to allow osmotic equilibrium to be reestablished in a more leisurely time frame.

If the total deficit of sodium is sufficiently excessive and if hypovolemia is great enough, glomerular filtration will decrease and the patient, formerly polyuric, will develop oliguria. If this shock-like state has lasted for several hours and there is acute tubular necrosis, treatment is markedly complicated and may require the use of central venous pressure catheters to monitor fluid needs as the patient is treated for renal failure. Patients with already existing cardiac or renal problems who present in ketoacidosis likewise require more intense intervention and monitoring which takes into account all these interdependent factors. Rarely, dialysis will be needed in such severely ill patients.

15.5 HYPOKALEMIA

Potassium should be given immediately if hypokalemia is suspected by electrocardiographic changes at presentation or if laboratory results confirm the presence of already low serum potassium; usually, however, potassium is added in the second to fourth hour of treatment. Early and vigorous treatment with potassium replacement may decrease mortality and morbidity. It has been suggested, therefore, that potassium be added to the initial intravenous solution as soon as a reliable history of polyuria has been obtained in a child, or once the first urine is voided.

Potassium can best be replaced at a rate of 40 mmol/l of solution without danger of a rapid rise in blood levels or of irritation at the intravenous site. Half should be given as potassium chloride (20 mmol/l KCl) and the other half as potassium phosphate (20 mmol/l K_2HPO_4) for the first 6–12 hours of replacement therapy. Thereafter, potassium chloride should be used so that iatrogenic hypocalcemia does not occur (section 15.6).

On rare occasions, more potassium is needed than can be supplied at 40 mmol/l. Continuous electrocardiographic monitoring then becomes a necessity as does frequent repeat serum determinations to guide therapy.

Administration of potassium via nasogastric tube should be considered if it becomes impossible to provide sufficient intravenous potassium for any reason. Multiple intravenous sites can also be used if local venous irritation develops.

Potassium values can plummet (Vignati *et al.*, 1985) from initial values as therapy proceeds because of increased glucose utilization secondary to insulin administration, acid-base shifts caused by decreased production of ketoacids as well as improved tissue perfusion (therefore less lactic acid production) and persistent urinary excretion of potassium by the kidney handling large loads of sodium (Bunge effect). Movement of potassium into cells may be quantitatively so great that life-threatening hypokalemia can occur despite simultaneous infusion of potassium. Special caution should be exercised when administering intravenous bicarbonate because of shifts in acid-base balance which might ensue (section 15.7). In oliguric or anuric patients, potassium administration may still be necessary especially if serum potassium levels are already low or a trend to hypokalemia levels becomes obvious.

Clinically significant hypokalemia can be characterized by the following:

(1) weakness of skeletal muscles progressing to frank paralysis
(2) rapid diminution or complete absence of deep tendon reflexes
(3) development of shallow gasping respirations especially in contrast to Kussmaul deep ventilatory efforts
(4) cyanosis
(5) abdominal distention and
(6) cardiac enlargement and failure.

Should such signs or symptoms occur, emergency evaluation of potassium status is warranted.

15.6 HYPOPHOSPHATEMIA AND OXYGEN STATUS

Patients with diabetic ketoacidosis sustain intracellular phosphate depletion and serum phosphate often follows a pattern similar to that of potassium. Although initial serum phosphate values may be normal or elevated, within 4–6 hours after insulin treatment has begun, these values may fall dramatically as glycogen deposition resumes. Significant hypophosphatemia can be observed within 30 minutes following onset of therapy. The consequences of hypophosphatemia may be reflected in red blood cell levels of 2,3 diphosphoglycerate (2,3 DPG), an intermediary metabolite of glycolysis. The role of red cell 2,3 DPG in diabetic ketoacidosis is important because 2,3 DPG has the capacity to alter the affinity of the hemoglobin molecule for oxygen and thus the delivery of oxygen to tissues. A fall in 2,3 DPG content may cause tissue and cerebral hypoxia in patients with diabetic ketoacidosis, hence the recommendation that most patients being treated for DKA should receive oxygen at least for the first few hours of treatment. If sodium bicarbonate is given in sufficient amounts to raise the pH of the blood rapidly, the protective Bohr effect which allows oxygen to be released in the face of acidosis is reversed and the sudden rise in hemoglobin affinity for oxygen might lead to tissue hypoxia and account for the sudden deterioration of some patients receiving bicarbonate. This sequence of events following the administration of sodium bicarbonate might contribute to cerebral edema.

This author suggests replenishment of phosphate losses by providing 50% of the needed potassium replacement and maintenance as phosphate salts and 50% as chloride salts (section 15.5). This is provided for the first 6–12 hours of intravenous fluid therapy so that changes in calcium–phosphate ratios are not excessive. Using this therapeutic approach, no problems with hypocalcemia or hypomagnesemia have been seen in over 10 years by this author. Oxygen is also recommended at low flow rates and usually delivered by nasal prongs.

15.7 ACIDEMIA AND ACIDOSIS: TREATMENT WITH SODIUM BICARBONATE?

Since acetoacetate and betahydroxybutyrate are metabolizable anions, restoration of serum bicarbonate concentration will follow insulin administration in the absence of treatment with alkali-containing solutions. As discussed earlier, acidosis results from a combination of release of fatty acids secondary to insulin deficiency, generation of 'ketone bodies' and starvation from poor food intake and, in some instances, excessive production of lactic acid because of plasma volume depletion, poor tissue perfusion and an increase in anaerobic glycolysis in muscles. The altered cardiovascular physiology during such systemic acidemia has been used as justification for rapid correction with bicarbonate but catastrophic complications such as cerebral edema and respiratory arrest have been attributed to this mode of therapy. Life-threatening hypokalemia (as potassium returns into the cell) as well as worsening tissue hypoxia affinity for oxygen can be added to this list of bicarbonate treatment complications (Table 15.6).

Treatment with sodium bicarbonate should be restricted to patients with a severe metabolic acidosis as indicated by an arterial pH of 7.0–7.1 or a bicarbonate value of less than 5 mmol/l and even then only on the advice of senior medical stalf. Rapid infusions or large amounts over a short time span should not be routinely ordered and should be reserved for acute and life-threatening cardiorespiratory arrest situations. If sodium bicarbonate is given, the amount of sodium should be subtracted from that amount of sodium contained in the replacement fluids to avoid exacerbation of the (already) hyperosmolar state. It is suggested that sodium bicarbonate not be given according to specified calculations of base deficits because of the likelihood of 'overdosage'. This can occur because insulin administration, better fluid balance and renal compensatory mechanisms all are working to rebalance the state of acidosis that existed. When sodium bicarbonate is used, it should be given by slow intravenous infusion over several hours. Frequent serial pH and/or bicarbonate determinations should be obtained so that the administration of bicarbonate can be discontinued when the pH reaches 7.2–7.25. It seems wise to allow normal body homeostatic mechanisms to take full responsibility to compensate for all such metabolic derangements as much as possible. Favorable results reported on low dose insulin protocols (Brink, 1987) without routine bicarbonate administration provide strong arguments against insulin resistance being common in patients with ketosis and acidosis despite earlier reports.

Table 15.6 Complications associated with bicarbonate administration in DKA.

1. Abrupt osmotic changes
2. Precipitous potassium changes
3. Overshoot alkalosis
4. Potential hypoxia with shift of oxyhemoglobin dissociation curve
5. Cerebral edema, coma and death

Deterioration of the clinical condition with rapid elevation of plasma pH accompanied by an exaggerated fall in cerebrospinal pH following the administration of sodium bicarbonate has been observed in patients with diabetic ketoacidosis. An increase in carbon dioxide (as respiratory effort decreases with an abatement of Kussmaul respirations) and the more slowly-moving bicarbonate diffusion across the blood-brain barrier may explain this paradoxical cerebrospinal acidosis. Cerebral vasodilatation and an increase in cerebral blood volume may contribute to an increase in cerebrospinal pressure and cerebral edema and account for changes in levels of consciousness in patients receiving sodium bicarbonate.

15.8 TRACE MINERALS

Little definitive work is available from which to offer therapeutic suggestions for use of trace minerals during ketoacidotic episodes. Calcium can be depressed transiently and may reflect a temporary state of hypoparathyroidism associated with fluxes in body phosphorus stores (section 15.6). In the past, replacement fluids have been used containing magnesium. Deficits of other minerals such as zinc, selenium and chromium may occur although no readily apparent clinical correlates can be documented. No recent work is available to document any changes in specific mineral replacement other than what has been stated above.

15.9 INSULIN TREATMENT

The route of administration and the dose of insulin necessary for treatment of diabetic ketoacidosis have been the subject of much disagreement in recent years. Successful results have been published with differing insulin regimes although most experts prefer continuous low dose infusion insulin as discussed below.

All patients in ketoacidosis have an immediate need for insulin; no matter which protocol is followed, fluid and electrolyte replacement as well as recognition of underlying precipitating events must remain high on the list of priorities to decrease morbidity and mortality. Close and repeated clinical as well as laboratory observations are mandatory to enable the wisest and safest therapeutic approaches and to allow for their modification once therapy ensues (Table 15.7).

The giving of 'enough' insulin should be one's aim and this should be guided by initial and subsequent blood sugar determinations and clinical condition of the patient. As a result of acid-base changes and insulin treatment, blood acetoacetate and acetone levels may rise initially despite a much greater fall in betahydroxybutyric acid. Consequently, blood and urine ketone determinations (which only measure acetone and acetoacetate, and not betahydroxybutyrate) may rise rather than fall as therapy starts to proceed. Blood and urine ketone determinations are therefore far less useful as an index of additional insulin requirement than is clinical response and blood glucose changes. Physicians should be wary of increasing insulin dosage solely because of worsening ketonemia and/or ketonuria; in fact, this should be expected over the first few hours of treatment. Too vigorous insulin administration may lead to rapid decreases in blood glucose and therefore excessive osmotic changes; the risks of cerebral edema increase if this crucial metabolic fact is ignored.

Table 15.7 When to modify insulin dose.

Increased dose	Decreased dose
Longer duration diabetes	Newly diagnosed patient
Severe infection	Not unconscious
Extreme obesity	Blood sugar below 24 mmol/l (400 h/mg/100 ml)
Insulin resistance	Very thin person
Severe acidosis	Young infant or child
History of skipping insulin	History of insulin sensitivity
	Renal insufficiency
	Hypokalemia
	Extreme hyperosmolality

Crystalline regular insulin should always be the type of insulin used in the treatment of coma patients so that adjustments made produce relatively quick results. Human insulin, because it is less allergenic than other preparations, should be the regular insulin of choice unless it is unavailable (or the patient is known to be using an alternative insulin product already). Many factors determine the amounts of insulin required. The largest doses are generally needed in older, more overweight patients who have had diabetes for some time, particularly when insulin has not been administered regularly or when insulin has not been given during the initial hours of an illness. Newly-diagnosed patients who are very acidotic may require very large amounts of insulin whereas others are exquisitively sensitive. Smaller children, infants and toddlers seem to be more sensitive to insulin than older children and teenagers. This is yet another example of the patient who does not need large doses of insulin but, rather, fluid and electrolyte replenishment with 'some insulin'.

At least one physician must at all times know the time of insulin administration, the relation of subsequent blood sugar determinations to each dosage, and the time of starting as well as the rate of flow of fluids and electrolytes. Keeping a flow sheet may be the single most important task once the diagnosis is established and treatment begun because of the dynamic state of affairs present in this condition and how much can change once treatment begins. There is no substitute formula to replace close hour-by-hour observation of the patient and supervision of treatment by the physician and the hospital team.

15.10 BOLUS INSULIN

In the past, traditional insulin therapy has been given by a combination of bolus intravenous as well as bolus subcutaneous regular insulin. Any possibility of decreased perfusion to a particular subcutaneous area, therefore, was eliminated because some insulin was available directly into the blood stream. Insulin was given according to a variety of guidelines which were related to body size, weight and/or habitus. Multiple decisions regarding initial and subsequent dosage amounts were required but most patients recovered without excess morbidity or mortality. In fact, with appropriate sequential blood sugar and electrolyte monitoring, mortality figures drastically decreased over the years that insulin has been available. Acknowledgment of the relative sensitivity of youngsters to insulin was made and most authors suggested that children receive most if not all of their insulin for treatment of ketoacidosis subcutaneously rather than intravenously. It was not infrequent to have the initial doses of insulin (given in this large bolus fashion) of sufficient magnitude so that no further insulin was needed for 16–24 hours after admission; hyperglycemia was rapidly corrected over a few hours.

15.11 INTRAMUSCULAR INSULIN

The earliest reports advocating the use of intramuscular insulin in the treatment of diabetic ketoacidosis were published in 1946 in the German literature (Katsch, 1946). Because intramuscular injection of insulin may produce a faster absorption of insulin and a greater drop in blood glucose levels when compared to subcutaneous doses, several investigators started to look at the use of frequent but smaller doses of intramuscular insulin injections. British diabetologists (Alberti, 1977) devised a treatment program which took into account the 'muscle half life of insulin' of about two hours and the relatively constant blood insulin levels which could be obtained by repeating such dosage at hourly intervals – for youngsters, a loading dose of 0.25 units of regular insulin per kilogram followed by 0.1 units per kilogram per hour intramuscularly.

The benefits of intramuscular treatment over intravenous plus subcutaneous treatment with insulin consist of the following:

(1) ease of protocol comprehension by staff
(2) no need for complex apparatus to deliver insulin

(3) no need for complicated calculations of insulin dose
(4) little risk of late hypoglycemia because of the near-normal blood insulin levels achieved
(5) smooth fall in blood lactate
(6) no major potassium fluxes and
(7) decreased potential for cerebral edema because of the slower falls in blood glucose and the slower resulting osmotic changes.

Potential problems utilizing intramuscular insulin protocols (apart from patient discomfort) arise when rehydration and electrolyte disturbances receive inadequate attention particularly if the patient is already hypotensive on admission. Another source of potential concern is the choice of injection site for the insulin; if the buttock is used, the insulin may be deposited in fat not muscle tissues. In order to avoid this, the recommendation has been to utilize a muscle such as the deltoid which is readily and predictably accessible despite obesity.

15.12 INTRAVENOUS LOW DOSE CONTINUOUS INFUSION

As with intramuscular protocols, intravenous low dose regular insulin infusion has become the standard method of treating diabetic ketoacidosis. Although the original reports were from Germany over 30 years ago (Vollm, 1960), it was not until 1972 that renewed enthusiasm was generated for low dose insulin infusions for ketoacidosis based on further British studies (Sonksen *et al.*, 1972) in the adult diabetes literature which 'rediscovered' this method for treating ketoacidosis (Page, 1974). The predictability of gently falling blood glucose values has been viewed as a marked improvement compared to larger bolus insulin treatments previously used. Generally, blood sugar falls by approximately 10% per hour once the initial 'dehydrated' blood glucose value is corrected (with the

Table 15.8 NEDEC DKA low-dose insulin infusion protocol for children and adolescents.

1. Maintain airway, breathing and circulation.
2. Confirm diagnosis of ketoacidosis at bedside.
3. Start intravenous infusion with normal saline 10–20 ml/kg to run over 1–2 hours.
4. Lead II EKG for potassium status (full EKG in adults).
5. Start flow sheet: weight, height, surface area calculations, pulse, BP, respiratory rate and effort, CNS status, baseline glucose, urine, electrolytes, calcium, acid-base data.
6. Determine estimated maintenance and deficit electrolyte and fluid orders.
7. Attach piggyback regular insulin infusion system to existing intravenous line:
   A. Prepare 100 units regular insulin (1 ml) in 100 ml of normal saline.
   B. Preflush intravenous tubing to allow adherence of insulin to plastic; no need for albumin.
   C. Set up piggyback system into existing IV line using available pump or pediatric drip-set.
   D. Give 0.1–0.2 units/kg of body weight as intravenous push of regular insulin stat as bolus.
   E. Start 0.1 unit/kg body weight/hr intravenously by continuous infusion.
   F. Expect initial drop from rehydration and then approximately 10% of blood sugar hourly (i.e., 50–70 mg/dl/hr [3–4 mmol/L/hr]).
   G. Monitor blood glucose at 1 hour and then every 2–4 hrs to make sure expected response occurs. Monitor urine for sugar and acetone at least every 3–4 hours.
   H. Double rate of infusion or switch to alternative insulin delivery protocol if no response.
   I. Calculate estimated time when blood glucose will reach 250–300 mg/dl (15–18 mmol/L) to avoid hypoglycemia.
   J. Stop insulin infusion when blood glucose reaches 250 mg/dl (15 mmol/L) and change intravenous solution to contain 5% dextrose with electrolytes.

Table 15.8 *Continued*

8. After initial 1–2 hours of normal saline infusion, switch to 0.5 normal saline plus 20 mmol/L KCl and 20 mmol/L K_2HPO_4 to avoid iatrogenic hypokalemia.
9. Check electrolytes at 2–4 hours and again as necessary according to clinical monitoring requirements, patient status, etc.
10. Must give subcutaneous insulin or intramuscular insulin 15 minutes before intravenous insulin is discontinued or if line no longer operational because of short half life of IV insulin to avoid recurrent ketoacidosis. Adjust dosage according to newness of IDDM, degree of ketosis and/or acidosis, age of patient, known sensitivity or other factors which will affect amount of insulin needed (pregnancy, renal failure, ongoing infection, etc.).
11. Identify and treat any underlying problem (i.e., continue antibiotics as needed for UTI, strep throat, etc.).
12. Keep flow sheet up to date and reassess frequently.
13. Pay attention to electrolyte changes and neurologic status including repeat fundus examination to detect and treat cerebral edema.
14. Educate patient and family to prevent recurrence: identify contributing psychosocial problems if present.

first few hours of hydration). Correction of acidemia and restoration of electrolyte status and lipid profiles presumably occurs at a slightly slower rate because of the smaller amounts of insulin being given; in some studies, no significant differences among the three types of insulin dosing protocols could be found (Fisher *et al.*, 1977). Early fears of insulin resistance have not been confirmed nor has there been any noticeable increase in mortality. One protocol for use of low dose continuous insulin infusion is presented in Table 15.8. Albumin is not needed to prevent insulin adsorption to glass and/or plastic bottles and tubing.

Infusing insulin at these rates allows for adequate blood insulin levels to correct hyperglycemia, inhibit lipolysis, inhibit glycogenolysis and correct abnormalities in counter-regulatory hormone levels found in ketoacidosis. Rarely, 'insulin resistance' will be discovered when no lowering of blood glucose occurs at the 1–2 hour check. If blood sugars do not respond as expected, the most common error is that the insulin was not started or was not connected properly to the infusion. If insulin was indeed delivered to the patient in DKA and the blood sugars remain elevated unexpectedly, the dose should either be doubled or an alternative protocol utilized. As in all other treatment regimes, dehydration remains a potential cause for non-response especially from underestimated ongoing losses. The presence of documented infection seems to slow down return of all parameters of metabolic control but there does not appear to be any significant difference clinically in low dose vs. high dose protocol comparisons (Balasse, 1976).

When blood sugar falls to approximately 15 mmol/l (250 mg/100 ml), 5% dextrose is added to the intravenous fluids being administered and subcutaneous insulin can be started. A potential problem occurs at this stage of treatment which has been called 'changing of the guard'. At shift-change times (for both nursing and physician staff), it is common to discontinue the insulin infusion but forget to order or give subcutaneous insulin! In order to avoid this type of error, it seems wise to specify in hospital DKA protocols that subcutaneous insulin be given one half-hour BEFORE the continuous insulin infusion is terminated. This allows sufficient time for absorption to occur from the subcutaneous site. Some authors recommend continuing intravenous insulin until ketonuria disappears or if the correction of hyperglycemia occurs more rapidly than the acidosis.

Some disagreement also exists as to the

necessity of a loading dose of insulin. Those favoring such an approach have suggested that maximum saturation of binding sites may occur slightly sooner than if the steady state were to occur over the first few minutes of infusion. Those opposed to the use of the 'bolus' loading dose feel that the rapid potential rate of change may be harmful and promote the secretion of the anti-insulin hormones (Alberti, 1977).

The benefits of continuous intravenous insulin treatment for diabetic ketoacidosis are the same as those for intramuscular treatment:

(1) more gentle osmotic correction of hyperosmolar state
(2) reduced risk of hypoglycemia because the decrease is more predictable
(3) decreased severe hypokalemia
(4) decreased theoretical risk of cerebral edema
(5) elimination of guessing the dose required.

Repeated intramuscular injections are obviously not necessary – an especially important benefit when dealing with small children scared of needles anyway. The major drawback may be the need to ensure a continuous intravenous route, especially a problem in the severely dehydrated patient or in the child who is difficult to restrain and keep quiet. Because of the very small amounts of insulin being given per hour, infusion pumps are often required; searching for special apparatus should not cause undue delays in beginning fluid and electrolyte therapy or in actually starting insulin replacement. Often a pediatric infusion set can serve the same purposes and not require specially trained personnel for monitoring.

One additional advantage of the insulin infusion method is that the infusion rate can be titrated against changes in the blood sugar in an almost instantaneous fashion because of the very short plasma half life of insulin and the fact that no depot insulin is in use. This can also be a disadvantage if the infusion is inadvertently discontinued. As a precaution against this occurring, the protocol used by this author stipulates that the insulin be hung in piggyback fashion and that the rate of delivery of insulin be controlled and ordered separately from that of the replacement fluids and electrolytes. In addition, the infusion is continued for 15–30 minutes after the dose of subcutaneous insulin is finally administered – as a safeguard to prevent omitting the subcutaneous dose but still discontinuing infused insulin.

With both the intramuscular and the continuous intravenous protocols, physician and staff complacency must be avoided. Insulin dosing should be made more simple with more predictable glucose changes as a result of both these newer treatments. The physician and ancillary personnel thus should have more time to consider precipitating factors and ongoing processes as well as to devote more attention to the fluid and electrolyte abnormalities which may be more lethal to the patient. It would be difficult to argue that low dose treatment methods are more effective than others, but they appear to be simpler to use, easier to teach, and for these reasons, better treatment for diabetic ketoacidosis.

15.13 CARBOHYDRATE ADMINISTRATION

Carbohydrate is necessary as substrate for insulin action if fatty acid breakdown is to be rapidly halted (Foster & McGarry, 1983). This author suggests that glucose be added to the intravenous fluids when the blood glucose is in the 15–18 mmol/l (250–300 mg/100 ml) range. For some patients whose problems of ketoacidosis are secondary to dehydration and vomiting, and who enter with blood sugars below this range, this means giving 5% dextrose with the initial fluid solution.

For other patients, this means adding 5–10% dextrose at 5–12 hours after initiating treatment with fluids, electrolytes and insulin. Deciding when to add glucose is facilitated with the more predictable decreases in glycemia that occur using low dose insulin infusion protocols and the availability of accurate bedside capillary blood glucose equipment.

15.14 SUBSEQUENT TREATMENT

Oral feeding should be reinstituted as soon as possible starting with clear liquids and progressing to soft solids and then more complex foods. For the severely-ill patient, this generally means no food for approximately 12–24 hours whereas many patients with only mild to moderate ketoacidosis can be fed four hours after initiation of treatment. This 'rule' must be flexible and change according to clinical consideration, state of consciousness, presence or absence of bowel sounds, emesis or nausea, diarrhea, etc. Early refeeding can hasten recovery as it may allow increased potassium replenishment in a safe manner in addition to avoiding the body's need to continue to break down fats and continue to make excess ketones. When youngsters start complaining that they are hungry ('starving'), it's usually prudent to begin refeeding!

Subsequent insulin dosage remains a clinical guess which takes into account many factors such as age and weight of the patient, duration of diabetes, prior usual dose of insulin (unless newly diagnosed), other potential confounding factors (pregnancy, renal failure, use of other drugs, etc.). Since average daily insulin doses are approximately 0.5–0.8 units per kilogram in the prepubertal and postpubertal periods and approximately 0.8–1.2 units per kilogram per day (or even higher) in the midst of the pubertal growth spurt, these values can be used to arrive at an estimated insulin dosage and can then be divided into morning and suppertime insulin. Newly-diagnosed patients may require much more insulin for several days to several weeks after diagnosis. Extra regular insulin may be needed for 24–48 hours after resolution of the ketoacidotic crisis.

Sequential blood sugar determinations are a guide to insulin dose and help determine when to change to intermediate acting insulin. Philosophy of insulinization dictates which protocols are to be considered for moving to BID, TID or QID insulin subcutaneously. Urinary ketones are not very helpful in making insulin dose decisions once clinical improvement is apparent. Some period of partial starvation is almost always part of the explanation for persistent mild ketonuria in addition to the fact that the largest proportion of ketoacid, betahydroxybutyric acid, is cleared to acetone and acetoacetate and this clearance takes place at a slow process for hours or days after the actual ketoacidotic crisis.

15.15 COMPLICATIONS

Complications during or as a result of treatment for diabetic ketoacidosis are listed in Table 15.9. Most of these have been discussed in preceding sections of this chapter. Missing the underlying precipitating factors whether due to lack of knowledge concerning home recognition of impending DKA, psychosocial turmoil at home (or at school) or truly organic events such as pyelonephritis or appendicitis can certainly increase morbidity and mortality significantly.

Gastric lavage should be considered for any patient truly unconscious because of the frequent association of gastric atony with ketoacidosis; the passing of a nasogastric tube should not be merely because it is listed as part of a protocol. Used judiciously, however, nasogastric tubes can certainly help to prevent aspiration in the patient who is critically ill at presentation.

Table 15.9 Frequent errors and complications of DKA.

1. Delay in diagnosis
2. Delay in instituting therapy
3. Inadequate fluid replacement
4. Unrecognized hypokalemia
5. Over-reliance on insulin
6. Overzealous bicarbonate usage
7. Hypoglycemia ('changing of the guard' syndrome)
8. Recurrent ketoacidosis ('changing of the guard' syndrome)
9. Overzealous phosphate replacement with resultant hypocalcemia
10. Aspiration
11. Unrecognized cerebral edema
12. Unrecognized acute tubular necrosis
13. Peripheral or pulmonary edema (insulin edema vs. fluid overload)
14. Not treating precipitating etiology of ketoacidosis
15. Neurologic handicap
16. Death

15.16 INSULIN EDEMA

The rapid appearance of edema, significant weight gain, abdominal bloating and blurred vision can occur shortly after treatment of DKA is begun. These clinical events are most often noted during or after aggressive treatment of patients with ketoacidosis or in a patient in whom the diagnosis of diabetes has been made recently but who has had symptomatic diabetes for a longer duration. Unless underlying cardiovascular or renal disease is present, not often the case in pediatric or adolescent IDDM, these symptoms usually abate spontaneously and have been called 'insulin edema' for lack of a better explanation (Vignati *et al.*, 1985). Any treatment protocol used which continually produced edema as its aftermath should be suspect until further work in this area can elucidate the possible causes of the edematous state.

15.17 CEREBRAL EDEMA

The patient with ketoacidosis who is unconscious or semiconscious when treatment is begun or becomes unconscious despite adequate treatment of the ketoacidosis continues to be a major therapeutic dilemma. While major treatment errors in fluid, electrolyte or insulin administration can and do occur, most cases of cerebral edema remain inexplicable (Rosenbloom, 1990). Clinical and laboratory parameters often cannot be correlated with the overall severity of the coma episode. Table 15.10 lists a series of clinical events which should lead one to be suspicious of the possibility of cerebral edema especially if the patient seems to be improving by laboratory criteria but worsening on clinical grounds.

Obviously any problem which leads to delay in diagnosis, an error in treatment, or a worsening of the acid-base, fluid and/or electrolyte status of the patient (if left unrecognized or if treated incorrectly) could be a

Table 15.10 Cerebral edema symptoms and signs.

1. Progressive CNS deterioration despite improvement of laboratory parameters
   (A) Headache
   (B) Increasing lethargy
   (C) Failure to regain consciousness
   (D) Increased CSF pressure
   (E) Abnormal reflexes
2. Eye changes
   (A) Papilledema
   (B) Unequal intraocular pressure
   (C) Increasing intraocular pressure
   (D) Decreasing pupillary light reflex
3. Hyperpyrexia
4. Hypertension
5. Diabetes insipidus
6. Abnormal electroencephalogram
7. Abnormal computerized tomography/magnetic resonance imaging of skull

possible explanation for inadequate delivery of oxygen to the brain. Those that might cause a cardiac arrhythmia or interfere with adequate respiratory efforts would be obvious candidates yet such findings are rarely documented as predisposing factors in the development of cerebral edema. Autopsy findings thought to be similar to those seen in the brains of victims of asphyxia and cerebral anoxia have been reported (Vignati *et al.*, 1985). Other investigators have been able to show some contribution to these changes by hyperosmolality *per se* and, because of these changes, recent recommendations have been to replace the overall fluid and electrolyte deficiencies in a slightly slower fashion (i.e., replacement over 36 rather than 24 hours) and with fewer drastic changes (i.e., avoiding boluses of sodium bicarbonate which might be associated with rapid pH changes and rapid movement of potassium and phosphorus; low dose insulin protocols rather than high dose bolus insulin to slow down the hyperglycemia-hyperosmotic changes over a somewhat more prolonged recovery period). The assumption that hypoxia is somehow the common final pathway has led to renewed interest in preventing rather than treating this problem. Studies demonstrating abnormalities of a non-specific nature in electroencephalograms during a variety of phases of diabetic ketoacidosis treatment and more recently, documentation of cerebral edema with the use of computerized tomography or magnetic resonance imaging of the head leads this author to the conclusion that cerebral edema, in admittedly milder forms, may be present in all patients with diabetic ketoacidosis (Brink, 1987). As a result of such findings, and with the hope of earlier recognition and therefore better treatment outcomes, the protocol being used suggests low flow oxygen delivery in addition to emphasizing detailed and sequential neurologic examination. This includes the ability to evaluate the presence or absence of venous pulsations and sharp disk margins on fundoscopy. Early consultation by a neurologist, neurosurgeon and/or ophthalmologist might be indicated if early recognition will lead to better treatment outcomes.

Treatment, once cerebral edema is recognized, is supportive and includes measures to maintain cardiorespiratory function and normal body temperature. The possible benefits of corticosteroids to reduce intracranial pressure and the use of other measures (usually felt to work through the induction of a therapeutic osmotic diuretic effect) have not been scientifically evaluated because of the small number of patients available at any single center.

Educating the general public to be aware of the signs and symptoms of diabetes, educating the patient and his or her family to the signs, symptoms and treatment of diabetic ketoacidosis – especially early in its inception – and educating the diabetes health professional to the proper diagnostic and treatment skills needed to adequately deal with this metabolic disaster will go far in preventing the morbidity and mortality of diabetic ketoacidosis.

15.18 RECURRENT DKA

DKA should, ideally, be prevented in the patient with an established diagnosis of diabetes mellitus. Ketoacidosis is not a sudden complication of IDDM and takes from hours to days to develop in the vast majority. Most cases can be recognized by well-educated younger patients if appropriate supervision by adult family members occurs. Telephone consultation with a member of the health care team, especially if an illness occurs shortly after IDDM is diagnosed, is an invaluable tool to help decide what is occurring at home and whether or not more detailed medical observation is necessary. A plan of action can be outlined with the family members 'serving as the eyes and ears' for the health care team and with defined criteria established which would require a different intervention strategy.

The extremely 'brittle' or 'labile' child or adolescent (approximately 2% of a general pediatric endocrinology or pediatric/adolescent diabetes practice) who presents with recurring DKA, often from a tumultuous family environment, may be the exception to this rule (Brink, 1987; Golden *et al.*, 1985). Such youngsters, usually around adolescence but occasionally a few years younger, seem to be enmeshed with parental and family issues that often demand that he or she 'be sick' in order to gain attention from other family members (Citrin *et al.*, 1987). Many episodes of diabetic ketoacidosis occur when insulin doses are 'forgotten' although stress-related crises are frequently part of the history obtained once a more honest assessment of the situation takes place. Sexual abuse, physical abuse, mental abuse, parents or family members who are drug or alcohol abusers or those family situations in which patients are neglected and left to care for themselves often are the true cause for recurrent DKA episodes. In these youngsters, on the basis of long-standing poorly controlled diabetes mellitus, ketoacidosis may be full blown within a few hours because of the chronic underinsulinized state that already exists.

15.19 OMITTED INSULIN – COMMONLY THE CULPRIT

Since omitted insulin was usually suspected in such patients, prevention involves awareness of the problem in those in the worst glucose control (highest glycosylated haemoglobin levels, for instance) and working out arrangements to have the most responsible adult at home actually inject insulin several times each day while psychological therapy is attempted. An extremely important question for the physician or nurse to determine is who is responsible for the daily administration of insulin. If, in fact, no adult supervision occurs routinely, a likely explanation for recurrent diabetic ketoacidosis is that the child or even the adolescent has not been getting sufficient insulin as prescribed. Such cases are more common than is generally acknowledged, are difficult to diagnose and tend to respond more quickly than other cases to routine fluid, electrolyte, and insulin administration because ongoing infection as a precipitant is not present.

15.20 PREVENTION OF KETOACIDOSIS

Teaching recognition of impending metabolic decompensation must remain a high priority for diabetes educators. Such recognition in the past depended on the patient's home urine testing program although, more recently, home blood glucose monitoring has replaced home urine testing. Such monitoring can signal a changing pattern of increasing glycemia as well as provide an awareness of such warning signs as increasing thirst, polyuria, nocturia, enuresis, malaise, weight loss, nausea, vomiting and ketonuria. Emphasis on identifying possible 'metabolic stresses' such as those occurring during intercurrent illnesses (respiratory and/or gastrointestinal) so as to foster increased monitoring during those times by responsible adults in the home is critical. A patient or family who does not regularly monitor their diabetes program and who does not keep good records of such monitoring does not have the ability to recognize a deteriorating pattern of glycemia and cannot intervene at an early time. Many intercurrent infections produce changes in insulin effectiveness for 8–24 hours prior to the onset of overt symptoms. Awareness of this can allow sufficient personal compensation to prevent further progression of the ketoacidotic state. We have not seen any episodes of ketoacidosis occurring because of overeating or other 'dietary indiscretions' although extremes of hyperglycemia as well as ketonuria do occur in many youngsters.

15.21 SICK DAY RULES

Preventive measures include the following 'Sick Day Rules' which are taught to all families and, as age-appropriate, to children and adolescents with IDDM. These sick day guidelines (Table 15.11) should be instituted whenever symptoms suggesting the possibility of DKA, with blood sugars more than 15 mmol/l (250 mg/100 ml) by capillary blood glucose monitoring by patient and/or family, with any unexplained weight loss or evidence for an intercurrent illness.

Table 15.11 Sick Day Rules for managing potential/actual DKA at home.

1. Home blood glucose monitoring (HBGM), with adult supervision – at least every 3–4 hours and occasionally every 1–2 hours and with results recorded in a log book
2. A minimum of urine ketone testing every 4 hours with results recorded in a log book
3. Continuation of such monitoring in the middle of the night (no matter how tired the patient or family is)
4. Increased salty fluid intake
5. Weight obtained 2–3× each 24-hour period
6. Treatment of underlying decompensating event (antibiotics for streptococcal pharyngitis, otitis media, urinary tract infection, etc.)
7. Antipyretics as appropriate
8. Anti-emetics if severe vomiting prevents adequate fluid intake
9. Continuation of insulin and usually administrating extra insulin 'booster shots' (10–20% extra) for as long as hyperglycemia and/or ketonuria persists
10. Recognition of when insulin dose (rarely) needs to be temporarily decreased
11. Contact with health care team especially if symptoms persist, get worse or resolution does not occur (especially persistent and severe abdominal pains, persistent emesis, deeper and/or more labored respirations, weight loss or change in neurologic status of any kind)

All too frequently a physician or nurse advises omission of insulin because the patient is ill and not eating. Under no condition should this be routinely done since most episodes of DKA require more insulin despite less food intake. On rare occasions, regular insulin may be temporarily discontinued or delayed with such decisions made after specific consultation with a member of the diabetes health care team. Mini-epidemics of certain viruses do seem to occur once every year or so and cause hypo- rather than hyperglycemic problems; once this pattern is recognized by the health care team, appropriate adjustment of insulin doses can be advised in other patients with the constant reminder to patients and family members that this dose decrease will be a transient one lasting only for a day or so when the illness is at its peak. Intermediate insulin is usually continued unchanged and more fluids with sugar content are prescribed for these few days.

REFERENCES

Alberti, K.G.M. (1977) Low dose insulin in the treatment of diabetic ketoacidosis. *Arch. Int. Med.*, **137**, 1367–70.

Balasse, E.O. (1976) Acid cetosi diabetique. Aspects de physiopathologiques et therapeutiques recents. *Diabete e Metabolisme*, **2**, 87–94.

Baum, J.D. and Kinmonth, A.L. (1985) *Care of the Child with Diabetes*. Churchill Livingstone, Edinburgh.

Bingley, P.J., Bonifacio, E., Shattock, M. *et al.* (1993) Can Islet Cell Antibodies Predict IDDM in the General Population? *Diabetes Care*, **16**, 45–50.

Botazzo, G.F. (June 1992) Speech to the American Diabetes Association, San Antonio, Texas.

Brink, S.J. (1987) *Pediatric and Adolescent Diabetes Mellitus*. Year Book Medical Publishers, Chicago.

Brink, S.J. (1992) 'Pediatric and Adolescent IDDM Meal Planning 1992: Our Best Advice to Prevent,

Postpone and/or Minimize Angiopathy', in B. Webers, W. Burger, and T. Danne, (eds). *Structural and Functional Abnormalities in Subclinical Diabetic Angiopathy. Pediatric and Adolescent Endocrinology, Vol. 22*, pp. 156–69. Karger, Basel.

Brink, S.J., Fleischnick, E., Srikanta, S. *et al.* (1986) 'Pre-Type I Diabetes Mellitus Detected in a Screening Program', in Z. Laron (ed.). *Pediatric and Adolescent Endocrinology, Vol. 15*, pp. 54–60. Karger, Basel.

Brink, S.J. and Stewart, C. (1986) Insulin Pump Treatment in Insulin Dependent Diabetes Mellitus. Children, Adolescents and Young Adults. *J. Am. Med. Assoc.*, **255**, 617–21.

Brink, S.J. and Wilson, D.P. (eds). (1990) Resource List, in *Day Camps for children with Diabetes, A Planning Guide*. American Diabetes Association, Alexandria, Virginia, USA. Appendix B.

Citrin, W., Tapp, J.T. and Wine, H.E. (1987) 'Diabetes Counseling Issue: The Patient and The Family', in S.J. Brink (ed.). *Pediatric and Adolescent Diabetes Mellitus*, pp. 369–90. Year Book Medical Publishers, Chicago.

The DCCT Research Group. (1993) The effects of intensive treatment of diabetes in the development and progression of long-term complications in insulin-dependent diabetes mellitus. *N. Eng. J. Med.*, **329**, 977–86.

De Beaufort, C. (1986) *Continuous Subcutaneous Insulin Infusion in Newly Diagnosed Diabetic Children*. Doctoral Thesis, Erasmus University, Rotterdam.

Drash, A.L. (1987) *Diabetes Mellitus In the Child and Adolescent*. Year Book Medical Publishers, Chicago.

Fisher, J.N., Shahshahani, M.N. and Kitabchi, A.E. (1977) Diabetic ketoacidosis treated by low dose insulin therapy by various routes. *N. Engl. J. Med.*, **297**, 238–41.

Foster, D.W. and McGarry, J.D. (1983) The metabolic derangements and treatment of diabetic ketoacidosis. *N. Engl. J. Med.*, **309**, 159–69.

Golden, M.P., Herrold, A.J. and Orr, D.P. (1985) An approach to prevention of recurrent diabetic ketoacidosis in the pediatric population. *J. Pediatr.*, **107**, 195–200.

Harris, G.D., Fiordalisi, I., Harris, W.L. *et al.* (1992) Minimizing Symptomatic Brain Swelling by Preventing Low Effective Osmolality During Repair of Diabetic Ketoacidemia. *Pediatr. Res.*, **31**, 185A.

Jackson, R.I. and Guthrie, R.A. (1986) *The Physiological Management of Diabetes in Children*. Elsevier Science Publishing Company, New York.

Katsch, G. (1946) Insulinbehand lung des Diabetischen Komas. *Deutsch Gesundheits*, **1**, 651.

Ludvigsson, J., Hermansson , G., Hager, A. *et al.* (1989) Adequate Substitution of Insulin is Fundamental in the Treatment of Diabetes in Childhood. *Diabetes in the Young*, **21**, 8–12.

Martin, A.M. (1986) *The Truth about Stacey*. Scholastic Inc., New York.

Page, M.McB. (1974) Treatment of diabetic coma with continuous low dose infusion of insulin. *Br. Med. J.*, **1**, 9–16.

Rosenbloom, A.L. (1990) Intracerebral Crises during Treatment of Diabetic Ketoacidosis. *Diabetes Care*, **13**, 22–33.

Sonksen, P.H., Srivastava, M.C., Tomkins, C.V. *et al.* (1972) Growth hormone and cortisol responses to insulin infusion in patients with diabetes mellitus. *Lancet*, **2**, 155–57.

Travis, L.B., Brouhard, B.H. and Schreiner, B.J. (1987) *Diabetes Mellitus in Children and Adolescents*. W.B. Saunders, Philadelphia.

Vardi, P., Crisa, L., Jackson, R.A. *et al.* (1991) Predictive value of intravenous glucose tolerance test insulin secretion less than or greater than the first percentile in islet cell antibody positive relatives of Type 1 insulin dependent diabetic patients. *Diabetologia*, **34**, 93–102.

Vignati, L., Asmal, A.C., Black, W.L. *et al.* (1985) 'Coma in Diabetes', in A. Marble, L.P. Krall, R.F. Bradley, *et al.* (eds). *Joslin's Diabetes Mellitus, Twelfth Edition*, pp. 526–52. Lea and Febiger, Philadelphia.

Volmm, K.R. (1960) On the preservation of insulin in a physiological sodium carbonate solution: on the problem of therapy of the diabetic comas with a continuous intravenous drip infusion of insulin. *Schweiz. Med. Wochenscr.*, **90**, 1080–83.

16

Long-term management: scope and aims

J.P.H. SHIELD and J.D. BAUM

16.1 INTRODUCTION

The incidence of insulin-dependent diabetes in children aged under 15 years in the United Kingdom has been estimated at 13.5/100 000/year (Metcalfe & Baum, 1991). Numerous studies have suggested an increasing incidence in northern Europe (Bingley & Gale, 1989; Burden *et al.*, 1989; Joner & Sovik, 1991; Tuomilehto *et al.*, 1991; Green *et al.*, 1992; Drykoningen *et al.*, 1992) (see also Chapter 10). Whether the increase is in total numbers of cases or due to an earlier age of presentation (Kurtz *et al.*, 1988) the fact remains that diabetes is likely to become more prevalent in childhood.

The introduction of insulin therapy in 1922 provided the treatment for an otherwise rapidly fatal wasting disease. However it gave rise to a new condition of insulin-dependent diabetes with its long-term burden of variable systemic and life-limiting complications. For those with insulin-dependent diabetes, prevention of microvascular disease, especially nephropathy, has become the most important long-term challenge of their health management. Type 1 diabetes seems to contain two populations, those with a poor prognosis who will die by the age of 45 and those whose disease, though disabling, has a much better prognosis (Deckert *et al.*, 1991). Nephropathy is responsible for a considerable proportion of the early deaths, in one study accounting for 54% of deaths within 35 years of diagnosis (Borch-Johnsen *et al.*, 1987).

Between 35 and 45% of patients with diabetes develop overt nephropathy; and diabetes is now the commonest cause of end stage renal failure in the US (Deckert & Poulsen, 1981; Andersen *et al.*, 1983; Viberti *et al.*, 1992). Nephropathy in itself accounts to a large degree for excess mortality in Type 1 diabetes; it also serves as a predictor of mortality from cardiovascular disease, with a relative mortality compared to nondiabetics of 37 times, non-nephropathic diabetics having only four times the risk (Borch-Johnsen & Kreiner, 1987). Nephropathy has also been shown to be predictive of neuropathy and retinopathy (Bell *et al.*, 1992; Barnett *et al.*, 1985). This has led the Steno Group to put forward the view that even microalbuminuria reflects widespread vascular damage in patients with Type 1 diabetes (Deckert *et al.*, 1989).

If we are to see significant improvements in the survival rates in diabetes it is to patients

Childhood and Adolescent Diabetes
Published in 1994 by Chapman & Hall, London
ISBN 0 412 48610 5

with evidence of renal involvement, that we must address renewed clinical efforts. This is not to say that the remaining 65% should be ignored but in general their life expectancy approaches normal with a lesser burden of morbidity.

16.2 FACTORS OF MICROVASCULAR DISEASE

Microvascular disease, the basis of diabetic glomerulopathy, is likely to be due to a combination of genetic, metabolic and hemodynamic factors. Before discussing how to arrest, reverse or prevent complications we must first assess the relative contributions made by each of the above and our ability to intervene.

16.2.1 GENETIC FACTORS

Strong positive associations between HLA antigens DR3 and DR4 and diabetes have been reported in numerous studies (see also Chapters 10, 11 and 13) and further work has found different frequencies in association with nephropathy, DR4 being significantly less common than DR3 and long-term survival being more common (Svejgaard *et al.*, 1986). Other evidence for genetic predisposition to microvascular disease has been gained from family studies in Denmark and the US showing familial clustering of diabetic nephropathy suggesting some hereditary influences (Borch-Johnsen *et al.*, 1992; Seaquist *et al.*, 1989).

16.2.2 METABOLIC FACTORS

Metabolic studies relating to nephropathy have mainly centered on basement membrane and mesangial composition and size. It has been shown that the content of heparin sulphate proteoglycan, which is felt to be a major determinant of glomerular permeability in the basement membrane by a charge selectivity effect (Groggel *et al.*, 1988), is decreased in both animal models and human diabetics (Rohrbach *et al.*, 1983; Parthasarathy & Spiro, 1982). Furthermore, the production of this proteoglycan appears to be inversely related to blood glucose levels (Rohrbach *et al.*, 1983). Another theory relates to laminin, a glycoprotein in the basement membrane that binds the other constituents together. Non-enzymatic glycosylation which is increased in diabetes reduces the affinity for binding between laminin and heparin sulphate leading to a reduction in heparin sulphate incorporation into the basement membrane (Tarsio *et al.*, 1988). Heparin sulphate has also been suggested to have various other roles in normal capillary function such as exerting an antithrombotic action (Marcum *et al.*, 1986) and influencing mesangial cell proliferation (Castellot *et al.*, 1985). In addition to the loss of the proteoglycan, compensatory increases in Collagen IV lead to the increase in width of the basement membrane seen in diabetes (Rohrbach *et al.*, 1983). Mesangial expansion, the other classic finding in nephropathy (Chavers *et al.*, 1989), may be due to the increased flux of macromolecules through the mesangium (Remuzzi & Bertani, 1990). It seems likely that mesangial expansion is one of the antecedents of glomerulosclerosis (Klahr *et al.*, 1988) and by reducing the glomerular filtration surface eventually reduces glomerular filtration rate (Steffes *et al.*, 1989).

Hyperglycemia also exerts an effect on sorbitol-inositol pathways. High blood glucose levels increase glucose conversion to sorbitol and also in some as yet undefined way decrease myo-inositol levels. Myo-inositol modulates sodium-potassium-ATPase activity in nerves and its depletion leads to impaired nerve conduction (Greene *et al.*, 1987). In 1976, Winegrad & Greene showed that achieving normoglycemia restored myo-inositol levels and nerve conduction velocities in diabetic rats (Winegrad & Greene, 1976).

16.2.3 HEMODYNAMIC FACTORS

In type 1 diabetes it is notable that glomerular filtration rate (GFR) is raised early in the disease (Morgensen & Andersen, 1973; Sandahl Christiansen *et al.*, 1981). This feature has been found in some studies to be predictive of later nephropathy (Rudberg *et al.*, 1992; Morgensen & Christensen, 1984), although other studies have challenged this link (Jones *et al.*, 1991; Lervang *et al.*, 1988). GFR is dependent on four factors: glomerular plasma flow, systemic oncotic pressure, glomerular transcapillary hydraulic pressure and finally, glomerular capillary ultrafiltration coefficient, the latter being a product of glomerular capillary hydraulic pressure and total surface area available for filtration (Hostetter, 1992). Part of the rise in the early stages of diabetes can be explained by the increase in observed kidney size leading to an increase in the glomerular capillary coefficient (Morgensen & Andersen, 1973; Sandahl Christiansen *et al.*, 1981). Hostetter *et al.* also demonstrated in streptozotocin-induced diabetic rats that increments in GFR were caused by two other changes, namely: an increase in single nephron plasma flow due to reductions in afferent and efferent arterial resistances and a rise in glomerular transcapillary hydraulic pressure difference. In these studies, no change was found in the glomerular ultrafiltration coefficient (Hostetter *et al.*, 1982; Hostetter *et al.*, 1981). The only factor not implicated therefore is the systemic oncotic pressure which has been found to be normal in diabetes (Mogensen, 1971). The state of hyperfiltration does not continue indefinitely but, in the Brenner hypothesis, leads to structural damage to the glomeruli and eventual sclerosis and loss of function: the greater the reduction of glomeruli the greater the hyperfiltration of those remaining (Brenner *et al.*, 1982).

16.2.4 HYPERTENSION

It is now almost certain that hypertension is not the initiating factor leading to microvascular disease but that it follows the onset of microalbuminuria (Mathiesen *et al.*, 1990; Norgaard *et al.*, 1990). It seems that only in the presence of albuminuria does elevated blood pressure increase the risk of organ damage significantly (Mogensen *et al.*, 1992).

At variance with this conclusion, other studies have shown that diabetic siblings with hypertensive parents have an increased incidence of nephropathy, linking these two factors together genetically (Viberti *et al.*, 1987; Krolewski *et al.*, 1988). However, Norgaard found the incidence of essential hypertension in a diabetic population to be the same as in the nondiabetic population, supporting the view that inherited hypertension was not the cause of diabetic nephropathy (Norgaard *et al.*, 1990).

16.3 AREAS FOR IMPROVEMENT

Having delineated the main group at risk as those with evidence of renal microvascular disease what treatment options are available?

16.3.1 GLYCEMIC CONTROL

The benefit of achieving tighter glycemic control has long been argued. Initial studies, mainly in adults, using various mechanisms to improve blood glucose control had mixed results: less deterioration in renal function and neuropathy but little effect on retinopathy (Reichard *et al.*, 1990; Feldt-Rasmussen *et al.*, 1986; Kroc Collaborative Study Group, 1984; Lauritzen *et al.*, 1985).

However, as the same studies have continued, it has now become apparent that good glycemia control has positive benefits on all the above complications, with retinopathy deteriorating less in strictly controlled groups when compared to normal clinic groups over a prolonged period of time (Reichard *et al.*,

1991; Feldt-Rasmussen *et al.*, 1991; Hanssen *et al.*, 1992; Dahl-Jorgensen, *et al.*, 1992). In animal experiments, in order for the control to be of most benefit, it should be near to normoglycemia and sustained from as early as possible following diagnosis, since strict control does not reverse established lesions (Kern & Engermann, 1990; Engermann & Kern, 1987). This has been confirmed in humans by Viberti *et al.* (1983) who showed that overt nephropathy was irreversible by strict control. In fact there is now evidence to show that microalbuminuria is an index of early established glomerulopathy which may not be reversible by tighter control (Walker *et al.*, 1992).

There are reasons to believe, however, that improved control is not the simple or practical solution to the problem of preventing diabetic microvascular disease in childhood onset diabetes. Tighter control leads to an increased incidence of hypoglycemia and ketoacidosis; it is moreover only an option for well-motivated children in stable supportive families (Strowig & Raskin, 1992; Jennings & Barnett, 1987; Baum, 1990). In addition, studies on the renal structure of kidneys transplanted into 'at risk' diabetes patients have shown differential progression of lesions suggesting intrinsic renal factors, in part at least, to be responsible for protection from microangiopathy (Mauer *et al.*, 1989).

16.3.2 ANTI-HYPERTENSIVE AGENTS

The treatment of hypertension in established diabetic nephropathy has been shown to arrest the decline into renal failure (Parving *et al.*, 1987; Mathiesen *et al.*, 1989). However, microvascular disease is well-established by the time nephropathy becomes overt and therefore recent trials have used anti-hypertensive agents at the microalbuminuric phase; specifically angiotensin converting enzyme (ACE) inhibitors have been used with some success to slow down the progression of renal disease. An animal study by Zatz *et al.* (1986) showed that Enalapril [an ACE inhibitor] reduced intraglomerular capillary pressure and consequently protected against the development of microalbuminuria regardless of poor glycemia control.

Human studies have all been conducted after microalbuminuria has developed but have consistently shown reduction in protein loss in normotensive patients (Mathiesen *et al.*, 1991; Cook *et al.*, 1990; Marre *et al.*, 1987; Wiegmann *et al.*, 1992). The suggestion is that these agents reduce intraglomerular pressure which is present even when systemic blood pressure is normal (Marre *et al.*, 1987; Wiegmann *et al.*, 1992). A further trial has suggested that Enalapril retards glomerular basement membrane thickening independent of its hemodynamic properties (Cooper *et al.*, 1989). An additional trial using Enalapril suggested that the drug diminished glomerular permeability by enhancing barrier size selectivity (Morelli *et al.*, 1990). This group of drugs seems therefore to modulate hemodynamic and structural abnormalities in patients with diabetes and offers the feasibility of arresting the otherwise inexorable progression towards frank nephropathy and renal failure.

16.3.3 SMOKING

Smoking is an independent risk factor for nephropathy (Telmar *et al.*, 1984), neuropathy (Cruickshanks *et al.*, 1989), retinopathy (Mulhauser *et al.*, 1986) and cardiovascular disease (Suarez & Barrett-Connor, 1984). Unfortunately, a recent study of young people with diabetes in Liverpool between 15 and 30 years of age found that 48% were smoking (Masson *et al.*, 1992). One long-term aim must be the elimination of cigarettes from all the diabetic community regardless of the need for society in general to recognize the serious nature of the health problem.

16.3.4 DIET

A study, including children, by Kupin *et al.* (1987) found that a reduced although nutritionally satisfactory protein intake in diabetic patients without nephropathy had a significant effect on reducing high glomerular filtration rates and renal plasma flow. Further studies have shown that dietary protein restriction has a beneficial role in treating patients with overt nephropathy by reducing the rate of GFR decline (Evanoff *et al.*, 1987). These findings were independent of blood glucose control or systemic blood pressure (Bending *et al.*, 1988). Apparently simple changes in lifestyle thus have the potential for retarding the progression of microvascular problems; but as with smoking habits, success with long-term changes in eating habits have been largely unsuccessful.

16.3.5 ANTI-THROMBOTIC AGENTS

Endothelial cell damage in diabetic patients results in the release of numerous factors including Von Willebrand's Factor and angiotensin converting enzyme (Jensen, 1989; Toop *et al.*, 1986). Von Willebrand's Factor is associated positively with platelet adhesion and this in conjunction with the finding that platelet aggregation is increased in diabetics, especially those with microangiopathy (Dallinger *et al.*, 1987), suggests that antithrombotic agents may have a future role in those patients exhibiting evidence of worsening microvascular disease.

16.4 DISEASE MARKERS

Accepting that various therapeutic measures may alter the natural history of complications, it is for the clinician to decide on the best treatment options for the individual child.

The onset of microalbuminuria was originally felt to be predictive of later overt nephropathy (Viberti *et al.*, 1982). However it seems likely now that, as well as being predictive, microalbuminuria equates with established glomerulopathy and with abnormalities of basement membrane thickness and mesangial matrix volume fraction compared with non-albuminuric patients (Walker *et al.*, 1992). As such, diabetic lesions are probably irreversible. It follows that potentially the most influential time for therapeutic intervention is prior to any clinical markers being positive. However, since 25% of diabetic subjects never develop significant complications (Borch-Johnsen *et al.*, 1987), it is vital that markers be established to identify those at risk prior to irreversible pathological lesions developing. Sodium/lithium countertransport rate (a genetic marker of essential hypertension [Hilton, 1986]) has been suggested as such a marker for nephropathy, and there is evidence for higher values in albuminuric as opposed to non-albuminuric patients with diabetes (Mangili *et al.*, 1988; Krolewski *et al.*, 1988). It has also been proposed that, as with essential hypertension, this could provide a genetic marker for nephropathy. A recent study, however, showed no increase in sodium/lithium countertransport in parents of nephropathic children thereby ruling this out as a genetic marker of the at-risk group (Jensen *et al.*, 1990).

16.5 CLINICAL PRACTICE

With no reliable markers available before the onset of clinical abnormalities, potential interventions can only be justified at the stage of incipient nephropathy (microalbuminuria). It seems sensible, though, to try and achieve as strict glycemic control as clinically possible for all patients, since improving glycemic control may offer some protection for adults with the potential for severe complications. Improved glycemic control has been reported with continuous subcutaneous insulin therapy and intensive conventional therapy with multiple insulin injection regimes (Pickup *et al.*, 1979; McCaughey *et al.*, 1986; Saurbrey *et al.*, 1988). But in children and adolescents, the demands of tighter control are very dependent on compliance and understanding: many efforts have resulted in a worsening of control in children and young adult patients in both conventional and pump insulin administration (Brink & Stewart, 1986; Hardy *et al.*, 1991; MacRury *et al.*, 1988). It has been suggested that in order to be successful both clinics and patients need to be well-organized, home glucose monitoring must be comprehensive, education full and 24-hour advice on clinical care available (De Beaufort & Bruining, 1986). There is no universally applicable and effective approach to glycemic control in children: better education and compliance may achieve improved control, but in themselves carry risks of long-term disordered psychological development (Pless *et al.*, 1988). Indeed in very young patients it has been suggested that looser control is justified in order to prevent intellectual defects associated with recurrent hypoglycemia (Rovet *et al.*, 1987).

Smoking appears to be an independent risk factor in the development of albuminuria and diabetic glomerulopathy, with a prevelance of increased albumin excretion 2.8 times higher in smokers than nonsmokers (Chase *et al.*, 1991). Interestingly, in a study from North America, only 58% of male and 38% of female diabetic smokers had ever been told to give up (Anda *et al.*, 1987). Although efforts to encourage giving up smoking have not been successful in adults (Fowler *et al.*, 1989), it seems possible that proper education of children prior to their experimentation with cigarettes may have more success.

16.5.1 ACE AND ALDOSE REDUCTASE INHIBITORS

At present the most effective therapeutic candidates for retarding the development of early microvascular disease (microalbuminuria) in children and young adults appear to be the ACE inhibitors: these agents are reported to have consistently protected against worsening proteinuria, at least in adults with Type 1 diabetes. Since patients with microalbuminuria but no hypertension have evidence of structural changes in the kidney it would seem logical to start treatment with such drugs as soon as microalbuminuria is detected. A review of the benefits of ACE inhibitors by Mogensen (1992) points out the problems that may be associated with treatment. There is a tendency for serum potassium levels to increase and these should be monitored and the addition of a potassium-losing diuretic considered. Small doses are advisable initally to prevent precipitous falls in blood pressure; larger doses may be needed subsequently to affect incipient nephropathy.

A reduction in dietary protein could also be attempted with careful assessment of a child's specific needs for growth and development. This implies the availability of good dietetic advice (Jones, 1986) (see Chapter 18), but begs the question of ascertaining and validating long-term dietary compliance.

Aldose Reductase inhibitors have yet to prove themselves in the prevention of diabetic complications. Numerous animal studies have shown protective effects against diabetic neuropathy associated with elevation of myo-inositol and reduction of sorbitol levels (Mayer & Tomlinson, 1983; Cameron *et al.*, 1986); however studies in humans have shown limited benefits or none at all (Judzewitsch *et al.*, 1983; Boulton *et al.*, 1990; Lewin *et al.*, 1984). Furthermore, recent animal studies have shown no effect at therapeutic doses, i.e., those that reduce sorbitol levels to normal, in preventing glomerular hyperfiltration or albuminuria (Daniels Hostetter, 1989; Korner *et al.*, 1992). At present there would seem to be only a case for using Aldose Reductase inhibitors in patients with chronic neuropathy.

The use of anti-thrombotic agents holds some potential for future studies. However a recent study has shown that aspirin does not have as good an anti-platelet function in diabetes as it does in controls (Mori *et al.*, 1992).

16.6 THE CHILD WITH DIABETES AS AN INDIVIDUAL

The aims of diabetes care in children should be to prevent acute biochemical and chronic microvascular complications without causing major psychological, intellectual or physical problems. The young child who develops recurrent hypoglycemic episodes, while under strict metabolic control, and later shows signs of cognitive dysfunction is not a therapeutic success story even if microvascular disease is prevented in later life. In children with diabetes, there is evidence that pre-pubertal disease duration is relatively unimportant to later onset microvascular complications (Kostraba *et al.*, 1989; Burger *et al.*, 1986). Because of this and the worries regarding hypoglycemia and neuropsychological dysfunction (Ryan *et al.*, 1985), it seems sensible to advocate less rigid glycemic control before puberty, concentrating more on diabetes education and self-awareness. A child with excellent diabetes control may find the struggle to maintain near-normoglycemia very wearing. One disturbing report indicates that in children between 9 and 18 years, those most likely to feel depressed, are those with better than average control (Close *et al.*, 1986).

Eating disorders, especially in girls, are more common in a diabetic population (Nielsen *et al.*, 1987) (see Chapter 27) as are feelings of social isolation and unhappiness (Gafvels *et al.*, 1991). It is too easy to forget the psychological burden of diabetes in childhood. It is not enough to set standard treatment guidelines for all children regardless of their individuality. Children must have their diabetes therapy molded for individual needs, considering domestic and psychological as well as physiologic health parameters.

16.7 CONCLUSION

A case can be made for routinely screening for microalbuminuria in diabetic clinics. Timed specimens are best and 24-hourly urine collections are the gold standard. This may not be practical, however, with children and therefore a spot early morning urine for albumin/creatinine ratio could be used as a primary screen with less than 3.5 mg/mmol being taken as normal (Marshall, 1991). However, once patients with glomerulopathy have been identified, it remains uncertain which intervention can be justified on current evidence. The hugely expensive DCCT trials in North America have defined the benefits of strict glycemic (DCCT Research Group, 1993; see addendum), but the application of these findings to children in routine clinical practice will be fraught with difficulties. It may well be more fruitful to treat normotensive and hypertensive microalbuminuric children with a single agent such as an ACE inhibitor, which in adults has already proved beneficial. The use of such agents in children will need careful evaluation and is probably only justified as part of a long-term, multicenter, placebo-controlled trial looking at benefits and side-effects. In respect of other therapeutic modalities, such as anti-platelet therapy and Aldose Reductase inhibitors, further fundamental work is needed prior to any recommendations for their use in childhood.

Smoking should be positively and effectively discouraged as it seems likely to be an important factor that could be removed from the pathophysiology of children with diabetes.

In the next few years, undoubtably, therapies will become available to modify or prevent the appalling consequences of long-term diabetes. At present, what is needed is the infrastructure of care and clinical observation in order to utilize new therapeutic modalities within the informative framework of a clinical trials network.

ADDENDUM

The DCCT has now reported its findings in a highly motivated group of volunteers of whom approximately 15% were between the ages of 13 and 18 years. It would appear that improving glycemic control is undoubtedly of benefit, not only for the primary prevention of nephropathy, neuropathy and retinopathy but also in slowing the progression of already manifest microvascular disease. However, the increased frequency of serious hypoglycemic events, weight gain in the intensively treated group and absence of children under 13 years, together with the unusual motivation of those in the DCCT, means that the translation of such care to a general pediatric population may be far more difficult in practice than in theory (DCCT Research Group, 1993).

REFERENCES

Anda, R.F., Remington, P.L., Sienko, D.G. *et al.* (1987) Are physicians advising smokers to quit? The patients' perspective. *J. Am. Med. Assoc.*, **257**, 1916–19.

Anderson, A.R., Sandahl Christiansen, J., Andersen, J.K. *et al.* (1983) Diabetic Nephropathy in Type 1 (Insulin dependent) Diabetes: An Epidemiological Study. *Diabetologia*, **25**, 496–501.

Barnett, A.H., Dallinger, K., Jennings, F. *et al.* (1985) Microalbuminuria and diabetic retinopathy. *Lancet*, **I**, 53–54.

Baum, J.D. (1990) Children with Diabetes. *Brit. Med. J.*, **301**, 502–503.

Bell, D.S., Ketchum, C.H., Robinson, C.A. *et al.* (1992) Microalbuminuria Associated with Diabetic Neuropathy. *Diabetes Care*, **15**:4, 528–31.

Bending, J.J., Dodds, R.A., Keen, H. *et al.* (1988) Renal Response to Restricted Protein in Diabetic Nephropathy. *Diabetes*, **37**, 1641–46.

Bingley, P.J. and Gale, E.A. (1989) Rising incidence of IDDM in Europe. *Diabetes Care*, **12**:4, 289–95.

Borch-Johnsen, K., Norgaard, K., Hommel, E., *et al.* (1992) Is diabetic nephropathy an inherited complication? *Kidney Internat.*, **41**, 719–22.

Borch-Johnsen, K. and Kriener, S. (1987) Proteinuria; value as a predictor of cardiovascular mortality in insulin dependent diabetes mellitus. *Brit. Med. J.*, **294**, 1651–54.

Borch-Johnsen, K., Nissen, H., Henricksen, E. *et al.* (1987) The natural history of insulin-dependent diabetes mellitus in Denmark: 1. Long-term survival with and without late diabetic complications. *Diabetic Med.*, **4**, 201–210.

Boulton, A.J.M., Levin, S. and Comstock, J. (1990) A multi-centre trial of the aldose-reductase inhibitor, tolrestat, in patients with symptomatic diabetic neuropathy. *Diabetologia*, **33**, 431–37.

Brenner, B.M., Meyer, T.W. and Hostetter, T.H. (1982) Dietary protein intake and the progressive nature of kidney disease: The role of hemodynamically mediated glomerular injury in the pathogenesis of progressive glomerular sclerosis in aging, renal ablation and intrinsic renal disease. *N. Eng. J. Med.*, **307**:11, 652–59.

Brink, S.J. and Stewart, C. (1986) Insulin Pump treatment in insulin-derendent diabetes mellitus. *J. Am. Med. Assoc.*, **255**:5, 617–21.

Burden, A.C., Hearnshaw, J.R. and Swift, P.G. (1989) Childhood diabetes mellitus: an increasing incidence. *Diabetic Med.*, **6**, 334–36.

Burger, W., Hovener, G., Dusterhus, R. *et al.* (1986) Prevalence and development of retinopathy in children and adolescents with Type 1 (insulin-dependent) diabetes mellitus. A longitudinal study. *Diabetologia*, **29**, 17–22.

Cameron, N.E., Leonard, M.B., Ross, I.S. *et al.* (1986) The effects of Sorbinol on peripheral nerve conduction velocity, polyol concentrations and morphology in the Streptozotocin-diabetic rat. *Diabetologia*, **29**, 168-74.

Castellot, J.J., Hoover, R.L., Harper, P.A. *et al.* (1985). Heparin and glomerular epithelial cell-secreted heparin species inhibit mesangial-cell proliferation. *Am. J. Pathol.*, **120**, 427–35.

Chase, H.P., Garg, S.K., Marshall, G. *et al.* (1991) Cigarette smoking increases the risk of albuminuria among subjects with Type 1 diabetes. *J. Am. Med. Assoc.*, **265**:5, 614–17.

Chavers, B.M., Bilous, R.W., Ellis, E.N. *et al.* (1989) Glomerular lesions and urinary excretion in Type 1 diabetes without overt proteinuria. *N. Eng. J. Med.*, **320**:15, 966–70.

Close, H., Davies, A.G., Price, D.A. *et al.* (1986) Emotional difficulties in diabetes mellitus. *Arch. Dis. Child.*, **61**, 337–40.

Cook, J., Daneman, D., Spino, M. *et al.* (1990) Angiotensin converting enzyme inhibitor therapy to decrease microalbuminuria in normotensive children with insulin-dependent diabetes mellitus. *J. Pediatr.*, **117**:1, 39–44.

Cooper, M.E., Allen, T.J., MacMillan, P.A. *et al.*

(1989) Enalapril retards glomerular basement membrane thickening and albuminuria in the diabetic rat. *Diabetologia*, **32**, 326–28.

Cruickshanks, K.J., Gay, E. and Hamman, R.F. (1989) Smoking is related to symptoms of neuropathy in a cohort of young subjects with insulin-dependent diabetes mellitus. *Diabetes*, **39**, 35A.

Dahl-Jorgensen, K., Bjoro, T., Kierulf, P. *et al.* (1992) Long-term glycaemic control and kidney function in insulin-dependent diabetes mellitus. *Kidney Internat.*, **41**, 920–23.

Dallinger, K.J.C., Jennings, P.E., Toop, M.J. *et al.* (1987) Platelet aggregation and coagulation factors in insulin dependent diabetics with or without microangiopathy. *Diabetic Med.*, **4**, 44–48.

Daniels, B.S. and Hostetter, T.H. (1989) Aldose reductase inhibition and glomerular abnormalities in diabetic rats. *Diabetes*, **38**, 981–86.

De Beaufort, C.E. and Bruining, G.J. (1987) Continuous subcutaneous insulin infusion in children. *Diabetic Med.*, **4**, 103–108.

DCCT Research Group (1993) The effects of intensive treatment of diabetes in the development and progression of long-term complications in insulin-dependent diabetes mellitus. *N. Eng. J. Med.*, **329**, 977–86.

Deckert, T. and Poulsen, J.E. (1981) Diabetic Nephropathy: Fault or destiny? *Diabetologia*, **21**, 178–83.

Deckert, T., Feldt-Rasmussen, B., Borch-Johnsen, K. *et al.* (1991) Natural history of diabetic complications: early detection and progression. *Diabetic Med.*, **8** (symposium), S33–S37.

Deckert, T., Feldt-Rasmussen, B., Borch-Johnsen, K. *et al.* (1989) Albuminuria reflects widespread vascular damage. The Steno Hypothesis. *Diabetologia*, **32**, 219–26.

Drykoningen, C.E.M., Mulder, A.L.M., Vaandrager, G.J. *et al.* (1992) The incidence of male childhood Type 1 (insulin-dependent) diabetes mellitus is rising rapidly in The Netherlands. *Diabetologia*, **35**, 139–42.

Engermann, R.L. and Kern, T.S. (1987) Progression of incipient diabetic retinopathy during good glycemic control. *Diabetes*, **36**, 808–812.

Evanoff, G.V., Thompson, C.S., Brown, J. *et al.* (1987) The effect of dietary protein restriction on the progression of diabetic nephropathy. *Arch. Intern. Med.*, **147**, 492–95.

Feldt-Rasmussen, B., Mathiesen, E.R. and Deckert, T. (1986) Effect of two years strict metabolic control on progression of incipient nephropathy in insulin-dependent diabetes. *Lancet*, **II**, 1300–1304.

Feldt-Rasmussen, B., Mathiesen, E.R., Jensen, T. *et al.* (1991). The effect of improved metabolic control on loss of kidney function in type 1 (insulin-dependent) diabetic patients; an update of the Steno studies. *Diabetologia*, **43**, 164–70.

Feldt-Rasmussen, B., Mathiesen, E.R., Hegedus, L. *et al.* (1986) Kidney function during 12 months of strict metabolic control in insulin-dependent diabetic patients with incipient nephropathy. *N. Eng. J. Med.*, **314**:11, 666–70.

Fowler, P.M., Hoskins, P.L., McGill, M. *et al.* (1989) Anti-smoking programme for diabetic patients; The agony and the ecstasy. *Diabetic Med.*, **6**, 698–702.

Gafvels, C., Borjesson, B. and Lithner, F. (1991). The social consequences of insulin treated diabetes mellitus in patients 20–50 years of age. An epidemiological case-control study. *Scand. J. Soc. Med.*, **19**, 86–93.

Green, A., Andersen, P.K., Svendsen, A.J. *et al.* (1992) Increasing incidence of early onset Type 1 (Insulin-dependent) diabetes mellitus: a study of Danish male birth cohorts. *Diabetologia*, **35**, 178–82.

Greene, D.A., Lattimer, S.A. and Sima, A.F. (1987) Sorbitol, Phosphoinositides, and Sodium-Potassium-ATPase in the pathogenesis of diabetic complications. *N. Eng. J. Med.*, **316**:10, 599–606.

Groggel, G.C., Stevensen, J., Hovingh, P. *et al.* (1988) Changes in heparan sulfate correlate with increased glomerular permeability. *Kidney Internat.*, **33**, 517–523.

Hanssen, K.F., Bangstad, H-J., Brinchmann-Hansen, O. *et al.* (1992) Blood glucose control and diabetic microvascular complications: long-term effects of near-normoglycaemia. *Diabetic Med.*, **9**, 697–705.

Hardy, K.J., Jones, K.E. and Gill, G.V. (1991) Deterioration in blood glucose control in females with diabetes changed to a basal-bolus regimen using a pen-injector. *Diabetic Med.*, **8**, 69–71.

Hilton, P.J. (1986). Cellular sodium transport in essential hypertension. *N. Eng. J. Med.*, **314**:4, 222–29.

Hostetter, T.H. (1992) Diabetic Nephropathy. Metabolic versus hemodynamic considerations.

Diabetes Care, **15**:9, 1205–1215.

Hostetter, T.H., Rennke, H.G. and Brenner, B.M. (1982) The case for intrarenal hypertension in the initiation and progression of diabetic and other glomerulopathies. *Am. J. Med.*, **72**:3, 375–79.

Hostetter, T.H., Troy, J.L. and Brenner, B.M. (1981) Glomerular hemodynamics in experimental diabetes mellitus. *Kidney Internat.*, **19**, 410–15.

Jennings, P.E. and Barnett, A.H. (1987) New approaches to the pathogenesis and treatment of diabetic microangiopathy. *Diabetic Med.*, **5**, 111–17.

Jensen, T. (1989) Increased plasma concentration of Von Willebrand factor in insulin dependent diabetics with incipient nephropathy. *Brit. Med. J.*, **298**, 27–28.

Jensen, J.S., Mathiesen, E.R., Norgaard, K. *et al.* (1990) Increased blood pressure and erythrocyte Sodium\Lithium countertransport activity are not inherited in diabetic nephropathy. *Diabetologia*, **33**, 619–24.

Joner, G. and Sovik, O. (1991) The incidence of Type 1 (insulin-dependent) diabetes mellitus 15–29 years in Norway 1987–1982. *Diabetologia*, **34**, 271.

Jones, A.M. (1986) Specialist diabetic dieticians – an essential part of the diabetic care team. *Practical Diabetes*, **3**:2, 81–83.

Jones, S.L., Wiseman, M.J. and Viberti, G.C. (1991) Glomerular hyperfiltration as a risk factor for diabetic nephropathy; five year report of a prospective study. *Diabetologia*, **34**, 59–60.

Judzewitsch, R.G., Jaspan, J.B., Polonsky, K.S. *et al.* (1983) Aldose reductase inhibition improves nerve conduction velocity in diabetic patients. *N. Eng. J. Med.*, **308**:3, 119–25.

Kern, T.S. and Engermann, R.L. (1990) Arrest of glomerulopathy in diabetic dogs by improved glycaemic control. *Diabetologia*, **33**, 522–25.

Klahr, S., Schreiner G. and Ichikawa, I. (1988) The progression of renal disease. *N. Eng. J. Med.*, **318**:25, 1657–66.

Korner, A., Celsi, G., Eklof, A.C. *et al.* (1992) Sorbinol does not prevent hyperfiltration, elevated ultrafiltration pressure and albuminuria in Streptozotocin-diabetic rats. *Diabetologia*, **35**, 414–18.

Kostraba, J.N., Dorman, J.S., Orchard, T.J. *et al.* (1989) Contribution of diabetes duration before puberty to the development of microvascular complications in IDDM subjects. *Diabetes Care*, **12**, 686–93.

Kroc Collaborative Study Group. (1984) Blood glucose control and the evolution of diabetic retinopathy and albuminuria. *N. Eng. J. Med.*, **311**:6, 365–71.

Krolewski, A.S., Canessa, M., Warram, J.H. *et al.* (1988) Predisposition to hypertension and susceptibility to renal disease in insulin-dependent diabetes mellitus. *N. Eng. J. Med.*, **318**:3, 140–45.

Kupin, W.L., Cortes, P., Dumler, F. *et al.* (1987) Effect of renal function of change from high to moderate protein intake in Type 1 diabetic patients. *Diabetes*, **36**, 73–79.

Kurtz, Z., Peckham, C.S. and Ades, A.E. (1988) Changing prevelence of juvenile-onset diabetes mellitus. *Lancet*, **II**, 88–90.

Lauritzen, T., Frost-Larsen, K., Larsen, H.-W. *et al.* (1985). Two-year experience with continuous subcutaneous insulin infusion in relation to retinopathy and neuropathy. *Diabetes*, **34**, 74–79.

Lervang, H.H., Jensen, S., Brochner-Mortensen, J. *et al.* (1988) Early glomerular hyperfiltration and the development of late nephropathy in Type 1 (insulin-dependent) diabetes mellitus. *Diabetologia*, **31**, 723–29.

Lewin, I.G., O'Brien, I.A.D., Morgan, M.H. *et al.* (1984) Clinical and neurophysiological studies with the Aldose reductase inhibitor, Sorbinil, in symptomatic diabetic neuropathy. *Diabetologia*, **26**, 445–48.

Mangili, R., Bending, J.J., Scott, G. *et al.* (1988) Increased sodium\lithium countertransport activity in red cells of patients with insulin-dependent diabetes and nephropathy. *N. Eng. J. Med.*, **318**:3, 146–50.

Marcum, J.A., Atha, D.A., Fritze, L.M.S. *et al.* (1986) Cloned bovine aortic endothelial cells synthesize anticoagulantly active Heparan Sulfate Proteoglycan. *J. Biol. Chem.*, **261**:16, 7507–7517.

Marre, M., LeBlanc, H., Suarez, L. *et al.* (1987) Converting enzyme inhibition and kidney function in normotensive diabetic patients with persistent microalbuminuria. *Brit. Med. J.*, **294**, 1448–52.

Marshall, S.M. (1991). Screening for microalbuminuria: Which measurement? *Diabetic*

Med., **8**, 706–711.

Masson, E.A., MacFarlane, I.A., Priestley, C.J. *et al.* (1992) Failure to prevent nicotine addiction in young people with diabetes. *Arch. Dis. Child.*, **67**, 100–102.

Mathiesen, E.R., Ronn, B., Jensen, T. *et al.* (1990) Relationship between blood pressure and urinary excretion in development of microalbuminuria. *Diabetes*, **39**, 245–49.

Mathiesen, E.R., Borch-Johnsen, K., Jensen, D.V. *et al.* (1989) Improved survival in patients with diabetic nephropathy. *Diabetologia*, **32**, 884–86.

Mathiesen, E.R., Hommel, E., Giese, J. *et al.* (1991) Efficacy of Captopril in postponing nephropathy in normotensive insulin dependent diabetic patients with microalbuminuria. *Brit. Med. J.*, **303**, 81–87.

Mauer, M.S., Goetz, F.C., McHugh, L.E. *et al.* (1989) Long-term study of normal kidneys transplanted into patients with type 1 diabetes. *Diabetes*, **38**, 515–23.

Mayer, J.H. and Tomlinson, D.R. (1983) Prevention of defects of axonal transport and nerve conduction velocity by oral administration of myo-inositol or an Aldose reductase inhibitor in streptozotocin-diabetic rats. *Diabetologia*, **25**, 433–38.

McCaughey, E.S., Betts, P.R. and Rowe, D.J. (1986) Improved diabetic control in adolescents using the Penject syringe for multiple insulin injections. *Diabetic Medicine*, **3**, 234–36.

MacRury, S.M., Small, M., Boal, A. *et al.* (1988) Diabetic ketoacidosis during Novopen therapy. *Diabetic Medicine*, **5**, 87–88.

Metcalfe, M.A. and Baum, J.D. (1991) Incidence of insulin dependent diabetes in children under 15 years in the British Isles during 1988. *Brit. Med. J.*, **302**, 443–47.

Mogensen, C.E. (1971) Glomerular filtration rate and renal plasma flow in short-term and long-term juvenile diabetes. *Scand. J. Clin. Lab. Invest.*, **28**, 91–100.

Mogensen, C.E. (1992) Angiotensin converting enzyme inhibitors and diabetic nephropathy. *Brit. Med. J.*, **304**, 327–28.

Mogensen, C.E., Osterby, R., Hansen, K. *et al.* (1992) Blood pressure elevation versus abnormal albuminuria in the genesis and prdiction of renal disease in diabetes. *Diabetes Care*, **15**:9, 1192–1204.

Mogensen, C.E. and Christensen, C.K. (1984) Predicting diabetic nephropathy in insulin-dependent patients. *N. Eng. J. Med.*, **311**:2, 89–93.

Mogensen, C.E. and Andersen, M.J.F. (1973) Increased kidney size and glomerular filtration rate in early juvenile diabetes. *Diabetes*, **22**:9, 706–712.

Morelli, E., Loon, N., Meyer, T. *et al.* (1990) Effects of converting-enzyme inhibition on barrier function in diabetic nephropathy. *Diabetes*, **39**, 76–82.

Mori, T.A., Vandongen, R., Douglas, A.J. *et al.* (1992) Differential effect of aspirin on platelet aggregation in IDDM. *Diabetes*, **41**, 261–66.

Mulhauser, I., Sawicki, P. and Berger, M. (1986) Cigarette-smoking as a risk factor for macroproteinuria and proliferative retinopathy in Type 1 (insulin-dependent) diabetes. *Diabetologia*, **29**, 500–502.

Nielsen, S., Borner, H. and Kabel, M. (1987) Anorexia nervosa/bulimia in diabetes mellitus. *Acta. Psychiatr. Scand.* **75**, 464–73.

Norgaard, K., Feldt-Rasmussen, B., Borch-Johnsen, K. *et al.* (1990) Prevelance of hypertension in Type 1 (insulin-dependent) diabetes mellitus. *Diabetologia*, **33**, 407–410.

Parthasrathy, N. and Spiro, R.G. (1982) Effect of diabetes on the glycosaminoglycan component of the human glomerular basement membrane. *Diabetes*, **31**, 738–41.

Parving, H.-H., Andersen, A.R., Smidt, U.M. *et al.* (1987) Effect of antihypertensive treatment on kidney function in diabetic nephropathy. *Brit. Med. J.*, **294**, 1443–47.

Pickup, J.C., Keen, H., Parsons, J.A. *et al.* (1979) Continuous insulin infusion; improved blood glucose and intermediary-metabolic control in diabetes. *Lancet*, **I**, 1225–57.

Pless, I.B., Heller, A., Belmonte, M. *et al.* (1988) Expected diabetic control in childhood and psychological functioning in early adult life. *Diabetes Care*, **11**, 387–92.

Reichard, P., Carlsson, B., Cars, I. *et al.* (1990) Metabolic control and complications over 3 years in patients with insulin dependent diabetes (IDDM); the Stockholm Diabetes Intervention study (SDIS). *J. Int. Med.*, **228**, 511–17.

Reichard, P., Berglund, B., Cars, I. *et al.* (1991) Intensified conventional insulin therapy retards the microvascular complications of insulin-dependent diabetes mellitus (IDDM): The Stockholm Diabetes Intervention Study (SDIS) after 5 years. *J. Int. Med.*, **230**, 101–108.

Remuzzi, G. and Bertani, T. (1990) Is glomerulosclerosis a consequence of altered glomerular permeability to macromolecules? *Kidney Internat.*, **38**, 384–94.

Rohrbach, D.H, Wagner, C.W., Star, V.L. *et al.* (1983) Reduced synthesis of basement membrane heperan sulfate proteoglycan in streptozotocin-induced diabetic rats. *J. Biol. Chem.* **258**:19, 11672–77.

Rovet, J.F., Ehrlich, R.M. and Hoppe, M. (1987) Intellectual deficits associated with realy onset of insulin-dependent diabetes mellitus in children. *Diabetes Care*, **10**, 510–15.

Rudberg, S., Persson, B. and Dahlquist, G. (1992) Increased glomerular filtration as a predictor of diabetic nephropathy – An 8 year prospective study. *Kidney Internat.*, **41**, 822–28.

Ryan, C., Vega, A. and Drash, A. (1985) Cognitive deficits in adolescents who develop diabetes early in life. *Pediatrics*, **75**, 921–27.

Sandahl Christensen, J., Gammelgaard, J., Frandsen, M. *et al.* (1981) Increased kidney size, glomerular filtration rate and plasma flow in short-term insulin-dependent diabetics. *Diabetologia*, **20**, 451–56.

Saurbrey, N., Arnold-Larsen, S., Moller-Jensen, B. *et al.* (1988) Comparison of continuous subcutaneous insulin infusion with multiple insulin injections using the Novopen. *Diabetic Med.*, **5**, 150–53.

Seaquist, E.R., Goetz, F.D., Rich, S. *et al.* (1989) Familial clustering of diabetic kidney disease. Evidence for genetic susceptibility to diabetic nephropathy. *N. Eng. J. Med.*, **320**:18, 1161–65.

Steffes, M.W., Osterby, R., Chavers, B. *et al.* (1989) Mesangial expansion as a central mechanism for loss of kidney function in diabetic patients. *Diabetes*, **38**, 1077–81.

Strowig, S. and Raskin, P. (1992) Glycaemic control and diabetic complications. *Diabetes Care*, **15**:9, 1126–40.

Suarez, L. and Barrett-Connor, E. (1984) Interaction between cigarette smoking and diabetes mellitus in the prediction of death attributed to cardiovascular disease. *Am. J. Epidem.*, **120**:5, 670–75.

Svejgaard, A., Jakobsen, B.K., Platz, L.P. *et al.* (1986) HLA associations in insulin-dependent diabetes; search for heterogenicity in different groups of patients from a homogenous population. *Tissue Antigens*, **28**, 237–44.

Tarsio, J.F., Reger, L.A. and Furcht, L.T. (1988) Molecular mechanisms in basement membrane complications of diabetes. Alterations in Heparin, Laminin and Type IV Collagen association. *Diabetes*, **37**, 532–39.

Telmar, S., Sandahl Christensen, J., Andersen, A.R. *et al.* (1984) Smoking habits and prevalence of clinical diabetic microangiopathy in insulin-dependent diabetics. *Acta. Med. Scand.*, **215**, 63–68.

Toop, M.J., Dallinger, K.J.C., Jennings, P.E. *et al.* (1986) Angiotensin Converting Enzyme (ACE); Relationship to insulin-dependent diabetes and microangiography. *Diabetic Med.*, **3**, 455–57.

Tuomilehto, J., Rewers, M., Reunanen, A. *et al.* (1991) Increasing trend in Type 1 (insulin-dependent) diabetes mellitus in childhood in Finland. *Diabetologia*, **34**, 282–87.

Viberti, G.C., Yip-Messant, J. and Morocutti, A. (1992) Diabetic Nephropathy. Future Avenues. *Diabetes Care*, **15**:9, 1216–25.

Viberti, G.C., Keen, H. and Wiseman, M.J. (1987) Raised arterial pressure in parents of proteinuric insulin dependent diabetics. *Brit. Med. J.*, **295**, 515–17.

Viberti, G.C., Bilous, R.W., Mackintosh, D. *et al.* (1983) Long term correction of hyperglycaemia and progression of renal failure in insulin dependent diabetes. *Brit. Med. J.*, **286**, 508–602.

Viberti, G.C., Hill, R.D., Jarrett, R.J. *et al.* (1982) Microalbuminuria as a predictor of clinical nephropathy in insulin-dependent diabetes mellitus. *Lancet*, **I**, 1430–32.

Walker, J.D., Close, C.F., Jones, S.L. *et al.* (1992) Glomerular structure in Type 1 (insulin-dependent) diabetic patients with normo- and microalbuminuria. *Kidney Internat.*, **41**, 741–48.

Wiegmann, T.B., Herron, K.G., Chonko, A.M. *et al.* (1992) Effect of Angiotensin-converting enzyme inhibition on renal function and albuminuria in normotensive Type 1 diabetic patients. *Diabetes*, **41**, 62–67.

Winegrad, A.I. and Greene, D.A. (1976) Diabetic polyneuropathy: the importance of insulin deficiency, hyperglycaemia and alterations in myo-inositol metabolism in its pathogenesis. *N. Eng. J. Med.*, **295**, 1416–21.

Zatz, R., Dunn, R., Meyer, T.W. *et al.* (1986) Prevention of diabetic glomerulopathy by pharmacological amelioration of glomerular capillary hypertension. *J. Clin. Invest.*, **77**, 1925–30.

17

Insulin: types and regimens

P.G.F. SWIFT

17.1 INSULIN: MIRACLES AND MIRAGES

Before 1922, childhood diabetes was a lethal disease. Dr Robin Lawrence, who received life-restoring insulin in 1923, wrote in the preface to *The Diabetic Life* (Lawrence, 1925) that only four years previously the book could have been entitled *The Diabetic Death*.

The famous author, H.G. Wells, in a letter to *The Times* (1934) described insulin as 'the very precise and beautiful treatment by which we have been restored to normality' (Lawrence, 1952). We realize now that although insulin rapidly restores health, its precision and ability to achieve normality as a replacement hormone is something of a mirage. Insulin transformed an acute lethal disease into a potentially disabling chronic condition.

A bewildering multiplicity of insulins, injection devices and regimens now exist. However, exogenous insulin still has to be administered into the wrong tissue space, at the wrong times and in the wrong doses. Injections cannot mimic endogenous insulin secretion and thus metabolic control can never be perfect.

17.2 INSULIN TYPES: A HISTORICAL PERSPECTIVE

As insulin became less contaminated, its action was noted to be more rapid and short-lived. The continuing evolution of insulin formulations has been driven by the demand for greater purity, better tolerated neutral (non-acidic) formulations, insulins with prolonged activity and, latterly, species similarity (Poulsen, 1985; Brange, 1987).

Although repeated crystallization increased insulin purity, readily detectable impurities, such as pancreatic polypeptide, glucagon and somatostatin remained (Bloom *et al.*, 1978). Antibodies to contaminants and insulin may have accounted for the common injection site complications, such as immune mediated allergic reactions and lipoatrophy (Reeves *et al.*, 1980). Removal of contaminated peptides has been achieved by processes based on molecular size (gel filtration) or charge (ion-exchange chromatography).

The latter process produced highly purified mono-component (MC) insulins introduced in the 1970s (Schlichtkrull, 1974) allowing children for the first time to receive insulin without provoking major insulin antibody production, and once again purer formulations were found to have a quicker, sharper

Childhood and Adolescent Diabetes
Published in 1994 by Chapman & Hall, London
ISBN 0 412 48610 5

activity with lower doses being required (Asplin *et al.*, 1978).

Human insulins introduced in the 1980s are now manufactured by several different processes and impurities are measured in decimals of parts per million (Owens, 1986). The porcine molecule B-chain alanine at position 30 when cleaved by trypsin and replaced by threonine produces the human insulin molecule. On the insulin bottle this semi-synthetic MC human insulin is designated 'emp' (enzymatically modified porcine). 'Emp' insulin is being replaced by genetically engineered human insulin. This may be synthesized by DNA programming of two *E. coli* lines producing separate A and B insulin chains followed by chemical recombination of the chains ('crb' – chain recombinant bacterial) or by a single *E. coli* line with the insertion of the whole proinsulin gene. Proinsulin is then enzymatically cleaved to human insulin and C-peptide ('prb' – proinsulin recombinant bacterial).

Genetically engineered human insulin is also produced using brewer's yeast, *Saccharomyces cerevisiae*, synthesizing a single chain precursor molecule containing a modified C-peptide region. This is enzymatically modified to the human insulin molecule ('pyr' – precursor yeast recombinant). Biosynthetic human insulins are identical to natural human insulin in physico-chemical structure (Owens, 1986).

Hagedorn *et al.* (1936) described various compounds used in the attempt to prolong the action of insulin. The small basic protein, protamine, derived from rainbow-trout sperm, proved the most successful. When added to insulin at neutral pH an amorphous precipitate formed and after injection was found to have a duration of effect about twice that of soluble insulin. In the same year, Scott and Fisher (1936) found that when excess zinc was added to protamine insulin it produced protamine-zinc-insulin (PZI) a compound with duration of effect up to 24 hours. PZI remained in common usage until the 1970s.

Hagedorn later perfected a chemical procedure which allowed complete binding of protamine to insulin in the presence of a small amount of zinc to form uniform size crystals. The exact chemical ratio of 10% protamine: 90% insulin at pH 7.3 is called the isophane (iso=same, phane=appearance) ratio. One of the first isophane insulins perfected in the US, Neutral Protamine Hagedorn (NPH), remains the most commonly used medium-acting insulin.

In 1951 the 'lente', slow-acting, insulins were produced (Hallas-Moller *et al.*, 1951) by allowing insulin to crystallize in the presence of excess zinc ions (without protamine). At different pH levels either an amorphous precipitate or crystalline particles form. Amorphous particles are smaller and are more quickly absorbed – the 'semi-lente' preparation. The larger crystalline form is the longer-acting 'ultra-lente'. A mixture of semi-lente (porcine) and ultra-lente (bovine) in the ratio 3:7 formed the basis of the popular 'Lente' insulin zinc suspension used for many years as a once-daily injection.

17.3 CURRENT INSULINS AND PHARMACOKINETIC STUDIES

World-wide, there are more than 300 insulin preparations in use, each one presumably having its advocates. Characteristics of commonly used insulins are shown in Table 17.1.

Soluble insulin is clear in solution and has many synonyms, such as 'regular', 'pure', 'crystalline', 'rapid-acting', etc. It may be injected on its own but is most often mixed with a prolonged-activity insulin when knowledge of compatibility is important. For instance, soluble mixed with the old PZI interacted with excess protamine and zinc, reducing its quick-acting efficacy. Insulin with phosphate buffer (e.g., Velosulin) mixed with lente formulation precipitates

Table 17.1 Guide to insulin preparations.

Activity profile	Type	Duration (hours) Onset	Peak	Maximum duration	Source and modern formulation (manufacture)
Short	Soluble regular, clear (Neutral or Acid)	0.25–1	2–4	5–8	H. Actrapid (pyr) H. or P. Velosulin (hp or emp) Humulin S (crb)
Medium	Biphasic (soluble: crystalline mixtures)	0.25–1	2–10	12–24	H. Mixtard (pyr) H. Actraphane (pyr) Humulin M1234 (prb)
	Isophane (Crystalline often NPH suspension)	2–4	6–10	12–24	H./P. Insulatard (emp) H. Protaphane (pyr) Humulin I (prb)
Long	Lente (Crystalline Amorphous Mixtures)	2–4	6–10	12–28	H. Monotard (pyr) P./B. Lentard MC (hp) Humulin Zn (prb)
Very long	Ultralente (Crystalline)	3–4	12–20	24–36	H. Ultratard (pyr)

NB This table only represents a small number of insulin preparations in common use in the UK.
Key to Table:
purity hp = highly purified
source H = human
P = pork
B = beef
mode of biosynthesis emp, crb, pyr, prb } see text

zinc and the retarded action of the suspension is lost. The significance of such incompatibilities have been highlighted by studies of insulin absorption and pharmacokinetics.

In contrast to the theoretically predictable rise and fall of insulin levels following an injection, endogenous insulin levels in non-diabetic persons rise from basal levels to a variable level dependent upon the size, quality and duration of the nutritional stimulus. Following the ingestion of 50 g glucose, plasma insulin increases about 5-fold (e.g., basal <10 mmol/L to peak >30 mmol/L) and returns to basal within 2 hours (Howell, 1991). After a substantial mixed meal, a more prolonged insulin surge is provoked which may not return to basal before the next meal (Figure 17.1). Holman and Turner (1985) point out that 40–50% of 24-hour insulin production is in the basal state which dominates the fasting (night-time) phase.

Theoretically, in C-peptide negative diabetes, provision of a steady basal insulin supply is the first objective in therapy, akin to 'replacement' therapy in other endocrine disorders. Preprandial increments should then be added to provide insulinemia for meals.

Insulin absorption profiles have been described quantitating the absorption of radio-labeled insulin from injection sites

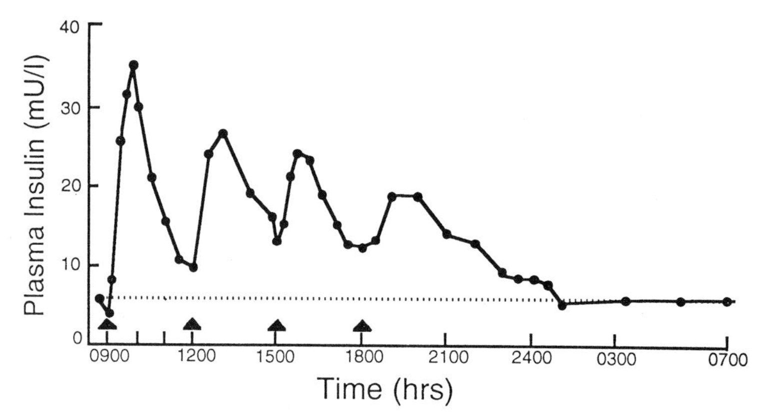

Figure 17.1 Endogenous plasma insulin values in nondiabetic adults after ingestion of four standardized 50 g carbohydrate meals (▲). The average plasma insulin level during the night is shown as a dotted line which encloses 44% of the total insulin area (basal secretion) (after Holman & Turner, 1985).

(Binder, 1969) or measuring plasma insulin levels under varying conditions (Galloway *et al.*, 1981; Berger *et al.*, 1982) or using euglycemic clamp techniques to avoid confounding counter-regulatory responses to hypoglycemia (Heine *et al.*, 1984). Most of these studies have been performed on nondiabetic adult volunteers. Absorption kinetics and activity profiles may well be different in children (Table 17.2).

17.3.1 ABSORPTION KINETICS AND ACTIVITY PROFILE OF SOLUBLE INSULIN

Plasma insulin levels and blood glucose responses to a standard subcutaneous injection of soluble insulin (Porcine Actrapid 10 units) into the thigh in a nondiabetic adult are shown in Figure 17.2 adapted from Berger, 1982.

The important features are:

1) At 10 minutes, a significant increase in insulin is measurable.
2) At 20 minutes, the insulin levels double.
3) At 60 minutes, the insulin level reached is over 80% of 'peak'.
4) At about 90 minutes, peak levels (more like a plateau) are reached.
5) A hypoglycemic effect is significant by 20 minutes.
6) The hypoglycemic effect is still apparent at 8 hours.

The most important finding in this and other studies (Binder, 1969; Galloway *et al.*, 1981) is the considerable intra-individual and even greater inter-individual variation. There are numerous other variables which substantially alter pharmacokinetic characteristics (Table 17.2).

17.3.2 ABSORPTION AND ACTIVITY PROFILES OF MIXED AND PROLONGED-ACTION INSULINS

Figure 17.3 is constructed from the results of various studies on insulin absorption (Galloway *et al.*, 1981; Berger *et al.*, 1982; Heine *et al.*, 1984) and illustrates the following points:

1) When soluble insulin is mixed with NPH there is a rapid absorption of insulin and a peak level is attained which is indis-

Table 17.2 Factors affecting absorption of insulin (key: quicker < slower).

					References
1) Site of injection					
	Abdomen <	Deltoid <	Buttock <	Thigh	
Time to peak (minutes)	63 ± 10	76 ± 9	–	92 ± 11	Berger *et al.*, 1982
	90	102	96	108	Galloway *et al.*, 1981
Importance of consistent anatomic region for injection					Bantle *et al.*, 1990
2) Depth					
	Deep intramuscular <	Superficial intramuscular <	Subcutaneous		Galloway *et al.*, 1981; Frid *et al.*, 1988; Spraul *et al.*, 1988
Peak (minutes)	30	60	90–120		
3) Skin quality: Lipohypertrophy slows absorption					Kolendorf *et al.*, 1983
4) Body weight: Lean patients (children) < fat patients					Kolendorf *et al.*, 1983
5) Exercise: Enhanced and more variable absorption after exercise					Galloway *et al.*, 1981; Thow *et al.*, 1989
6) Massage: enhanced absorption					Berger *et al.*, 1982
7) Temperature and skin blood flow: Increased temperature of skin enhances absorption					Berger *et al.*, 1982; Kolendorf *et al.*, 1983
8) Intra-individual variation: Coefficient of variation about 25%					Galloway *et al.*, 1981
9) Inter-individual variation: Coefficient of variation up to 50%					Kolendorf *et al.*,1978
10) Insulin characteristics					
a) Formulation – different types of soluble					Binder, 1969
NPH					Berger *et al.*, 1982
Mixtures					Davis *et al.*, 1991
b) Degradation in tissues					Berger *et al.*, 1982
c) Concentration					Galloway *et al.*, 1981
U10 < U1000 but no difference between . . . U40–U100					Swift *et al.*, 1983
d) Volume: Small volume < large volume					Binder, 1979
Small multiple injections < large bolus					
e) Species – Human < pork ≪ beef					Owens, 1986

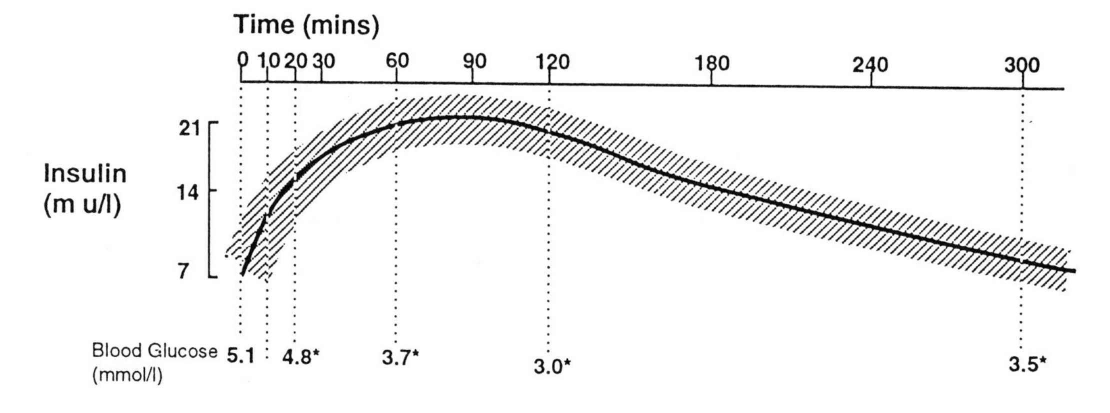

Figure 17.2 Insulin absorption and hypoglycemic effect following standard injection of soluble insulin (after Berger *et al.*, 1982).

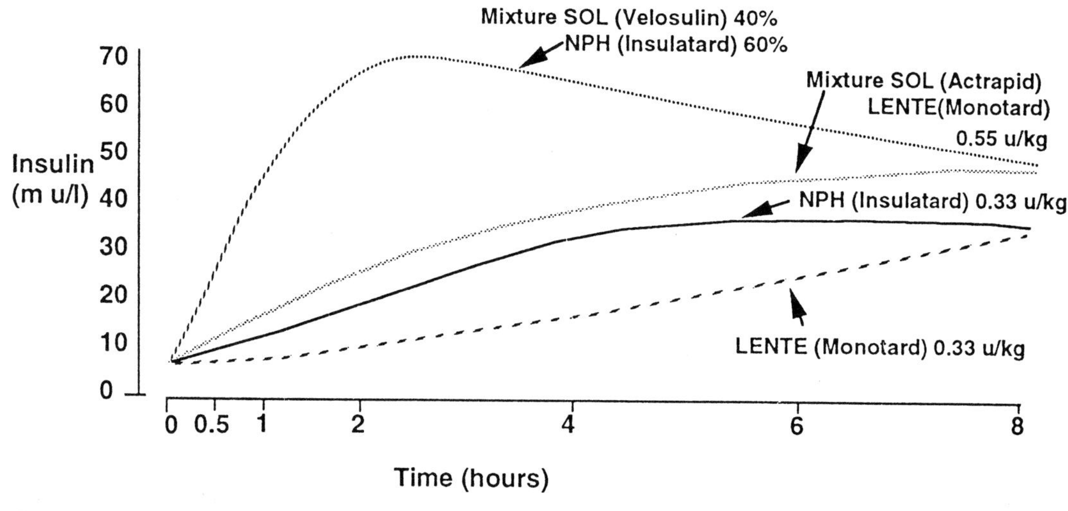

Figure 17.3 Absorption profiles of prolonged action insulin.

tinguishable from soluble insulin alone. Indeed, insulin action during the first 4 hours after injection is determined mainly by soluble components.

2) NPH has a slightly quicker absorption than lente (but their activity profiles are indistinguishable).
3) When soluble is mixed with insulin zinc suspension (such as Monotard) and injected immediately, there is a significant delay in insulin absorption and activity. This delayed absorption is exaggerated if the injection of the mixture is delayed.

Davis *et al.* (1991) have looked at the absorption and metabolic effects of three ready-mixed human insulins. Mixtard insulin which has a different isophane formulation from Actraphane and Humulin M3, produced significantly higher levels of insulin but all three provoked similar metabolic effects. Standardized absorption studies of bovine, pork and human ultra-lente preparations have shown discernible differences between the preparations but all exhibit extremely slow absorption. The hypoglycemic effect of human ultratard occurs within 4–6 hours and lasts a variable time, up to 32 hours (Owens, 1986).

17.3.3 THE PHARMACOKINETICS OF HUMAN INSULIN

In the UK there has been an almost universal acceptance of human insulin as the species of choice for children. The evidence that human insulin provokes even less antibody formation than pork MC insulin (Heding *et al.*, 1984; Luyckx *et al.*, 1986) and that antibody formation might be associated with a reduced C-peptide production and a shorter 'honeymoon period' (Ludvigsson, 1984) added scientific credibility to the use of human insulin in children. Comparisons have been made in the absorption and activity of bovine, porcine and human soluble insulins producing contradictory findings but general conclusions have been made (Owens, 1986). Insulin levels are marginally higher 30–60 minutes after human, rather than porcine, injections. Human insulin possesses a relatively quicker and less prolonged hypoglycemic action relative to bovine with porcine occupying an intermediate position.

There are physicochemical differences between human and porcine insulin. Human insulin is a more hydrophilic molecule allowing more rapid absorption from injection sites (Home *et al.*, 1984; Galloway *et al.*, 1981) whereas porcine being more lipophilic may enter brain tissue more rapidly.

These findings may be of importance in view of the suggestion that some adult patients transferred from animal to human insulin experienced a significant loss in the hypoglycemic warning signs (Teuscher & Berger, 1987). Pediatricians will view with interest the outcome of carefully designed comparative studies which so far do not seem to confirm the human insulin/loss of awareness hypothesis (Maran *et al.*, 1993) (see also Chapter 25). Some children undoubtedly experience sudden hypoglycemic attacks without warning. This phenomenon existed before the advent of human insulin and it is debatable whether it is now more common. A small number of children probably absorb soluble (particularly human) insulin very rapidly, thus appearing to be exquisitely 'sensitive'. They may be more comfortably managed on slower acting (perhaps porcine) preparations. The current debate (Teuscher, 1992; Patrick, 1992) serves to emphasize the principles that:

a) If a child's diabetes is under satisfactory control, the insulin regimen (including the insulin species) should not be changed.
b) If diabetes control problems do exist, a change in insulin formulation or species might be beneficial.

The preceding discussion and the contents of Table 17.2 emphasize the variability of absorption from the sites of injection. How much does this variability actually affect glycemic control? In a carefully managed study of patients in hospital given standardized injections and regular patterns of meals and exercise, there was 100% variability of measured insulin levels which correlated with mean blood glucose concentration (Lauritzen *et al.*, 1979). Such extreme variability offers an explanation for the apparently 'inexplicable' swings of blood glucose concentration which are the subject of frustrated debate in so many diabetic clinics.

17.4 PRACTICAL ADMINISTRATION OF INSULIN

17.4.1 STARTING CHILDREN ON INSULIN

The first insulin injection carries with it enormous emotional and practical significance. For the child this is the first in a lifelong experience of injections. For parents it signifies the loss of a normal child, the realization that their child has to be subjected to, and is totally dependent on, the discomforting administration of an injectable medication for the rest of childhood. It is important, therefore, that the demonstration and administration of the first injection is performed in a quiet, unhurried, confident manner by an experienced member of the diabetes team (Swift, 1991). If the child is frightened, insecure and unsupported and the injection happens to be painful, there is more likelihood that there will be subsequent injection difficulties.

Years later, adults describe the trauma of childhood injections but it is interesting that the majority of children seem to cope with injections or at least do not report problems (Lindsay, 1985). Injections may be given by a child with supervision from a surprisingly early age. Recently in a group of over 200 children who had developed diabetes aged less than 2 years, 45% were injecting themselves by 7 years, 87% by 10 years. However, as several authors have cautioned, it is unwise to expect children to manage self-care before knowledge and understanding of their disease is adequately established (Etzwiler, 1962; Johnson *et al.*, 1982; see also Chapters 7 and 20). It remains important that supervision of dosage, accuracy and precision is a

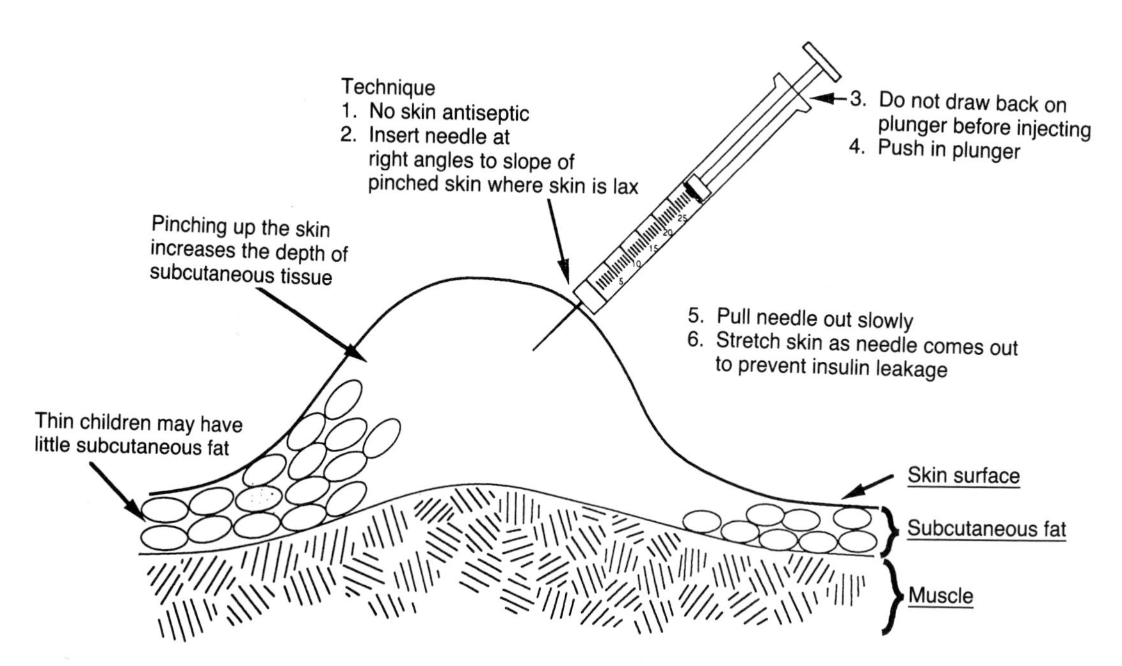

Figure 17.4 Standardized insulin injection technique.

shared responsibility throughout childhood (Follansbee, 1989). Modern equipment has undoubtedly improved acceptance of injections and in the UK and US advice on injection technique (Craddock, 1989; American Diabetes Association, 1992) has become standardized (Figure 17.4).

The depth and angle of injection in children is important (Galloway *et al.*, 1981; Thow & Home, 1990), especially as many young, slim children have such shallow subcutaneous fat spaces that perpendicular injections may become intramuscular or intraperitoneal (Smith *et al.*, 1991).

17.4.2 PROBLEMS WITH INJECTIONS

17.4.2.1 Pain

A minority of children find injections very painful or difficult and never overcome the fear and anxiety of the needle. Injection phobia undoubtedly affects attempts at obtaining glycemic control. The insulin injection technique should be observed and advice offered. The newer pain-reducing injector guns (e.g., Auto-injector™) are helpful in young children and in some cases help has been obtained by psychotherapeutic approaches (Lindsay, 1985) and hypnotherapy (Ratner *et al.*, 1990).

17.4.2.2 Leakage, bleeding and bruising

These are common and cannot be completely avoided and are further reasons for the variability of insulin action. Stretching the skin after the needle is withdrawn or firm finger pressure over the site of injection helps.

17.4.2.3 Bubbles in the insulin

Small bubbles difficult to see in cloudy insulin are not harmful. Bubbles big enough to alter the dose of insulin in small children should be carefully expelled.

17.4.2.4 Infections

Skin infections, although reported (Anonymous, 1981), are rare and previously reported abscesses were probably caused by sterilizing fluids, such as surgical spirit. Insulin preparations contain antimicrobial preservatives (Paraben M-cresol or Phenol) which greatly reduce the possibility of contaminated insulin being injected.

17.4.2.5 Subcutaneous atrophy and hypertrophy

Disfiguring lipoatrophy occurred commonly with older insulins (Reeves *et al.*, 1980) and even with modern highly purified insulins this problem has not disappeared (Jones *et al.*, 1981). Equally unpleasant hypertrophic fibrotic lumps are still common (Young *et al.*, 1981) to which some children seem particularly prone and are a major cause of erratic insulin absorption (Kolendorf *et al.*, 1983). They can only be avoided by assiduous attention to regular rotation of injection sites.

17.4.2.6 Insufficient or excess insulin

The commonest reasons for diabetic ketoacidosis (DKA) in a child are injections which are occasionally forgotten, more often avoided or wilfully neglected. This is not a new phenomenon as emphasized by R.D. Lawrence (1925) when he pointed out that advice by medical personnel to omit insulin in a stressed child with an intercurrent infection may be described as 'a medical crime'.

Occasionally parents or children mistakenly give a double or additional dose of insulin.

When insufficient or excess insulin is given, this is rectified by additional doses of insulin or extra carbohydrate with frequent blood glucose monitoring. Attempts at suicide by excess insulin administration unfortunately occur and have been aborted by excision of the subcutaneous insulin depot.

17.4.2.7 Storage of insulin

Insulin is a stable protein but it may be denatured by extremes of temperature (above 30°C or below 0°C) or exposure to direct sunlight for days. It is recommended by insulin manufacturers that the bottle is kept in a refrigerator at 4°C or at room temperature for up to one month.

17.4.3 ALTERNATIVE INSULIN INJECTION DEVICES

17.4.3.1 Pen injectors

The earliest pen injectors, devised to simplify transport and multiple injection therapy, used a modified plastic syringe (Paton *et al.*, 1981), but have been superceded by a family of devices from the classic push-button Novopen™ 1 to numerous dial-a-dose pens. A fully disposable pre-filled plastic pen from Novo Nordisk containing either soluble or premixed insulins is now available in some countries, having undergone trials which suggest popularity and practicality for children. As with all mechanical devices a number of infrequent technical problems have been described (Dahl-Jorgensen *et al.*, 1986; Patel & Crowley, 1990). A small 'airshot' should be performed before each injection to confirm patency of the needle and expulsion of air bubbles.

17.4.3.2 Insulin infusion pumps

Continuous subcutaneous insulin infusion (CSII) was introduced at Guy's Hospital (Pickup *et al.*, 1978) and assumed considerable popularity.

Reviews were written on pump therapy in children (Greene, 1985; de Beaufort & Bruining, 1987) but it became apparent that only a small number of children could realistically benefit (Pickup *et al.*, 1981; Davies *et al.*, 1984). In a large clinical study (Knight *et al.*, 1986) only 29% of 45 adolescents chose CSII and 64% of these discontinued it rapidly. Improvement in control was achieved by some groups (Schiffrin *et al.*, 1983) but often not sustained and clinical problems were commonly described (Becker *et al.*, 1984; Brink & Stewart, 1986).

Numerous complications, technical failures and mishaps began to be reported, including a number of deaths (Anonymous, 1982 & 1985). Even short-term CSII required more motivation than intelligence (Pickup *et al.*, 1981) and rigorous behavioral demands of pump treatment caused discontinuations (Becker *et al.*, 1984; de Beaufort & Bruining, 1987). This is particularly so in CSII management of children of pre-school age (Brambilla *et al.*, 1987). However, CSII is still recognized as the only method of achieving normoglycemia (Hirsch *et al.*, 1990) and continues to be the chosen modality of insulin administration in some young people. It may be useful in some other situations, such as surgery, acute infections and DKA although much more easily applicable as an IV rather than subcutaneous infusion (Boulton & Penfold, 1981; Smail, 1986). Currently, in the UK, few pediatricians recommend domiciliary CSII (Johnston, 1989) and in major units in the US, CSII is rarely thought to be practicable (Drash, 1986).

17.4.3.3 Jet injectors

High-pressure devices forcing insulin through a fine nozzle enabling it to penetrate the skin without a needle injection are available. They are not entirely painless and are bulky, expensive and unsuitable for mixtures of insulins. Their safety is not yet proven (Sonksen *et al.*, 1991) and the speed of absorption is different than that from a syringe (Selam & Charles, 1990). Jet injectors have not gained widespread acceptance (MacPherson & Feely, 1990).

17.4.3.4 Subcutaneous cannulae

In parts of Sweden the majority of children with IDDM are on multiple daily injection regimens, giving as many as 6 injections a day. To ease the injections, a Teflon cannula with an injection port (Insuflon™) is inserted under the skin (Hanas & Ludvigsson, 1990). At diagnosis children are offered the Insuflon™ and 25% continue to use this at home (Hanas, 1991). This technique has been used in other countries with varying success (Long & Hughes, 1991; Schober, 1991).

17.4.4 CHOICE OF INSULIN REGIMEN

Where there is an unlimited supply of highly purified insulin, the choice of a particular regimen is embarrassingly large. The choice is often based more on prejudice than scientific evaluation. Particular insulin regimens are favoured in certain countries but insulin preferences may even vary between doctors within the same clinic. In the US, the most widely used regimen is twice-daily individualized mixes of regular and isophane (the 'split-mix' regimen). In Scandinavia, multiple injection treatment (MIT) regimens using pen injectors are popular. In the UK, a variety of regimens are used with an increasing number of advocates for ready-mixed insulins and a continuing use of regular-insulin zinc suspension mixtures.

17.4.4.1 One or two injections a day?

In the 1920s, the inconvenience of multiple injections of acid-soluble insulin gave rise to the search for longer acting insulins. Between 1936 and the early 1980s, single dose PZI or lente insulins were commonly used but as time has progressed the quest for postprandial and early morning normoglycemia has led to an almost universal swing in favor of at least two injections a day, each one containing at least a proportion of quick-acting soluble insulin. It has been surprisingly difficult to prove in study groups of all ages that twice-daily is superior to once-daily insulin.

Early studies concluded that twice-daily injections gave better control than once-daily (Åkerblom & Hiekkala, 1970; Aagenes, 1975), but the experimental design of these studies (selected groups, non-randomized, with no cross-over) would nowadays be unacceptable. Not surprisingly, the expected intervention effect seemed to prove efficacy (Worth *et al.*, 1982). In a randomized crossover trial once or twice-daily pork MC insulin regimens were compared (Werther *et al.*, 1980) but the study is open to the criticism of potential interaction between soluble and insulin zinc suspensions and the twice-daily insulin had too short an activity profile. Not surprisingly the once-daily soluble-monotard regime showed a significantly lower fasting blood glucose but higher evening postprandial levels, but overall no significant difference in control. A further study in adolescents (Langdon *et al.*, 1981) showed that twice-daily insulin was not statistically distinguishable in terms of glycemic control from once-daily. Individually some children seemed better on one than the other. It was concluded that any advantage of a split dose regimen was small in comparison with other factors, such as residual insulin secretion, diet, methods of monitoring control and compliance. Despite these findings most pediatricians advocate, on clinical and physiologic grounds, more than one injection per day.

17.4.4.2 Twice daily therapy

In the world-wide context, the most common insulin regime is the individualized twice-daily soluble-isophane mixture enabling patients to vary the ratio of insulins. Recently, because of evidence that varying ratios of quick and slower insulin made little impact on insulin and glucose levels

(Galloway *et al.*, 1981), fixed-mixture insulins have been gaining popularity, particularly now that soluble-isophane ratios from 10:90 to 50:50 are available and may be given in pen injectors. For children and parents, such mixtures have the potential advantage of simplicity of use, avoiding the time, effort and inaccuracy of drawing up small volumes of soluble or isophane insulins. These practical difficulties have been confirmed in a clinical study by home nursing personnel (McEvilly *et al.*, 1990) showing no HbA_1 change over three months but increased acceptability, self-confidence, involvement in self-injections and accuracy of drawing up. In the original double blind cross-over investigation in adults (Roland, 1984) equally acceptable stable control was achieved by a fixed 30:70 mixture compared with individualized split-mix regimens. Similar results have been obtained by others (Cucinotta *et al.*, 1991) including a comparison with MIT (Corcoran & Yudkin, 1986) and a study confirming the greater accuracy of drawing up fixed mixtures by both professionals and patients (Bell *et al.*, 1991). The convenience of pre-mixed insulins, therefore, may be an important bonus for certain groups, such as the young, the visually impaired and those who do not wish to use MIT.

17.4.4.3 Multiple injection therapy (MIT)

Free-insulin levels are of paramount importance in controlling overnight blood glucose and intermediary metabolism (Gale *et al.*, 1980; Malone & Root, 1981). Levels fall significantly on most insulin regimens (Edge *et al.*, 1990). Methods of sustaining free-insulin levels overnight should diminish the so-called 'dawn phenomenon' that is, the physiologic increase in insulin resistance during the dawn hours which is accentuated in diabetes, particularly during puberty (Amiel *et al.*, 1991; Dunger, 1992). This phenomenon probably partly accounts for the Somogyi effect, an original clinical observation (Somogyi, 1959) of rebound morning hyperglycemia and ketosis following injection of excess amounts of soluble insulin and in response to counter-regulatory mechanisms. This explanation is only part of the story and the maintenance of adequate levels of biologically-active insulin throughout the night, particularly before breakfast, is of crucial importance. Thus studies have been conducted using combinations of medium or long-acting insulins given before bedtime rather than earlier in the evening. In children such strategies are important because many younger European children eat their main evening meal in the late afternoon (4:30–5 p.m.) with supper at about 7:30 p.m. and then are fasting until 8 a.m.

This is different in other cultures. For example, the children of parents of Asian origin in the UK usually eat an evening meal with high carbohydrate content about at 7 or 8 p.m. with no supper to follow.

In a one-year cross-over study, a comparison between a conventional twice-daily and thrice-daily regimen, delaying the intermediate acting insulin until bedtime, showed a significant decrease in the fasting blood glucose and post breakfast hyperglycemia (Hinde & Johnston, 1986), but HbA_1 control remained poor. This group of 18 adolescents was reviewed frequently over 12 months but not intensively monitored. An important conclusion stated that the season or month of the year seemed to account for substantially more variation in HbA_1 than the change in insulin regimen. Hocking *et al.* (1986) also commented that

> although intensified monitoring and treatment may improve metabolic status, it remains abnormal (in adolescents). The main stumbling block is difficulty in obtaining normal pre-breakfast blood

glucose and without attention to factors other than monitoring and insulin only a modest improvement can be expected.

MIT involving pre-meal boluses of insulin and night-time prolonged action insulin (the so-called 'basal-bolus regimen') has been given extra stimulus by the availability of pen injector devices.

Some would describe pen injectors as a gimmick rather than a therapeutic advance (Anonymous, 1989) but patients report that pen injectors have revolutionized their lives and after study trials many continue to choose them. Some professionals consider that such ultra-flexible regimens may be counter-productive (Anonymous, 1989).

Early short trials in children and adults (Jefferson *et al.*, 1985; Walters *et al.*, 1985) with Novopen™ 1 suggested improved metabolic control but, as in the once/twice-daily studies, they were almost certainly influenced by an intervention effect. A later evaluation (Dahl-Jorgensen *et al.*, 1986) in a group of strictly controlled adults already on MIT with syringes showed a significant increase in HbA_1 when switched to Novopen™ 1, but all patients wished to continue with pens because of simplicity of use and increased flexibility. A comparison of MIT and twice-daily mixed insulins showed no difference in diabetic control as assessed by HbA_1 or hypoglycemic reactions, but patients using the pen felt it added flexibility to their lifestyle (Small *et al.*, 1988). Close supervision of patients in a trial setting often improves glycemic control but intensifying therapy with MIT may fail to make a further impact despite making significant positive contributions to lifestyle. A large Danish study (Gall *et al.*, 1989) of 168 unselected patients (with a sub-group aged under 18 years) offered the Novopen™ and followed for 12 months showed no change in HbA_1 but frequency of DKA and severe hypoglycemia diminished and 90% of patients reported improvement in well-being.

The number of insulin injections *per se* is not the most important factor in improving metabolic control (Agardh & Tallroth, 1985). Other factors such as intensive attention by the health care team (Worth *et al.*, 1982), psychosocial factors (Belmonte *et al.*, 1988) or dedicated patient blood glucose self-monitoring (Schiffrin & Belmonte, 1982) are more important whatever insulin regime is adopted.

17.5 WHAT REGIMEN AND HOW

Hirsch *et al.* (1990) have produced a very persuasive paper in favor of intensive insulin therapy, arguing against a narrow view of using a single modality of therapy, such as insulin, in attempting to achieve normoglycemia. Their view is a broad-based multicomponent management program with the patient and management team forming a cooperative partnership. Emphasis is placed on achieving 'effective insulinemia' by MIT or CSII but also a recognition that for many individuals acceptable rather than meticulous control can be achieved with twice-daily insulin so long as other elements of management are utilized, such as self-management strategies, careful food balance, understanding of activity programs and, in particular, defined goals, comprehensive education and psychological support. Such a philosophy will be welcomed by most pediatricians and the term 'intensive insulin treatment' might be better expressed as 'personal comprehensive management' emphasizing the 'personal' with respect to:

a) close interaction between a small experienced diabetes team and the child,
b) individualized insulin regimens and
c) promotion of self management.

The author's personal preference is to teach all children how to use the syringe and insulin vial techniques and initiate therapy with regular (soluble) or ready-mixed 30:70 insulin. If this is started during a brief hospital admission or on a domiciliary, outpatient basis the dose is likely to be 0.25–0.30 units per kilogram twice daily, slowly increasing until blood glucose shows either acceptable levels or a need to switch from soluble to a longer acting ready-mixed formulation, often introducing pen injection devices. Such a graduated increasing dosage introduction to insulin therapy allows the family to feel in control of the regimen from the outset and see clearly the relationship between dosage changes and blood glucose levels (Swift *et al.*, 1993). Guidelines have been proposed for the proportions of different insulins in split-mixed regimens, for example, two-thirds of the total daily insulin given in the morning and one-third in the evening. Similarly it has been suggested that with MIT, the proportion of prolonged action insulin at bedtime might be 40% with 20% of soluble injected before each main meal.

It is certainly a practical necessity to find the bedtime insulin preparation and dose which achieves the most effective overnight control and then adjust preprandial doses through the day. In practice, however, it becomes clear that an infinite variety of individual dosage patterns evolve and the proportions of insulin change throughout the year and as the child matures. Adequate control in the preschool child might be obtained at least temporarily on once- or twice-daily intermediate-acting insulins with no soluble component (except for crises) whereas prepubertal children (particularly during the 'honeymoon period') might be best served by a twice-daily fixed-mixture, only to find that in puberty split-mixed or MIT regimens become more effective and acceptable.

17.6 SUMMARY

The practice of medicine is both an art and a science. Art is emotive, subjective and often controversial, whereas science is based on logic, hypothesis and controlled experiment. Diabetes and its control cannot be tested with total scientific precision because there are too many variables. The art of diabetes management is, therefore, very influential.

Insulin remains the indispensable factor in crude control of diabetes. Precision-tuning with manipulation of insulin cannot, as yet, maintain long-lasting normoglycemic and perfect intermediary metabolism. Accepting these limitations, it is of paramount importance for professionals involved in diabetes care to be able to initiate children into a lifetime of insulin use with a regimen involving not only a knowledge of pharmacokinetic and endocrine replacement therapy but a deep understanding of diabetes, children's developmental needs and family dynamics. From the outset, the children and family need to feel a sense of control over their own diabetes, to feel comfortable with the available advice and to be able to call on expert help when needed. The patient's attitude, motivation and behavior towards diabetes (Lockington *et al.*, 1987) is far more important than a doctor's preconceived and prejudiced ideas about insulin regimens.

In 1960, Michael Somogyi wrote, 'Insulin therapy is still beset with grave difficulties'. Some of those difficulties have diminished and some remain. Fortunately the majority of children with informed, consistent and uncomplicated advice are able to maintain excellent health and acceptable glycemic control. As a consequence, the prognosis has improved (McNally, 1991; Borch-Johnsen *et al.*, 1986 & 1987) enabling many young people to benefit from advances in the future.

REFERENCES

Aagenes, O. (1975) 'Insulin once or twice daily', in Z. Laron and M. Karp (eds). *Modern Problems in Paediatrics* Vol. 12., p. 136. Karger, Basel.

Agardh, C.-D. and Tallroth, G. (1985) Lack of relation between glycosylated haemoglobin concentrations and number of daily insulin injections: cross sectional study in care of ambulatory diabetes. *Brit. Med. J.*, **291**, 622.

Åkerblom, H.K. and Hiekkala, H. (1970) Diurnal blood and urine glucose and acetone bodies in labile juvenile diabetes on one and two injection therapy. *Diabetologia*, **6**, 130.

American Diabetes Association Recommendations. (1992) Insulin administration. *Diabetes Care*, **15** (suppl. 2), 30–33.

Amiel, S.A., Caprio, S., Sherwin, R.S. *et al.* (1991) Insulin resistance of puberty: a defect restricted to peripheral glucose metabolism. *J. Clin. Endocrin. and Metab.*, **72**, 277–82.

Anonymous. (1981) Insulin injections and infections. *Brit. Med. J.*, **282**, 340.

Anonymous. (1982) Deaths in diabetics using insulin infusion pumps. *Lancet*, **I**, 636.

Anonymous. (1985) Acute mishaps during insulin pump treatment. *Lancet*, **I**, 911–12.

Anonymous. (1989) Insulin pen: mightier than syringe? *Lancet*, **I**, 307–308.

Asplin, C.M., Hartog, M. and Goldie, D.J. (1978) Change of insulin dosage, circulating free and bound insulin and insulin antibodies on transferring diabetics from conventional to highly purified porcine insulin. *Diabetologia*, **14**, 99–105.

Bantle, J.P., Weber, M., Rao, S.M.S. *et al.* (1990) Rotation of anatomic regions used for insulin injections and day-to-day variability of plasma glucose in Type 1 diabetic subjects. *J. Am. Med. Assoc.*, **263**, 1802–1806.

Becker, D.J., Kerensky, K.M., Transue, D. *et al.* (1984) Current status of pump therapy in childhood. *Acta Paed. Japan*, **26**, 347–58.

Bell, D.S.H., Clement, R.S., Perentesis, G. *et al.* (1991) Dosage accuracy of self-mixed versus premixed insulin. *Arch. Int. Med.*, **151**, 2265–69.

Belmonte, M., Shiffrin, A. and Dufresne, J. (1988) Impact of SMBG on control of diabetes as measured by HbAl. *Diabetes Care*, **11**, 484–88.

Berger, M., Cuppers, H.J., Hegner, H. *et al.* (1982) Absorption kinetics and biologic effects of subcutaneously injected insulin preparations. *Diabetes Care*, **5**, 77–91.

Binder, C. (1969) Absorption of injected insulin. *Acta Pharmacologica and Toxicologica*, **27** (suppl. 2), 1–87.

Bloom, S.R., West, A.M., Polak, J.M. *et al.* (1978) 'Hormonal contaminants of insulin', in S.R. Bloom S.R. (ed.). *Gut hormones*, pp. 318–22. Churchill Livingstone, Edinburgh.

Borch-Johnsen, K., Kreiner, S. and Deckert, T. (1986) Mortality of Type 1 (insulin dependent) diabetics in Denmark: a study of relative mortality in 2930 Danish Type 1 diabetic patients diagnosed from 1933 to 1972. *Diabetologia*, **29**, 767–72.

Borch-Johnsen, K., Nissen, H., Salling, N. *et al.* (1987) The natural history of IDDM in Denmark: long-term survival with and without late diabetic complications. *Diabetic Med.*, **4**, 201–210.

Boulton, J. and Penfold, J. (1981) Insulin infusion for diabetic children. *Med. J. Austral.*, **2**, 474–76.

Brambilla, P., Artavia-Loria, E., Chaussain, J.-L. *et al.* (1987) Risk of ketosis during intensive insulin therapy in pre-school-age children. *Diabetes Care*, **10**, 44–48.

Brange, J. (1987) *Galenics of Insulin*. Springer-Verlag, Berlin.

Brink, S.J. and Stewart, C. (1986) Insulin pump treatment in insulin dependent diabetes mellitus. *J. Am. Med. Assoc.*, **255**, 617–21.

Corcoran, J.S. and Yudkin, J.S. (1986) A comparison of premixed with patient-mixed insulins. *Diabetic Med.*, **3**, 246–49.

Craddock, S. (1989) The ABC of insulin injections. *Balance* (magazine of British Diabetic Association), **iii**, 22–25.

Cucinotta, D., Mannino, D., Lasco, A. *et al.* (1991) Premixed insulin at ratio 3/7 and regular plus isophane insulins at mixing ratios from 2/8 to 4/6 achieve the same metabolic control. *Diabete et Metabolisme* (Paris), **17**, 49–54.

Dahl-Jorgensen, K., Hanssen, K.F., Mosand, R. *et al.* (1986) The 'insulin pen': Comparison with multiple injection treatment with syringes. *Practical Diabetes*, **3**, 90–91.

Davies, A.G., Price, D.A., Houlton, C.A. *et al.* (1984) Continuous subcutaneous insulin infusion in diabetes mellitus. *Arch. Dis. Child.*, **59**, 1027–33.

Davis, S.N., Thompson, C.J., Brown, M.D. *et al.* (1991) A comparison of the pharmacokinetics and metabolic effects of human regular and NPH insulin mixtures. *Diabetes Res. and Clin. Prac.*, **13**, 107–18.

de Beaufort, C.E. and Bruining, G.J. (1987) Continuous subcutaneous insulin infusion in children. *Diabetic Med.*, **4**, 103–8.

Drash, A.L. (1986) 'Approaches to the prevention and cure of insulin dependent diabetes mellitus', in *Clinical Care of the Diabetic Child*, p. 114. Year Book Medical Publishers, Chicago.

Dunger, D.B. (1992) Diabetes in Puberty. *Arch. Dis. Child.*, **67**, 569–70.

Edge, J.A., Matthews, D.R. and Dunger, D.B. (1990) Failure of current insulin regimes to meet the overnight insulin requirements of adolescents with insulin dependent diabetes. *Diabetes Res.*, **15**, 109–12.

Etzwiler, D.D. (1962) What the juvenile diabetic knows about his disease. *Pediatrics*, **29**, 135–41.

Follansbee, D.S. (1989) Assuming responsibility for diabetes management: What age? *Diabetes Educ.*, **15**, 347–53.

Frid, A., Gunnarsson, R., Guntner, P. *et al.* (1988) Effects of accidental intramuscular injection on insulin absorption in IDDM. *Diabetes Care*, **11**, 41–45.

Gale, E.A.M., Kurtz, A.B. and Tattersall, R.B. (1980) In search of the Somogyi effect. *Lancet*, **ii**, 279–82.

Gall, M-A., Mathiesen, E.R., Skott, P. *et al.* (1989) Effect of multiple insulin injections with a pen injector on metabolic control and general well-being in IDDM. *Diabetes Res.*, **11**, 97–101.

Galloway, J.A., Spradlin, C.T., Nelson, R.L. *et al.* (1981) Factors influencing the absorption, serum insulin concentration and blood glucose responses after injections of regular insulin and various insulin mixtures. *Diabetes Care*, **4**, 366–76.

Greene, S.A. (1985) Insulin pump therapy, in J.D. Baum and A.-L. Kinmonth, (eds). *Care of the Child with Diabetes*, pp. 85–91. Churchill Livingstone, Edinburgh.

Hagedorn, H.C., Jensen, B.N., Kratup, N.B. *et al.* (1936) Protamine Insulinate. *J. Am. Med. Assoc.*, **106**, 177–80.

Hallas-Møller, K., Peterson, K. and Schlichtkrull, J. (1951) Crystalline and amorphous insulin-zinc compounds with prolonged action [in Danish]. *Ugeskrift for laeger*, **113**, 1767–71.

Hanas, R. (1991) *Insuflon Guide*. Department of Pediatrics, Uddevalla Hospital, S451 80 Sweden.

Hanas, R. and Ludvigsson, J. (1990) Side effects and indwelling times of subcutaneous catheters for insulin injections. *Diabetes Res. in Clin. Prac.*, **10**, 73–83.

Heding, L.G.H., Marshall, M.O., Persson, B. *et al.* (1984) Immunogenicity of monocomponent human and porcine insulin in newly diagnosed type 1 (insulin dependent) diabetic children. *Diabetologia*, **27**, 96–98.

Heine, R.J., Bilo, H.J.G., Fonk, T. *et al.* (1984) Absorption kinetics and action profiles of mixtures of short and intermediate acting insulins. *Diabetologia*, **27**, 588–62.

Hinde, F.R.J. and Johnston, D.I. (1986) Two or three insulin injections in adolescence. *Arch. Dis. Child.*, **61**, 118–23.

Hirsch, I.B., Farkas-Hirsch, R. and Skyler, J.S. (1990) Intensive Insulin Therapy for Treatment of Type 1 Diabetes. *Diabetic Care*, **13**, 1265–83.

Hocking, M.D., Rayner, P.H.W. and Nattrass, M. (1986) Metabolic rhythms in adolescents with diabetes. *Arch. Dis. Child.*, **61**, 124–29.

Holman, R.R. and Turner, R.C. (1985) A practical guide to basal and prandial insulin therapy. *Diabetic Medicine*, **2**, 45–53.

Home, P.D., Mann, N.P., Hutchinson, A.S. *et al.* (1984) A fifteen-month double-blind cross-over study of the efficacy and antigenicity of human and pork insulins. *Diabetic Med.*, **1**, 93–98.

Howell, S.L. (1991) 'Insulin biosythesis and secretion' in J.C. Pickup and William, G. (eds). *Textbook of Diabetes*, p. 76. Blackwell Scientific Publications, London.

Jefferson, I.G., Marteau, T.M., Smith, M.A. *et al.* (1985) A multiple injection regimen using an insulin injection pen and pre-filled cartridged soluble human insulin in adolescents with diabetes. *Diabetic Med.*, **2**, 493–95.

Johnson, S.B., Pollak, T., Silverstein, J.H. *et al.* (1982) Cognitive and behavioural knowledge about insulin-dependent diabetes among children and parents. *Pediatrics*, **69**, 708–713.

Johnston, D.I. (1989) Management of diabetes mellitus. *Arch. Dis. Child.*, **64**, 622–28.

Jones, G.R., Statham, B., Owens, D.R. *et al.* (1981) Lipoatrophy and monocomponent porcine insulin. *Brit. Med. J.*, **282**, 190–91.

Knight, G., Boulton, A.J.M. and Ward, J.D. (1986) Experience of continuous subcutaneous insulin infusion in the outpatient management of diabetic teenagers. *Diabetic Med.*, **3**, 82–84.

Kolendorf, K., Aaby, P., Westergaard, S. *et al.* (1978) Absorption effectiveness and side-effects of highly purified procine NPH-insulin preparations. *Eur. J. Clin. Pharmacol*, **14**, 117–24.

Kolendorf, K., Bojsen, J. and Deckert, T. (1983) Clinical factors influencing absorption of ^{125}I-NPH insulin in diabetic patients. *Horm. and Metab. Res.*, **15**, 274–78.

Langdon, D.R., James, F.D. and Sperling, M.A. (1981) Comparison of single and split dose insulin regimens with 24 hour monitoring. *J. Pediatr.*, **99**, 854–61.

Lauritzen, T., Faber, O.K. and Binder, C. (1979) Variations in ^{125}I-insulin absorption and blood glucose concentration. *Diabetologia*, **17**, 291–95.

Lawrence, R.D. (1925) *The Diabetic Life – its control by diet and insulin*. J and A Churchill Ltd., London.

Lawrence, R.D. (1952) 'The beginning of the diabetic association in England', in D. Ven Engelhardt (ed.). *Diabetes: its medical and cultural history*, p. 452. Springer-Verlag, Berlin.

Lindsay, M. (1985) 'Emotional management', in J.D. Baum and A.-L. Kinmonth (eds). *Care of the Child with Diabetes*, pp. 41–63. Churchill Livingstone, Edinburgh.

Lockington, T.J., Meadows, K.A. and Wise, P.A. (1987) Compliant behaviour: relationship to attitudes and control in diabetic patients. *Diabetic Med.*, **4**, 56–61.

Long, A.R. and Hughes, I.A. (1991) Indwelling cannula for insulin administration in diabetes mellitus. *Arch. Dis. Child.*, **66**, 348–49.

Ludvigsson, J. (1984) Insulin antibodies in diabetic children treated with monocomponent porcine insulin from the outset: relationship to B-cell function and partial remission. *Diabetologia*, **26**, 138–43.

Luyckx, A.S., Daubresse, J.C., Jaminet, C. *et al.* (1986) Immunogenicity of Semi Synthetic human insulin in man. Long term comparison with porcine mono-component insulin. *Acta Diabetologia (Lat)*, **23**, 101–106.

McEvilly, E.A., Eccles, L. and Rayner, P.H.W. (1990) An assessment of the benefits of premixed insulins in childhood diabetes. *Practical Diabetes*, **7**, 122–24.

McNally, P.G. (1991) Childhood-onset diabetes: is the prognosis improving? *Practical Diabetes*, **8**, 133–36.

MacPherson, J.N. and Feely, J. (1990) Insulin. *Brit. Med. J.*, **300**, 731–36.

Malone, J.I. and Root, A.W. (1981) Plasma free insulin concentrations: keystone to effective management of diabetes mellitus in children. *J. Pediatr.*, **99**, 862–67.

Maran, A., Lomas, J., Archibald, H. *et al.* (1993) Double blind clinical and laboratory study of hypoglycaemia with human and porcine insulin in diabetic patients reporting hypoglycaemia unawareness after transferring to human insulin. *Brit. Med. J.*, **306**, 167–71.

Owens, D.R. (1986) *Human Insulin: clinical and pharmacological studies in normal man*. MTP Press Ltd, Lancaster.

Patel, S. and Crowley, S. (1990) My pen ran cold (Horace Walpole). *Practical Diabetes*, **7**, 16.

Paton, J.S., Wilson, M., Ireland, J.T. *et al.* (1981) Convenient pocket insulin syringe. *Lancet*, **i**, 189–90.

Patrick, A.W. (1992) Human insulin and loss of hypoglycaemia awareness: much ado about nothing? *Practical Diabetes*, **9**, 178–79.

Pickup, J.C., Keen, H., Parsons, J.A. *et al.* (1978) Continuous subcutaneous insulin infusion: an approach to achieving normoglycaemia. *Brit. Med. J.*, **i**, 204–207.

Pickup, J.C., Keen, H., Viberti, G.C. *et al.* (1981) Patient reactions to long-term outpatient treatment with continuous subcutaneous insulin infusion. *Brit. Med. J.*, **282**, 766–68.

Poulsen, J.E. (1985) *50 years experience of Protamine insulin*, issued by Nordisk Gentofte A/S, Denmark.

Ratner, H., Gross, L., Casas, J. *et al.* (1990) A hypnotherapeutic approach to the improvement of compliance in adolescent diabetes. *Am. J. Clin. Hypnosis*, **32**, 154–59.

Reeves, W.G., Allen, B.R. and Tattersall, R.B. (1980) Insulin induced lipoatrophy: evidence for an immune pathogenesis. *Brit. Med. J.*, **280**, 1500–1503.

Roland, J.M. (1984) Need stable diabetics mix their insulins? *Diabetic Med.*, **1**, 51–53.

Schiffrin, A. and Belmonte, M. (1982) Multiple daily self-glucose monitoring: its essential role in long-term glucose control in insulin dependent diabetes patients treated with pump and multiple subcutaneous injections. *Diabetic Care*, **5**, 479–84.

Schiffrin, A., Desrosiers, R.N., Moffatt, M.D. *et al.* (1983) Feasibility of strict diabetic control in insulin dependent diabetic adolescents. *J. Pediatr.*, **103**, 522–27.

Schlichtkrull, J. (1974) Antigenicity of monocomponent insulins. *Lancet*, **ii**, 1260–61.

Schober, E. (1991) Indwelling cannula for insulin administration in diabetes. *Arch. Dis. Child.*, **66**, 1261–62.

Scott, D.A. and Fisher, A.M. (1936) Studies on insulin with protamine. *J. Pharmacol. and Exper. Therapeutics*, **58**, 78–92.

Selam, J-L. and Charles M.A. (1990) Devices for insulin administration. *Diabetic Care*, **13**, 955–79.

Smail, P. (1986) Children with diabetes who need surgery. *Arch. Dis. Child.*, **61**, 413–14.

Small, M., MacRury, S., Boal, A. *et al.* (1988) Comparison of conventional twice daily subcutaneous insulin administration and a multiple injection regimen using Novopen in insulin dependent diabetes mellitus. *Diabetes Res.*, **8**, 85–89.

Smith, C.P., Sargent, M.A., Wilson, B.P.M. *et al.* (1991) Subcutaneous or intramuscular insulin injections. *Arch. Dis. Child.*, **66**, 879–82.

Somogyi, M. (1959) Exacerbation of diabetes by excess insulin action. *Am. J. Med.*, **26**, 169–91.

Somogyi, M. (1960) Exacerbation of diabetes by excess insulin action. *Diabetes*, **9**, 328–30.

Sonksen, P., Fox, C. and Judd, S. (1991) *Diabetes at your fingertips*, p. 65. Class publishing Ltd., London.

Spraul, M., Chantelau, E., Koumoulidou, J. *et al.* (1988) Subcutaneous or Non-subcutaneous injection of insulin. *Diabetes Care*, **11**, 733–36.

Swift, P.G.F. (1991) Starting children on insulin. *Maternal and Child Health*, **16**, 361–66.

Swift, P.G.F., Kennedy, J.D. and Gerlis, L.S. (1983) Change to U-100 insulin does not appear to affect insulin absorption. *Brit. Med. J.*, **286**, 1015–17.

Swift, P.G.F., Hearnshaw, J.R., Botha, J.L. *et al.* (1993) A decade of diabetes: keeping children out of hospital. *Brit. Med. J.*, **307**, 96–98.

Teuscher, A. (1992) Human insulin 1992: a significant independent risk factor for sudden hypoglycaemia. *Practical Diabetes*, **9**, 174–76.

Teuscher, A. and Berger, W.G. (1987) Hypoglycaemia unawareness in diabetics transferred to human insulin. *Lancet*, **ii**, 382–85.

Thow, J.C., Johnson, A.B., Antsiferov, M. *et al.* (1989) Exercise augments the absorption of Isophane (NPH) insulin. *Diabetic Med.*, **6**, 342–45.

Thow, J. and Home, P. (1990) Insulin injection technique – depth of injection is important. *Brit. Med. J.*, **301**, 3–4.

18

Dietary management of children with diabetes

S. BRENCHLEY and A. GOVINDJI

18.1 INTRODUCTION

Insulin replacement may remain the ideal treatment for IDDM but optimum control depends on a careful balance of food, physical activity and insulin. In few conditions are food and nutrition as important as in the management of diabetes. Unfortunately, diet is often the most misunderstood and undermined area of diabetes and at the diagnosis of their child, many parents have preconceived ideas of what this will entail.

Dietary advice for individuals with diabetes has changed significantly over the last ten years and current advice is based on healthy eating guidelines (British Diabetic Association, 1992a). Although the basis for dietary advice given to adults, these recommendations need to be amended to take into account the specific dietary requirements of children.

Why are dietary measures employed in the treatment of diabetes? First, they aim to avoid the primary symptoms by helping to maintain blood glucose levels within the normal range and avoid swings between hypo- and hyperglycemia. A child with diabetes has the same basic nutritional requirements as any other child so the diet should ensure normal growth and development and in addition help to avoid obesity. Finally and most importantly, via the long-term control of blood lipids and glycemia, dietary manipulation may help to reduce the incidence of long-term complications of diabetes (D'Antonio *et al.*, 1989).

18.2 DIETARY COMPOSITION

18.2.1 ENERGY REQUIREMENTS

An adequate energy intake is needed to achieve and maintain normal growth and the energy needs of children with diabetes are similar to that of their nondiabetic counterparts. Prescribing an appropriate energy intake can be difficult as individual energy needs vary tremendously, especially during periods of rapid growth or during high levels of physical activity. Initially, energy requirements are estimated by a review of the child's usual eating habits. It is vital that changes in eating patterns are assessed together with height and weight on a regular basis. Often when children are newly diagnosed, they may be in a negative energy balance and will need additional energy for catch-up growth.

This must be taken into account at diagnosis and reviewed subsequently. The energy content of the diet is probably the most relevant

Childhood and Adolescent Diabetes
Published in 1994 by Chapman & Hall, London
ISBN 0 412 48610 5

to overall control and no longer is a child with diabetes given such an energy-reduced eating plan that they are constantly hungry. Both the parents and the child must be reassured that the diet plan is flexible and will change with increasing or decreasing energy needs. Sometimes, parents withhold food when the child's blood sugar levels are high. Parents should be advised that adequate energy intake is the most important principle for the child and if they do need more food, the insulin dosage can be adjusted to allow for increased nutritional needs. Exercise should be encouraged and the child's exercise profile should be taken into account when developing an appropriate eating plan.

18.2.2 CARBOHYDRATE

In adults with diabetes, a dietary carbohydrate intake of approximately 50–55% daily calories is recommended and this should mainly be in the form of high-fiber, complex varieties. The inclusion of high-fiber foods in experimental diets of adults with diabetes improves both blood glucose and lipid control (Reckless, 1984). Data also suggest that the use of high carbohydrate foods in combination with foods high in soluble fiber may decrease post-prandial blood glucose levels in children with diabetes (Kinmonth *et al.*, 1982; Simpson *et al.*, 1981). In addition, children with diabetes who eat more fiber experience better blood glucose control than those with a low-fiber intake (American Academy of Pediatrics, 1981).

It would therefore appear that the incorporation of fiber into the diet would be advantageous, and leguminous and wholegrain cereal foods should be chosen in preference to their low-fiber processed alternatives. The use of soluble fiber (i.e., oats, beans, legumes, citrus fruits) should be emphasized as this seems to be the most effective component in the modulation of blood glucose and lipid levels (Vinik, 1988). A fiber intake of 2 g per 100 kcals each day is a suggested target in school children with diabetes (Kinmonth *et al.*, 1982). However, this will result in substantial changes to the diet of some children and their families. It is therefore recommended that a reasonable first step should be 1 g fiber per 100 kcals each day with particular emphasis on soluble fiber (Kinmonth, 1983). Any increase in the fiber content of the diet should be made gradually to limit flatulence and abdominal distension (Table 18.1).

Many children, especially the younger ones, experience difficulties attaining 50% energy from carbohydrate. Parents should therefore offer what is practically acceptable. Where possible however, dietary carbohydrate intake should not be restricted below the usual average family intake of about 40–45% energy. Caution is necessary when recommending increased fiber consumption for children below 5 years of age. Young children have a smaller physical capacity of food and require a more energy-dense diet

Table 18.1 Suggestions for increasing the fiber content of the diet.

- Use more wholewheat, wholegrain or high-fiber white bread.
- Try a wholewheat or oat-based breakfast cereal – there are a wide variety available in all supermarkets and grocery stores.
- Make more use of beans and legumes, i.e., add beans to stews and casseroles. Beans on toast make an excellent high fiber meal.
- Eat plenty of fruit and vegetables. Try eating potatoes in their skins.
- Experiment using wholewheat flour in baking. Many children do not enjoy the taste of cakes and biscuits made with 100% wholewheat flour so 50% white, 50% wholewheat may be more acceptable.
- Try using brown rice and pasta.

NB It is important to remember that it is not necessary to make all the above changes. The family should be encouraged to chose those which are acceptable to them.

than adults. Overemphasis on bulky high-fiber foods may result in a reduced intake of energy and important nutrients. In addition, there may be impaired mineral absorption (Bindra, 1985). Food refusal, food fads and unconventional eating patterns are extremely common in preschool children and such behavior will cause great anxiety to parents of a child with diabetes. Again, it should be stressed that although fiber intake can be increased gradually in this group, it should only be increased to a level which is practical for that particular child.

In older children, consumption of high-fiber complex carbohydrate in preference to their more refined counterparts should be encouraged. Emphasis on more fruit and vegetables, wholewheat bread, wholewheat breakfast cereals, beans and legumes would substantially increase fiber intake. Potatoes, pasta, rice and baked beans tend to be enjoyed by children and these can contribute to the daily fiber and carbohydrate intake. Children's particular preferences should be taken into account and more refined foods such as white bread and white pasta are still perfectly acceptable and nutritious foods. It is the overall fiber intake which is important and such children can obtain fiber from other sources.

18.2.3 SUCROSE

Many parents believe that it was the sugary foods eaten by their child prior to diagnosis which caused the diabetes. In actual fact, there is no evidence that sucrose is an etiological factor in the development in diabetes (Dept. of Health, 1989). Candy and sugary foods are enjoyed by all children and the total exclusion of dietary sugar is unnecessary. For many years, sugar was proscribed in the diet for individuals with diabetes because it was believed to be rapidly absorbed and thus cause a large rise in the blood glucose level. However, studies have shown that eating small amounts of sucrose does not worsen glycemic control in well-controlled IDDM patients (Bantle *et al.*, 1986). It has also been suggested that allowing modest amounts of sucrose in the diet may enhance palatability and improve compliance with a high-fiber, low-fat diet (Mann, 1987). The British Diabetic Association recommends that small amounts of sucrose can be taken as part of an overall healthy diet, particularly if taken as part of or after a meal. Although total sucrose intake should be kept to a sensible level, there are other important areas in the diet to emphasize such as eating regular meals and cutting down on fatty foods.

For many years, fructose (fruit sugar) was advocated for use in home baking in preference to sucrose. This product can be expensive and has inferior baking properties. More importantly, fructose has not been shown to have any definite advantages over sucrose in long-term use (Anderson *et al.*, 1989). It is now recommended that sucrose is used in home baking (up to 25 g per day), in conjunction with high-fiber, low-fat ingredients. Recipes can easily be adapted to include substantially less sucrose than traditionally advocated with perfectly acceptable results. Such a move has resulted in the baking of 'healthy' cakes, which can be prepared for the whole family rather than 'diabetic' cakes which are specifically made for the child with diabetes (Table 18.2).

Specially-formulated diabetic foods, i.e., cakes, cookies and candy have been available for many years and originated in a era where sucrose consumption was virtually forbidden and carbohydrate intake was regulated at unduly low levels. Today, children can incorporate ordinary cakes and cookies into their diet plan and the need for such specialized products is no longer considered to be necessary (British Diabetic Association, 1992b). In addition, many products have a high fat and calorie content which does not make them compatible with healthy eating

Table 18.2 Suggestions for reducing the sugar content of the diet.

- Substitute high-sugar foods and drinks with the reduced-sugar or sugar-free varieties readily available in the shops, i.e., reduced sugar jams and marmalades, sugar-free jello, yogurts, desserts and drinks.
- Try to take tea, coffee and breakfast cereals without added sugar. If sweetness is still required, artificial sweeteners can be used. Artificial sweeteners can also be used to sweeten many puddings and desserts.
- Reducing the amount of sugar used in home-baked cakes and cookies can result in perfectly satisfactory results. Often the amount of sugar can be reduced by one-half of that traditionally used.

advice. The sweetening agents usually used, i.e., fructose, isomalt and sorbitol, can have a laxative effect especially in young children. Today, there is a growing range of reduced-sugar/sugar-free products such as jams, yogurts, jello and soft drinks readily available in the shops. These foods can be enjoyed by the whole family without the child with diabetes being singled out as requiring special products.

Artificial sweeteners (e.g., aspartame, acesulphame K and saccharin) can be used in preference to sugar for sweetening custards, puddings, drinks and cereals. In addition, they are now used in a wide variety of commercially prepared sugar-free or 'diet' products. Guidelines on the acceptable daily intake (ADI) of the three above mentioned sweeteners have been defined. In the UK, the ADI for saccharin is up to 5 mg/kg body weight, for aspartame 40 mg/kg body weight and for acesulfame potassium, 9 mg/kg body weight. Unfortunately, there are very little data pertaining to sweetener intake in children. One study showed that adults with diabetes were not exceeding the ADIs for the above sweeteners except for a small minority who were exceeding the ADI for saccharin (MAFF, 1990). Due to their smaller body size, and possibly greater consumption of sugar-free products, children with diabetes may be potentially more likely to exceed the ADIs for the various sweeteners than adults and further consumption studies are needed. It would therefore appear prudent to advise that sweetener consumption in children be maintained within the acceptable level and that a variety of sweeteners be used to decrease the possibility of excessive use of any one variety.

18.2.4 FAT

After the child reaches two years of age, the diet should be slowly changed to one which is lower in fat. However, as previously indicated, young children have a smaller food capacity than adults and need a more energy-dense diet. Overemphasis on fat restriction can lead to a reduction in energy intake. Food fads in the under 5s may be exaggerated by the impalatability of low-fat foods. In addition, diarrhea in this group may be caused by the more rapid gastric emptying caused by a diet low in fat (Cohen *et al.*, 1979). Fully-skimmed cows' milk should not be given to under 5s as it contains insufficient vitamin A and too little fat (and therefore energy). If desired, semi-skimmed (lower-fat) milk can be introduced after the age of two providing the child's diet is nutritionally adequate.

Adults with diabetes have an increased risk of cardiovascular disease compared with age and sex-matched peers (Dorman *et al.*, 1984). In addition, there is evidence that adolescents with IDDM have mildly disturbed cardiovascular risk profiles compared with nondiabetic siblings (Cruickshanks *et al.*, 1985). Such a finding emphasizes the fact that diabetes is a disorder of carbohydrate and lipid metabolism and reduction of fat intake in the schoolchild with diabetes should be a priority. The diet advocated should aim to keep low, very low and high density lipoprotein (LDL, VDL and HDL) cholesterol levels as close to normal as possible for age and sex. The British Diabetic Association (1992a) recommend that fat intake be reduced to 30–35% energy with saturated fats contributing less then 10%, polyunsaturated fats contributing less then 10% and mono-unsaturated fats 10–15% of energy intake.

An emphasis on increased consumption of high-fiber starchy foods has enabled reductions in fat intake to be made without resulting in hunger. Potato chips, French fries and other fatty foods tend to be popular with children and adolescents, and it is not appropriate to omit such foods from the diet altogether. Compromises should be made where possible (for example halving the number of bags of potato chips eaten each week); such a move may achieve more success than if inflexible, dogmatic advice is given (Table 18.3).

Table 18.3 Suggestions for reducing the fat content of the diet.

- Cut down on high-fat snack foods such as French fries, potato chips, nuts and burgers.
- Try to avoid frying foods – where possible, cook by some other method which does not include adding fat such as baking, boiling and grilling.
- In older children, cut down on the amount of full-fat dairy products eaten, i.e., butter, cream and full-fat cheese. There are many reduced fat varieties available in the shops. Use skimmed or semi-skimmed milk instead of full fat.
- Watch the amount of cakes, cookies and pastries eaten as these tend to be high in fat.
- Choose leaner cuts of meat when possible and remove the skin from poultry. Try to eat more fish.

NB It is important to note that it is not necessary to make all the above changes. The family should be encouraged to choose those which are acceptable to them.

18.2.5 PROTEIN

Children with diabetes do not have increased protein requirements when compared with their nondiabetic peers. The protein requirements of children have been documented in the report *Dietary Reference Values for Food Energy and Nutrients for the United Kingdom* (Department of Health, 1991). Until recently, protein foods were often referred to as 'free foods' and as a consequence of a fairly restricted carbohydrate intake, children were encouraged to fill up on these foods. This resulted in many children eating well over the recommended level of protein. High-protein foods, especially those of animal origin (meat, cheese and milk) tend to be high in saturated fat. Whole-protein foods of vegetable origin, such as beans and legumes, have the advantage of being associated with dietary fiber and complex carbohydrate.

Some studies have indicated that in the early stages of renal damage, a reduction in protein intake may reduce albuminuria and glomerular filtration rate (Viberti, 1988). Present evidence for this is not conclusive but does support the view that individuals with diabetes should avoid higher than average protein intakes (British Diabetic Association, 1992a).

18.2.6 SALT

Although it is not clear whether sodium restriction will help to decrease the prevalence of hypertension in children and adolescents with diabetes, avoidance of excessive salt intake is probably a good nutritional principle. Children with diabetes may have a higher sodium intake than their peers because of an emphasis on salty rather then sweet foods (Hackett *et al.*, 1988). A small but significant relationship has been shown between sodium intake and blood pressure in infancy (Hofman *et al.*, 1983) and therefore, moderation in salt intake should be the aim for people with diabetes of all ages. There are no clear guidelines for children with diabetes but adults with diabetes are advised to restrict salt intake to 6 g/day and reduce it further to 3 g/day if hypertension is present (European Association for the Study of Diabetes, 1988).

18.2.7 ALCOHOL

Some adolescents do drink underage, albeit illegally, so it is vital that all young adults be given sensible advice about drinking alcohol. Many people mistakenly believe that since many drinks contain carbohydrate, alcohol will increase the blood glucose level. In fact, hypoglycemia is the most common danger in combining alcohol with IDDM. Alcohol metabolism impairs gluconeogenesis. It also suppresses the release of the counter-regulatory hormones which promote glycogenolysis and inhibits hepatic conversion of glycogen to glucose. Such actions block the body's ability to raise its own blood glucose levels. General guidelines on alcohol consumption are given in Table 18.4.

Table 18.4 General guidelines for alcohol consumption.

- It is illegal to sell alcohol to persons under the age of 18 years in the UK (21 in the USA).
- Never drink and drive.
- Alcohol should be restricted to 3 units per day for men and 2 units per day for women and it is advisable to have 2–3 alcohol-free days each week (1 unit of alcohol equals ½ pint beer/lager or cider, 1 pub measure spirit, 1 small glass of sherry, 1 standard glass of wine or 1 pub measure liqueur).
- Don't drink on an empty stomach. Always have something to eat with your drink or shortly afterwards. Alcohol should not be substituted for your usual meals and the carbohydrate content of alcohol should not be counted into the diet.
- All types of alcohol drinks tend to be high in calories so bear this in mind if you are watching your weight.
- If drinking beer or lager, choose the ordinary varieties (preferably those with an alcohol content of less than 5%). Low-sugar beers tend to be higher in alcohol and are best avoided. Low-alcohol beers and lagers are useful, especially when driving. However, some varieties can be very high in sugar and should be taken in moderation.
- Dry/medium wines are preferable to the sweet varieties. If drinking liqueurs or spirits, add sugar-free mixers.
- Always wear some form of diabetes identification – you and others may confuse a hypo with drunkenness.

18.2.8 EXERCISE

Children with diabetes should be encouraged to exercise, both as a means of improving general fitness but also to aid weight control. Of particular relevance to diabetes, exercise improves insulin sensitivity (Yki-Jarvinen *et al.*, 1984) and improves lipoprotein levels (Franz, 1987) (see also Chapter 19).

Parents and children need advice on how to minimize the risk of hypoglycemia during and after exercise. When physical activity is planned, the insulin dose can be reduced or the carbohydrate intake increased at the previous meal or snack. A child may still need a boost of quick-acting carbohydrate such as a small chocolate bar immediately prior to strenuous exercise. Unfortunately, however, physical activity in children is often spontaneous and energetic. To help prevent hypoglycemia, children should be encouraged to carry a source of quick-acting carbohydrate with them at all times (for example, glucose tablets). Hypoglycemia can occur up to several hours after the exercise has taken place, so extra carbohydrate with the following meal or snack may be necessary.

Some children will be keen to take up specific sports and train on a regular basis e.g., swimming or tennis. It is very difficult to give general advice and a specific daily regimen of insulin and food should be devised after careful monitoring of blood glucose levels and with liaison between the child with diabetes and his or her medical advisers.

18.2.9 RELIGIOUS AND CULTURAL CONSIDERATIONS

Diabetes occurs in all cultures so, to be effective, dietary advice must be sensitive to an individual's cultural and religious practices. It has been well-documented that the incidence of diabetes is higher in adults of Afro-Caribbean origin and from the Asian subcontinent than in the indigenous population (Mather & Keen, 1985). However, it is unclear whether there is an increased incidence of diabetes in the children from these communities.

Most work on ethnic communities has been directed at adults and whether the findings can be extrapolated to children is debatable. British Asian adults with diabetes have been shown to have poorer blood glucose control, awareness of diabetes management and knowledge of complications (Hawthorne, 1990). This finding could be explained by a combination of environmental and genetic factors, poor housing, stress, unemployment, poverty, poor dietary education and communication difficulties.

In the Asian community, there is a wide diversity of language, tradition, religion, origin and class. All the above factors will influence dietary practices but care must be taken not to make generalizations.

The religious beliefs of the parents will influence the dietary practices of their children. For example, Jains (a Hindu sect) are strict vegetarians whereas Mirpuri Pakistanis will eat meat as long as it is Halal and not pork. Ramadan, the Moslem religious fast may also affect dietary intake. During Ramadan, individuals are expected to fast during the hours of daylight. Pregnant women, children and the sick are exempt from the fast but are expected to make up the days missed at a later stage. In practice, many prefer to fast with everyone else.

Rastafarianism and Seventh Day Adventists are more common in the Afro-Caribbean community and each religion has their own beliefs surrounding food. Rastafarians believe in consuming 'Ital' foods which are naturally unprocessed foods, grown and prepared without chemicals and additives. Some Rastafarians may be vegetarian or lacto-ovo-vegetarian. Seventh Day Adventists do not eat fish without fins or scales, pork or pork products. They do not drink alcohol or drinks which are regarded as stimulants, such as tea or coffee. Many are vegetarian.

Within the Asian community, although the children may be able to speak and read English, their parents and in particular their mothers may not. They will rely on other family members to interpret written material and the spoken word and this is not always ideal, especially if the interpreter is a child. It is therefore advantageous if diet information can also be presented in the appropriate language.

In both the Asian and Afro-Caribbean communities, food traditions are strong. Many families still eat traditional meals, even if the parents were born in the UK. Obviously, some Westernized foods will be consumed but the extent of this varies between families. Where possible, health professionals should emphasize the positive attributes of the traditional diet rather than suggest changes more appropriate to a Westernized diet. It is important to remember that actual dietary intake may be influenced to a large extent by poverty and socioeconomic deprivation and should not be automatically attributed to religious and cultural practices.

18.3 PRACTICAL CONSIDERATIONS

After a child has been diagnosed, parents are often bombarded with information on insulin injections and blood-testing techniques. Although it is important that the parents see a dietitian quite soon after diagnosis to alleviate any fears or misconceptions, it is vital that any information given is short and practical. This advice should aim to avoid large swings in the blood glucose level and should therefore emphasize eating regular meals, eating complex carbohydrate at each meal and avoiding concentrated sugary foods and drinks.

Subsequent consultations with the dietitian will help build up a clearer picture of the family's and child's normal eating habits and lifestyle. Do the parents work and will this influence meal timing and composition? What time are lunch and breaks at school? Does the child participate in after-school activities? Are there any foods which the family will not eat due to religious beliefs? The ethnic origin of the family will have a particular effect on the eating habits of the child and this must be taken into account.

Where possible, the family should be encouraged to adopt a similar eating pattern so that the child with diabetes is not having to eat specially-prepared meals. Initially, meals and snacks should remain familiar and simple. Once the family is more comfortable with the diabetes, further advice on incorporating more fiber and less fat into the diet can be given. Regularity of meals should be stressed and food intake matched to the anticipated rise and fall in insulin levels. Chaotic schedules and irregular meal times make it very difficult to control blood glucose levels.

Ideally, carbohydrate intake should provide approximately 50% of daily energy intake. Table 18.5 shows the grams of carbohydrate required to be eaten each day to provide 50% of the energy intake for a child at a given age. As previously discussed, many children find it difficult to consume this amount of carbohydrate, especially younger children, and advice should be amended accordingly.

Once an acceptable carbohydrate intake has been determined, the dietitian must translate this information into a format which is meaningful to the parents and the child. The carbohydrate exchange system is widely taught in the UK. Major sources of carbohydrate in the diet are tabled in quantities which provide approximately 10 g of carbohydrate (Table 18.6). One 'exchange' is equivalent to 10 g of carbohydrate. The carbohydrate for the day will be distributed be-

Table 18.5 Amount of carbohydrate (CHO) to provide 50% daily energy intake based on expected average requirements for energy.

	Boys		Girls	
Age in years	EAR (kcals/day)	CHO (g/day)	EAR (kcals/day)	CHO (g/day)
1–3	1230	164	1165	155
4–6	1715	228	1545	206
7–10	1970	262	1740	232
11–14	2220	296	1845	246
15–18	2755	367	2110	281

NB Expected Average Requirements (EARs) for energy based on Department of Health's Dietary Reference Values. EARs are based on present lifestyles and activity levels.

Table 18.6 Approximate amounts of food containing 10 g carbohydrate.

Food items	Approximate measure
Wholewheat bread	1 thin slice
Potato	1 small
Shredded Wheat	1 biscuit
Bran Flakes	5 tablespoons
Digestive type biscuit	1
Crackers, plain	2
Rice	3 tbsp (cooked)
Apple	1
Orange	1
Banana	1
Milk	⅓ pint
Fruit yogurt (diet)	1 small carton

tween main meals and snacks and the actual distribution will depend on the child's life-style and the duration and mode of action of the insulin injected. Such a system has attracted considerable debate recently, mainly in response to work on the glycemic index which shows that foods containing similar amounts of carbohydrate may produce different effects on the blood glucose level (Jenkins *et al.*, 1981).

The blood glucose response to a food is governed by many factors apart from actual carbohydrate content such as the fat, protein or dietary fiber content, the physical form of the food and the water content. In addition, it has been estimated that the food tables from which the carbohydrate value of various foods is calculated are likely to be accurate only to within 10–20% (Stockley, 1988). It would therefore appear to be unnecessary and impractical to advise strict weighing-out of foods and many centers now advocate that household measures be used instead, i.e., cupfuls, spoonfuls, whole potatoes, whole slices of bread.

Children's appetites do vary on a day-to-day basis so specified amounts of carbohydrate for each meal are often unacceptable. It is preferable to advocate an upper and lower limit for each meal and snack which would take into account normal fluctuations in appetites. This will alleviate problems at mealtimes where parents try to force their reluctant child to eat the extra slice of bread or potato to make up their carbohydrate allowance. Worse still, a genuinely hungry child may be denied some extra potato because his or her carbohydrate allowance does not allow for this.

Some centers use very simplified versions of the carbohydrate exchange system and do not teach in terms of carbohydrate. In contrast they may encourage the child to choose a certain number of foods at each meal (i.e., 4–5) from a simple list of common carbohydrate-containing foods. The list may consist of foods such as slice of bread, a medium-size potato, a small bowl of cereal, or a piece of fruit. However, no single technique of teaching diet is superior and the choice of method used should be based on the individual's needs.

Both the parents and child should be reassured that the dietary regime given is flexible and can be changed in accordance with the child's individual requirements. The insulin regimen should fit the child's eating habits as far as possible and not vise versa as in the past. A more relaxed attitude to carbohydrate-containing foods may help provide a more balanced view of good nutrition.

18.3.1 BABIES AND INFANTS

The diagnosis of diabetes in a baby is uncommon but when it does occur it poses specific problems in dietary management. Babies with diabetes have the same basic nutritional requirements as other infants. A mother who wishes to breast feed should be encouraged to do so and the normal night-feed will help to prevent nocturnal hypoglycemia. Once the infant is sleeping throughout the night, expert advice regarding the insulin regimen may be needed to prevent hypoglycemia.

After the age of 3 months, babies may require solid foods and commonly accepted weaning foods such as rice-based cereals and fruit purees can be given. Many parents understandably worry about hypoglycemia but the regular meal pattern will help maintain acceptable blood glucose control.

As the child develops, both the parents and the child will be faced with issues which test their confidence in coping with diabetes. Food fads and food refusal are notoriously common in toddlers, and parents need information, reassurance, support and most importantly flexible, practical, and realistic meal-planning advice.

18.3.2 SCHOOL CHILDREN

Schoolchildren are naturally anxious for peer approval and may be reluctant to eat meals and foods different to their friends. Advice should be realistic. Suggesting that a child has fruit every day at mid-morning break when everyone else is eating potato chips will result in the fruit piling up in the child's locker and the child using their money to buy the potato chips anyway. Compromises must be made. Children should be taught to make good food choices from school lunches but unfortunately, in many schools the opportunity for healthy choices is limited. Parents may have to accept that the school lunch is not going to be ideal but they can try to ensure that the breakfast and evening meal compensates for this.

Birthday parties are a common and extremely enjoyable social event in the young schoolchild's life. The child with diabetes should be encouraged to join in the fun and as these events are usually very energy-intensive, there will be some flexibility to eat the party goodies which are presented there. Often the birthday cake and candy are given to the children to take home with them and these can be incorporated into the child's diet at a later stage.

Children with diabetes (and their parents) should see a dietitian every 2–3 months to discuss progress and to make any necessary adjustment to the diet plan. These visits also provide an opportunity for ongoing education and reinforcement of advice.

18.3.3 TEENAGERS

Teenage years can be very difficult for any adolescent and the dietitian will need to be able to teach these young people how best to fit such typical teen activities such as late-night snacking, eating fast foods, and erratic mealtimes into their lifestyle. Many younger children are managed on two insulin injections a day. However, as they move towards adolescence many require a more flexible insulin regime (see Chapter 17). Multiple injection regimens allow greater flexibility with meal timing and quantities. However, such a regimen does require commitment to blood glucose monitoring and a good understanding of insulin and dietary interaction.

18.4 CONCLUSION

In summary, it is vital that the dietary plan be compatible with the child's lifestyle. More importantly, it should be realistic and flexible. Where possible, the whole family should be encouraged to adopt a healthy diet rather then the child with diabetes being singled out for separate meals.

Food is to be enjoyed and it is only through a realistic and consistent approach to diet, that the child will grow up to regard the food he or she eats as making a valuable contribution to diabetes control and well-being.

REFERENCES

American Academy of Pediatrics, Committee on Nutrition. (1981) Plant fibre intake in the pediatric diet. *Pediatrics*, **67**, 572–75.

Anderson, J.W., Story, L.J., Zettwoch, N.C. *et al.* (1989) Metabolic effects of fructose supplementation in diabetic individuals. *Diabetes Care*, **12**, 337–44.

Bantle, J.P., Laine, D.C. and Thomas, J.W. (1986) Metabolic effects of dietary fructose and sucrose in types 1 and 11 diabetic subjects. *J. Am. Med. Assoc.*, **256**, 3241–46.

Bindra, G. (1985) Fibre and phytate. *Nutrition and Food Science*, **95**, 20–21.

British Diabetic Association. (1992a) Dietary recommendations for people with diabetes: An update for the 1990s. *Diabetic Med.*, **9**, 189–202.

British Diabetic Association. (1992b) Discussion paper on the role of 'diabetic' foods. *Diabetic Med.*, **9**, 300–306.

Cohen, S.A., Hendricks, K.M. and Eastham, E.J. *et al.* (1979) Chronic non-specific diarrhea: A complication of dietary fat restriction. *Am. J. Dis. in Child.*, **133**, 490–92.

Cruickshank, K.J., Orchard, T.J. and Becker, D.J. (1985) The cardiovascular risk profile of adolescents with insulin-dependent diabetes mellitus. *Diabetes Care*, **8**, 118–24.

D'Antonio, J.A., Ellis, D., Doft, B.H. *et al.* (1989) Diabetes complications and glycemia control. The Pittsburgh prospective insulin depdendent diabetes cohort study status report after 5 years of IDDM. *Diabetes Care*, **12**, 694–700.

Department of Health, Committee on Medical Aspects of Food Policy. (1989) *Dietary Sugars and Human Disease*. Report on health and social subjects 37. HMSO, London.

Department of Health. (1991) *Dietary Reference Values for Food Energy and Nutrients for the United Kingdom*. Report on Health and Social Subjects 41. HMSO, London.

Dorman, J.S., Laporte, R.D., Kuller, L.H. *et al.* (1984) The Pittsburgh insulin-dependent diabetes mellitus (IDDM) morbidity and mortality study: mortality results. *Diabetes*, **33**, 271–76.

European Association for the Study of Diabetes, Nutrition Study Group. (1988) Nutritional recommendations for individuals with diabetes mellitus. *Diabetes, Nutrition and Metabolism*, **1**, 145–49.

Franz, M.J. (1987) Exercise and the management of diabetes mellitus. *J. Am. Dietetic Assoc.*, **87**, 872–80.

Hackett, A.F., Court, S., McCowen, C. *et al.* (1988) Urinary sodium excretion in diabetic children. *Acta Paed. Scand.*, **77**, 757–58.

Hawthorne, K. (1990) Asian diabetics attending a British hospital clinic: a pilot study to evalulate their care. *Brit. J. Gen. Pract.*, **40**, 243–47.

Hofman, A., Hazebroek, A. and Valkenburgh, H.A. (1983) A randomised trial of sodium intake and blood pressure in newborn infants. *J. Am. Med. Assoc.*, **250**, 370–73.

Jenkins, D.J.A., Wolever, T.M.S., Taylor, R.H. *et al.* (1981) Glycaemic index of food: a physiological basis for carbohydrate exchange. *Am. J. Clin. Nutrition*, **34**, 362–66.

Kinmonth, A.L. (1983) 'Studies on diet and diabetic control in childhood'. MD Thesis, Cambridge University, 1–318.

Kinmonth, A.L., Angus, R.M., Jenkins, P.A. *et al.* (1982) Whole foods and increased fibre improves blood glucose control in diabetic children. *Arch. Dis. Child.*, **57**, 187–94.

Mann, J.I. (1987) Simple sugars and diabetes. *Diabetic Med.*, **4**, 135–39.

MAFF (Ministry of Agriculture, Fisheries and Food). (1990) *Intakes of Intense and Bulk Sweeteners in the UK 1987–1988*. Food surveillance paper No. 29. HMSO, London.

Mather, H.M. and Keen, H. (1985) Southall Diabetes Survey: prevalence of known diabetes. *Brit. Med. J.*, **291**, 1081–84.

Reckless, J.P.D. (1984) 'Fibre in the diet of the diabetic and its effects on blood lipids', in *Dietary fibre in the management of the Diabetic*, pp. 15–20. Medical Education Services, Oxford.

Simpson, H.C.R., Mann, J.I., Lousley, S. *et al.* (1981) A high carbohydrate leguminous fibre diet improves all aspects of diabetic control. *Lancet*, **1**, 1–5.

Stockley, L. (1988) Food composition tables in the calculation of the nutrient content of mixed diets. *J. Hum. Nutr. and Diet.*, **1**, 187–95.

Viberti, G.C. (1988) Low-protein diet and progression of diabetic kidney disease. *Nephrology Dialysis Transplant*, **3**, 334–39.

Vinik, A.L. and Jenkins, D.J.A. (1988) Dietary fibre in the management of diabetes. *Diabetes Care*, **11**, 160–73.

Yki-Jarvinen, H., Defronzo, R.A. and Koivisto, V.A. (1984) Normalization of insulin sensitivity in type 1 diabetic subjects by physical training during insulin pump therapy. *Diabetes Care*, **7**, 520–27.

19

Exercise

S.A. GREENE and C. THOMPSON

Exercise in children and adolescents with type 1 insulin-dependent diabetes mellitus (IDDM) is associated frequently with disturbance of metabolic control, often producing clinical symptoms. This chapter describes these clinical problems, reviewing their physiologic and metabolic basis. A strategy of management is outlined for the routine type of exercise seen in childhood and practical suggestions are given for the approach to sporadic exercise.

19.1 CLINICAL PROBLEMS

Exercise, frequently intense in its nature and random in its timing, features a great deal in children's lives and constitutes an additional dimension in the task of controlling blood glucose concentration. In the nondiabetic child, blood glucose remains in the physiologic range throughout a period of exercise, regardless of its intensity or duration. The blood glucose may rise (Richter *et al.*, 1992) or fall to the lower range of normal during severe prolonged exercise but without affecting physical performance (Felig *et al.*, 1982). This is in marked contrast to diabetic children in whom the blood glucose response to physical exercise is variable, giving rise to different clinical reactions. Hypoglycemia is the commonest unwanted reaction, and may occur during or shortly after a severe bout of exercise, or several hours later. Hyperglycemia can also occur, especially if blood glucose and total ketones are abnormally high at the start of the exercise (Berger *et al.*, 1977).

19.1.1 HYPOGLYCEMIA

The fall in blood glucose in association with exercise in diabetic children can produce clinical symptoms which may be severe, especially if initially overlooked or disregarded due to the excitement of the exercise event. The predisposition to this fall in blood glucose is influenced by several factors:

- Pre-exercise blood glucose concentration
- Pre-exercise plasma free insulin concentration
- Workload performed – duration and intensity
- Timing of exercise in relation to
  - insulin injection
  - intake of carbohydrate
- Physical fitness.

Hypoglycemia may also develop several hours after the exercise, with a fall in blood glucose concentration during the following night and early the next morning presenting a particular problem (MacDonald, 1987)

Rapid onset of hypoglycemia is seen in

Childhood and Adolescent Diabetes
Published in 1994 by Chapman & Hall, London
ISBN 0 412 48610 5

sudden exercise of high intensity. Most children will stop with the onset of symptoms or be recognized to be hypoglycemic by parents or carers. The association of hypoglycemia with the exercise is made quickly and evasive action can be taken. This contrasts with the post-exercise hypoglycemia which occurs several hours (even up to 24 hours) after the event. The connection between exercise and the hypoglycemia is frequently not made and the child may 'drift' into the problem with often a more severe clinical outcome.

19.1.2 HYPERGLYCEMIA AND KETOSIS

High blood glucose indicates relative insulin deficiency, particularly in association with an elevation of total ketones. In this situation the metabolic response to exercise (in the child with diabetes) may be a rise in blood glucose and a further increase in total ketones, blood lactate and pyruvate. Ketoacidosis may follow, particularly in the poorly-controlled diabetic (Berger *et al.*, 1977). This response may be seen more frequently in the adolescent with diabetes, where erratic insulin administration is a known phenomenon (see Chapter 26).

19.1.3 ATTITUDES TO EXERCISE

During the child's progression from school-age to adolescence, exercise is performed on an increasingly regular basis for some teenagers and becomes the central feature in their daily life. This offers an opportunity for the well-organized and suitably motivated diabetic youth to plan his or her daily routine to accommodate a period of exercise with particular reference to the avoidance of extremes of hyperglycemia or hypoglycemia. For the majority of children, there is a decrease in participation in sports as they become older (Boreham *et al.*, 1993). Exercise in this age group when it does occur is unplanned and an unusual phenomenon.

We assessed the daily activity in our clinic of 50 diabetic children and adolescents, comparing them with 50 nondiabetic subjects. While reassuringly most diabetic subjects and their families undertook similar activities, with an expected difference in their dietary habits around the exercise, disappointingly, fewer diabetic children were involved in team sports and there was less participation in parties with difficulty in making friends. Parents of young diabetic children socialized less frequently outside of the family environment. These aspects mitigate even more against diabetic children and teenagers pursuing sporting activities into young adult life.

For other children and their families the uncertainty of the metabolic effects of exercise may introduce additional anxieties and conflicts, further disturbing the so-called 'normality' of their lifestyle. The unpredictable effects of exercise on the metabolic state of the diabetic child make its use as a therapeutic tool in the control of blood glucose difficult, despite the traditional belief that it constitutes a cornerstone in the therapeutic 'triad' of diabetes (insulin, diet and exercise). An understanding of the physiologic and biochemical reactions to exercise, both in nondiabetic and diabetic children, may explain some of the apparently erratic metabolic reactions to exercise, in addition to providing a guide to its practical management.

19.2 METABOLIC AND HORMONAL RESPONSE TO PHYSICAL EXERCISE

19.2.1 REGULATION OF FUEL SUPPLY IN NORMAL CHILDREN

The sources of energy used during exercise depend on the intensity and duration of the exercise and the physical fitness of the child. The small energy requirement for resting muscles is supplied mostly in the form of free fatty acids (FFA), derived from the oxidation of fat. The much greater requirement of exercising muscle is supplied for the first 2 or 3 minutes only by energy stores in the muscle itself. The first few contractions of the muscle are sustained by a small intracellular depot of adenosine triphosphate (ATP) and the following few minutes of muscular work are maintained by endogenous stores of muscle glycogen. After this the muscle relies on the availability of additional fuels derived from other body stores.

As intensity and duration of the exercise increase, the relative importance of the different fuel sources varies (Ahlborg *et al.*, 1974). During exercise at less than 75% of the individual's maximum work capacity, the utilization of glucose for energy is as great or often greater than that of fat. The peak of glucose utilization is reached at about 1–2 hours and fat then becomes the predominant fuel. Fat is available to muscle either as triglyceride stored within muscle (endogenous), or as one of the fat fuels present in the blood. These include long chain fatty acids, betahydroxybutyrate and acetoacetate, triglycerides and glycerol. Fatty acids in the blood are derived from triglyceride stored in adipose tissue and ketones are formed from the partial oxidation of fatty acids in the liver. Triglyceride is present in the blood predominantly in the form of very low density lipoproteins (VLDL) from which triglycerides can be made available for oxidation to supply energy in the muscle by the enzyme lipoprotein lipase (Marette *et al.*, 1992). The percentage contribution of these various fuel sources can be altered by the physical fitness of the individual. With physical training, various enzymatic changes occur which allow the subject to utilize substrates derived from fat more efficiently and over a longer period of time (Richter *et al.*, 1992).

Exhaustion of the muscle may depend upon several factors. Depletion of ATP and an accumulation of lactate within the muscle are likely to be of prime importance. Lactate production develops from the anaerobic oxidation of carbohydrate secondary to lack of oxygen; the subsequent rise in intracellular pH secondary to the increased lactate concentration may impede muscle cell performance. Stored muscle glycogen is rapidly depleted and circulating blood glucose must be replenished from hepatic reserves of glycogen. It is possible that a local reduction in stored muscle glycogen may affect transmission of nerve impulses to the muscle fibers (Newsholme & Start, 1981); this would further add to the metabolic changes within the muscle cells leading to an inability to perform further muscular work.

Thus, continuing muscular exercise requires the mobilization of both free fatty acids from triglyceride stores and increased glucose production from the liver, coupled with a continuing supply of oxygen to muscle mitochondria. The mobilization of these fuels is secondary to intricate hormonal changes that occur during exercise. The result is a blood glucose concentration that remains steady within the normal physiologic range, despite the enormous flux of glucose from liver to muscle that occurs during and following exercise.

19.2.2 HORMONAL CHANGES DURING EXERCISE IN NORMAL SUBJECTS

Exercise induces a dramatic rise in the glucose utilization by the working muscle. The increased supply of glucose necessary to maintain a steady supply of this important fuel is derived from an increased hepatic production of glucose (Wasserman & Zinker, 1992). During exercise, plasma levels of insulin decrease whereas levels of epinephrine are increased (Zinman *et al.*, 1977; Christensen *et al.*, 1979). These changes augment the hepatic content of cyclic AMP and consequently stimulate gluconeogenesis. There is also a rise in concentration of growth

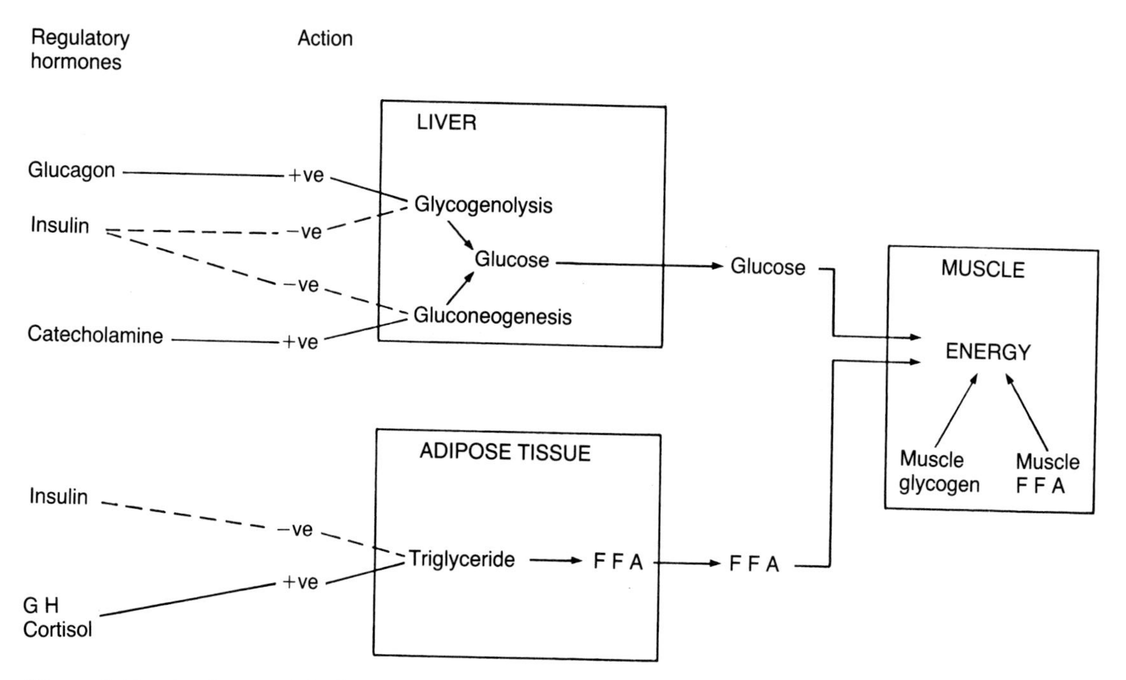

Figure 19.1 A scheme of the hormonal changes known to occur during exercise in normal nondiabetic subjects.

hormone and glucocorticoids (Hartley *et al.*, 1972) which stimulates increased lipolysis in adipose tissue. A scheme of the hormonal changes known to occur during exercise is shown in Figure 19.1.

Although hepatic glycogenolysis accounts for glucose production in the initial exercise phase, gluconeogenesis from lactate, alanine and glycerol becomes the major source of glucose in the blood as exercise proceeds (Wahren, 1979). Insulin and glucagon do not appear to have a direct influence on this process as gluconeogenesis can still proceed despite the abolition of insulin and glucagon actions by somatostatin (Bjorkmen *et al.*, 1981). Catecholamines, however, do appear to be of importance; stimulation of the splanchnic nerves increases hepatic glucose production and blockade with propranolol prevents glucose production and release from the liver despite catecholamine stimulation (Galbo *et al.*, 1976).

19.2.3 METABOLIC AND HORMONE RESPONSE IN INSULIN DEPENDENT DIABETES

In insulin-dependent diabetes, the normal intricate hormonal balance is disturbed, with inappropriately high or low insulin levels at various times throughout the day and night. Consequently, the metabolic and hormonal responses to exercise of children with diabetes are variable and differ from those of their normal peers (Table 19.1).

Well-insulinized children with diabetes respond to exercise with an increase in plasma free insulin (Figure 19.2; Greene *et al.*, 1985). This is secondary to an increased mobilization of insulin from injection sites which may vary

Table 19.1 Major fuel and hormone changes during exercise in healthy and diabetic children (well-insulinized and insulin-deficient).

		Diabetic	
	Normal	Well-insulinized	Insulin-deficient
Insulin	↓	↑	→
Glucose	→	↓	↑
Total ketones	↓	↓	↑
Glucagon Catecholamines Growth hormone Cortisol	↑	↑	↑

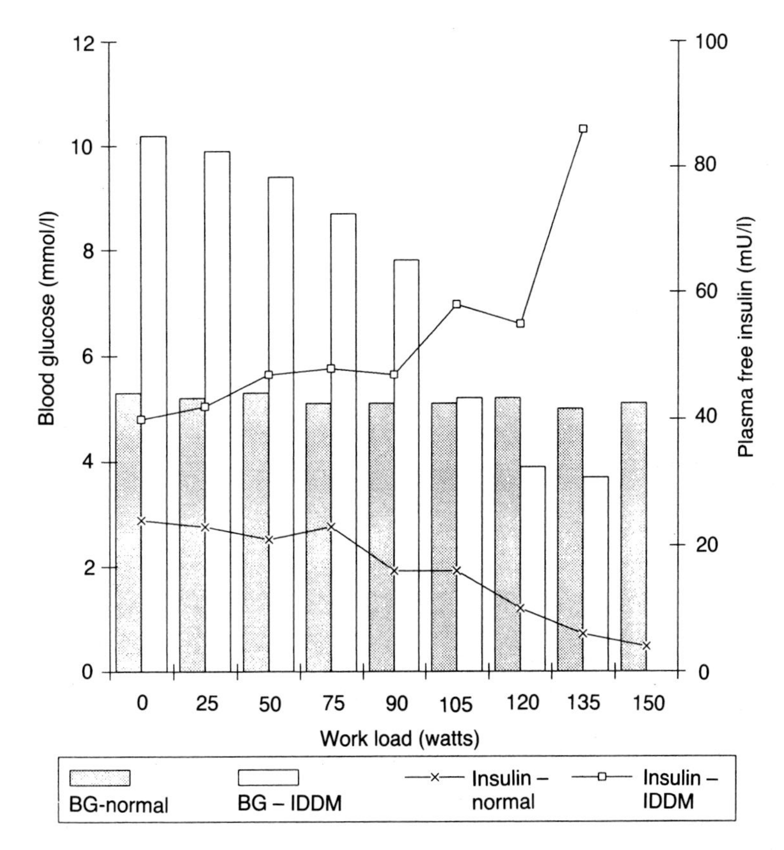

Figure 19.2 The changes in blood glucose and plasma free insulin concentrations in diabetic (n = 9) and normal nondiabetic age-matched controls (n = 9). All subjects exercised to exhaustion in a step-wise program on a bicycle ergometer, with incremental changes in work every four minutes.

Plasma-free insulin fell in all of the normal subjects, whereas there was an increase in insulin in all of the diabetic children. Their diabetes was treated with conventional twice-daily insulin preparations and the exercise took place between 16.00 and 17.00 h, 4–5 hours after lunch, prior to the evening insulin injection.

Blood glucose remained constant in the nondiabetic subjects but dropped precipitately in the diabetic group. One subject became clinically hypoglycemic at the end of the exercise period.

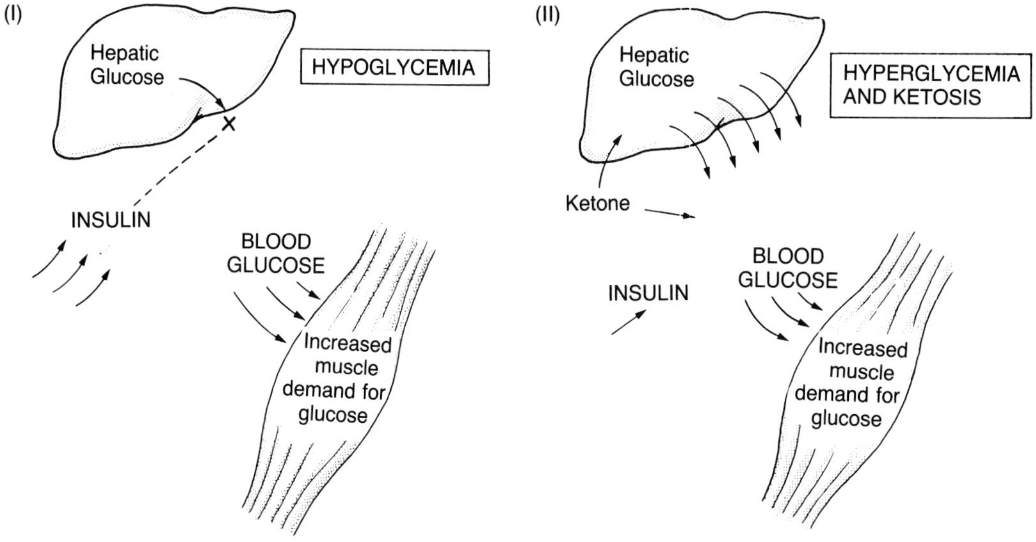

Figure 19.3 Schematic presentation of the consequence of exercising in the well-insulinized (I) and the insulin-deficient state (II).

with the nature of the exercise itself and the anatomical position of the depot of injected insulin (Wahren *et al.*, 1975); the latter, however, has been questioned (Kemmer *et al.*, 1979), and appears in clinical practice to make little difference to blood glucose changes with exercise (Susstrunk *et al.*, 1981). High circulating plasma insulin levels suppress hepatic glucose production. In the face of an increased rate of glucose uptake by working muscles, blood glucose falls. Despite these large differences in blood glucose response to exercise between well-insulinized diabetic children and normal nondiabetic children, the response to maximum exercise of lactate and total ketones is similar for both groups (Greene *et al.*, 1983).

A hypoglycemic response to exercise is not seen in diabetic children with low insulin levels. If insulin levels are low enough to be associated with a high blood glucose and ketone concentration (in one study glucose greater than 18 mmol/l and a total ketone concentration greater than 2 mmol/l; Berger *et al.*, 1977), then exercise may result in hyperglycemia and increasing ketosis. This appears to be due to the lower circulating insulin levels allowing continuous hepatic production of glucose and increased lipolysis which yields free fatty acids for muscle energy production but leads to the accumulation of ketones (Figure 19.3).

Blood glucose levels in insulin-treated children fluctuate considerably throughout the day (Griffin *et al.*, 1980). Part of this fluctuation may relate to a circadian rhythm in insulin sensitivity at a cellular level. The 'dawn phenomenon' of the rising insulin requirement before breakfast (Schmidt *et al.*, 1982) is an example of such a rhythm. As a result, exercise at different times of the day in a diabetic child may produce differing blood glucose reactions despite a similar rise in plasma free insulin (Greene, 1985). Post-breakfast exercise does not produce a fall in blood glucose; indeed the level of blood glucose may continue to rise despite the exercise.

The response to exercise in patients receiving continuous subcutaneous insulin infusion (pump insulin) may differ from that in subjects on conventional therapy. Insulin levels do not appear to rise so strikingly and consequently post-exercise hypoglycemia in this well-insulinized group is less of a clinical problem (Greene *et al.*, 1983).

19.3 PHYSICAL TRAINING AND DIABETES

Several changes occur following a period of sustained regular physical exercise over a period of three months or more. Skeletal muscle undergoes both enzymatic and structural changes. These have been studied in adults with diabetes using muscle biopsy techniques. Succinate dehydrogenase, a marker of mitochondrial activity, increases with training (Costill *et al.*, 1979), and a rise in other muscle mitochondrial enzymes has also been noted, in association with decreased plasma cholesterol and increased peripheral insulin sensitivities (Wallberg-Henriksson *et al.*, 1982). Although the fiber composition of skeletal muscle is normal in subjects with long-standing diabetes, the increase in capillary density which occurs in normal adults following physical training appears to be lacking (Saltin *et al.*, 1979).

Oxygen supply to working muscle increases with training partly due to the improved blood supply, but also reflecting in part an increase in the maximal ability of muscle to take up oxygen; this ability to increase maximum oxygen uptake appears intact in diabetic subjects (Wallberg *et al.*, 1981). Therefore, a limiting step in the oxidation of the various fuels in diabetic adults may be a failure to increase the muscle capillary bed following a period of physical training.

The effects of training upon lipid metabolism (a fall in plasma cholesterol and a rise in high density lipoproteins) are similar in diabetic and normal subjects. Furthermore, prolonged physical training leads to a reduction in basement membrane thickening in diabetic subjects similar to that seen in normal adults. These observations suggest that diabetic subjects may be able to respond to physical training in a manner similar to healthy subjects in the prevention of macrovascular disease (Peterson *et al.*, 1980).

There is good evidence to suggest that physical training can improve insulin sensitivity in insulin-treated diabetes (Wallberg & Henriksson *et al.*, 1982; Yki-Jarvinen *et al.*, 1984; Landt *et al.*, 1955) and increased insulin receptor numbers have been reported (Pederson *et al.*, 1980). With increased insulin sensitivity there is a concomitant fall in total daily insulin requirements (Yki-Jarvinen *et al.*, 1984), but there have been conflicting data regarding the effects on glycemic control. Ludvigsson (1980) has suggested that prolonged training could result in an improvement in blood glucose control, but the weight of evidence indicates that even training sufficient to improve insulin sensitivity and physical fitness, and reduce daily insulin requirements is not associated with a sustained improvement in glycemic control (Dahl-Jorgensen *et al.*, 1980; Wallberg-Henriksson *et al.*, 1982; Zinman *et al.*, 1984; Landt *et al.*, 1985). It has been proposed that the lack of improvement in control may be due to the rise in blood glucose which accompanies intense, short-duration exercise (Mitchell *et al.*, 1988) but is far more likely to reflect increased appetite and calorie consumption (Åkerblom *et al.*, 1980; Zinman *et al.*, 1984). However, the availability of home blood glucose monitoring now allows the possibility for a motivated diabetic patient to incorporate exercise and training into their daily routine. Blood glucose control may then be improved by changes in insulin and dietary management in response to the blood glucose control obtained with various exercise patterns.

Many diabetic athletes on conventional diabetic therapy have achieved success on a par with nondiabetic competitors. It remains to be seen whether improved control increases the motivation of children with diabetes to perform exercise by removing the uncertainty of post-exercise hypoglycemia.

19.4 PRACTICAL MANAGEMENT

The clinical advice given to diabetic subjects revolves around two different patterns of exercise: acute random exercise and regular physical training programs.

19.4.1 ACUTE EXERCISE

In children the metabolic response to the exercise will vary depending on the type of exercise, its intensity and duration, relationship to meals, injection time and the time of day at which the exercise is performed. Given these variables it is not surprising that the response appears to be widely different and unpredictable.

Consequently the all-encompassing advice of 'sugar before exercise' seems inappropriate. A more satisfactory approach would include knowledge of the blood glucose and plasma insulin at the time of exercise. An awareness of the potentially different effects of exercise at different times of the day should help the subject understand his own response and react appropriately to avoid extreme symptoms.

Anticipating the exercise with extra carbohydrate, preferably in the form of high-fiber starchy foods, in the meal prior to exercise is easy to accomplish for most children and their families. This will minimize the special precautions or preparations required immediately before or during an exercise period. However, occasionally fast-acting glucose (e.g., dextrose tablets, sweet drinks, chocolate bars) is necessary, especially during a prolonged or intense exercise period. Previous reactions together with observations of the subject's own blood glucose response should identify when this is necessary.

Whether it is usually required or not, the child and his or her family should have fast-acting glucose available for emergency use during and following periods of exercise. Advice should include such details as sewing pockets into sports clothing for carrying glucose tablets and informing school sports staff and school friends about the action to take in the event of hypoglycemia. Manipulation of the daily insulin dose is usually unhelpful in the general management of exercise although reduction in insulin dose may be useful on days when particularly severe exercise is anticipated, e.g., school sports tournaments followed by swimming, or an energetic vacation activity.

Continuous insulin infusion pumps require no alteration for mild exercise and, perhaps surprisingly, the removal of the needle for two hours or so of intense exercise appears to be compatible with the maintenance of blood glucose control (Greene *et al.*, 1983). A summary of a practical approach to the

Table 19.2 A guide to the practical management of exercise in children with insulin-dependent diabetes mellitus.

Exercise Prescription	
Planned	Spontaneous
Monitor response	Monitor response
Alteration of carbohydrate prescription: time, amount, type	
Alteration of insulin regimen: dose, type	
Consider pre/post loading with 'sugar'	Consider pre/post loading with 'sugar'

management of exercise in children with diabetes is given in Table 19.2.

19.4.2 TRAINING PROGRAM

Many of the potentially advantageous metabolic changes that follow physical training in normal people also occur in diabetic subjects. Regular physical activity sustained over many weeks alters the insulin sensitivity and even in the face of increased energy intake the insulin dose may need to be reduced (Larsson, 1980). Disappointingly, perhaps, the limited studies that have been published have not shown sustained improvement in blood glucose control with training (Wallberg *et al.*, 1981). However, other changes have been noted, in particular improvement in blood lipid profiles (Wallberg *et al.*, 1981). In view of this, and in particular of the positive effects of training upon lipid metabolism and the potential reduction in the risk of developing atherolsclerotic disease, we should encourage all diabetic children and teenagers to establish habits of participation in regular sporting activity.

Many studies have reported a general sense of well-being and good health among people undertaking regular exercise. Such feelings may help to motivate patients with diabetes to train in the face of a natural initial concern that such training may put them at an extra risk of hypoglycemia. This concern can be further alleviated by the self-knowledge of the individual's response to exercise which can be obtained from home blood glucose measurements. This is to be encouraged among children wishing to gain the maximum pleasure and benefit from physical sports and games. For many children, exercise itself can act as an introduction to the use of blood glucose monitoring; the association between the need for good control and good athletic performance is readily grasped by most youngsters. The broadening of the concept of athletics to include, for example, disco dancing and roller skating together with all-night parties is useful for the less sportingly inclined!

Table 19.3 Sports which restrict participation for people with insulin-dependent diabetes.

Some restrictions	Total ban on participation
Ballooning	Bobsleigh
Gliding	Boxing
Martial arts	Flying
Motorcycling	Horse racing (jockey)
Parachuting	Motor racing
Power boat racing	Paragliding
Rowing	
Underwater swimming	

19.4.3 CHOICE OF SPORTS

Children and young adults with insulin-dependent diabetes, once they have achieved a degree of independence and conquered the fear of hypoglycemia, are often keen to try a wide variety of sports. There are some sports however, which for predominantly medico-legal reasons, present restrictions to participation of insulin-treated diabetics. A list of such sports is shown in Table 19.3; further details on precise restrictions are available from national diabetic associations. Excluding those sports which place restrictions on participation however, youngsters should be encouraged to pursue their interest in whichever sport they enjoy.

19.5 SUMMARY

With an improvement in the knowledge of the control of blood glucose during exercise and the possibility of documenting the children's personal reactions to exercise, the extremes of blood glucose variably after exercise can be prevented. Used sensibly as a therapeutic tool, exercise can serve as a cornerstone in the management of diabetes in childhood. In view of the changes in blood lipids, blood rheology and the reduction in capillary basement membrane thickening, it may well be that long-term physical training will be shown to be useful in the prevention of diabetic macrovascular disease.

In the future it seems reasonable to suppose that the therapeutic prescription for diabetes will include a defined amount of regular exercise (Larsson, 1980). For the present it would seem wise to encourage physical activity together with an improvement in the patient's use of blood glucose monitoring to rationalize this aspect of diabetes management.

REFERENCES

Ahlborg, G., Felig, P., Hagenfeldt, L. *et al.* (1974) Substrate turnover during prolonged exercise in man: splanchnic and leg metabolism of glucose, free fatty acids and amino acids. *J. Clin. Invest.*, **53**, 1078–84.

Åkerblom, K.H., Koivakangas, T. and Ilkag, J. (1980) Experiences from a winter camp for teenage diabetics. *Acta Paed. Scand.* (suppl. 2832), 50–52.

Berger, M., Berchtold, P., Cüppers, H.J. *et al.* (1977) Metabolic and hormonal effect of muscular exercise in juvenile type diabetes. *Diabetologia*, **13**, 355–65.

Bjorkman, O., Felig, P., Hagenfeldt, L. *et al.* (1981) Influence of hypoglycaemia on splanchnic glucose output during leg exercise in man. *J. Clin. Physiol.*, 43–58.

Boreham, C., Savage, J.M., Primrose, D. *et al.* (1993) Coronary risk factors in school children. *Arch. Dis. Child.*, **68**, 182–86.

Christensen, N.J., Galbo, H., Hansen, J.F. *et al.* (1979) Catecholamines and exercise. *Diabetes*, **28** (Suppl.) **1**, 58–62.

Costill, D.L., Cleary, P., Fink, W.J. *et al.* (1979) Training adaptations in skeletal muscle of juvenile diabetics. *Diabetes*, **28**, 818–22.

Dahl-Jorgensen, K., Meen, H.D., Hanssen, Kr. F. *et al.* (1980) The effects of exercise of diabetic control and haemoglobin A (HbA1) in children. *Acta Paed. Scand.*, **283** (Suppl.) 53–56.

Felig, P., Cherif, A., Minagawa, A. *et al.* (1982) Hypoglycaemia during prolonged exercise in normal man. *N. Eng. J. Med.*, **306**:15, 895–900.

Galbo, H., Holst, J., Christensen, N. *et al.* (1976) Glucagon and plasma catecholamines during beta receptor blockade in exercising man. *J. App. Physiol.*, **40**, 855–63.

Greene, S.A. (1985) Exercise and diabetes, in J.D. Baum and A.-L. Kinmonth (eds). *Care of the Diabetic Child*, Churchill Livingston, Edinburgh, pp. 94–105.

Greene, S.A., Smith, M.A. and Baum, J.D. (1983) Clinical application of insulin pumps in the management of insulin dependent diabetes. *Arch. Dis. Child.*, **58**, 578–81.

Griffin, N.K., Spanos, A., Turner, R. *et al.* (1980) Twenty-four hour metabolic profiles in diabetic children. *Arch. Dis. Child.*, **55**, 112–17.

Hartley, L.H., Mason, J.W. and Hogan, R.P. (1972) Multiple hormonal responses to prolonged exercise in relation to physical training. *J. App. Physiol.*, **33**, 602–606.

Kemmer, F.W., Berchtold, P., Berger, M. *et al.* (1979) Exercise induced fall of blood glucose in insulin treated diabetes in unrelated to alteration of insulin mobilisation. *Diabetes*, **28**, 1131–37.

Landr, K.W., Campaigne, B.N., James, F.W. *et al.* (1985) Effects of exercise training on insulin sensitivity in adolescent with Type 1 diabetes. *Diabetes Care*, **8**, 461–65.

Larsson, Y. (1980) Physical exercise and juvenile diabetes – summary and conclusions. *Acta Paed. Scand.* (Suppl.) **283**, 120–22.

Ludvigsson, J. (1980) Physical exercise in relation to degree of metabolic control in juvenile diabetes. *Acta Paed. Scand.* (Suppl.) **283**, 45–49.

MacDonald, M.J. (1987) Post-exercise late-onset hypoglycaemia in insulin-dependent diabetic patients. *Diabetes Care*, **10**, 584–88.

Marette, A., Hundal, H.S. and Klip, A. (1992) 'Regulation of glucose transporter proteins in skeletal muscle', in J. Devlin, E.S. Horton and M. Vranic (eds). *Diabetes mellitus and exercise*, pp. 27–43. Smith Gordon, Nishimura.

Mitchell, T.H., Abraham, G., Schiffrin, A. *et al.* (1988) Hyperglycaemia after intense exercise in IDDM subjects during continuous subcutaneous insulin infusion. *Diabetes Care*, **11**, 311–17.

Newsholme, E.A. and Start, C. (1981) *Regulation in Metabolism*. Wiley, Chichester.

Pederson, O., Beek-Nielsen, H. and Heding, L. (1980) Increased insulin receptors after exercise in patients with insulin-dependent diabetes mellitus. *N. Eng. J. Med.*, **302**, 886–92.

Peterson, C.M., Jones, R.L., Esterly, J.A. *et al.* (1980) Changes in basement membrane thickening and pulse volume concomitant with improved glucose ccontrol and exercise in patients with insulin-dependent diabetes mellitus. *Diabetes Care*, **3**, 586–89.

Richter, E.A., Turcotte, L., Hespel, P. *et al.* (1992) 'Regional substrate metabolism during exercise in humans', in S. Devlin, E.S. Horton and M. Vramic (eds). *Diabetes mellitus and exercise*, pp. 129–38, Smith Gordon, Nishimura.

Saltin, B., Houston, M., Nygaard, E. *et al.* (1979) Muscle fibre characteristics in healthy men and patients with juvenile diabetes. *Diabetes*, **23** (Suppl. 1), 30–32.

Schmidt, M.I., Hadfi-Georgopoulos, A., Renden, M. *et al.* (1982) The dawn phenomenon, an early-morning glucose rise: implications for diabetic intraday blood glucose variation. *Diabetes Care*, **4**:6, 679–88.

Susstrunk, H., Morell, B., Ziegler, W.H. *et al.* (1981) Insulin absorption from the abdomen and the thigh to healthy subjects during rest and exercise. *Diabetologia*, **22**, 171–74.

Wahren, J. (1979) Glucose turnover during exercise in healthy man and in patients with diabetes mellitus. *Diabetes*, **28** (suppl. 1), 82–88.

Wahren, J., Hagenfeldt, L. and Felig, P. (1975) Spanchnic and leg exchange of glucose, amino acids and free fatty acids during exercise in diabetes mellitus. *J. Clin. Invest.*, **55**, 1303–1304.

Wallberg, H., Gunnarsson, R., Henriksson, J. *et al.* (1981) Physical training in diabetes: dissociation between changes in insulin sensitivity and blood glucose regulation. *Clinical Res.*, **29**, 426A.

Wallberg-Henriksson, H., Gunnarsson, R., Henriksson, J. *et al.* (1982) Increased peripheral insulin sensitivity and muscle mitochondrial enzymes but unchanged blood glucose control in Type 1 diabetes after physical training. *Diabetes*, **31**, 1044–50.

Wasserman, D.H. and Zinker, B.A. (1992) 'Hormonal regulation of glucose fluxes during exercise', in J. Devlin, E.S. Horton and M. Vranic (eds). *Diabetes meelitus and exercise*, pp. 113–28. Smith Gordon, Nishimura.

Yki-Jarvinen, H., de Fronzo, R. and Koivisto, V.A. (1984) Normalisation of insulin sensitivity in Type 1 diabetic subjects by physical training during insulin pump therapy. *Diabetes Care*, **7**, 520–27.

Zinman, B., Murray, F.T., Vranic, M. *et al.* (1977) Glucoregulation during moderate exercise in insulin treated diabetes. *J. Clin. Endocrin. Metab.*, **45**, 641–52.

Zinman, B., Zuniga-Guajardo, S. and Kelly, D. (1984) Comparison of the acute and long-term effects of exercise on glucose control in Type 1 diabetes. *Diabetes Care*, **7**, 515–19.

20

Psychological management of diabetes

A.M. LA GRECA and J.S. SKYLER

20.1 INTRODUCTION

For children and adolescents with insulin-dependent diabetes mellitus (IDDM), a major goal of the therapeutic regimen is the attainment of normal or near-normal levels of glycemic control. Adequate glycemic control is achieved by a balance between the availability and expenditure of energy and the action of injected insulin necessary for effective utilization of energy. As outlined in preceding chapters, the three traditional components of treatment management include insulin, diet, and exercise. It is only recently that health care professionals have come to recognize the important contributions of behavior and psychological factors to diabetes care (Hamburg *et al.*, 1979; Hauser & Pollets, 1979; La Greca *et al.*, 1991b).

Given the complex demands of daily diabetes management, efforts to promote, reward, and support good self-care are essential to long-term adherence. Moreover, psychological factors play a substantial role in glucose regulation, either directly or indirectly. Psychological stress may disrupt the individual's eating habits, exercise program or daily routine, thereby altering insulin requirements and daily diabetes management. Alternatively, stress-induced secretion of counter-regulatory hormones can alter the individual's insulin needs and produce an acute hyperglycemic state (Peyrot & McMurry, 1992; Surwit *et al.*, 1992).

In the present chapter, we highlight the role of behavioral and psychological factors in diabetes management, with an emphasis on how this information can be used to improve the quality of health care provided for youngsters with IDDM and their families. Before doing so, we will briefly consider two key issues that will help to establish a context for understanding psychological management: the chronicity and course of diabetes, and the importance of a developmental perspective.

20.1.1 DIABETES AS A CHRONIC DISEASE

Diabetes management imposes demands that alter the individual's lifestyle forever; it requires a detailed and lifelong commitment to a complex treatment regimen. Coping with a chronic disease, such as diabetes, is not a static process, but rather one that evolves over time. As such, there are several pre-

Childhood and Adolescent Diabetes
Published in 1994 by Chapman & Hall, London
ISBN 0 412 48610 5

dictable phases that accompany the individual's adjustment to the disease.

20.1.1.1 Onset of diabetes

The first phase occurs at the time of initial onset of IDDM. In most cases, this crisis affects the entire family. In addition to the demands and complexities of daily management, concerns about serious health complications (both acute and chronic) may seem overwhelming. Not surprisingly, many children and families report feeling anxious and depressed (Jacobson *et al.*, 1986; Kovacs *et al.*, 1986). Kovacs and colleagues (Kovacs *et al.*, 1985a) evaluated children following their initial diagnosis with IDDM, finding that 64% reported mild symptoms of distress, such as sadness, social withdrawal, or feeling friendless. The remaining children (36%), a substantial minority, reported more severe psychological symptoms. Similar results were obtained for mothers' adaptation following their child's diagnosis of IDDM (Kovacs *et al.*, 1985b), although fathers reported little initial distress.

Such findings emphasize that the period immediately following the initial diagnosis of diabetes is a time when many children and families are distressed. Because of this, the education and support of the health care team is essential for promoting successful diabetes management and disease adaptation. Intensive interventions, that involve the child and family, are appropriate during this phase. Efforts to reduce youngsters' and parents' psychological distress should be incorporated into initial diabetes education programs (Marrero, 1989). In fact, multidisciplinary programs with newly-diagnosed youngsters, which involve medical, educational, dietary and psychological components, have a long-lasting, positive impact on youngsters' treatment adherence, family relations, and sociability (Galatzer *et al.*, 1982).

20.1.1.2 Maintenance phase

Within a year of diagnosis, most children and families make a satisfactory adjustment to the disease (Kovacs *et al.*, 1986; Kovacs *et al.*, 1990), and enter the maintenance phase. However, parents (especially mothers) who exhibit severe stress at the time of the child's diagnosis, may continue to experience difficulty for an extended period of time (Kovacs *et al.*, 1990). Furthermore, deterioration in youngsters' and families' levels of adherence have been observed within a year after the initial diagnosis (Allen *et al.*, 1992; Kovacs *et al.*, 1986). Because of these changes, throughout the course of diabetes, continued support and intervention may be critical for maintaining adequate levels of self-care.

Even after a prolonged period of stable diabetes management, major events and stressors in the lives of children and families (e.g., starting a new school, relocating, divorce, etc.) are likely to disrupt daily management and glycemic control. For these reasons, periodic reassessment of the child's and family's coping with the disease and their strategies for disease management are important throughout the course of the disease. Most of the interventions described in this chapter have been implemented with youngsters and families who are in the maintenance phase of diabetes.

20.1.1.3 Medical complications

Yet a third major phase of diabetes occurs when disease-related complications become evident. Although most children and adolescents with IDDM do not develop severe health complications before their adult years, early signs of diabetic retinopathy can be evident among poorly controlled adolescents. Research indicates that diabetes-related complications impose additional stresses for the individual and family, and may lead to feelings of depression, anger, and hostility (La

Greca *et al.*, 1991b; Wulsin *et al.*, 1987). Extensive support and attention from the health care team may be essential when disease-related complications arise (Rubin & Peyrot, 1992).

20.1.2 DEVELOPMENTAL CONTEXT

In addition to predictable phases associated with the course of diabetes, developmental transitions occur throughout childhood and adolescence that require adjustments on the part of youngsters and their families. Perhaps the greatest challenge for children and families is the shift in responsibility for diabetes care from a parent-managed to a child-managed approach. Prior to early adolescence, family members (especially mothers) assume most or all of the responsibility for daily diabetes care (Etzwiler & Sines, 1962; Follansbee, 1989; La Greca *et al.*, 1990). However, most children gradually assume responsibility for daily management, so that by mid to late adolescence they are primarily responsible for their own care. This transition of responsibility from parent to child can be a difficult and frustrating process (Anderson *et al.*, 1990). Children and families may benefit from the support and assistance of the health care team during this transition period (Follansbee, 1989; La Greca, 1991).

Marked physical, cognitive, and social changes that accompany the onset and course of puberty further complicate the difficult task of coping with diabetes. For example, the physical growth and hormonal changes associated with puberty may lead to increased insulin resistance (Bloch *et al.*, 1987) and attendant difficulties in daily glucose regulation. As adolescents gain more independence from thier families, and seek greater involvement with peers, social pressures to 'be like everyone else' may interfere with daily demands of diabetes care, such as glucose testing or dietary regulation. Typical adolescent concerns regarding body shape and size may also lead some youngsters to develop patterns of eating and insulin use that are detrimental to their glycemic control (Rodin & Daneman, 1992).

Given the tremendous changes and challenges that confront an adolescent with IDDM, it is not surprising that adolescents typically have poorer treatment adherence and worse metabolic control than younger children (e.g., Jacobson *et al.*, 1987; Johnson *et al.*, 1986 & 1990; La Greca *et al.*, 1990; Lorenz *et al.*, 1985). Adolescence is a particularly difficult time for diabetes management, and a period during which heath care professionals may need to work with youngsters and families in a new more intensive manner.

20.2 A MODEL FOR BEHAVIORAL AND PSYCHOLOGICAL MANAGEMENT

With the above concerns in mind, we will provide a heuristic framework for behavioral and psychological management of childhood diabetes. Figure 20.1 depicts a model that we have found extremely useful in guiding intervention efforts. Three levels of the model are depicted: diabetes knowledge and management skills, self-care behaviors, and psychological factors. These levels are organized so that diabetes-specific factors precede more complex psychological variables. All factors in the model might be considered to be essential, but not sufficient in and of themselves, for achieving good metabolic control. In terms of developing appropriate interventions, as one progresses through the levels of the model, greater involvement from mental health professionals, with expertise in behavioral and psychological issues, becomes critical.

In order to develop a plan for psychological management, health care professionals should begin their assessment at Level I. When problems arise with metabolic

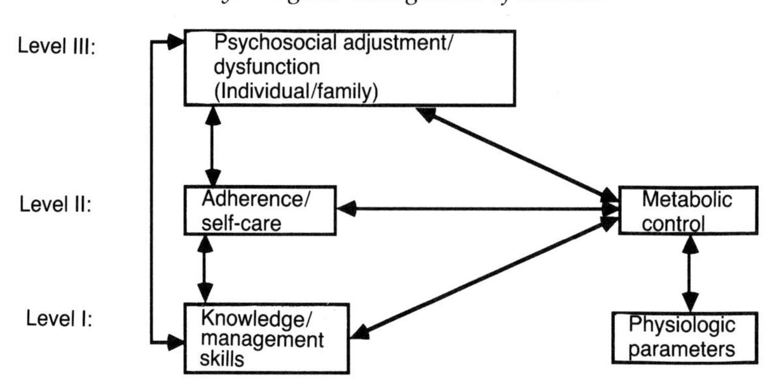

Figure 20.1 Multivariate model of behavioral and psychological factors in diabetes (modified from La Greca & Skyler, 1991).

Table 20.1 Intervention strategies for diabetes.

	Stage of diabetes	
Area for intervention	Newly diagnosed	Long-term course
Level I:		
Knowledge and Management Skills	• Standard inpatient education • Intensive outpatient program for child and family (e.g., Self Management Training)	• Periodic reassessment of skills and knowledge • Intensive outpatient program for child and family when transition in daily self-care responsibility occurs
Level II:		
Adherence/Self-Care Behavior	• Provision of support and reinforcement for self-care • Child and family programs that combine self-management and behavioral principles	• Continued support and reinforcement for self-care • When problems arise: goal setting, identifying barriers to self-care, problem-solving, reinforcing self-care efforts • Peer and family groups to promote communication, problem-solving skills
Level III:		
Psychological Issues (subclinical)	• Support groups for newly diagnosed children and families (can be combined with Level I or II interventions)	• Periodic support groups for children and families (can be combined with Level I or II interventions)
Psychological Dysfunction	• Referral to mental health specialist who understands diabetes if problems are severe	• Referral to mental health specialist who understands diabetes if problems are severe

control, it will be helpful to first consider whether problems exist with the most basic, disease-specific factors, before proceeding to psychological interventions. For example, interventions for improving diabetes knowledge and management skills should be considered prior to efforts to alter family functioning. Table 20.1 lists each level of the model and suggests appropriate interventions corresponding to each level. These intervention approaches will be described in the following sections.

20.2.1 LEVEL I: DIABETES KNOWLEDGE AND MANAGEMENT SKILLS

Given the complexities of daily diabetes care, the child or family must have at least a basic working knowledge of diabetes management if good control is to be achieved. This means knowing how to execute daily management tasks effectively and make adjustments when problems arise. With intensified insulin regimens, diabetes knowledge also includes the youngster's ability to make adjustments in insulin or food intake based on target glucose values. Thus, when a child or adolescent is experiencing problems with glucose control, an initial step may entail assessing whether the child and family have the necessary knowledge and skills to manage diabetes effectively. Does the child or parent test blood glucose correctly? Does he or she know how to make adjustments in the regimen when glucose levels are too high or too low?

One question that may arise is whose knowledge and skills should be assessed, the parent's or the child's? Our recommendation is to evaluate both. Research has revealed marked developmental differences in children's and parents' knowledge of diabetes. Typically, mothers are more knowledgeable than their children, but as children get older, their knowledge of diabetes increases substantially (Johnson *et al.*, 1982; La Greca *et al.*, 1990). For preadolescent children (i.e., <12 years of age), parents' knowledge of diabetes care may be more directly related to treatment adherence and glycemic control than children's knowledge, because parents are largely responsible for the diabetes management of young children. During adolescence, this relationship changes, so that it is the adolescent's knowledge of diabetes management, and not the parents', that relates to disease management and control (La Greca *et al.*, 1990).

With the advent of intensified insulin regimens and methods for self monitoring of blood glucose (SMBG) comes a greater potential for youngsters to achieve near-normal glucose control. Unless glucose values are used to make adjustments in the treatment regimen, however, SMBG appears to have little effect on glycemic control (Wing *et al.*, 1985; Wysocki *et al.*, 1992a). Thus, the child's and family's ability to use the information for self-management appears to be the key factor.

20.2.1.1 Educational interventions

Numerous programs have been developed for teaching diabetes knowledge and management skills to children, adolescents, and families. (See Glasgow & Osteen, 1992 and Padgett *et al.*, 1988, for reviews.) Research suggests that didactic education alone is not sufficient for promoting adequate levels of treatment adherence and metabolic control among children and adolescents (Delamater, 1993; Glasgow & Osteen, 1992). In contrast, programs that stress problem-solving and the active use of management skills coupled with reinforcement for daily management tasks have been successful with children and families (e.g., Anderson *et al.*, 1989; Delamater *et al.*, 1990), leading to improvements in youngsters' self-care and metabolic functioning.

Teaching active disease knowledge and

management skills is especially important for newly-diagnosed children and adolescents. Consonant with this view, Delamater *et al.* (1990) developed a program for teaching self-management skills to youngsters with IDDM and their families during the first six months after initial diagnosis of IDDM. Following hospital admission for diagnosis and standard inpatient education, 36 children (3–16 years) were randomly assigned to conventional treatment (CT), supportive counseling (SC), or self-management training (SMT). Children in the CT group were seen on an outpatient basis at one and three months post-diagnosis, and were contacted by telephone on an as-needed basis. Children and parents in the SC group received the same conventional medical care, but in addition met with a counselor for supportive treatment on nine occasions over six months. Those in the SMT group also received conventional medical treatment, but additionally met for nine sessions of self-management training that stressed the use of SMBG, reinforcement of accurate monitoring and recording, and use of SMBG data for making adjustments in the daily regimen. Homework assignments were given to provide the children and families with active opportunities to develop problem-solving strategies and to integrate the information from the SMBG into their daily decisions for self-care. Parents were also instructed to praise their child for appropriate self-management behavior. With this type of active learning environment, combined with incentives for good self-care, children in the SMT group achieved significantly better metabolic control one and two years post-diagnosis than those receiving only the conventional treatment. (The metabolic functioning of those in the SC group was intermediate to the other groups.) These results suggested that SMT can help prevent the common deterioration in metabolic control seen in children with IDDM during the first two years post-diagnosis.

Although the Delamater *et al.* program was designed for newly-diagnosed children and adolescents, similar interventions that combine self-management training with reinforcement and support for self-care activities are likely to be useful for adolescents as they assume increasing responsibility for their own diabetes care. Deficiencies in adolescents' management skills have been documented for insulin administration (Ingersoll *et al.*, 1986), diet regulation (Delamater *et al.*, 1988), and use of blood glucose data (Wing *et al.*, 1985; Delamater *et al.*, 1989). Furthermore, recent surveys indicate that professionals tend to overestimate adolescents' competence in self-care skills (Wysocki *et al.*, 1990, 1992b). Parents report lower levels of mastery of certain diabetes management skills for their adolescents relative to the expectations of health care professionals. These management skills include ones that are either used infrequently (e.g., urine-ketone testing), require extensive planning or anticipation (e.g., preventing hyperglycemia, adjusting insulin dose acutely), or have no immediate aversive consequences for an error (e.g., using a meal plan in a restaurant) (Wysocki *et al.*, 1992b). Such findings indicate that it is not safe to assume that, just because an adolescent has had diabetes for several years, he or she has adequate self-management skills. Given the complexity of diabetes care, it would be advisable for health care professionals to periodically assess adolescents' management skills, and to provide instruction, feedback, and support for their accurate implementation.

20.2.2 LEVEL II: SELF-CARE BEHAVIORS/TREATMENT ADHERENCE

Effective diabetes knowledge and management skills, although important, are not sufficient for achieving good glycemic control. Even if the child and family are very knowledgeable, problems will arise if they do not maintain adequate levels of self-care. Consequently, the second step for assessment and intervention is to determine the extent to which children and families actively engage in self-care activities. How often does the child monitor blood glucose? How is exercise incorporated into daily activities? Is a regular meal plan maintained?

Adherence is complex to evaluate, as there are numerous tasks involved in daily self-care. Furthermore, adherence is not an 'all or none' phenomenon. Many youngsters follow some aspects of their treatment plan well, but have problems with others. Substantial research indicates that the various components of the diabetes regimen are not strongly related to one another (Johnson, 1992), so that an individual's self-care behavior in one area (e.g., diet) is not necessarily predictive of that person's behavior in another area (e.g., glucose monitoring). Appreciating the complexity of diabetes management means that health care professionals must systematically assess and discuss each area of self-care when reviewing youngsters' diabetes management.

Another general point to consider is that adherence and glycemic control are not interchangeable (Johnson, 1992). Many health care professionals use measures of metabolic control to assess adherence; when a youngster's metabolic control is poor they may (erroneously) assume that poor adherence is the cause. Although important, adherence is but one factor among many that influences glycemic control.

In general, children tend to have better levels of treatment adherence than adolescents (Jacobson *et al.*, 1987; Johnson *et al.*, 1986, 1990; Lorenz *et al.*, 1985), perhaps because parents are more actively involved in the diabetes management activities of younger children. Moreover, some aspects of the diabetes regimen are easier to follow than others. Children and adolescents report greater adherence to insulin administration than any other aspect of the regimen. In addition, adherence to glucose testing is higher than for the more complex lifestyle aspects of the regimen, such as food regulation and exercise (La Greca *et al.*, 1990). Furthermore, as previously noted, treatment adherence appears to be highest during the period following initial diagnosis with IDDM, and deteriorates thereafter (Allen *et al.*, 1992; Jacobson *et al.*, 1987; Kovacs *et al.*, 1986).

Given the multiple demands of the diabetes regimen, health care professionals should view periodic non-compliance as the rule rather than the exception. Disruptions to self-care should be expected and children's and families' efforts to maintain good levels of self-care should be recognized and supported. In fact, preventive interventions, such as self-management training with newly-diagnosed youngsters (Delamater *et al.*, 1990; described in the previous section), may be useful for strengthening self-care activities before treatment adherence becomes problematic. Another strategy for intervention entails monitoring youngsters' treatment adherence during routine visits for medical care, so that problems can be identified and treated before they beome entrenched and resistant to change.

20.2.2.1 Intervention strategies for increasing self-care

Once problems with treatment adherence have been identified, what can be done to help the child and family? On an individual basis, a problem-solving approach may be most effective. After pinpointing the specific areas of self-care that are problematic, it will be useful for the health care professional to identify the specific barriers or obstacles to adherence and to develop strategies for reducing or ameliorating these barriers. Reasons for nonadherence can be quite varied and idiosyncratic. For example, children and adolescents have reported many different obstacles to maintaining a regular meal plan, including: social interference (e.g., eating too much when out with friends), appetite problems (e.g., not feeling hungry at a meal time), scheduling difficulties (e.g., disruption of regular routine when traveling), and emotional distress (e.g., eating too much when depressed or anxious) (La Greca *et al.*, 1990). Adolescent concerns about body weight and dieting may also be an impediment to maintaining a regular meal plan (Rodin & Daneman, 1992). Delamater *et al.* (1988) found that adolescents reported non-adherence to be most frequent in social situations – at school, with friends, and at restaurants.

By examining these specific barriers to self-care, an effective intervention plan can be developed. If social barriers exist, for example, the youngster might be taught how to make adjustments in insulin to accommodate certain social occasions without embarrassment or, alternatively, encouraged to be more assertive about his or her own health care needs when out with friends (Follansbee *et al.*, 1983; Gross *et al.*, 1983; Kaplan *et al.*, 1985). The solution will depend on the type of problem presented.

In addition to effective problem-solving, providing support and reinforcement for self-care activities is an important aspect of improving treatment adherence. Parents, peers, and health care providers can all be utilized as effective sources of support and encouragement for diabetes care activities. Adolescents with high levels of support and encouragement from family members for diabetes management activities have better treatment adherence (La Greca *et al.*, 1991a). Furthermore, behavioral interventions have documented the importance of reinforcement for improving treatment adherence (Carney *et al.*, 1983; Epstein *et al.*, 1981; Gross, 1982; Lowe & Lutzker, 1979).

Several behavioral intervention programs have been designed specifically for improving youngsters' and families' treatment adherence. These programs share several elements in common: (a) they focus separately on distinct aspects of the treatment regimen (e.g., glucose testing, dietary adherence, exercise, etc.), (b) they identify specific problems or barriers to adherence, and plan the intervention to resolve these difficulties, (c) they set specific goals for improvement, and (d) they monitor adherence and provide reinforcement for self-care. Although these programs have been done both individually as well as in groups, the group-oriented programs have the advantage of providing social/emotional support for children and parents.

In general, programs for preadolescent children stress parental involvement in daily care, and provision of reinforcement for the child's self-care activities; these programs involve both children and families. With adolescents, in addition to parental reinforcement or support for self-care behaviors, there appears to be a greater emphasis on teaching communication skills and problem-solving, so that adolescents and families develop the skills needed for negotiating the complex demands of diabetes care during this difficult developmental period. Emphasis on adolescents assuming increasing responsibility for self-care, but still having parents involved in treatment, are important aspects of the intervention process for this age group. As with younger children, programs for adolescents typically involve both the youngster and family, although some programs target adolescents alone. Also, with adolescents, the use of peer groups in the intervention process has been explored. In general, these programs illustrate that behavioral interventions can effectively improve treatment adherence, and in some cases also improve metabolic control, among children and adolescents with IDDM. Several examples are provided below.

Using an individualized approach that entailed goal-setting and behavioral contracts (i.e., establishing consequences for self-care behaviors), Schafer and colleagues (1982) improved the treatment adherence of three adolescents with IDDM (ages 16–18 years) in the course of an eight-week program. Several aspects of the treatment regimen were targeted: urine testing, exercise, insulin administration, and wearing an identification bracelet. With the introduction of goal setting for these behaviors, treatment adherence and metabolic control improved in two of the three adolescents. The third adolescent required the addition of behavioral contracting before improvements in adherence were apparent. Two of the three adolescents continued to maintain improvements in metabolic control at the two-month follow-up assessment; however, the remaining subject's gains were limited by family conflict. Similar programs have been used successfully by Lowe and Lutzker (1979), Gross (1982), and Carney *et al.* (1983), with youngsters ranging in age from 9 to 18 years.

As another example, a group-oriented program for children (8–12 years) with IDDM and their families was designed by Epstein and colleagues (Epstein *et al.*, 1981). This 12-week program emphasized comprehensive diabetes education and behavior management. Children and parents negotiated behavioral contracts for urine testing, dietary adherence, and exercise; parents were also taught how to contingently reinforce the targeted adherence behaviors. Both treatment adherence and percentage of negative urine tests (an index of glycemic control) improved as a result of this family-based intervention, although no improvements were observed in glycosylated hemoglobin levels.

With adolescents, group-oriented interventions have focused on adolescents in a family context (Satin *et al.*, 1989), or in peer groups with parallel parent groups (Anderson *et al.*, 1989). As evidenced by these programs, as well as from considerable research on factors related to adherence among adolescents (Hanson, 1992; La Greca & Skyler, 1991), parental involvement in diabetes care continues to be important. Balancing parental involvement with increasing adolescent autonomy and responsibility for self-care requires clear parent–adolescent communication regarding diabetes management and effective problem-solving skills (Anderson *et al.*, 1990; Follansbee, 1989; La Greca, 1991).

In one of the few family-based intervention programs, Satin *et al.* (1989) evaluated the effects of a six-week multifamily intervention for improving adolescents' treatment adherence and metabolic control. Adolescents (12–19 years) and their parents were randomly assigned to one of the following groups: Multifamily, Multifamily plus Parent Simulation of Diabetes, and Wait-list Control. For the two Multifamily conditions, adolescents and their parents met in small groups with other families; these sessions stressed effective communication skills around diabetes-specific situations, problem-solving strategies for diabetes management, and parents' support for the adolescents' self-care. In one treatment condition, parents also simulated diabetes for a one-week period. Each parent completed all aspects of a diabetes treatment regimen (e.g., daily injections [of saline], multiple daily glucose tests and recording of results, dietary plan, exercise prescription, blood drawn for HbA_1 assessment), and adolescents 'coached' their parents in how to manage their diabetes. The goal of the simulation exercise was to heighten parents' awareness and understanding of the difficulties of daily diabetes care. Adolescents who participated in the multifamily intervention demonstrated significant improvements in metabolic control six months post-intervention, and were rated as more adherent with daily self-care than were control youngsters. This program emphasizes the importance of family involvement in diabetes care and communication regarding daily management activities.

An alternative strategy for family intervention is illustrated by Anderson and colleagues (1989), who used peer groups and group-oriented parent training to improve adolescents' treatment adherence – particularly for glucose testing and diet. Adolescents (11–14 years) met in peer groups to learn how to use self-management of blood glucose (SMBG) for solving diabetes management problems and adjusting their regimen. Parallel parent groups focused on similar educational issues, as well as ways to improve family communication skills and family involvement in diabetes care. Some improvement in treatment adherence was apparent for participating adolescents relative to control subjects receiving standard care. Adolescents also demonstrated significantly better metabolic functioning than controls at the end of treatment.

One noteworthy aspect of the Anderson *et al.* study was that the six intervention sessions took place immediately prior to quarterly outpatient appointments for diabetes care, and extended over an 18-month period. Thus, this intervention was integrated into the adolescents' routine medical care, and did not require additional meetings for participation. This factor may be important for gaining the full cooperation and participation of adolescents and families.

In summary, interventions demonstrated to be effective in improving treatment adherence and metabolic control among children and adolescents with diabetes typically involve the youngster and the family. The interventions primarily stress the following elements: (a) education and problem-solving for diabetes care activities, (b) reinforcement for good treatment adherence, (c) good communication between youngster and family, as well as between youngsters and health care professionals, (d) family involvement in diabetes care, and (e) social support and encouragement. The behavioral and psychological components of these interventions typically require input from mental health professionals (e.g., psychologists, social workers), in collaboration with nutritionists, nurses, or clinical health care specialists. The programs described in this section do not typically include youngsters and families with severe psychopathology or family conflict. Psychological management of those with more severe dysfunction will be considered in the following section.

20.2.3 LEVEL III: PSYCHOLOGICAL FACTORS – INDIVIDUAL AND FAMILY DYSFUNCTION

For a number of years, researchers considered the possibility that personality factors contributed to the etiology and course of diabetes. Recent investigations have refuted this position; in general, no support has been found for a 'diabetic personality' (Hauser & Pollets, 1979). Moreover, beyond the period of initial diagnosis of IDDM, psychological disorders do not appear to be more prevalent in children with diabetes. Most studies find that the psychological functioning of children and adolescents with diabetes is comparable to that of healthy controls. (See Johnson, 1980; Fisher *et al.*, 1982; Rubin & Peyrot, 1992, for reviews.) When diabetes occurs in the context of personal or family dysfunction, however, severe disruption in adherence and metabolic control is likely. Psychological problems and family dysfunction have been widely recognized as factors in brittle diabetes and recurrent ketoacidosis (Nathan, 1985; Orr *et al.*, 1983; Schade *et al.*, 1985; White *et al.*, 1984).

Although cases of frank psychopathology will be the exception rather than the rule, and will require assistance from mental health specialists when they occur, even subclinical levels of psychological or family dysfunction can have implications for glycemic control. In numerous investigations (Anderson *et al.*, 1981; Koski, 1969; La Greca & Skyler, 1991), youngsters in poor glycemic control demonstrated greater psychological distress, such as symptoms of anxiety, depression, and poor self-esteem, than well-controlled youths with diabetes. Parallel findings have been observed for family functioning; youngsters with cohesive and supportive families have better treatment adherence and metabolic control than those with less supportive family situations (Anderson *et al.*, 1981; Hanson, 1992; La Greca *et al.*, 1991a). Furthermore, high levels of family conflict have repeatedly been associated with diabetes management problems, especially among adolescents (Bobrow *et al.*, 1985; Schafer *et al.*, 1986). One study of mother–daughter interactions found that poor adherence was related to more emotionally charged, confrontive interactions between adolescents and their mothers (Bobrow *et al.*, 1985). Parents who are critical and nag their adolescents regarding their diabetes care have adolescents with poorer adherence to glucose testing and dietary management in comparison to families in which such non-supportive behaviors are less common (Schafer *et al.*, 1986).

20.2.3.1 Psychological interventions (subclinical)

The association between youngsters' poor metabolic control and the presence of at least subclinical levels of psychological and family dysfunction, suggests that health care professionals must consider psychological factors as important components of diabetes management. From the standpoint of prevention, it may be helpful to establish diabetes support groups for youngsters and families. Support groups provide children and families with a network of others who understand the frustrations of managing a chronic disease and who can offer suggestions and encouragement for new ways of handling everyday situations related to diabetes care. As discussed previously, it is unreasonable to expect that children and families will always cope effectively with the demands of daily diabetes. Efforts to promote youngsters' and families' sharing of ideas, feelings, and coping strategies may facilitate overall adjustment to diabetes, and prevent more serious problems from developing.

A related strategy for enhancing the psychological functioning of children and families with diabetes, is to incorporate social support into other types of interventions, such as those designed to improve diabetes management, SMBG, or levels of self-care. In general, the family- and group-oriented interventions described in the previous sections (Anderson *et al.*, 1989; Delamater *et al.*, 1990; Satin *et al.*, 1989), incorporated psychological support into the overall treatment approach.

20.2.3.2 Psychological interventions (clinical)

Most of the interventions described thus far do not include children and families who exhibit clinical levels of psychological dysfunction. What interventions are appropriate when youngsters or families exhibit severe psychopathology or family conflict? Although such youngsters and families constitute a small proportion of those with IDDM, they may tax the health care system and utilize an inordinate proportion of available resources. In such cases, the services of mental health professionals who are knowledgeable about diabetes, for conducting individual or family therapy, may be needed to supplement diabetes-specific interventions.

For example, Snyder (1987) reported a case study involving a 14-year-old boy who demonstrated problems with treatment adherence and serious antisocial behavior. Behaviorally-oriented family therapy was used to improve noncompliance, as well as reduce antisocial behavior and family conflict. Treatment occurred over an extended period of time – 21 weeks – as might be expected with a more intensive psychological intervention. Intervention gains were maintained at follow-up, two-months post-treatment.

As noted above, severe psychopathology and family dysfunction often coincide with brittle diabetes (i.e., frequent episodes of severe hypo- and hyperglycemia) and recurrent diabetic ketoacidosis (RDKA). In such cases, intensive, long-term treatment of the child and family, by an experienced mental health professional, is usually part of the overall intervention approach (e.g., Gray *et al.*, 1988; Golden *et al.*, 1985; Nathan, 1985; White *et al.*, 1984). In some instances of severe noncompliance, residential care may be needed for the child or adolescent (Buithieu *et al.*, 1987; Henderson, 1991; Rosenbloom, 1982).

Systematic referral of youngsters and families for psychotherapy, when severe psychosocial problems are apparent, may be a useful approach to preventing episodes of RDKA (Golden *et al.*, 1985). Recent studies suggest that individuals who receive psychotherapy, in addition to medical assistance for diabetes-related medical crises, fare better than those who do not receive such therapeutic assistance (Golden *et al.*, 1985; Moran *et al.*, 1991).

20.3 CONCLUSION

In conclusion, a multilevel approach to conceptualizing behavioral and psychological factors in diabetes care is important. By examining youngsters' and families' knowledge of diabetes, adherence or self-care strategies, and psychological adjustment, a plan for intervention can be developed.

Given the importance of insulin, diet, exercise, and psychological factors in diabetes management, a complex array of health care professionals is needed to effectively deal with the demands of diabetes care. It is essential for health care teams to include professionals with expertise in behavior and psychological management. Prescribing a detailed and demanding diabetes regimen, without adequate attention to the psychological needs of the child and family, may lead to problems with diabetes management and poor metabolic control.

REFERENCES

Allen, C., Zaccaro, D.J., Palta, M. *et al.* (1992) Glycemic control in early IDDM. *Diabetes Care*, **15**, 980–87.

Anderson, B.J., Auslander, W.F., Jung, K.C. *et al.* (1990) Assessing family sharing of diabetes responsibilities. *J. Pediatr. Psych.*, **15**, 477–92.

Anderson, B.J., Miller, J.P., Auslander, W.F. *et al.* (1981) Family characteristics of diabetic adolescents: Relationship to metabolic control. *Diabetes Care*, **4**, 586–94.

Anderson, B.J., Wolf, F.M., Burkhart, M.T. *et al.* (1989) Effects of peer-group intervention on metabolic control of adolescents with IDDM: Randomized outpatient study. *Diabetes Care*, **3**, 179–83.

Bloch, C.A., Clemons, P. and Sperling, M.A. (1987) Puberty decreases insulin sensitivity. *J. Pediatr.*, **110**, 481–87.

Bobrow, E.S., AvRuskin, T.W. and Siller, J. (1985) Mother-daughter interaction and adherence to diabetes regimens. *Diabetes Care*, **8**, 146–51.

Buithiev, M., Geffken, G., Silverstein, J.H. *et al.* (1987) Evalvation of a residential program for youngsters with insulin-dependent diabetes mellitus (IDDM). *Diabetes*, **36** (suppl. 1), 19A.

Carney, R.M., Schechter, D. and Davis, T. (1983) Improving adherence to blood glucose testing in insulin-dependent diabetic children. *Behavior Therapy*, **14**, 247–54.

Delamater, A.M. (1993, in press) Compliance interventions for children with diabetes and other chronic disease, in N.A. Krasnegor, L. Epstein, S.B. Johnson *et al.* (eds). *Developmental aspects of health compliance behavior*, pp. 335–54. Lawrence Erlbaum, Hillsdale, NJ.

Delamater, A.M., Bubb, J., Davis, S.G., *et al.* (1990) Randomize prospective study of self-management training with newly diagnosed diabetic children. *Diabetes Care*, **13**, 492–98.

Delamater, A.M., Davis, S., Bubb, J. *et al.* (1989)

Self-monitoring of blood glucose in adolescents with diabetes: Technical skills and utilization of data. *Diabetes Educator*, **15**, 491–502.

Delamater, A.M., Kurtz, S., Smith, J. *et al.* (1988) Dietary skills and adherence in children with insulin-dependent diabetes mellitus. *Diabetes Educator*, **14**, 33–36.

Epstein, L.H., Figueroa, J., Farkas, G.M. *et al.* (1981) The short-term effects of feedback on accuracy of urine glucose determinations in insulin-dependent diabetic children. *Behavior Therapy*, **12**, 560–64.

Etzwiler, D.D. and Sines, L.K. (1962) Juvenile diabetes and its management: Family, social, and academic implications. *J. Am. Med. Assoc.*, **181**, 304–308.

Fisher, E.B., Jr., Delamater, A., Bertelson, A. *et al.* (1982) Psychological factors in diabetes and its treatment. *J. Consul. and Clin. Psychol.*, **50**, 993–1003.

Follansbee, D.M. (1989) Assuming responsibility for diabetes care: What age, what price? *Diabetes Educator*, **15**, 347–52.

Follansbee, D.M., La Greca, A.M. *et al.* (1983) Coping skills training for adolescents with diabetes. *Diabetes*, **32** (suppl. 1), 147.

Galatzer, A., Amir, S., Gil, R. *et al.* (1982) Crisis intervention program in newly diagnosed diabetic children. *Diabetes Care*, **5**, 414–19.

Glasgow, R.E. and Osteen, V.L. (1992) Evaluating diabetes education: Are we measuring the most important outcomes? *Diabetes Care*, **15**, 1423–32.

Golden, M.P., Herrold, A.J. and Orr, D.P. (1985) An approach to prevention of recurrent diabetic ketoacidosis in the pediatric population. *J. Pediatr.*, **107**, 195–200.

Gray, D.L., Marrero, D.G., Godfrey, C. *et al.* (1988) Chronic poor metabolic control in the pediatric population: a stepwise intervention program. *Diabetes Educator*, **14**, 516–20.

Gross, A.M. (1982) Self-management training and medication compliance in children with diabetes. *Child and Fam. Behav. Ther.*, **4**, 47–55.

Gross, A.M., Heimann, L., Shapiro, R. *et al.* (1983) Social skills training and hemoglobin A1c levels in children with diabetes. *Behav. Mod.*, **7**, 151–64.

Hamburg, B.A., Lipsett, L.F., Inoff, G.E. *et al.* (1979) *Behavioral and psychosocial issues in diabetes: Proceedings of the National Conference.* National Institutes of Health, Washington, DC. Publication Number 80–1993.

Hanson, C.L. (1992) Developing systemic models of the adaptation of youths with diabetes, in A.M. La Greca, L.J. Siegel, J.L. Wallander *et al.* (eds). *Stress and Coping in Child Health*, pp. 212–41. Guilford Press, New York.

Hauser, S.T. and Pollets, D. (1979) Psychological aspects of diabetes mellitus: A critical review. *Diabetes Care*, **2**, 227–32.

Henderson, G. (1991) The psychosocial treatment of recurrent diabetic ketoacidosis: An interdisciplinary team approach. *Diabetes Educator*, **17**, 119–23.

Ingersoll, G.M., Orr, D.P., Herrold, A.J. *et al* (1986) Cognitive maturity and self-management among adolescents with insulin-dependent diabetes mellitus. *J. Pediatr.*, **108**, 620–23.

Jacobson, A.M., Hauser, S.T., Wertlieb, D. *et al.* (1986). Psychological adjustment of children with recently diagnosed diabetes mellitus. *Diabetes Care*, **9**, 323–29.

Jacobson, A.M., Hauser, S.T., Wolfsdorf, J.I. *et al.* (1987) Psychological predictors of compliance in children with recent onset of diabetes mellitus. *J. Pediatr.*, **108**, 805–811.

Johnson, S.B. (1980) Psychological factors in juvenile diabetes. *J. Behav Med.*, **3**, 95–116.

Johnson, S.B. (1992) Methodological issues in diabetes research: Measuring adherence. *Diabetes Care*, **15**, 1658–67.

Johnson, S.B., Freund, A., Silverstein, J. *et al.* (1990) Adherence-health status relationships in childhood diabetes. *Health Psychol.* **9**, 606–631.

Johnson, S.B., Pollack, R.T., Silverstein, J. *et al.* (1982) Cognitive and behavioral knowledge about insulin-dependent diabetes among children and parents. *Pediatrics*, **69**, 708–713.

Johnson, S.B., Silverstein, J., Rosenbloom, A. *et al.* (1986) Assessing daily management of childhood diabetes. *Health Psychol.*, **5**, 545–64.

Kaplan, R.M., Chadwick, M.W. and Schimmel, L.E. (1985) Social learning intervention to promote metabolic control in Type I diabetes mellitus: Pilot experimental results. *Diabetes Care*, **8**, 152–55.

Koski, M.L. (1969) The coping process in childhood diabetes. *Acta Paed. Scand.*, **198**, 1–56.

Kovacs, M., Brent, D., Steinberg, T.F. *et al.* (1986) Children's self-reports of psychologic adjustment and coping strategies during first year of insulin-dependent diabetes mellitus. *Diabetes Care*, **9**, 472–79.

Kovacs, M., Feinberg, T.L., Paulauskas, S. *et al.* (1985a) Initial coping responses and psychosocial characteristics of children with insulin-dependent diabetes mellitus. *J. Pediatr.*, **106**, 827–34.

Kovacs, M., Finkelstein, R., Feinberg, T.L. *et al.* (1985b) Initial psychologic responses of parents to the diagnosis of insulin-dependent diabetes mellitus in their children. *Diabetes Care*, **8**, 568–75.

Kovacs, M., Iyengar, S., Goldston, D. *et al.* (1990) Psychological functioning among mothers of children with insulin-dependent diabetes mellitus: A longitudinal study. *J. Consult. and Clin. Psychol.*, **58**, 189–95.

La Greca, A.M. (1991) Assessing family sharing of diabetes responsibilities: Commentary. *Diabetes Spectrum*. **4**, 269–71.

La Greca, A.M., Follansbee, D. and Skyler, J.S. (1990) Developmental and behavioral aspects of diabetes management in youngsters. *Children's Health Care*, **19**, 132–39.

La Greca, A.M., Greco, P., Auslander, W. *et al.* (1991a) Assessing family and peer support of diabetes. Paper presented at the Florida Conference on Child Health Psychology, Gainesville, FL, April.

La Greca, A.M., Rapaport, W. and Skyler, J.S. (1991b) 'Emotions: A critical factor in diabetes control', in M.B. Davidson (ed.). *Diabetes Mellitus* (3rd edn.). Churchhill Livingstone, New York.

La Greca, A.M. and Skyler, J.S. (1991) 'Psychosocial issues in IDDM: A multivariate framework', in P. McCabe, N. Schneiderman, T. Field *et al.* (eds). *Stress, Coping and Disease*, pp. 169–90. Erlbaum, Hillsdale, NJ.

Lorenz, R.A., Christensen, N.K. and Pichert, J.W. (1985) Diet-related knowledge, skill, and adherence among children with insulin-dependent diabetes mellitus. *Pediatrics*, **75**, 872–76.

Lowe, K. and Lutzker, J.R. (1979) Increasing compliance to a medical regime with a juvenile diabetic. *Behav. Ther.*, **10**, 57–64.

Marrero, D. (1989) Commentary. *Diabetes Spectrum*, **2**, 241–42.

Moran, G., Fonagy, P., Kurtz, A. *et al.* (1991) A controlled study of psychoanalytic treatment of brittle diabetes. *J. Am. Acad. Child. Adol. Psychiatry*, **30**, 926–35.

Nathan, S.W. (1985) Psychological aspects of recurrent diabetic ketoacidosis in preadolescent boys. *Am. J. Psychother.*, **39**, 193–205.

Orr, D.P., Golden, M.P., Myers, G. *et al.* (1983) Characteristics of adolescents with poorly controlled diabetes referred to a tertiary care center. *Diabetes Care*, **6**, 170–75.

Padgett, D., Mumford, E., Hynes, M. *et al.* (1988) Meta-analysis of the effects of educational and psychosocial interventions on management of diabetes mellitus. *J. Clin. Epidemiol.*, **41**, 1007–1030.

Peyrot, M.F. and McMurry, J.F. (1992) Stress buffering and glycemic control: The role of coping styles. *Diabetes Care*, **15**, 842–46.

Rodin, G.M. and Daneman, D. (1992) Eating disorders and IDDM: A problematic association. *Diabetes Care*, **15**, 1402–1412.

Rosenbloom, A.L. (1982) Need for residential treatment for children with diabetes mellitus. *Diabetes Care*, **5**, 545–54Pa.

Rubin, R.R. and Peyrot, M. (1992) Psychosocial problems and intervention in diabetes: A review of the literature. *Diabetes Care*, **15**, 1640–57.

Satin, W., La Greca, A.M., Zigo, M.A. *et al.* (1989) Diabetes in adolescence: Effects of multifamily group intervention and parent simulation of diabetes. *J. Pediatr. Psychol.* **14**, 259–76.

Schade, D.S., Drumm, D.A., Duckworth, W.C. *et al.* (1985) The etiology of incapacitating, brittle diabetes. *Diabetes Care*, **8**, 12–20.

Schafer, L.C., Glasgow, R.E. and McCaul, K.D. (1982) Increasing the adherence of diabetic adolescents. *J. Behav. Med.*, **5**, 353–62.

Schafer, L.C., McCaul, K.D. and Glasgow, R.E. (1986) Supportive and nonsupportive family behaviors: relationships to adherence and metabolic control in persons with Type I diabetes. *Diabetes Care*, **9**, 179–85.

Snyder, J. (1987) Behavioral analysis of poor diabetic self-care and antisocial behavior: A single-subject experimental study. *Behavior Therapy*, **18**, 251–63.

Surwit, R.S., Schneider, M.S. and Feinglos, M.N. (1992) Stress and diabetes mellitus. *Diabetes Care*, **15**, 1413–21.

White, K., Kolman, M.L., Wexler, P. *et al.* (1984) Unstable diabetes and unstable families: A psychosocial evaluation of diabetic children with recurrent ketoacidosis. *Pediatrics*, **73**, 749–55.

Wing, R.R., Lamparski, D.M., Zaslow, S. *et al.* (1985) Frequency and accuracy of self-monitoring of blood glucose in children: Relationship to glycemic control. *Diabetes Care*, **8**, 214–18.

Wulsin, L.R., Jacobson, A.M. and Rand, L.I. (1987) Psychosocial aspects of diabetic retinopathy. *Diabetes Care*, **10**, 367–73.

Wysocki, T., Hough, B.S., Ward, K.M. *et al.* (1992a) Use of blood glucose data by families of children and adolescents with IDDM. *Diabetes Care*, **15**, 1041–44.

Wysocki, T., Meinhold, P.A., Abrams, K.C. *et al.* (1992b) Parental and professional estimates of self-care independence of children and adolescents with IDDM. *Diabetes Care*, **15**, 43–52.

Wysocki, T., Meinhold, P., Cox, D.J. *et al.* (1990) Survey of diabetes professionals regarding developmental changes in diabetes self-care. *Diabetes Care*, **13**, 65–68.

21

Testing for control – home and hospital

M. SILINK

21.1 INTRODUCTION

The aim of 'diabetes control' is the maintenance of metabolic homeostasis as close to the nondiabetic state as is practically possible. More pragmatically, the term is generally used to indicate how close to a specified target range blood glucose levels are maintained. The target range in childhood diabetes has to take into account a variety of clinical parameters. The chief parameter to be considered is the age of the child. For the child <5 years of age, a pre-prandial target range of 5–12 mmol/l is generally regarded as reasonable whereas for adolescents this is compressed to 4–8 mmol/l. A 2-hour post-prandial level should ideally remain <10 mmol/l or a little higher in the very young. If hypoglycemia unawareness with recurrent neuroglycopenia (causing focal or generalized seizures) is present, then a higher target range may be the safest compromise.

It should be stated that families object to the term 'diabetes control' when descriptive and judgmental adjectives such as 'good' or 'bad' are used. A family struggling to maintain reasonable glucose levels in their child who, despite all their efforts has erratic ('brittle') control, will be justifiably hostile when told by insensitive health professionals that their child has bad control.

In practice, the judgement of how well the diabetes is controlled is complex and the physician makes use of a cluster of symptoms and signs as well as other clinical and laboratory data (Table 21.1). This would explain the published studies showing wide scatter of glycosylated hemoglobin and fructosamine values for a given clinical rating of control.

Often unstable or chronically high glucose levels are associated with less than optimal health, but occasionally this is not so.

21.2 DIABETES CONTROL AND COMPLICATIONS

There is generally an acceptance that diabetes complications are largely consequences of the deranged metabolic control present in patients with insulin-dependent diabetes mellitus (see also Chapters 39 and 41). This acceptance is based on indirect evidence, on animal experiments and on the demonstration that other causes of diabetes such as non-insulin dependent diabetes mellitus and hemochromatosis are also associated with

Childhood and Adolescent Diabetes
Published in 1994 by Chapman & Hall, London
ISBN 0 412 48610 5

Table 21.1 Indicators of poor diabetes control.

1. Polyuria and polydipsia
2. Enuresis and nocturia
3. Blurred vision
4. Skin infections (staphylococcus and candida)
5. Weight loss
6. Poor growth
7. Pubertal delay
8. Deteriorating school performance and school absenteeism
9. Signs of diabetes complications
10. Blood lipid abnormalities
11. Elevated glycosylated hemoglobin
12. Elevated fructosamine

classical diabetes complications (Galton, 1965). More recently, a landmark study, the Diabetes Control and Complications Trial (DCCT) conducted in 29 centers in North America, has convincingly demonstrated that maintenance of near-normoglycemia compared with poorer metabolic control over an average period of 6.5 years reduced by 35–76% the development and/or the progression of the classical microvascular complications of insulin dependent diabetes (DCCT Research Group, 1993).

In the various studies relating diabetes control to the development of complications, animal models have proved to be very useful. These models have included models of spontaneous diabetes (e.g., non-obese diabetic (NOD) mouse, Bio-Breeding Worcester (BBW) rat), diabetes after partial or complete pancreatectomy (dogs, rats), and chemically-induced diabetes (alloxan- or streptozotocin-induced diabetes in mice, rats, dogs, monkeys and baboons). In each of these, microvascular lesions which resemble those occurring in human diabetes have been found in the kidneys and the eyes. Treatment of diabetes in these models has either prevented or retarded the progress of these lesions, and in some instances reversal has been noted (e.g., insulin therapy of alloxan-diabetic dogs can reduce the severity of retinopathy (Engerman & Kern, 1987) and nephropathy, islet transplantation can reverse renal lesions in streptozotocin diabetic rats (Mauer *et al.*, 1975)).

In humans, there are also many observations relating degree of control to the occurrence and the progression of diabetic complications (Feldt-Rasmussen *et al.*, 1986). Normal kidneys when transplanted into diabetic recipients develop nephropathic changes (Mauer *et al.*, 1976) and there has been at least one report of a diabetic kidney when transplanted into a nondiabetic recipient showing remarkable morphologic resolution of the characteristic nephropathic lesions of diabetes (Abouna *et al.*, 1983).

Against the concept that the abnormal diabetic milieu has been responsible for the development of the diabetic lesions (the metabolic hypothesis), has been the genetic hypothesis that the complications may be concurrent genetic manifestations of diabetes. Certainly the animal models have helped to counter this concept as a primary cause of the complications as have the previously mentioned observations that similar or identical lesions occur in other forms of diabetes (Type 2 diabetes, hemochromatosis, hemosiderosis) (Deckert, 1960).

Yet the concept of poor diabetes control causing diabetic complications is clearly more than one of harmful glucose levels being the only cause, as there are patients (more than 60%) who never develop diabetic nephropathy whilst others develop nephropathy with seemingly similar degrees of control (Seaquist *et al.*, 1989). For certain needs such as general health, growth and development, perfect or near-perfect 'control' is not an absolute prerequisite. There are obviously modulatory influences which may be genetic, environmental as well as the effects of co-morbidities such as hypertension and dyslipidemias (Garber *et al.*, 1992) which may adversely affect organ function.

Following analysis of the data generated by the DCCT the aim of modern management for the adolescent and young adult with diabetes is to maintain the blood glucose levels as close to the nondiabetic range as often as possible without unduly exposing the patient to the possible adverse effects of intensive therapy (DCCT Research Group, 1993).

The DCCT studied 1441 subjects, aged 13–39 years for a mean of 6.5 years. The patients were randomized into intensive therapy (either three or more injections of insulin daily or continuous subcutaneous insulin infusion, frequent monitoring and comprehensive management by a multidisciplinary team) and conventionally treated groups. The median glycosylated hemoglobin levels for the two groups were 7.2% and 9.0% respectively, in an assay with an upper limit of normal of 6.05% whilst the mean blood glucose levels obtained from regular glucose profiles for the two groups were 8.6 mmol/l and 12.8 mmol/l respectively. The two groups maintained their 'glycemic separation' for the duration of the study. The intensive therapy group demonstrated the following outcomes: a) 62% reduction in progression of retinopathy, b) 27% reduction in the appearance of retinopathy in the cohort with no retinopathy at entry, c) 56% reduction in the development of clinical albuminuria (daily excretion >300 mg), and d) 61% reduction in clinically significant neuropathy. The major adverse outcomes were a 300% rise in severe hypoglycemic episodes and a 4.6 kg weight gain. The DCCT investigators also concluded that the risk: benefit ratio for intensive therapy may be less favorable in children <13 years, in patients with hypoglycemia unawareness or recurrent severe hypoglycemia, and, in patients with advanced diabetic complications, coronary or cerebrovascular disease.

It should be emphasized that the DCCT did not study children under the age of 13 years. Because of concerns of the effects of recurrent hypoglycemia on neuropsychological development and the fact that young children do not develop micro- or macrovascular complications of diabetes in childhood, there should be caution in implementing intensive therapy in the very young.

Despite the large amount of data now available there remain many questions:

- How close to the nondiabetic state does diabetes control need to be to prevent, delay or reverse diabetic complications? Analysis of the DCCT data did not reveal a specific value of glycosylated hemoglobin at which risks were minimized or the benefits maximized and for every degree of improvement in the glycosylated haemoglobin there was a reduction in the risks. This implies that the target should be the achievement of normoglycemia.
- Is hyperglycemia the only cause of microvascular complications and does the degree of control affect the development of complications to the same extent in all patients? Current data suggests that even intensive management is unable to guarantee freedom from complications. This may be due to the near impossibility of achieving normoglycemia by present methods or perhaps to genetic, environmental and other factors. There are good data indicating that factors other than glycemic control are also of major importance (genetic, presence of hypertension, dyslipidemias, family history of diabetic complications, etc.).
- Does improved control have an effect on complications already present? In some studies in patients with established diabetic complications, short-term changes have been documented following improved glycemic control (reduction of microalbuminuria, reduction in glomerular hyperfiltration, improvement in retinal capillary leakage, improved nerve conduction parameters, improved lipid and rheological parameters, etc.). However, the long-term results as yet are not known. In other studies, established complications such as retinopathy may actually worsen (Dahl-Jorgensen *et al.*, 1985) or remain unchanged (e.g., nephropathy) with improved control (Dahl-Jorgensen *et al.*, 1986; Reichard *et al.*, 1988). The DCCT did not

study patients with severe complications. Those with early retinopathy on entry demonstrated a 54% reduction in progression of retinopathy with intensive therapy (DCCT Research Group, 1993).

- Are there stages in the development of complications which are clearly irreversible? The available data suggest that this indeed may be the case; however, more data are needed.
- Is intensive therapy indicated for all people with diabetes? Common sense and clinical judgement need to be exercised in making this decision. If the patient is a child, or elderly, or with hypoglycemia unawareness, or has established complications, the risk: benefit ratio may not be favorable and conventional management may be the correct decision.
- What resources are necessary to implement intensive management? The answer to this is far from clear. Certainly the experience from the DCCT indicates that patients need better and more frequent access to a multidisciplinary team consisting of diabetes educators, nutritionists and mental health workers, as well as doctors trained in diabetes management. More frequent consultations together with telephone advice given to a better informed and motivated patient would seem the key.

Despite the research already undertaken, the fact remains that diabetes mellitus remains a difficult disorder associated with increased mortality at all ages and with complications that can cause blindness, renal failure and neuropathy. In addition, it is associated with macrovascular diseases such as myocardial infarction, cerebral thrombosis and peripheral gangrene. Thus, in the early 1990s, until all the issues concerning diabetes control and complications are resolved most diabetologists would like their adolescent and adult patients to achieve normoglycemia or near-normoglycemia providing the risk: benefit ratio of such intensive management is favorable. For younger children there is concern about the widescale application of intensive management because of the deleterious effects of recurrent hypoglycemia on the developing brain and the psychological stresses of intensive therapy.

We have at least reached the stage of being able to better define relevant questions and have better tools to quantify degrees of diabetes control (Strowig & Raskin, 1992). The remainder of this chapter explores the practical methods available to health professionals and indeed also the patient with diabetes in assessing how well the diabetes is controlled both at home or in hospital.

However, an important caveat needs to be stated here. Diabetes control is dependent on much more than having access to a particular insulin regimen and the means to monitor glucose levels by direct or indirect means. Some patients have an inherent brittleness to their diabetes and this should be accepted without apportioning blame. Some patients choose not to follow the medical guidelines and whilst they need to be counseled this is their right. Others may wish for better control but fail because of lack of knowledge, or social or psychological reasons. Patients and families in this latter group will be more successful if they receive appropriate support from diabetes educators, social workers, dietitians and other health professionals. Indeed one of the messages of the DCCT study was that intensive therapy was only possible by having appropriate support services including frequent (monthly) multidisciplinary clinic visits with even more frequent telephone contacts from health professionals.

21.3 WHAT DOES GOOD CONTROL MEAN?

Diabetes mellitus is a complex disorder in which the deficiency of insulin (action) results in more than an elevation of the blood glucose. Insulin is the hormone of energy

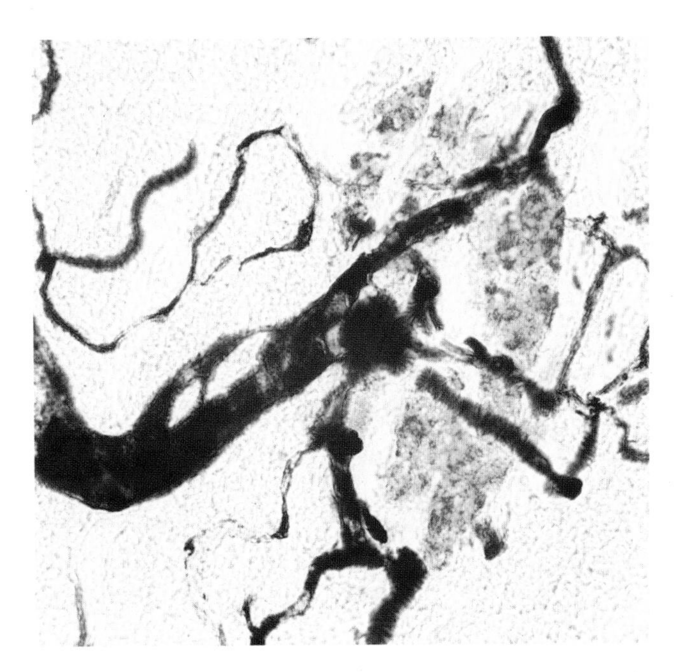

Plate 1 The arterial system of this normal pancreas was injected with India ink. The pancreas was subsequently sectioned and the islets immunostained brown. An arteriole enters the islet from the left, breaks up into intra-islet sinusoids which then ramify in the surrounding exocrine tissue. Islet sinusoids are not directly drained by veins (×400)

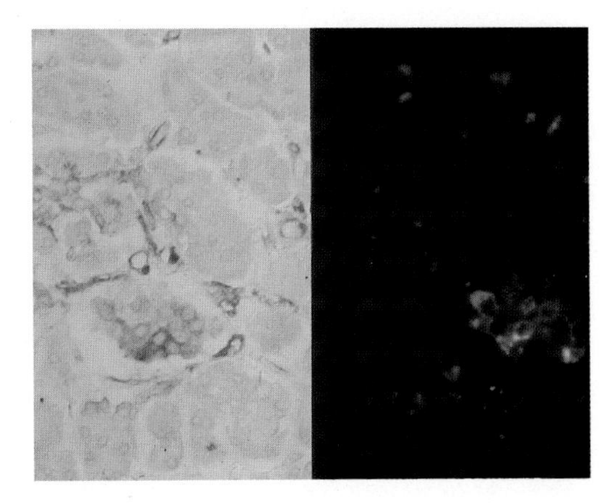

Plate 2 This islet has been double-stained to show class II MHC expression by light microscopy (left) and insulin by immunoflourescence (right). Note that several insulin-containing B cells express class II MHC (×400)

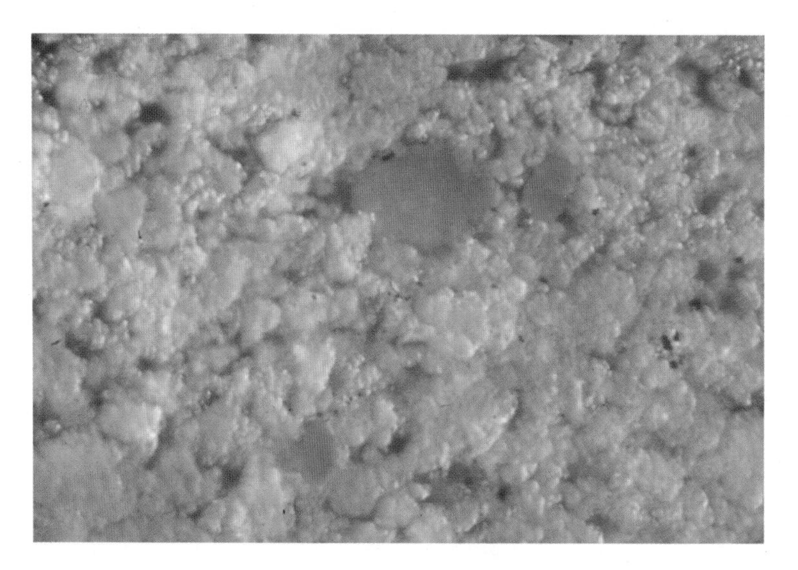

Plate 3 Photomicrograph of human pancreatic digest before purification. The islets are stained red by dithizone.

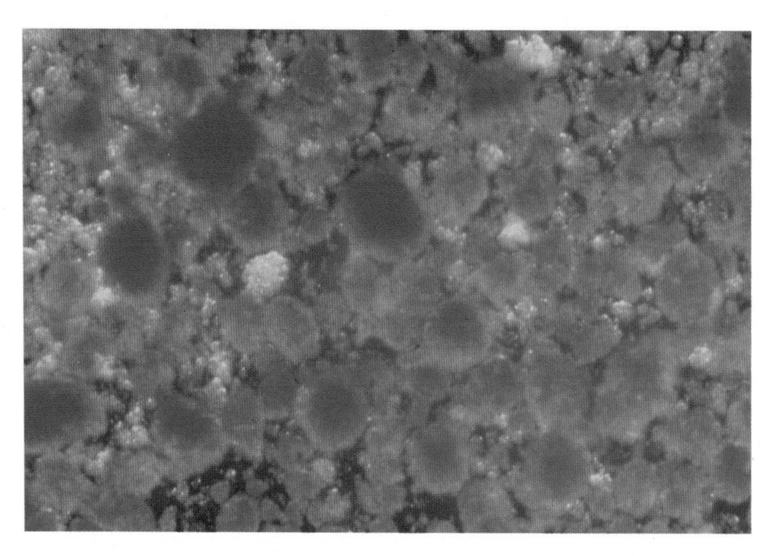

Plate 4 Photomicrograph of dithizone-stained purified human islets. The purity of this preparation was estimated at 90%. The islets range in diameter from 50–450 μm.

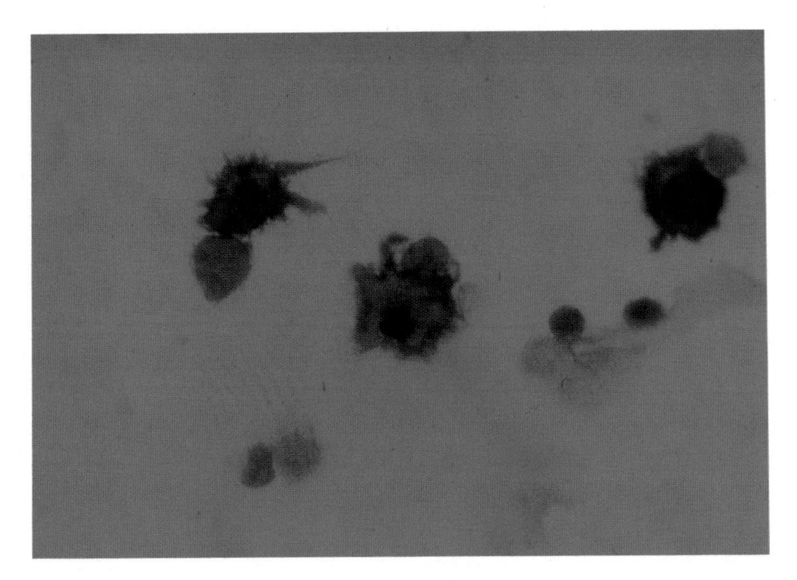

Plate 5 Photomicrograph of human dendritic cells (isolated from the spleen). The dendritic cells are stained red by an anti-class II monoclonal antibody. Each human islet contains between 5 and 20 of these powerful antigen presenting cells.

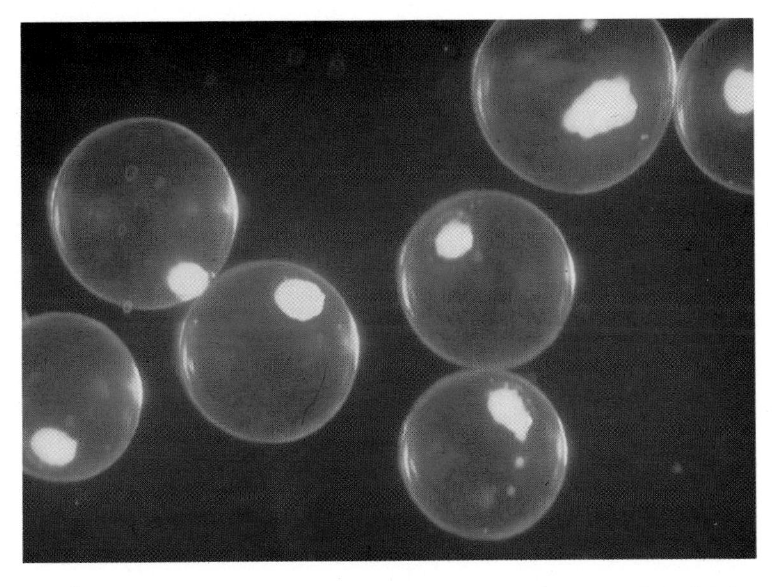

Plate 6 Photomicrograph of alginate/poly-l-lysine microencapsulated islets. Each capsule contains one islet and the capsules range in diameter from 400–500 μm.

storage and is profoundly anabolic. Deficiency of insulin action has an impact on lipid metabolism, prostaglandin effects, cytokine actions, local vascular changes, changes in the oxygen-carrying capacity of red blood cells, on rheological parameters, on the function of various enzymes and proteins as well as many other interrelated parameters. As an approximation of overall metabolic control the measurement of blood glucose levels has been a practical but vastly simplistic concept. Whilst this may be true of normoglycemia, the further the blood glucose deviates from the nondiabetic range the more likely and the more unpredictable will be the effects on other aspects of 'metabolic control'. The complexity and the interrelationships of these various parameters are only now being appreciated.

21.4 MEASUREMENT OF BLOOD GLUCOSE

Modern analytical methods can now measure glucose in a few microliters of blood and provide results in less than a minute. Accuracy (ability to obtain true values) and precision (ability to obtain reproducible results) in the measurement of glucose concentrations in the circulation are the cornerstones of clinical practice and research into diabetes. Accuracy and precision are important in the monitoring of therapy be it during surgery (see Chapter 24), acute diabetic emergencies (see Chapter 15), or in the home. Imprecise measurements can lead to incorrect and at times, disastrous adjustments to therapy.

Blood glucose estimations at home or by the bedside are predominantly based on the glucose oxidase/peroxidase method. In reality, these methods measure plasma glucose concentrations. Test strips, used in these methods, are impregnated with the bacterial enzymes glucose oxidase and peroxidase (Burrin & Alberti, 1990).

When a drop of blood is placed on the strip, the plasma permeates into the strip and the glucose in the plasma is converted by glucose oxidase to d-gluconic acid and hydrogen peroxide. The latter is converted by the enzyme peroxidase to nascent oxygen which can then oxidize a chromagen system. The reaction is stoichiometric (i.e., for every mole of glucose reacted one mole of chromogen is oxidized) and hence the change in color of the chromogen can be directly related to the glucose concentration. The change in color can be read visually against standard color blocks or read automatically by a reflectance meter, the read-out of which is calibrated in mmol/l of glucose. Providing the manufacturer's instructions are followed these systems have acceptable accuracy for clinical purposes. The early meters were mains-operated and cumbersome but were soon replaced by a variety of small portable battery-operated meters.

Other systems, still utilizing the glucose oxidase system, incorporate an electrochemical measurement system (electrode), rather than a chromogen.

Test strips and meters are sufficiently accurate and precise under controlled situations when appropriate training and instructions are given (North *et al.*, 1987). However, it is an almost universal experience that with routine use poor results are the rule rather than the exception. Coefficient variations of well over 10% have been reported, far removed from 1–3% which can be obtained with the same meters under laboratory conditions (Burrin & Alberti, 1990). Misuse led the United Kingdom Department of Health to issue a health hazard warning with regard to extra laboratory meter use (NHS Procurement Directorate, 1987).

Newer models include microprocessor-controlled meters with integral bar code calibration. Memory-chip logbook meters which can accept data on insulin dosage, variations in diet, exercise or other special events such as hypoglycemia are now available and can provide comprehensive data that can be down-loaded to a computer data system in the form of a summary statement. Some meters can be coupled to a modem so that stored information can be directly transmitted to a diabetes center through the telephone system (Ahring *et al.*, 1992).

The future development of glucose measuring systems is awaited with great keenness. Experimental continuous glucose-measuring systems have been devised using indwelling needle-electrodes impregnated with glucose oxidase. These remain active for several days before requiring replacement. Great interest is being shown in a transcutaneous infra-red system in which glucose levels are estimated on the basis of absorption of infra-red light at a very specific wave-length.

21.4.1 GLUCOSE MEASUREMENT AT HOME OR BY THE BEDSIDE

The measurement of blood glucose by test strips has been available since the 1960s. The introduction of a reflectance meter in 1970 encouraged widespread use, predominantly in hospitals. In 1978, clinical trials indicated patients were able to use the meters themselves (Sonksen *et al.*, 1978; Walford *et al.*, 1978).

The ability of the patient to measure the blood glucose at home has been the single most important advance in the treatment of diabetes in the 1980s and is referred to as either SBGM (self-blood glucose monitoring) or HBGM (home-blood glucose monitoring) (McCall & Mullin, 1987). SBGM is recommended for all patients using insulin and has given the patient, the family and the physician the opportunity for more rational management of the diabetes (ADA Position Statements, 1989; ADA Consensus Statements, 1987). It has also opened the way to more intensive insulin regimens (basal-bolus regimens involving multiple injections or insulin pump therapy) to achieve more physiologic insulin delivery and subsequent better glucose homeostasis. Self-monitoring is of great benefit in the routine adjustment of daily insulin dosages, in the management of recurrent asymptomatic hypoglycemia, in suspected hypoglycemia, in the management of 'sick days', in all patients with unstable diabetes and in those with abnormal renal glucose thresholds.

One of the outstanding benefits of SBGM or HBGM is the psychological empowerment that the ability to monitor progress at home gives to the patient and family. Diabetes is unique among all the chronic disorders in that it demands so much of the patient and family. SBGM at least provides some rational basis to the daily management decisions.

Another benefit of SBGM is the educational value and the fact that patient and families are able to learn about their diabetes (e.g., At what level does hypoglycemia cause symptoms? What is the effect of 5–7 jelly beans on blood glucose levels? What is the effect of exercise on blood glucose levels? etc.). The availability of rapid, reasonably accurate blood glucose estimations has revolutionized the emergency care of the diabetic patient in the consulting rooms, ward, operating theaters, recovery rooms and casualty departments. Most large institutions offer a 24-hour emergency hotline service for the management of sick days at home and the ability of the family to monitor their child's diabetes at home has led to major reductions in hospitalization frequency.

The number of tests done is determined by the physician taking into account the individual needs of the clinical situation. In general, more tests are needed in the very young (who are unable to express their needs) and during times of illness. Most families tend to test two to four times a day with the majority of the tests being done before breakfast and before the evening meal. This routine will allow adjustment of long-acting insulin dosages if on a standard twice-daily insulin routine. In particularly stable patients it may be possible to reduce the testing so that a complete pre- and postprandial profile is only done every few days.

It is a common fault not to test post-prandially after breakfast and the evening meal (i.e., before morning snack or lunch and before supper) so that short-acting insulin can be adjusted optimally. Families need constant reinforcement to vary the time of testing so that a realistic profile of the glycemic excursions throughout the day can be obtained. The special problem of unsuspected nocturnal hypoglycemia means that occasional blood glucose levels need to be measured between midnight and 2 a.m.

21.4.2 ACCURACY OF BEDSIDE GLUCOSE METHODS

It should be remembered that all strips are quantitative for glucose over only a limited range of blood glucose concentrations and that at the extremes of the range, unreliability has been reported which can be clinically important (Southgate & Marks, 1986).

In general, the various commercially available strips and meters are accurate and reproducible enough for clinical use. There are, however, caveats to their use and these are largely covered by the manufacturer's instructions (Table 21.2). Whenever the meters and strips are used in hospitals, quality assurance schemes and training schemes must also be introduced. All patients need to use control samples to monitor their technique and have a yearly review with a diabetes educator.

The process of obtaining the capillary blood has been simplified by the development of blood-letting devices which puncture the skin at predetermined distances using spring-loaded lancets. Some of these devices incorporate shields that hide the lancet and the travel of the lancet can be adjusted by the use of appropriate spacers. It is indeed remarkable that so many young children tolerate this process up to several times a day with such little objection. Clearly the perceived advantages of SBGM outweigh the negative aspects of the trauma.

Table 21.2 Factors interfering with accurate glucose measurements.

1. High hematocrit (>50%) samples give falsely low reading.
2. Inaccurate timing – allowing the reaction to proceed for longer or shorter periods overestimates and underestimates the true result respectively.
3. Non-compliance with operating instructions.
   - Insufficient blood on the strip.
   - Use of strip after the expiry date.
   - High environmental temperatures.
   - Inadequate cleaning of the meter.
   - Nonadherence to calibration procedures.
   - Storage of strips under incorrect conditions.

Unfortunately, it is becoming apparent that the limiting factor for current blood glucose measurements techniques is no longer technical but human. Simultaneous recordings of glucose levels by the patient and by a memory-chip built into the meter, have shown a significant incidence of fabrication of results (Mazze *et al.*, 1984). When this is compounded by failure to comply with the manufacturer's instructions, studies have revealed 30–40% of blood glucose results to be reported wrongly (usually more favorably) (Colaguiri *et al.*, 1990).

21.4.3 MEASUREMENT OF URINARY GLUCOSE

Glycosuria occurs only if the renal threshold (usually 10 mmol/l) is exceeded (Skyler, 1988). Thus urinary glucose testing cannot give any information about possible hypoglycemia. With age the renal threshold rises. The relationship between the blood glucose level and the degree of glycosuria is not linear, even allowing for the fact that urine collected in the bladder may represent urine produced over several hours. To improve the accuracy, double voided specimens have been used in which the patient discards the first voided specimen and then tests the second voided specimen passed 30 minutes later. Clearly any degree of urinary retention invalidates this method. Despite the use of double voided specimens, the poor correlation with blood glucose values has resulted in routine urinary glucose testing being virtually completely replaced by blood glucose monitoring in all patients requiring insulin.

The historical method for urinary glucose testing is based on the Benedict's test in which an alkaline copper solution is boiled in the presence of glucose. This results in the formation of cuprous ions which react with phosphomolybdate to form colored compounds (blue → green → brown → orange) depending on the amount of glucose present. These tests are still used in developing countries because of expense.

The Clinitest™ tablet is a modification of the Benedict test and contain anhydrous copper sulphate, anhydrous sodium hydroxide, citric acid and sodium bicarbonate. The standard test uses 5 drops of urine, 10 drops of water and 1 reagent tablet. The reaction between water and the sodium hydroxide is sufficiently exothermic to boil the tube. The colors generated are similar to those in the Benedict's test with blue being negative and orange 2% glycosuria.

Higher degrees of glycosuria (5%) can be measured using only 2 drops of urine together with the 10 drops of water, however a different color chart needs to be used.

In most developed countries, urinary glucose methods have largely been replaced with glucose oxidase-based test strips. These are convenient and specific for glucose. They are, however, interfered with by salicylates and ascorbic acid which, when present in the urine in large amounts, may cause false negative results.

21.4.4 MEASUREMENT OF URINARY GLUCOSE AT HOME

It is clear that urinary glucose levels (even double voided collections) cannot be used to predict blood glucose levels at any given time. However, they do have a place in being able to cross-check the validity of blood glucose tests. The presence of glycosuria in the face of a blood glucose profile <10 mmol/l is helpful in alerting the health professional to a serious problem in the technique of blood glucose measurement or the fabrication of results by a non-compliant patient. In these circumstances, any information is better than no information.

The measurement of the total amount of glucose excreted over a period time was used as a measure of glucose control before glycosylated hemoglobin measurement became available. Good control was felt to be present if glycosuria was <20 gm/day. The amount of glycosuria could be estimated using the semi-quantitative Clinitest™ reagents and the test could be further refined in collecting the urine over shorter periods of time (e.g., 6 hours) and obtaining a better idea of when the glycosuria occurred.

Urinary glucose measurements have been simplified by the introduction of urinary glucose reagent strips which frequently have an indicator system for ketone as well. This is a most useful indicator system which has proved invaluable in the management of illnesses at home. The occurrence of glycosuria and ketonuria indicates a major insulin deficiency. Under these circumstances frequent monitoring and additional insulin is required until the ketonuria disappears. If untreated the ketosis could proceed to ketoacidosis. If the combined urinary glucose and ketone strip indicates ketonuria but no glycosuria, then ketosis of starvation (or deficient energy intake) is present. This can occur in diabetes in prolonged hypoglycemia or when gastritis or food poisoning has prevented intake of food in an otherwise healthy individual. Measurement of the blood glucose would reveal it to be low. If needed, a 5% Dextrose (glucose) infusion may have to be given.

21.5 MEASUREMENT OF KETONE BODIES

Unlike urinary glucose tests, urinary ketone testing remains important in monitoring diabetes control (ADA Position Statement, 1992).

Ketone bodies (acids) include acetoacetic acid and beta-hydroxybutyric acid. Acetoacetic acid spontaneously degrades to form a molecule of acetone and carbon dioxide. The currently available clinical tests only measure acetoacetate, yet the levels of beta-hydroxybutyrate are usually four times that of acetoacetate. During hypoxia or when there is lactic acidosis, this ratio may be greatly increased and a measure of the acetoacetate levels may greatly underestimate the actual total level of ketone bodies.

Ketone acids are quickly and conveniently measured in the urine by the use of special reagent strips which often combine a reagent pad for the measurement of glycosuria. Their availability has greatly enhanced the monitoring of ketosis and the management of sick days at home (see Chapter 15). Prior to the availability of the strips, tablets incorporating the same Rothera nitroprusside reagents were in common use (e.g., Acetest™).

Acetoacetate can be semiquantitatively measured in the blood at the bedside by making 1:2 to 1:32 dilutions of plasma and using either the reagent strips (e.g., Ketostix™) or Acetest™ tablets. From a practical point of view, most institutions that have access to the measurement of blood gases do not measure blood ketone levels at the bedside in the management of diabetic ketoacidosis. Blood gas measurements provide more information (pH, pCO_2, HCO_3 and base deficit) about the total acid-base status.

21.6 MEASUREMENT OF GLYCOSYLATED HEMOGLOBIN

Currently the best index of glycemic control is provided by the measurement of glycosylated hemoglobin (also known as GHb, glycated hemoglobin, glycohemoglobin, HbA_1 or fast hemoglobin).

The reaction in which glucose binds to hemoglobin is non-enzymatic. The higher the blood glucose concentration and the longer the red blood cells are exposed to it, the higher the HbA_1, which is usually expressed as a fraction of total Hb (usually <7.5% in nondiabetic individuals). Because of the long lifespan of the red cells (120 days), HbA_1 levels will provide an index of diabetes control over the preceding 1–2 months. From a clinical point of view glycosylated hemoglobin measurements should be done every 3–4 months. This will give a good evaluation of glycemic control over the year.

Prospective studies in Type 1 patients have shown that the level of glycosylated hemoglobin is a significant parameter associated with the development of future complications and is regarded as the most clinically useful test to monitor diabetes control (Brownlee *et al.*, 1988).

Rahbar in 1962 discovered increased concentration of glycosylated hemoglobin in the blood of diabetic individuals (Rahbar, 1962). The structure of glycosylated hemoglobin was identical to that of the early products of the Maillard or browning reaction.

The initial event in the Maillard reaction is the condensation of the free aldehyde group of any sugar with amino groups on proteins to form a labile aldimine (Schiff base). This subsequently rearranges to form a stable ketoamine linkage (Amadori product) (Figure 21.1).

The general term describing the Amadori product of any sugar with hemoglobin is Hemoglobin A_1 (Trivelli *et al.*, 1971). This has been subdivided into 3 or more subfractions, HbA_{1a}, HbA_{1b} and HbA_{1c}. HbA_{1a} has at least 2 subfractions called HbA_{1a1} and HbA_{1a2}. When glucose reacts with hemoglobin, Hemoglobin A_{1c} is formed (Bunn *et al.*, 1976). Because of the abundance of glucose, HbA_{1c} is the major component of

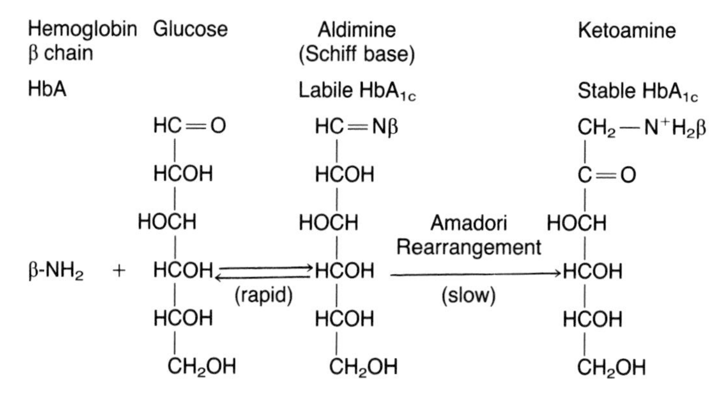

Figure 21.1 Formation of glycosylated hemoglobin (HbA_1c) by the Maillard reaction.

Table 21.3 The HbA_1 or glycosylated hemoglobins.

HbA + Reducing Sugar	→	HbA_1
HbA + Hexose-6-Phosphate	→	HbA_{1a}
HbA + Fructose	→	HbA_{1b}
HbA + Glucose	→	HbA_{1c}
HbA + ?	→	HbA_{1d}

HbA_1. Glucose-6-phosphate and fructose react with hemoglobin to form HbA_{1a1} and HbA_{1b} respectively (Table 21.3). Of all the forms of glycosylated hemoglobin, it is HbA_{1c} which best reflects glycemic levels over the preceding 2–3 months and laboratory methods measuring this are now preferred in the clinical management of diabetes.

Analogous glucose-protein adducts form on most proteins (e.g., albumin, collagen, etc.) (Hamlin *et al.*, 1975) and it is now thought that the products of the Maillard reactions play a central role in the process of ageing and in the development of the complications of diabetes mellitus (Dominiczak, 1991).

Until recently, the HbA_1 or HbA_{1c} results have generally been available after the clinic visit unless special arrangements had been made for the patient to visit the pathologist prior to the consultation. In some centers, a dried blood method for glycosylated hemoglobin has allowed the blood sample to be posted to the laboratory prior to the clinic visit (Eross *et al.*, 1984).

Newer, more rapid analytical methods using HPLC or monoclonal antibodies have allowed the estimation of the HbA_1 or HbA_{1c} on the day of the clinic visit.

Does knowing the HbA_1 or HbA_{1c} significantly alter the nature of the consultation? In several studies it was demonstrated that this knowledge caused a significant change in the management of the diabetes in 17–25% of patients with IDDM. The most obvious benefit of knowing the HbA_1 or HbA_{1c} level is when there is a major discrepancy between the glucose profile in the patient's logbook and the HbA_1 or HbA_{1c} level. In one study, the relationship between HbA_1 and SBGM values over the preceding six weeks revealed that in 41% there was a discrepancy between assigned categories of blood glucose control with all patients having better SBGM than HbA_1 values (Rumley *et al.*, 1990).

Discrepancy between glycosylated hemoglobin values and reported blood glucose profiles would occur if:

1. SBGM values had been falsified.
2. A major problem exists with either the meter or the SBGM technique leading to falsely low glucose levels.
3. Peaks of elevated blood glucose values

had been occurring unknown to the patient because of a failure to monitor blood glucose levels at those times. This most frequently occurs when patients fail to test their blood glucose levels postprandially.

21.7 MEASUREMENT OF FRUCTOSAMINE

Johnson *et al.* (1983) described a simple colorimetric fructosamine assay for the determination of glycosylated serum proteins. The method is based on reduction of nitro blue tetrazolium chloride (NBT) in alkaline solution and has been adapted for use by automated analytical systems. Assay refinements reduced the initial interference caused by lipemic serum and uric acid but problems in fructosamine measurements occur in hypoproteinemia, dysproteinemia, renal failure, thyrotoxicosis and dehydration.

Because the turnover of albumin is considerably more rapid than that of hemoglobin, HbA1 and fructosamine measurements reflect different periods of blood glucose control (John *et al.*, 1985). In pediatric practice, most physicians still tend to use the glycosylated hemoglobin measurements for monitoring glycemic control.

Fructosamine values essentially follow a Gaussian distribution with the reference range for adults being 200–280 mmol/l. Providing serum albumin and protein concentration are within reference ranges no corrections are necessary for variations in protein concentrations. Under stable diabetes control, fructosamine correlates well with HbA1c and glycemic control (Cefalu *et al.*, 1988). Under unstable metabolic conditions, the different kinetic behavior of glycosylated plasma proteins and HbA_1 would be expected to cause scattering of correlations. Thus, following a recent episode of hyperglycemia the ratio of fructosamine to glycosylated hemoglobin rises and subsequently falls during restabilization.

REFERENCES

Abouna, G.M., Al-Adnani, M.S., Kremer, G.D. *et al.* (1983) Reversal of diabetic nephropathy in human cadaveric kidneys after transplantation into nondiabetic recipients. *Lancet*, **ii**, 1274–76.

ADA Consensus Statement. (1987) Self-monitoring of blood glucose. *Diabetes Care*, **10**, 95–99.

ADA Postion Statement. (1989) Standards of medical care for patients with diabetes mellitus. *Diabetes Care*, **12**, 365–68.

ADA Position Statement. (1992) Urine and ketone measurements. *Diabetes Care*, **15** (suppl. 2), 38.

Ahring, K.K., Ahring, J.P.K., Joyce, C. *et al.* (1992) Telephone modem access improves diabetes control in those with insulin-requiring diabetes. *Diabetes Care*, **15**, 971–75.

Brownlee, M., Cerami, A. and Vlassara, H. (1988) Advanced glycosylation end products in tissue and the biochemical basis of diabetic complications. *N. Eng. J. Med.*, **318**, 1315–21.

Bunn, H.F., Haney, D.N., Kamin, S. *et al.* (1976). The biosynthesis of human hemoglobin A1c. Slow glycosylation of hemoglobin *in vivo*. *J. Clin. Invest.*, **57**, 1652–59.

Burrin, J.M. and Alberti, K.G.M.M. (1990) What is blood glucose: can it be measured? *Diabetic Med.*, **7**, 199–206.

Cefalu, W.T., Parker, T.B. and Johnson, C.R. (1988) Validity of serum fructosamine as index of short-term glycemic control in diabetic outpatients. *Diabetes Care*, **11**, 662–68.

Colaguiri, R., Colaguiri, S., Jones, S. *et al.* (1990) The quality of self-monitoring of blood glucose. *Diabetic Med.*, **7**, 800–804.

Dahl-Jorgensen, K., Brinchmann-Hansen, O., Hanssen, K.F. *et al.* (1985) Rapid tightening of blood glucose control leads to transient deterioration of retinopathy in insulin dependent diabetes mellitus: the Oslo study. *Brit. Med. J.*, **290**, 811–15.

Dahl-Jorgensen, K., Brinchmann-Hansen, O., Hanssen, K.F. *et al.* (1986) Effect of near normoglycaemia for two years on progression of early diabetic retinopathy, nephropathy and neuropathy: the Oslo study. *Brit. Med. J.*, **293**, 1195–99.

The DCCT Research Group. (1993) The effect of intensive treatment of diabetes on the development and progression of long-term complications in insulin-dependent diabetes mellitus.

N. Eng. J. Med., **329**, 977–86.

The DCCT Research Group. (1986) The Diabetes Control and Complications Trial (DCCT): design and methodologic considerations for the feasability phase. *Diabetes*, **35**, 530–45.

The DCCT Research Group. (1991) Epidemiology of severe hypoglycemia in the Diabetes Control and Complications Trial. *Am. J. Med.*, **90**, 450–59.

Deckert, T. (1960) Late diabetic manifestations in 'pancreatogenic' diabetes mellitus. *Acta Med. Scand.*, **168**, 439–46.

Dominiczak, M.H. (1991) The significance of the products of the Maillard (browning) reaction in diabetes. *Diabetic Medicine*, **8**, 505–16.

Engerman, R.L. and Kern, T.S. (1987) Progression of incipient diabetic retinopathy during good glycemic control. *Diabetes*, **36**, 808–12.

Eross, J., Kreutzmann, D., Jimenez, M. *et al.* (1984) Colorimetric measurement of glycosylated protein in whole blood, red blood cells, plasma and dried blood. *Ann. in Clin. Biochem.*, **21**:6, 477–83.

Feldt-Rasmussen, B., Mathiesen, E. and Deckert, T. (1986) Effect of two years of strict metabolic control on progression of incipient nephropathy in insulin-dependent diabetes. *Lancet*, **ii**, 1300–1304.

Galton, D.J. (1965) Diabetic retinopathy and haemochromatosis. *Brit. Med. J.*, **1**, 1169.

Garber, A.J., Vinik, A.I. and Crespin, S.R. (1992) Detection and management of lipid disorders in diabetic patients: a commentary for clinicians. *Diabetes Care*, **15**, 1068–74.

Hamlin, C.R., Kohn, R.R. and Luschin, J.H. (1975) Apparent accelerated aging of human collagen in diabetes mellitus. *Diabetes*, **24**, 902–904.

John, W.G., Webb, A.M. and Jones, A.E. (1985) Glycosylated haemoglobin and glycosylated albumin in non-diabetic and diabetic mothers and their babies. *Diabetic Med.*, **2**, 103–104.

Johnson, R.N., Metcalf, P.A. and Baker, J.R. (1983) Fructosamine; a new approach to the estimation of serum glycoprotein. *Clinica Chimica Acta*, **127**, 87–95.

Mauer, S.M., Steffes, M.W., Sutherland, D.E.R. *et al.* (1975) Studies on the rate of regression of the glomerular lesions in diabetic rats treated with pancreatic islet transplantation. *Diabetes*, **24**, 280–85.

Mauer, S.M., Barbosa, J., Vernier, R.L. *et al.* (1976) Development of diabetic vascular lesions in normal kidneys transplanted into patients with diabetes mellitus. *N. Eng. J. Med.*, **295**, 916–20.

Mazze, R., Shannon, H., Pasmmantier, R. *et al.* (1984) Reliability of blood glucose monitoring by patients with diabetes mellitus. *Am. J. Med.*, **77**, 211–17.

McCall, A.L. and Mullin, C.J. (1987) Home blood glucose monitoring: keystone for modern diabetes care. *Med. Clinics of N. Amer.*, **71**, 763–87.

NHS Procurement Directorate, DHSS. (1987) *Blood glucose measurements: reliability of results in extra-laboratory areas.* Health Notice (Hazard) 87/13. DHSS, London.

North, D.S., Steiner, J.F., Woodhouse, K.M. *et al.* (1987) Home monitors of blood glucose: comparison of precision and accuracy. *Diabetes Care*, **10**, 360–66.

Rahbar, S. (1962) An abnormal haemoglobin in red cells of diabetics. *Clinica Chimica Acta*, **22**, 296–98.

Reichard, P., Britz, A., Cars, I. *et al.* (1988) The Stockholm diabetes intervention study (SDIS): 18 months' results. *Acta Med. Scand.*, **224**, 115–22.

Rumley, A.G., Carlton, G. and Small, M. (1990) Within-clinic glycosylated haemoglobin measurement. *Diabetic Med.*, **7**, 838–40.

Seaquist, E.R., Goetz, F.C., Rich, S. *et al.* (1989) Familial clustering of diabetic kidney disease: evidence for genetic susceptibility to diabetic nephropathy. *N. Eng. J. Med.*, **320**, 1161–65.

Skyler, J.S. (1988) 'Monitoring diabetes mellitus', in J.H. Galloway, J.H. Potvin and, C.R. Shuman (eds). *Diabetes Mellitus*, 9th edn, pp. 160–73. Lilly, Indianopolis, IN.

Sonksen, P.H., Judd, S.K. and Lowy, C. (1978) Home monitoring of blood glucose: method for improving laboratory control. *Lancet*, **i**, 729–35.

Southgate, H.J. and Marks, V. (1986) Measurement of hypoglycaemia by Reflocheck. *Practical Diabetes*, **3**, 206–207.

Strowig, S. and Raskin, P. (1992) Glycemic control and complications. *Diabetes Care*, **15**, 1126–40.

Trivelli, L.A., Ranney, H.M. and Lai, H.-T. (1971) Hemoglobin components in patients with diabetes mellitus. *N. Eng. J. Med.*, **284**, 353–57.

Walford, S., Gale, E.A.M., Allison, S.P. *et al.* (1978) Self-monitoring of blood glucose: improvement of diabetic control. *Lancet*, **i**, 732–35.

22

Children's diabetes clinics

D.I. JOHNSTON

22.1 INTRODUCTION

An effective children's diabetes service provides a continuum of care between inpatient episodes, outpatient clinic supervision and community support. As the management of diabetic children has evolved, and specialist liaison staff have been recruited, the focus of care has shifted away from ward and clinic activities towards less formal guidance in the home and at school. This altered emphasis does not subtract from the role of the diabetes clinic but provides the opportunity for reappraisal of clinic objectives, structure and function. The total care of a diabetic child and family is ill-served by the traditional clinic setting dominated by time and staff constraints. A brief two- or three-monthly encounter between child and doctor can do little to clarify problems, and is a mere gesture when attempting to promote education and kindle motivation. The challenge is to provide a clinic process that generates enthusiastic participation from children, adolescents and families as well as meeting the requirements of structured monitoring and continuing education.

Different clinic populations and geographical settings dictate a flexible approach and various successful models have emerged. Clinics, whether catering for small or large populations, need to provide a service whose quality can be judged against nationally agreed criteria. Families prefer access to and are potentially better served by local clinics. However, they also have the right to expect expertise. In the UK, health authorities are incorporating increasingly detailed service specifications in their contracts for diabetes care. Children's diabetes services must not only be active in promoting optimal care, they must also be seen to have a structure and process capable of meeting these quality standards (BPA, 1990; BDA, 1990). The majority of principles discussed here are applicable to European and North American health systems.

22.2 OBJECTIVES

22.2.1 CHILD AND FAMILY EDUCATION

Education is recognized as very important at the time of diagnosis but there is less emphasis on reinforcement in the diabetes curriculum. In an audit conducted in northeast England, knowledge about diabetes and practical skills was very variable (McCowen *et al.*, 1986). Of the factors that might influence metabolic control, only the family's knowledge appeared amenable to improvement.

Childhood and Adolescent Diabetes
Published in 1994 by Chapman & Hall, London
ISBN 0 412 48610 5

Ideally, there should be a program of continuing education aimed not only at reinforcement but also at ensuring transfer of knowledge from parents to child. The diabetes team also needs to examine its own capacity for informing families, and for answering queries about progress in research or about issues highlighted by the media.

22.2.2 DIABETES REVIEW

Clinic visits provide a regular opportunity for monitoring general health, growth, injection procedures, metabolic control and complications. Not all of these aims have to be serviced at every visit. One option is to set aside one visit each year for a thorough physical review, and another for a focus on education. The remaining visits can follow a flexible approach with scope for general discussion and the fostering of a good working relationship.

Scrutiny of the home blood sugar monitoring diary takes on almost ritualistic significance in clinic. Examination of its contents can certainly be revealing and provides a focus for discussion of diabetic control during good and poor phases. However the emphasis must be on how the child or family interprets tests rather than on summary inspection and judgement by the doctor. The review process depends on long-term collection of useful and retrievable data. This requires structure and discipline. Checklists and computerization are invaluable aids in achieving this objective but data collection procedures must be robust, user-friendly and preferably compatible with that used by the rest of the District Diabetes Service.

22.2.3 PROBLEM-SOLVING RESOURCE

Readmission due to hyper- or hypoglycemia can be interpreted as a failure of prevention. The telephone, supported by a medical or nursing member of the diabetes team, is the main instrument of prevention but there are grumbling issues that are better tackled by direct confrontation in the clinic. The team may not always come up with an immediately successful solution, but the child and family will be reassured by this demonstration of team involvement. Testing problems emerge in almost every clinic and reinforce the case for experienced, authoritative staff.

22.2.4 GROUP ACTIVITIES

In spite of diabetes being relatively common, diabetic youngsters and their families can feel isolated and victimized. The clinic can be a vehicle for promoting contact but it is inadequate to rely upon spontaneous demonstrations of companionship in the waiting area. Useful group activity requires skilled leadership, careful targeting of potentially compatible youngsters, and protected time. A modest package of educational aims linked to small group activity appears popular with families and can improve control in the short and medium term (Hackett *et al.*, 1989). However, an intensive education program is expensive in terms of time and personnel and may not achieve long-term sustained improvement in control (Bloomfield *et al.*, 1990).

22.2.5 TEACHING, AUDIT AND RESEARCH

Students of various disciplines are attracted by childhood diabetes as a topic, but are largely divorced from its increasingly community-orientated approach to management. A good learning experience is to accompany the specialist nurse but there are obvious limitations to this resource. Clinics have therefore to accommodate teaching both at undergraduate and postgraduate levels. This should not be an excuse for denying patients their privacy or for asking junior doctors to reveal their relative ignorance at the hands of parents who have been immersed in diabetes for years. Successful audit and research flourish in a setting where expertise coexists with careful observation and record-keeping.

22.3 STRUCTURE: THE DIABETES TEAM

22.3.1 CONSULTANT STAFF

In every district there should be at least one pediatrician with expertise in diabetes. Where two or more pediatricians provide diabetes care, they should develop an integrated service and consolidate resources. Geography and provider pressures may dictate that they operate clinics in more than one location but there are strong care and economic arguments for sharing community liaison and support staff. It is also valuable to develop common treatment protocols spanning inpatient care, clinic monitoring and instructions to liaison staff. Agreed protocols reduce uncertainty when diabetic children are managed by less experienced medical and nursing staff. They also provide a uniform database for population research and audit.

The pediatrician must also forge close links with adult diabetic specialists. This may extend to having a shared care approach to adolescents. Some clinics benefit from the presence of an adult physician in the children's diabetic clinic. A more widespread practice is for there to be a handover clinic, and for there to be agreed management approaches so that the changeover is straightforward.

22.3.2 OTHER DOCTORS IN THE DIABETES TEAM

The relationship between health professionals and the young diabetic person is long-term but mere duration does not ensure a productive association. Success hinges on bilateral commitment. A diabetic child or adolescent needs to relate to a doctor or nurse who can speak with both authority and understanding. Families coping with the daily pressure of diabetes should have confidence in their advisers; they are well-versed in the potential deficiencies of inexperienced doctors. The clinic must therefore contain a core of experienced staff. The consultant usually provides the permanent component of this core but increasingly important aspects of monitoring, advice and education can be delegated to specialist nurses. Larger clinics needing two or more committed doctors can draw from the community pediatric sector, and therefore reinforce the contact with the school health service. Family practitioner clinical assistants provide another valuable input into this core team.

22.3.3 DIABETES SPECIALIST NURSES

Specialist diabetes nurses and health visitors have totally transformed the concept of total diabetes care. The availability of specialist nursing is probably the single most important criterion of an effective diabetes clinic. The size of the young diabetes population will determine whether it is appropriate to have a specific pediatric specialist nurse or to share staff with the adult service. The former has the advantage that the nurse will also develop expertise in child and family care. In either event there must be a commitment to full participation in the children's clinic. As doctors have gained confidence and respect for their nursing colleagues' skills they have also evolved strategies for delegating areas of clinic practice.

22.3.4 OUTPATIENT NURSES

The smooth running and efficiency of any clinic is dependent on the enthusiasm of involved nursing staff. Hospital management needs to be constantly reminded that outpatient nurses have a role far beyond that of merely directing patients to the consulting room. Nurses can maximize the value of the time spent before and after interviews with doctors. They can convert an arid waiting room into a fruitful area for education, friendship and informal counselling. They should contribute to the development of clinic protocols, and see themselves as active participants in the total diabetes team. Within the general pediatric outpatient team, one or two nurses can be given special responsibility for diabetes.

22.3.5 DIETITIANS

An understanding of nutrition and its place in diabetes is an essential foundation for good metabolic control. It is vital therefore that diet is a regular topic for review and information (see Chapter 18). There is an unfortunate tendency for superficial dietary assessment in clinics and for recourse to the dietitian only when more florid problems arise. Dietitians need to be part of an organized regular review, reinforcing healthy eating and advising on the all-too-frequent diet problems of the young. They need to take a proactive approach to the common eating disorders of adolescence, especially the drift of many teenage girls towards obesity.

22.3.6 CLINICAL PSYCHOLOGISTS

The interplay between behavior, mood and diabetes control is well-recognized if ill-understood. Needle phobia, rebellion, and sullen hostility are just some of the more readily recognized behavior problems encountered in the clinic. Ideally, a clinical psychologist or child and family psychiatrist is part of the regular team rather than a resource to be summoned in desperation. Health professionals immersed in the supervision of chronic disease are themselves subject to considerable emotional pressure. There are inevitable situations in which difficulties and frictions arise at the interface between carer and recipient. An experienced psychologist can be a guide to patients, families and staff.

22.3.7 OTHER PROFESSIONALS

The infrequency of eye and foot complications in the young diabetic population lessens the case for regular participation of ophthalmic and chiropody staff (but see Chapter 40). Eye and foot examination are essential components of annual review but the skills can be acquired by core medical and nursing staff. Chiropodists are available in some centers and provide a useful educational role as well as dealing with the more mundane foot disorders that occur in any young population.

22.3.8 CLINICAL CHEMISTRY

It is essential that the Children's Diabetes Service has a clear pathway by which blood samples can be collected and analyzed for either glycosylated hemoglobin (HbA_1) or fructosamine. Capillary HbA_1 measurement can be performed before or during clinic attendance (see Chapter 21). While there are enthusiastic advocates for real time HbA_1 results within clinic, most children show tracking with predictable levels, and such immediacy is of debatable cost-effectiveness. More important is for the clinic HbA_1 results to be considered as part of clinic review some days later. Patients or parents also need to learn of their results promptly.

22.3.9 SUPPORT STAFF

In this era of the Patient's Charter and total quality management, it is essential that all components of the child and family's encounter with hospital and clinic are examined. Poor clinic attendance may reflect unsympathetic car parking lot attendants or over-taxed clinic receptionists rather than the specialist's personal qualities! This wider team includes play leaders and volunteers.

22.4 STRUCTURE: CLINIC ACCOMMODATION

Most clinics use existing outpatient facilities. It is desirable that the diabetic clinic is allocated specific sessions, and that nursing staff are allocated to the clinic without competition from an adjacent baby or asthma clinic. Total quality management should follow the path of families and assess the standard of access routes, signposting, reception, waiting areas, measuring room, blood and urine testing facilities, toilets and changing rooms, and all this is before they reach the consulting room. The modern multidisciplinary approach to diabetes care demands more space; few of us work optimally in a consulting room so full of staff that there is hardly room for patient and family. We also have to be sensitive to those occasions when a young person or parent requires private time, and this includes providing a mechanism by which the youngster can enter the consulting room without an obligatory parental escort.

A number of districts have created Diabetes Day Centers combining the resources of clinic supervision with the option of informal visits for treatment and education (Day & Spathis, 1988; Day *et al.*, 1992). Inevitably the main preoccupation of such centers is the care of adult diabetics, but modern customized design and the ready availability of specialist staff makes them attractive for children's clinics. A little planning and room adjustment can ensure that areas are attractive to the young. Pediatricians are naturally anxious about exposing vulnerable diabetic youngsters to a procession of blind and elderly amputees in such shared facilities. The reality is that diabetes centers are more likely to be full of 'normal' people and they are certainly less awe-inspiring than the average general hospital main entrance.

Day centers are one solution to the quest for a territory more likely to appeal to teenagers. There are compelling reasons to attempt age-stratification of the pediatric diabetic clinic. The disillusioned adolescent may be interested in fast cars but not when they are being pushed between his legs by a tiresome toddler who just happens to have the same disease. Again, clinic numbers will determine the best approach; setting aside time after school, finding friendlier age-matched accommodation or sharing facilities with an adult colleague and younger clients. Beware of creating too informal a setting for your teenage patients; they may conclude that you are not really interested in their diabetes either! (see Chapter 26).

22.5 THE CLINIC PROCESS

The following model has emerged from the author's experience in both teaching hospital and district general hospital settings. The scale of activity is of less importance than issues relating to quality. The model reflects both achievement and ambition and owes much to the advice of colleagues and clients. It is unrealistic to expect that children and adolescents should look forward to attending a diabetic clinic, but a criterion of success might be that the doctors and nurses judge it to be their favourite clinic.

A flow diagram helps in planning the logistics of a clinic (Figure 22.1). An annual review of clinic numbers and age profile will determine the best policy for age stratification, either within clinic sessions or between clinics. High school children can then be accommodated after school or at clinics which coincide with school vacations. Interestingly not all youngsters welcome the option of not disrupting school attendance. It may be fea-

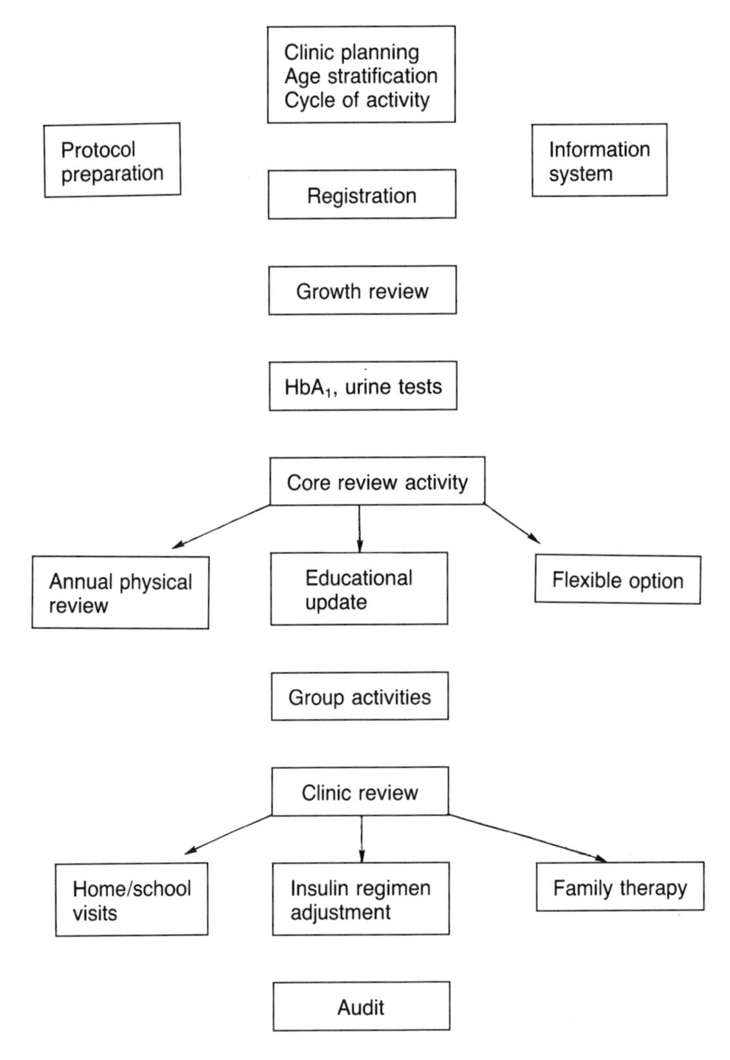

Figure 22.1 Flow chart for use in planning logistics of a diabetes clinic.

sible to keep compatible groups in phase with each other; this can foster friendships and allow a more promising setting for group education. This group cohesion can be taken a step further by organizing trips and camps.

In a diabetic service supported by specialist nurses and with ongoing family support, clinic visits for most children need be no more frequent than 3–4 monthly. Within each yearly cycle, visits can have different objectives as listed above. Each attendance also has to provide time for core activities: growth measurement, capillary blood sampling (if not organized beforehand), inspection of injection sites, and discussion of diabetes management.

Reception desk or appointment staff play a key role in facilitating this organized flow of activity. Together with the liaison nurses they have to be alert to persistent nonattenders, and sympathetic to parents whose concerns and life pressures demand flexibility.

Information technology has gained ground more rapidly in diabetes clinics than in most other areas of medicine. The pressure for innovation has been immense in adult diabetic clinics where large clinic numbers and the chaos of bulky patient files denies organized review and data retrieval. Children's clinics are spared some of these rigors but ten or fifteen years later even the best-kept case-notes can become impenetrable. There is now a choice of well-proven computer software to facilitate clinic organization (Williams *et al.*, 1988). These encompass appointment planning, examination and an investigation checklist as well as the option for clinic letters. They can generate updated patient summaries for filing in the notes; edited versions being available for family practitioners and families. The resulting case-notes are slimmer, more amenable to rapid inspection and are disciplined. Scope for limited but adequate freehand notes can be retained. Modern software can focus on the requirements of the adult diabetes service but contain sufficient flexibility to allow for a customized children's version. Compatibility with adult systems provides a comprehensive district diabetes register as well as the potential for population analyses. A well-founded concern is that information technology creates an interface with data at the expense of the doctor–patient relationship. Piloting of data input sheets must take account of their intrusion into clinic time. Questions have to be limited to those of proven value and designed in an easy-to-answer format. Computer consoles in the clinic cut out the paper phase of data collection, and enthusiasts claim that they promote patient involvement.

A key component of clinic organization is

Table 22.1 Summary of structure and process measures applicable to children's diabetes clinics. (Derived from Williams *et al.*, 1992.)

Structure	Staffiing
	Pediatrician with a special interest
	• Specialist nurse
	• Dietitian
	• Clinical psychologist
	Designated Diabetes Clinic
	Education area/resource
	HbA1 or fructosamine testing available
Process	Clinic appointments, missed or cancelled
	Waiting times in clinic
	Completion of annual physical review:
	• Growth
	• Injection sites
	• Optic fundi (with pupils dilated if aged over 12 years)
	• Blood pressure
	• Urine for microproteinuria
	Completion of family and child education review
	Dietary review

an opportunity for the team to meet in order to review patients, evaluate measurements of metabolic control and incorporate information gathered by liaison nurses during home and school visits. The return of HbA_1 results determines when this is best planned. It is often more logical to decide on insulin regimens adjustment in the light of this review process rather than to attempt manipulation within the clinic. Such meetings can also guide the liaison nurses on how they should best target their efforts over the following weeks. The group can also use the time to discuss clinic management, broader issues of diabetes care, and audit (Table 22.1).

REFERENCES

Bloomfield, S., Calder, J.E., Chisolm, V. *et al.* (1990) A project in diabetes education for children. *Diabetic Med.*, **7**, 137–42.

British Diabetic Association. (1990) What diabetic care to expect. *Diabetic Med.*, **7**, 554–55.

British Paediatric Association Working Party. (1990) The organisation of services for children with diabetes in the United Kingdom. *Diabetic Med.*, **7**, 457–64.

Day, J.L. and Spathis, M. (1988) District diabetes centres in the United Kingdom. *Diabetic Med.*, **5**, 372–80.

Day, J.L., Metcalfe, J. and Johnson, P. (1992) Benefits provided by an integrated education and clinical diabetes centre: A follow-up study. *Diabetic Med.*, **9**, 855–59.

Hackett, A., Court, S., Matthews, J. *et al.* (1989) Do education groups help diabetics and their parents? *Arch. Dis. Child.*, **64**, 997–1003.

McCowen, C., Hackett, A., Court, S. *et al.* (1986) Are families of diabetic children adequately taught? *Brit. Med. J.*, **292**, 1361.

Williams, C., Harvey, F. and Sonksen, P. (1988) A role for computers in diabetes care? *Diabetic Med.*, **5**, 177–99.

Williams, D.R.R., Home, P.D. and Members of a Working Group of the Research Unit of the Royal College of Physicians and British Paediatric Association. (1992) A proposal for continuing audit of diabetes services. *Diabetic Med.*, **9**, 759–64.

23

Hospital nursing care

R.M. MITCHELL, S.C. BROWN, S. FALLON and L. SMITH

23.1 INTRODUCTION

The management of newly-diagnosed insulin dependent diabetics has changed over the last 10–15 years. The principal reasons for the changes in management are the result of an increased awareness of the condition in society and early detection of the condition and referral by general practitioners.

Nowadays, it is not always necessary to admit children to hospital for initial stabilization; in some instances, stabilization is possible and desirable within the community (Young & Greenhalgh, 1992; McEvilly, 1991; Legge, 1993; Swift *et al.*, 1993). For details of the nursing care for a child admitted in ketoacidosis, see Table 23.1.

Children who are admitted to hospital spend on average 5–7 days for the initial period of stabilization. The length of stay depends on several factors e.g., the severity of onset, the emotional impact of the diagnosis on the family and the parents'/caregivers' understanding of the condition. Some centers contend that admitting the child to hospital allows the parents a period of readjustment following the initial emotional shock of the diagnosis.

Helping the child and parents to accept the diagnosis of insulin dependent diabetes mellitus and initiating the process of enabling them to live with it on a day-to-day basis, is a major role for the nurse during the first few days following diagnosis.

Successful management of children with diabetes is nowadays recognized to depend on the effective transfer of skills and information to the diabetic child and the family (Young & Greenhalgh, 1992). Nurses with specialist skills are required and it is not sufficient to have information passed on by nurses who themselves have received the information by 'passive absorption' (Shillitoe, 1988). Nurses themselves require specialist training and it might be argued that they require counselling skills in order to work effectively with children and their parents. The transfer of knowledge and skills may take place in the hospital environment or at home, depending on local policies and practices.

The length of stay in hospital varies from child to child as many aspects of management have to be explored with the parents. However, time spent by the child in hospital at the time of diagnosis has been reduced as home support has increased (McEvilly, 1991). Before any education can begin, the child, if old enough, and the parents have to be receptive to the exchange of information. For the older child there is the 'dawning realization that the disease is lifelong. The mixed emotions, behavioral disturbance and confused feelings

Childhood and Adolescent Diabetes
Published in 1994 by Chapman & Hall, London
ISBN 0 412 48610 5

about oneself and others both individually and in relation to the family' (Shillitoe, 1988, p. 144).

The intense emotional impact on the child and parents should never be underestimated (Eiser, 1985). The nurse can expect parents' and children's reactions to be varied but often similar to those associated with bereavement or any other sudden unwelcome life event (Kübler-Ross, 1970; Young & Greenhalgh, 1992). During the initial denial stage, only limited benefit can be expected from an education program, because many factors (such as guilt feelings and anxiety) have an inhibitory effect on memory and concentration (Shillitoe, 1988).

It is during this stage that the nurse must use skill and judgement to decide when it is right to begin teaching and what form it should take. Emotional and intellectual factors in both child and parents have to be considered. In particular, the child's understanding of the problems, of how the body works, their capacity to acquire new knowledge and requisite fine motor skills must be taken into account. It is essential to involve other key individuals who care for the child in the education program e.g., members of the extended family and school teachers. Variations in how children acquire knowledge should also be taken into consideration when establishing individual teaching programs. For example, there is evidence that mothers acquire more information about diabetes than do fathers (McCowen *et al.*, 1986). The creation of a friendly, relaxed, informal atmosphere during the child's stay in hospital is of benefit to both child and family, by helping them to feel more relaxed and facilitating information exchange with the members of the multidisciplinary team.

Few studies have been carried out which attempt to evaluate the effectiveness of diabetes education programs. Brandt and Magyary (1993) investigated the effect of a diabetes education program for school-aged diabetic children and their mothers. All the participants had previously received some basic instruction about diabetic management at the time of diagnosis. The primary goals of the program were to improve the child's and parents' knowledge of skills for diabetes management at home. The secondary goals were to improve the child's feelings of competence and the parents' supportive network. The program for the parents consisted of eleven sessions, each one lasting approximately 50 minutes. A variety of teaching methods were used.

At the three-month follow-up, diabetic knowledge and skills in children and their mothers had improved and the program appeared to be beneficial to the majority. However, the researchers themselves comment that the study design makes it impossible to know whether increased knowledge and skills can be attributed solely to the program. The secondary goals were not achieved as successfully as the primary goals and the researchers suggest that mothers and children might have been able to learn more if they had felt supported by others, for example, their family network (Brandt & Magyary, 1993). Studies such as this highlight the importance of evaluating existing programs if the needs of the parents and children are to be identified and met effectively.

There are many books and leaflets which may be additional sources of information for parents (see pp. 342 and 475). These can be complemented by the nurse sharing knowledge and demonstrating aspects of management e.g., insulin administration, blood glucose monitoring. The books and leaflets given to parents should contain the type of information parents will require at home. These booklets often serve as a reference source as parents begin to take on the daily responsibility for decision-making in relation to the management of their child.

The child and parents should themselves determine the depth of information provided and the rate at which it is imparted by the nurse. Initially, a small amount of information is given to enable the child and parents to cope on a day-to-day basis. Care is taken to avoid overwhelming the family with large quantities of information. Additional knowledge and skills are acquired gradually over the forthcoming months. Education of the family begins in hospital and is completed in the community.

23.2 THE NATURE OF THE DISEASE AND ITS MANAGEMENT

During the first few days after admission many parents feel very guilty about what has happened to their child. They may experience guilt if they delayed taking their child to hospital or to the general practitioner or for not recognizing the signs and symptoms of diabetes mellitus. Some parents may feel that their actions are directly responsible for causing their child to develop diabetes mellitus. There are many parental misconceptions about the causes of diabetes in childhood, for example giving a child too many sweets or the wrong diet. Nursing and medical staff are constantly required to reassure the parents that they are in no way to blame. An outline plan of the child's management is given to the parents and in due course each aspect is discussed in greater detail. An uncomplicated explanation of the nature of the disease and its immediate implications should be offered.

A selection of books which parents and older children may find beneficial is given at the end of this chapter.

23.3 TECHNIQUE AND TIMING OF INSULIN INJECTIONS

Most children and parents are daunted by the prospect of daily insulin injections. If the child is old enough and shows a willingness to learn about the injection technique, the educational approach is geared to the needs of that individual child. In this situation, the parents take on an advisory role. However, the parents are still taught the necessary skills in case they are required to administer the insulin in the event of future ill health or non-compliance on the part of the child (see also Chapters 7 and 15).

The types of insulin available and their modes of action and storage of insulin are discussed with the child's parents. Opportunities are given for the parents to draw up insulin, to mix insulin and to administer it, in accordance with the child's requirements. Advice is given about future changes in insulin requirements, e.g., the child may initially only require one injection of medium acting insulin per day if very young or very active and subsequently the requirement may increase to twice-daily injections.

Many circumstances in childhood bring about alterations in insulin requirements, e.g., illness, surgery, stress, growth and puberty and these will need to be discussed. The importance of injection site rotation is emphasized. This can be made more interesting for the young child by providing a life-sized poster on which stickers are placed when different injection sites are used (Henderson, 1992). Rates of absorption from different injection sites are discussed as is the timing of injections and advice is offered on the interval between administration of insulin and mealtimes – approximately 30–40 minutes (see also Chapter 15).

Recent advice issued by Gill (1991) on behalf of the British Diabetic Association recommends that patients commencing insulin treatment should inject into a pinched fold of skin at an angle of 90 degrees, with the raised skin-fold maintained during the injection (see Fig. 17.4, p. 260). Comparatively little research has been carried out into children's injection techniques but Noyer highlights the fact that an unacceptably high proportion of children (21%) aged 10–16 years drew up an inaccurate dose of insulin (Noyer & Tomlinson, 1992).

In general, no specific skin preparation is advocated prior to the insulin injection as, in the past, problems have been encountered, such as alteration in skin texture and delayed absorption from the site of injection, following the repeated use of alcohol wipes on the skin.

23.4 BLOOD MONITORING

From the time the child is admitted to hospital parents observe the monitoring of blood glucose levels and their early participation is actively encouraged. Whether or not the family will be using a glucose meter, the visual method is taught during the initial education in order that the family are competent in this method in the event of meter failure in the future.

Correct technique is emphasized, as faulty monitoring at home could result in inappropriate insulin dosage or dietary change. When a meter is used, the importance of regular cleaning and calibration is explained. The calibration checks are essential both to verify accurate functioning of the machine and correct technique on the part of the user. Parents can be advised to measure and record blood glucose results once or twice a day and to vary the times on a day-to-day basis. Many children with diabetes resent most the need for finger-prick home blood glucose monitoring and recent research (Willey *et al.*, 1993) suggests that once-daily home blood glucose monitoring, at a variable time each day gives adequate information for clinical interventions and reduces the heavy demand on individuals with diabetes.

Bedlow (1988) highlights a range of circumstances when more intensive monitoring may be required which include:

- confirmation of suspected nocturnal hypoglycemia
- when ill, especially in the presence of vomiting or diarrhea
- persistent symptoms of high or low blood glucose
- ketonuria
- unusual activity
- traveling through time-zones or changing meal times.

In addition, when a diabetic child complains of abdominal pain, the blood glucose level should be checked as this symptom may be indicative of hyperglycemia. Guidelines are given to the parents as to the necessary action required if serial readings are outwith the accepted range of 4–9 mmol/l.

In some centers it is the practice to 'induce' a hypoglycemic episode in the child prior to discharge home. The normal dose of insulin is given and breakfast withheld. This is done in a closely controlled environment within the ward (Estridge & Davies, 1992). This experience enables the parents to observe the physical and behavioral changes which occur as their child becomes hypoglycemic. The older child is encouraged to recognize the feelings associated with a hypoglycemic episode thereby allowing them to take the necessary steps, on a future occasion, to correct hypoglycemia at an early stage. When the induced hypoglycemic episode occurs, steps are taken immediately to restore the child's blood glucose levels to within normal limits. The child is given an exchange in the form of a glucose drink followed by further exchanges of a longer-acting carbohydrate. (An exchange is equivalent to 10 g of carbohydrate.) The experience is used as a teaching situation for the child and parents.

Initially, parents are encouraged to contact the ward directly for guidance regarding the adjustment of insulin dosages and an experienced doctor should always be available to give advice if required. The liason diabetic nurse who visits the child prior to and following discharge can also be contacted for advice and support. In due course many parents acquire the necessary knowledge, skills and confidence to make adjustments to insulin dosage at home, although often after telephone discussion and advice.

23.5 URINE TESTING

The value of testing for glycosuria is much debated. Research has indicated that urine glucose correlates very poorly with blood glucose levels (Daly *et al.*, 1988). The major disadvantage of this type of monitoring from a parent's point of view, is that urine testing indicates what has already happened to the child and does not reflect the present situation, and all our patients are doing home blood glucose monitoring (see above). However the method of, and indications for, testing urine for ketones, must be taught (see Chapter 21).

23.6 DIETARY ADVICE

The main aims of dietary control are to ensure that the child's blood glucose levels are maintained within normal limits and that the child grows appropriately throughout childhood. In the initial stages the dietician spends considerable time with the family explaining the dietary aspects of care. Discussion includes the child's dietary requirements in health and illness and the implications that exercise may have on dietary and insulin requirements (see Chapter 18).

Brenchley (1993) highlights the importance of dietary advice by stating 'suggested changes in the diet must be appropriate to the needs of child and family and should be adapted to take on board the changing circumstances in the child's life'.

23.7 IMPACT OF THE DIAGNOSIS ON THE FAMILY UNIT

In the initial stages and after the devastating shock of diagnosis, Hodges and Parker (1987) identified four main areas which cause parents concern:

1. Managing the diabetic regimen, including acquiring the necessary knowledge and understanding to do so
2. Coping on a daily basis with the restraints imposed by diabetes
3. Dealing with school problems
4. Working with the health care team.

In supporting the family, the nurse should attempt to appreciate and understand their concerns and be prepared to address any issues they raise. The type of support which is appreciated and reported useful by parents is advice, encouragement and regular opportunities to discuss problems (Challen *et al.*, 1990). This can be facilitated by:

1. increased and more intensive support at the time of diagnosis (Bradford & Singer, 1991; Kenneth, 1991)
2. identification of families who may require extra special attention and support
3. easy access to professional advice
4. clear and consistent advice, which may need to be repeated and key issues reinforced
5. introductions to other parents of diabetic children
6. liaison with school teachers to improve support while at school
7. provision of a diabetic home care nurse service (Moyer, 1989).

Although having diabetes is not necessarily associated with adjustment problems, children that experience psychological difficulties during the initial phase of diabetes are more prone to have long-term problems (see Chapters 7 and 20).

23.8 SIBLINGS

The impact of the diagnosis on other family members can be considerable (see Chapter

32) and it is the responsibility of the nurse to ensure that parents appreciate the potential effects on non-diabetic siblings. Sibling reaction is well-documented in many chronic illnesses or disabilities (e.g., asthma, cardiac and hematological problems, cystic fibrosis or cerebral palsy) but less well for diabetes (Lavigne & Ryan, 1979; Taylor, 1980; Doyle, 1987; Breslau, 1981; Kanfl, 1982; Walker, 1988). It is likely that the well sibling of a diabetic child may react in similar ways.

The feelings of the well sibling at diagnosis are many and varied and may include: worry of responsibility for the illness, fear of catching it and a mixture of feelings of jealousy, anger, sadness and guilt (Brenner, 1984; Taylor, 1980; Lynn, 1989). Extreme feelings of guilt may be suppressed but the sibling may attempt to compensate for this by trying to be good and helping their ill sibling and parents as much as possible (Campion, 1991). If unexplored, the feelings of guilt which are secondary to resentment may intensify and may contribute a moderate or even severe degree of emotional deprivation. The signs of this may be withdrawal, hostility, behavior problems and delinquency (Steinhauer *et al.*, 1974; Taylor, 1980; Lavigne & Ryan, 1979).

Isolation is documented as the single most common feeling experienced by well siblings, saying they often felt alone, ignored, uninvolved and left outside family relationships. Compounding this, many siblings reported they were very interested in their ill sibling's diagnosis and care (Taylor, 1980). Conversley, many well siblings conveyed positive feelings such as sensitivity, compassion and demonstrated increased maturity (Tizza, 1962).

It has been documented (Knafl, 1982) that siblings are not 'infinitely adaptable'. With this in mind the following list taken and modified from Rosen and Stearns (1979) (cited by Brenner, 1984), offers simple practical suggestions on how the nurse can help parents support the well sibling in adapting to the stresses and changes in family life:

1. Ensure siblings have accurate but simple information about the illness and know they did not cause it and will not catch it.
2. The information given should be updated regularly.
3. Encourage the sibling to ask questions and try to answer truthfully.
4. Use understandable language – appropriate for stage of cognitive development.
5. Ensure the children's (patient's and sibling's) close friends have accurate information.
6. Bring siblings to the hospital and clinic visits if possible.
7. Help siblings choose tasks they can do to help care for the patient.
8. Explain what the ill sibling will and will not be able to do (i.e., diet restriction, daily injections, etc).
9. Support siblings' feelings of sadness, fear, and expressions of those feelings (crying etc.) and be prepared to share your feelings with them.
10. Help siblings to accept their negative feelings about being deprived of the patient's companionship and their parents' attention and care.
11. Continue normal daily routines and activities as much as possible (sports activities, visits to friends, parties, etc.).

23.9 SUBSEQUENT HOSPITAL ADMISSIONS

The child with insulin dependent diabetes mellitus may require subsequent admission with one of the problems outlined below:

Diabetic ketoacidosis – potentially a serious and life-threatening complication of diabetes in childhood (Table 23.1)
Hypoglycemia (Table 23.2)
Emergency/routine Surgery (see also Chapter 24)
Intercurrent illness
Re-education

Table 23.1 Nursing care of a child admitted in ketoacidosis.

Problem	Nursing/family goal	Nursing/family action	Rationale
Decreased Conscious Level	1. Maintain a safe enviroment. 2. Assess conscious level.	1. Nurse patient in semi-prone position. 2. Nurse patient beside oxygen and suction equipment. 3. Insert nasogastric tube/nil by mouth. 4. One-hourly neurological observations using the Glasgow Coma Scale. 5. EKG monitor *in situ*.	1. To maintain airway. 2. To maintain airway. 3. Child may be vomiting, stomach may be dilated, therefore a nasogastric tube will reduce the risk of aspiration during semi-conscious state. 4. To assess level of consciousness and detect signs of cerebral edema (raised intracranial pressure). 5. Urea and electrolyte imbalance may cause cardiac ectopics and arrhythmias.
Dehydration and Electrolyte Imbalane and Possible Acidosis	1. Rehydrate and restore normal fluid and electrolyte balance.	1. One-hourly observations of pulse and respirations (rate, rhythm and depth). 2. Assist the doctor with gaining venous access and taking blood samples for urea electrolyte and glucose levels. 3. Intravenous fluids as prescribed, Care of IV Site.	1. Possibility of Kussmaul breathing – which is part of the body's mechanism to eliminate excess ketones. 2. To minimize the trauma to the child, of repeated blood sampling during the period of stabilization. 3. Rehydrate *gradually* to reduce the risk of cerebral edema. A possible intravenous regime may be i. Plasma – depending on patient's condition (i.e., in shock).

Table 23.1 *Continued*

Problem	Nursing/family goal	Nursing/family action	Rationale
			ii. 0.9% saline until blood glucose below or equal to 13 mmol/l + soluble insulin IV. If necessary, potassium may be given to correct hypokalemia. iii. When blood glucose ≤13 mmol/l, fluids changed to 0.45% saline + 5% dextrose. Insulin infusion will be titrated accordingly. iv. If blood glucose falls, 10% dextrose intravenously or one oral carbohydrate exchange may be given. Recommended type of exchange e.g. cereal, toast. v. Potassium will be added to infusion when patient has passed urine.
		4. Fluid balance chart.	4. To maintain an accurate record of input and output.
		5. Weigh patient if possible (or as soon as possible).	5. To assess degree of dehydration.
		6. Test all urine for glucose and ketones.	6. To assess response to treatment.
		7. Nasogastric tube/nil by mouth.	7. To reduce risk of vomiting/aspiration.

Raised blood glucose level and inability to maintain levels within normal limits.	1. Reduce blood glucose and return to normal limits. Normal: 4–7 mmol/l.	1. Intravenous insulin as prescribed. Syringe – Change 6-hourly; dose 0.05 U/kg/hr 2. Hourly blood glucose monitoring. 3. Intravenous fluids + IV Regimen as above.	1. Reduces blood glucose. Insulin allows the utilization (uptake) of glucose by the cells to provide the body with energy. Continuous intravenous insulin as this reduces blood glucose steadily thus avoiding the peaks and troughs which may be associated with subcutaneous administration of insulin. 2. Allows accurate recording of response to treatment
Child and Family Anxiety	1. To provide a calm and supportive atmosphere. 2. To reduce stress and anxiety. 3. To reassure the child and explain all procedures, giving a better understanding of the child's condition.	1. Introduce self and relevant team members. 2. Orientate to ward and facilities within the hospital. 3. In the initial stage give uncomplicated explanations of all procedures and care. 4. Answer all questions. 5. Ensure education is pitched at appropriate level and pace for parents and child. 6. Play – Provide appropriate play activities.	1. Gradually increase parents'/child's confidence so that they can function independently of the hospital staff.

Table 23.2 Nursing a child admitted with hypoglycemia.

PROBLEM	Nursing/family goal	Nursing/family action	Rationale
Low Blood Sugar	1. Determine cause. 2. Restore to normal blood glucose 4–7 mmol/l.	Nursing actions will depend on severity of hypoglycemia. SEVERE (i.e., unconscious or fitting) 1. Obtain history from parents. 2. Take an initial blood glucose measurement. 3. Assist doctor with the insertion of an IV cannula and either: Give IV Dextrose as prescribed IM Glucagon as prescribed Hypostop gel 4. Maintain a safe environment Airway Oxygen Suction 5. Check blood glucose 30 minutes after IV Dextrose/IM Glucagon/or Oral Hypostop and when the child is awake give × 1 exchange of a long-acting carbohydrate (starch, i.e., bread as opposed to a glucose drink). 6. Observe for potential effects of severe hypoglycemia, i.e., transient hemiparesis, hemianopia, headaches.	IV DEXTROSE raises blood glucose instantly. IM GLUCAGON converts glycogen in the liver to glucose thereby increasing blood glucose. Side-effect of Glucagon is vomiting, therefore there may be a problem introducing oral carbohydrate. HYPOSTOP used for rapid increase in blood glucose levels (Savage, 1992). To assess oral response to IV Dextrose, IM Glugagon or Oral Hypostop and to maintain blood glucose within normal limits.

		MILD TO MODERATE 1. Take an initial blood glucose measurement. 2. Recognize possible signs of hypoglycemia, i.e., hunger, pallor, sweating, irritability. 3. Give one exchange of a fast-acting carbohydrate (i.e., glucose drink or glucose tablets). If not improved in 5–10 minutes give another fast-acting exchange. If Hypo is pre-snack or pre-meal, give an extra exchange of a fast-acting carbohydrate followed by the normal number of exchanges.	
Parental Anxiety Due to Hypoglycemic Episode	1. Reduce anxiety by promoting understanding of cause for hypoglycemic episode. 2. Offer advice of ways to prevent further episodes.	1. Find out why hypo occurred by obtaining history of events leading up to the event. 2. By knowing the above and understanding why the above caused the drop in blood glucose, parents and child can prevent hypo happening in the future.	Possible Reasons: 1. Too much insulin. Delayed snack/missed meal. Over-exercise.

23.9.1 THE CHILD WITH DIABETES REQUIRING SURGERY (SEE CHAPTER 24)

It is the practice within some hospitals to admit the child to the ward appropriate to their presenting problem. Other centers elect to admit all diabetics directly to the specialist diabetic endocrine ward. There are obvious benefits in admitting children to specialist wards where staff have the necessary knowledge, skill and attitudes to provide holistic care. Admission to a specialist ward allows staff to reinforce the philosophy of care that children with diabeties can lead near to normal lives without diabetes dominating their day-to-day lives in hospital or at home.

23.10 SUMMARY

Nursing care of the child is family-centered and parents are encouraged to be involved in the care of their child from the time of admission until discharge (Foster *et al.*, 1989).

On admission, the child and family are assessed and a profile of the child is obtained. This information enables the nurse to identify actual and potential problems for each indi-vidal child. Care is then planned and implemented and it is at this point that many parents become active participants in the care of their child. They learn many complex skills in the process, e.g., insulin administration and adjustment of insulin dosage which equip them to cope with their child at home following discharge.

Many parents take on this role with great courage and enthusiasm and there is no doubt that parental presence is of great benefit to the child in providing reassurance and continuity at a time of great practical upheaval and emotional stress.

Communication is a key component of successful partnership with parents. The atmosphere must exist where parents are free to express their fears and anxieties and where they can question aspects of care which they may not fully understand. Evaluation of the care provided is essential and often at this point the value of group support for parents is highlighted.

Local and national support groups exist which provide considerable reassurance for worried and naturally anxious parents (see Chapter 37).

In due course, the children themselves derive benefit from meeting up with members of their peer group who are also diabetic. This may be arranged while the child is still in hospital or may be arranged when the child subsequently attends the clinic at the outpatient department.

APPENDIX: FURTHER READING

Books useful to older newly-diagnosed diabetic children and their parents:

Braithwack, A. (1992) *I Have Diabetes.* Dinosaur Publications: HarperCollins with Lilly Diabetes Care Division, London.
Hilson, R. (1988) *Diabetes – a Young Person's Handbook.* McDonald and Co., London.
Sonksen, P. *et al.* (1992) *Diabetes at your Fingertips.* Class Publishing, London.
Steel, J. (1987) *Coping with Life on Insulin.* Chambers, London.

REFERENCES

Bedlow, J. (1988) Blood Glucose Monitoring. *Nursing Standard,* May 28, 24–25.
Bradford, R. and Singer, J. (1991) Support and Information for Parents. *Paediatric Nursing,* **3**:4, 18–20.
Braithwack, A. (1992) *I Have Diabetes,* Dinosaur Publication and Lilly Diabetes Care Division, London.
Brandt, P.A. and Magyary, D.L. (1993) The Impact of a Diabetes Education Programme on Children and Mothers. *J. Paed. Nurs.,* **8**:1, 31–40.
Brenchley, S. (1993) Children with Diabetes:

Current Dietary Advice. *Professional Care of Mother and Child*, **3**:2, 32–34.

Brenner, A. (1984) *Helping Children Cope with Stress*, 2nd edn, pp. 72–74. Lexington Books, Toronto.

Breslau, N. (1981) Psychologic Functioning of Siblings of Disabled Children. *Paediatrics*, **67**:3, 344–53.

Campion, J. (1991) *Counselling Children*, 1st edn, pp. 74–75. Whiting and Birch, London.

Challen, A.H., Davies, A.C., Williams, R.J.W *et al.*, (1990) Support for Families with Diabetic Children: Parent's View. *Practical Diabetes*, **7**:1, 26–31.

Daly, H., Clarke, P. and Field, J. (1988) 'What is Diabetes?', in T. Doman (ed.). *Diabetes Care. A Problem Solving Approach*, pp. 23–24. Heineman, London.

Doyle, B. (1987) I Wish You Were Dead. *Nursing Times*, **85**:45, 44–46.

Eiser, C. (1985) *The Psychology of Childhood Illness*, pp. 94–115. Springer-Verlag, New York.

Estridge, B. and Davies, J. (1992) *So Your Child Has Diabetes*, p. 46. Vermillion, London.

Foster, R., Hunsberger, M. and Anderson, J. (1989) *Family Centered Nursing Care of Children*. W.B. Saunders, Philadelphia.

Gill, G. (1991) Injection Technique. *Practical Diabetes*, **8**:6, 242.

Henderson, G. (1992) Life-Size Body Drawings: A Psychoeducational tool for Children with IDDM. *J. Diabetes Educ.*, **18**:2, 158–60.

Hilson, R. (1988) *Diabetes – A Young Person's Handbook*, McDonald and Co., London.

Hodges, L.C. and Parker, J. (1987) Concerns of Parents with Diabetic Children. *Paediatric Nursing*, **13**:1, 22–24.

Kenneth, A. (1991) Communicating with Care. *Paediatric Nursing*, **3**:3, 24–27.

Knafl, K.A. (1982) Parents' Views of the Response of Siblings to a Paediatric Hospitalization. *Res. in Nurs. and Health*, **5**: 13–20.

Kübler-Ross, E. (1970) *On Death and Dying*. Tavistock Publications, London.

Lavigne, J.L. and Ryan, M. (1979) Psychological Adjustment of Siblings of Children with Chronic Illness. *Paediatrics*, **63**:4, 616–27.

Legge, A. (1993) Care at Home is Best for Diabetic Children. *Mims Magazine Weekly*, July 7th, p. 2.

Lynn, M.R. (1989) Siblings' Response in Illness Situations. *J. Paediatr. Nurs.*, **4**:2, 127–29.

McCowen, C., Hackett, A.F., Court, S. *et al.* (1986) Are Families of Diabetic Children Adequately Taught? *Brit. Med. J.*, **292**, 1361.

McEvilly, A. (1991) Tailoring a Lifestyle for Diabetic Child. *Midwife, Health Visitor and Community Nurse*, **27**:2, 39–41.

Noyer, A. (1989) Caring for a Child with Diabetes: The Effects of Specialist Nurse Care on Patients' Needs and Concerns. *J. Adv. Nurs.*, **14**, 536–45.

Noyer, A. and Tomlinson, D.A. (1992) Injections Giving Children with Insulin Dependent Diabetes Mellitus: Responsibility and Performance. *Practical Diabetes*, **9**:5, 185–88.

Rosen and Stearns (1979) cited Brenner (1984) *Temporary Separation: Sibling Illness Helping Children Cope with Stress*, 2nd edn. Lexington Books, toronto.

Savage, D. (1992) Diabetic Emergencies in Children. *Post Graduate Update*, **45**:7, 487–96.

Shillitoe, R.W. (1988) *Psychology and Diabetes*. Chapman & Hall, London.

Sonkenson, P., Fox, P. and Judd, S. (1992) *Diabetes at Your Fingertips*. Class Publishing, London.

Steel, J. (1987) *Coping with Life on Insulin*. Chambers Ltd., London.

Steinhauer, P.D., Mushin, D.N. and Rae-Grant, Q. (1974) Psychological Aspects of Chronic Illness. *Paediatr. Clin. N. Amer*, **21**:4, 825–40.

Swift, P.G.F., Hearnshaw, J.R., Botha, J.L. *et al.* (1993) A Decade of Diabetes: Keeping Children out of Hospital. *Brit. Med. J.*, **307**, 96–98.

Taylor, S.C. (1980) The Effects of Chronic Childhood Illness Upon Well Siblings. *Maternal and Child Nursing J.*, **9**:2, 109–116.

Tizza, V.B. (1962) Management of the Parents of the Chronically Ill Child. *Am. J. Orthopsychiatry*, **32**, 53–59.

Walker, C.L. (1988) Stress and Coping in Siblings of Childhood Cancer Patients. *Nursing Res.*, **37**, 208–12.

Willey, K.A., Twigg, S.M., Yue, D.I.C. *et al.* (1993) Home Blood Glucose Monitoring: How Often? *Practical Diabetes*, **10**:1, 22–25.

Young, R.J. and Greenhalgh, S. (1992) The New Diabetic Child. *Diabetes Care*, **1**:2, 4–5.

24

Peri-operative management of the diabetic child

R.M. MILASZKIEWICZ and G.M. HALL

24.1 INTRODUCTION

It appears that even in specialized children's hospitals there are few children with diabetes per year presenting for surgery. Unlike adult patients who may need surgery for complications of their diabetes, children usually have diabetes as a coincident disease. Therefore, there are no controlled trials comparing different methods of management of diabetes in children undergoing surgery, and much of the data about glucose metabolism and the 'stress response' to surgery has been extrapolated from adult work.

24.2 STRESS RESPONSE TO SURGERY AND ANESTHESIA

In the peri-operative period, additional metabolic demands contributing to the potential instability of the child with IDDM are (a) pre-operative starvation and dehydration, (b) the 'stress response' to surgery and anesthesia, and (c) post-operative food and fluid deficit.

In adults, hyperglycemia after major surgery is common, even in nondiabetic patients. This is due mainly to initial relative insulin hyposecretion, followed by post-operative insulin resistance. Insulin resistance is thought to result from elevated concentrations of counter-regulatory hormones, cortisol, glucagon and growth hormone. The overall picture is one of hyperglycemia, increased catabolism and protein breakdown, known as the 'stress response'. Children and neonates also show a stress response to surgery, and it has been suggested that neonates have augmented catabolic hormone secretion (Anand *et al.*, 1990).

It is thought that modification of the stress response may lead to fewer complications in the postoperative period, however, the evidence at present is not conclusive. Anand *et al.* (1987, 1988, 1992) have shown that amelioration of the stress response by anesthetic techniques, such as either high-dose opioids or the use of inhalational anesthetic agents where previously none would have been used, improved the outcome of neonates undergoing major surgery. Nakamura and Takasaki (1991) showed that caudal anesthesia suppressed the humoral responses associated with lower abdominal surgery in young children, although they did not comment on differences in outcome. Murat *et al.* (1988) found that small doses of epidural bupivacaine were effective in

Childhood and Adolescent Diabetes
Published in 1994 by Chapman & Hall, London
ISBN 0 412 48610 5

decreasing the stress response to surgery in children.

In adults, however, it appears that the only successful way of preventing the stress response is by complete afferent neuronal blockade of both somatic and autonomic nerves. The only operative sites in which this can be achieved are limbs, pelvis, and eyes. Unless the block is complete, the effect on the stress response will be variable (Kehlet *et al.*, 1979). For extradural and spinal anesthesia, plasma concentrations of epinephrine and norepinephrine decrease with the height of the sensory blockade (Pflug & Halter, 1981). Insulin response to hyperglycemia is affected by a high extradural blockade (T2–T6), but not by a low blockade (T9–T12) (Halter & Pflug, 1980), suggesting that resting neuronal input to the pancreas is necessary for a normal insulin response.

The diabetic patient is more at risk than a nondiabetic patient of metabolic decompensation. Although glycemic control may appear satisfactory, a situation can arise where insulin and fluids have been given in sufficient quantities to prevent hyperglycemia, but insufficient to prevent lipolysis and ketosis. In patients with IDDM it is likely that the management of the diabetes is of greater importance in determining postoperative outcome than the anesthetic technique.

An important point to remember is that diabetic children can rapidly develop ketoacidosis, but ketoacidosis may mimic an abdominal emergency. If hyperglycemia and ketoacidosis are present, these should be corrected before any surgical intervention takes place both because the child's life could be at risk and unnecessary surgery may be avoided.

24.3 PERI-OPERATIVE MANAGEMENT

Due to the lack of controlled trials, there is little evidence to support any particular method of management of diabetic children in the peri-operative period. However, pediatric patients are liable to be more unstable than adults and therefore any regimen chosen should allow a great deal of flexibility. Patient safety is of major importance. Frequent measurements of blood glucose concentrations should be made throughout the peri-operative period. In ideal circumstances, the child should be looked after by a team including the clinician in charge of the diabetes, the admitting surgical team and the anesthetist. The psychological needs of the child and family, as well as the physical needs of the child, should be taken into consideration when deciding on the duration of the hospital stay. With the increased trend towards day-stay surgery, it may be possible to consider admitting children with IDDM as day-cases if they have very stable diabetes, are undergoing minor surgery and will be able to eat, drink and to take insulin as usual soon after surgery. However, the safety of this has yet to be evaluated. Many children will not fulfil the criteria for day-stay surgery, or they may suffer from vomiting postoperatively and will require a longer period of admission and intravenous insulin and glucose.

24.4 PRE-OPERATIVE ASSESSMENT

The pre-operative assessment should be performed in the outpatient clinic. A glycosylated hemoglobin level will reflect the glycemic control in the preceding 6–8 weeks. If grossly elevated there may be time before elective procedures to adjust the child's insulin to improve control. It has been the practice in the past to admit these patients to hospital 36–72 hours pre-operatively in order to stabilize the diabetes. This is no longer practical unless the glycemic control is very deranged. A careful history should be obtained about the duration and severity of the diabetes. Although complications are rare they should be sought. Hypoglycemia, if asymptomatic, may indicate the presence of autonomic neuropathy which may cause cardiovascular instability or delayed gastric emptying. An inability to approximate the hands in the 'prayer sign' should alert the clinician to the possibility of a difficult introbation or other microvascular complications. All children must have their blood glucose concentration checked on more than one occasion pre-prandially. Urinalysis for glucose, ketones and protein should also be undertaken on more than one occasion and plasma urea and electrolyte concentrations must be measured.

24.5 PREMEDICATION

For elective procedures normal insulin injections should continue until the night before surgery. The stress of surgery may begin in the pre-operative period, especially in older children who are very anxious. These children benefit from sedative premedication (Lindahl *et al.*, 1985). Ideally the child should be first on the operating list in the morning to minimize any metabolic disturbance resulting from a prolonged period of starvation (and it is important to ensure that full laboratory facilities are available if metabolic control proves difficult to achieve). In this situation, the insertion of an intravenous cannula may be deferred until the child is anesthetized. However, if there is likely to be any delay, an intravenous infusion providing glucose, potassium and insulin should be started. This is also the most reliable way of providing glucose and insulin for children whose operations are not scheduled until the afternoon. Flexibility is necessary, and for these children it may be acceptable to give half the usual dose of insulin with breakfast and then to monitor blood glucose very carefully, starting an infusion immediately if there are any problems in maintaining normoglycemia.

24.6 INSULIN AND GLUCOSE THERAPY

A recent review article has discussed the controversy surrounding the management of adults with diabetes, and also considered the key issues in pediatric management (Hirsch *et al.*, 1991). While there is a great deal of debate about the preferred regimen for adult patients, children are best managed with separate infusions of glucose and insulin. The ideal is to maintain metabolism as near as possible to normal in order to minimize morbidity, avoiding hypoglycemia, hyperglycemia, ketogenesis, protein catabolism, and electrolyte disturbance.

There has been some controversy regarding the use of glucose containing solutions for nondiabetic children. Hyperglycemia has been noted in neonates in the peri-operative period and fluid replacement with non-glucose containing solutions recommended (Srinivasan *et al.*, 1986). Nilsson *et al.* (1984) failed to observe hypoglycemia in otherwise healthy children presenting for surgery, whereas other groups found hypoglycemia to be present (Kelnar, 1976; Payne & Ireland, 1984; Welborn *et al.*, 1986 & 1987). It has been recommended that glucose should be administered at a rate of 5 mg/kg/min to healthy children. In the absence of studies to help resolve the controversy this is also the suggested rate of glucose infusion for diabetic children. It is unclear which solution is preferable, however, the commonest ones used are either 5% dextrose or dextrose 4% with sodium chloride 0.18%. Ellis (1987) recommended the addition of sodium chloride to infusions of glucose. The amount suggested varies with age, and in children under 6 years she recommended 0.20–0.25% sodium chloride should be given with the glucose, while in older children 0.25–0.3% should be given. There is a potential risk of water overloading and hyponatremia if glucose alone is used. Potassium chloride will be required in children, provided renal function is normal. The suggested amount is 10 mmol per 500 mls of 5% dextrose.

Insulin may be given in a variety of ways either subcutaneously, intramuscularly, or intravenously as a bolus or an infusion.

There is evidence that in circumstances where epinephrine levels are high, such as may occur during surgery, the absorption of insulin from subcutaneous sites is unreliable (Fernqvist *et al.*, 1988). The use of intravenous boluses is unphysiologic as the half-life of intravenous insulin is 5 minutes and its biological half-life is 20 minutes. Giving insulin in this way causes greater metabolic derangement as the blood glucose concentration swings rapidly between hyperglycemia and hypoglycemia resulting in greater lipolysis and ketogenesis. With the development of newer, more reliable infusion pumps the delivery of insulin using a continuous infusion is probably the most flexible and safe method. It minimizes perturbations in blood glucose which often occur using other methods. However, if separate infusions of glucose and insulin are used, there is always a possibility of one infusion not running. Careful, regular monitoring of blood glucose concentrations is vital.

The usual requirement for insulin in diabetic children is 0.8–1.0 units/kg/day (Kelnar, 1992). The suggested starting rate for an infusion of insulin is 0.1 units/kg/hour (Lindahl, 1989), and this is adjusted, as required, on the basis of frequent blood glucose measurements. The addition of protein to the infusion is not necessary if the solution is concentrated and the first few milliliters are run through the giving set. The frequency of blood glucose estimations will depend on the severity of the diabetes and the nature of the surgery. In certain circumstances it may be necessary to check the blood glucose every 30 minutes intra-operatively. This will be adjusted according to the clinical progress of the patient, and may be up to two-hourly in the stable patient postoperatively.

There is no consensus on what constitutes good peri-operative control of blood glucose. Whichever method of insulin delivery is used, both hypo- and hyperglycemia must be avoided. A blood glucose concentration within the range 6–12 mmol/l is a safe target figure. If the regimen is too strict there is a danger of hypoglycemia occurring. Intermittent laboratory blood glucose determinations should be performed as the use of test strips may not always be reliable (Hutchinson & Shenkin, 1984). Urinalysis should be performed, where feasible, to assess ketoacidosis; it is not however, a reliable monitor of glycemic control as it correlates poorly with blood glucose concentrations and depends on renal function. In the peri-operative period, the renal threshold for glucose is altered (Keon & Templeton, 1987).

Fluid and electrolyte balance should be carefully monitored and other losses replaced as appropriate. If giving blood, it is necessary to take into consideration the high glucose concentrations contained in stored blood. Glucose and insulin infusions should be continued until the child is able to return to a normal diet. Insulin infusions must not be terminated abruptly as rebound hyperglycemia is common.

24.7 SUMMARY OF SUGGESTED MANAGEMENT OF CHILDREN WITH IDDM

Pre-operatively:

Check: Glycosylated hemoglobin
Fasting blood glucose
Plasma urea and electrolytes
Urinalysis for ketones and protein

Prepare: Intravenous infusion: Glucose 5% with KCl 10 mmol per 500 mls. +/− NaCl. Rate according to weight. (Table 24.1)
Insulin via syringe pump: 1 unit soluble human insulin per ml. Rate adjusted, using sliding scale guidelines (Table 24.2) if necessary, so as to maintain

blood glucose concentration of 6–12 mmol/l.

Peri-operatively:
Frequency of blood glucose monitoring depends on stability of patient. Up to every 30 minutes intra-operatively, up to two hourly post-operatively. Start insulin and glucose infusions when blood glucose is >10 mmol/l.

Post-operatively:
Check laboratory glucose and potassium post-operatively. Continue infusion and sliding scale insulin until oral intake established. Gradually wean insulin infusion.

24.8 CONCLUSION

Although there is little specific research on the management of diabetic pediatric patients undergoing surgery, much of the treatment is based on general principles. With sensible pre-operative care and peri-operative fluid and insulin regimens with careful, frequent monitoring of blood glucose concentrations, few patients should experience problems.

Table 24.1 Rate for maintenance fluids.

Body weight	Fluid volume
1st 10 kg	4 ml/kg/hr
10–20 kg	add 2 ml/kg/hr
>20 kg	add 1 ml/kg/hr

Table 24.2 Sliding scale for insulin.

Blood glucose (mmol/l)	Insulin Infusion (units/kg/hr)
0–5	0
6–10	0.05
11–15	0.1
16–20	0.15
>20	0.2

The mortality and morbidity of children with diabetes should be no more than in their nondiabetic peers.

REFERENCES

Anand, K.J.S., Sippell, W.G. and Aynsley-Green, A. (1987) Randomised trial of fentanyl anaesthesia in pre-term babies undergoing surgery: Effects on the stress response. *Lancet*, **i**, 243–48.

Anand, K.J.S., Sippell, W.G., Schofield, N.M. *et al.* (1988) Does halothane anaesthesia decrease the metabolic and endocrine stress response of newborn infants undergoing operation? *Brit. Med. J.*, **296**, 668–72.

Anand, K.J.S., Hansen, D.D. and Hickey, P.R. (1990) Hormonal-metabolic stress responses in neonates undergoing cardiac surgery. *Anesthesiology*, **73**, 661–70.

Anand, K.J.S. and Hickey, P.R. (1992) Halothane-morphine compared with high-dose sufentanil for anaesthesia and postoperative analgesia in neonatal cardiac surgery. *N. Eng. J. Med.*, **326**, 1–9.

Ellis, E.N. (1987) 'Management before and after surgery', in L.B. Travis, B.H. Brouhard and B.J. Schreiner (eds). *Diabetes mellitus in children and adolescents* (Major problems in Clinical Pediatrics, Vol. 29), pp. 201–204. W.B. Saunders Company, Philadelphia.

Fernqvist, E., Gunnarsson, R. and Linde, B. (1988) Influence of circulating epinephrine on absorption of subcutaneously injected insulin. *Diabetes*, **37**, 694–701.

Halter, J.B. and Pflug, A.E. (1980) Effect of sympathetic blockade by spinal anaesthesia on pancreatic islet cell function in man. *Am. J. Physiol.*, **239**, E150–55.

Hirsch, I.B., McGill, J.B., Cryer, P.E. *et al.* (1991) Perioperative management of surgical patients with diabetes mellitus. *Anesthesiology*, **74**, 346–59.

Hutchinson, A.S. and Shenkin, A. (1984) BM Strips: How accurate are they in general wards? *Diabetic Med.*, **1**, 225–26.

Kehlet, H., Brandt, M.R., Prange-Hansen, A. *et al.* (1979) Effect of epidural anaesthesia on metabolic profiles during and after surgery. *Brit. J. Surg.*, **66**, 543–46.

Kelnar, C.J.H. (1976) Hypoglycaemia in children undergoing adenotonsillectomy. *Brit. Med. J.*, **1**, 751–52.

Kelnar, C.J.H. (1992) 'Endocrine gland disorders: Diabetes mellitus', in A.G.M. Campbell and N. McIntosh (eds). *Forfar and Arneil's Textbook of Paediatrics*, 4th edn, pp. 1146–54. Churchill Livingstone, Edinburgh.

Keon, T.P. and Templeton, J.J. (1987) 'Diseases of the endocrine system: Diabetes Mellitus', in J. Katz and D.J. Steward (eds). *Anaesthesia and Uncommon Pediatric Diseases*, pp. 338–42. W.B. Saunders Company, Philadelphia.

Lindahl, S.G.E. (1989) Pre-operative physical assessment and preparation for surgery, in E. Summer and D.J. Hatch (eds). *Textbook of Paediatric Anaesthetic Practice*, p. 16. Balliere Tindall, London.

Lindahl, S.G.E., Charlton, A.J., Hatch, D.J. *et al.* (1985) Endocrine response to surgery in children after premedication with midazolam or papaveretum. *Eur. J. Anaesthesiol.*, **2**, 369–77.

Murat, I., Walker, J., Esteve, C. *et al.* (1988) Effect of lumbar epidural anaesthesia on plasma cortisol levels in children. *Can. J. Anaesthesia*, **35**, 20–24.

Nakamura, T. and Takasaki, M. (1991) Metabolic and endocrine responses to surgery during caudal analgesia in children. *Can. J. Anaesthesia*, **38**, 969–73.

Nilsson, K., Larsson, L.E., Andreasson, S. *et al.* (1984) Blood glucose concentrations during anaesthesia in children. Effects of starvation and peri-operative fluid therapy. *Brit. J. Anaesthesia*, **65**, 375–79.

Payne, K. and Ireland, P. (1984) Plasma glucose levels in the peri-operative period in children. *Anaesthesia*, **39**, 868–72.

Pflug, A.E. and Halter, J.B. (1981) Effect of spinal anaesthesia on adrenergic tone and the neuroendocrine response to surgical stress in humans. *Anesthesiology*, **55**, 120–26.

Srinivasan, G., Jain, R., Pildes, R.S. *et al.* (1986) Glucose homeostasis during anaesthesia and surgery in infants. *J. Paed. Surg.*, **21**, 718–21.

Welborn, L.G., McGill, W.A., Hannallah, R.S. *et al.* (1986) Peri-operative blood glucose concentrations in pediatric outpatients. *Anesthesiology*, **65**, 543–47.

Welborn, L.G., Hanallah, R.S., McGill, W.A. *et al.* (1987) Glucose concentrations for routine intravenous infusion in pediatric outpatient surgery. *Anesthesiology*, **67**, 427–30.

25

Hypoglycemia – practical and clinical implications

A.E. GOLD and B.M. FRIER

25.1 INTRODUCTION

The development of acute hypoglycemia presents an alarming problem to the parents and carers of children with diabetes. This dangerous and potentially life-threatening side-effect of insulin therapy is the most feared metabolic disturbance associated with diabetes. The risk of developing hypoglycemia may provoke chronic anxiety, especially in the parents of young children with diabetes, on whom the child is usually dependent for its recognition and treatment. Hypoglycemia can disrupt family life and interfere with the child's education. Although the morbidity associated with severe hypoglycemia may be more apparent in adult diabetic patients treated with insulin, evidence is accumulating that recurrent severe hypoglycemia may have potentially deleterious effects on the immature brain of the child.

The clinical manifestations of hypoglycemia in diabetic children are similar in many ways to the effects of hypoglycemia in adults, but some important differences can be identified. These include definition, counter-regulatory and metabolic responses, symptomatology and presentation, and long-term sequelae on the 'developing' brain.

Childhood and Adolescent Diabetes
Published in 1994 by Chapman & Hall, London
ISBN 0 412 48610 5

25.2 DEFINITION OF HYPOGLYCEMIA IN CHILDHOOD

Severe hypoglycemia in children has usually been defined as an episode which causes coma, neurological deficit and/or a convulsion (Bergada *et al.*, 1989; Daneman *et al.*, 1989; Egger *et al.*, 1991), but some studies have widened the definition to include any episode which requires external assistance to resuscitate the patient with hypoglycemia (Aman *et al.*, 1989). This definition is more commonly used in adult patients as it emphasizes the development of neuroglycopenia, but it is difficult to apply to infants and young children, most of whom require external help from parents for every episode of hypoglycemia, irrespective of severity. In addition, young children cannot usually interpret or express subjective alterations in sensations which may herald acute hypoglycemia, so that identification depends upon observation of their altered behavior by adult carers who can recognize the underlying metabolic cause.

It is very difficult to provide a definition of mild and moderate hypoglycemia. The presence or absence of symptoms cannot be used as a guide as this is clearly impractical in neonates and is unreliable in young children. Many observations in this area have been extrapolated from studies of spontaneous neonatal hypoglycemia, which may not be relevant to insulin-induced hypoglycemia in diabetic children (Aynsley-Green, 1991). This problem was highlighted by Koh and colleagues (1988a) who conducted a survey of the definition of neonatal hypoglycemia in the UK. This revealed that a blood glucose value ranging from 1.0–4.0 mmol/l was used to define hypoglycemia in 30 different textbooks and wide differences in definition were obtained on questioning 242 pediatricians. Many of the management policies in neonatal units had been influenced by the erroneous belief that 'asymptomatic' hypoglycemia was not harmful to the infant, although this assumption has since been refuted (Aynsley-Green, 1991). In a follow-up study of 661 surviving preterm infants by Lucas *et al.* (1988), 67% had experienced hypoglycemia as defined by a plasma glucose concentration which was lower than 2.6 mmol/l, and in 25% of the infants hypoglycemia had recurred on separate days. The frequency with which hypoglycemia had occurred was closely related to a lower neonatal development score at 18 months. It is not known whether permanent neurological impairment in neonates can occur at a plasma glucose concentration greater than 2.6 mmol/l, and whether diabetic infants who are exposed to recurrent hypoglycemia are affected to the same degree, although Type 1 diabetes is rare in infancy.

An alternative method of defining hypoglycemia may be based on the glucose concentration at which impairment of neuropsychological function occurs. This is discussed in detail later.

25.3 SYMPTOMS AND SIGNS OF HYPOGLYCEMIA IN CHILDREN

In adult humans the symptoms of hypoglycemia can be divided into those resulting from the direct effects of glucose deprivation on the brain, causing neuroglycopenia and those resulting from activation of the autonomic nervous system (Hepburn *et al.*, 1991). Although some of the symptoms of hypoglycemia in adult diabetic patients also occur in children (e.g., trembling, sweating, hunger, weakness) the frequency and intensity with which they occur are different. For example, sweating is a common symptom of hypoglycemia in insulin-treated diabetic adults but is reported less frequently by children. Hypoglycemia in children is often recognized by parents or carers and is not identified by the child, and warning signs are usually more important than symptoms in the young child (McCrimmon *et al.*, 1994). The symptoms and signs of hypoglycemia in children are detailed in Table 25.1. The most frequently reported symptoms and signs of hypoglycemia in children are tremor, pallor, weakness, dizziness and sweating (Aman *et*

Table 25.1 Features of hypoglycemia in diabetic children.

Tremor	Hunger	Convulsions
Pallor	Headache	Transient hemiparesis
Sweating	Irritability	Coma
Naughtiness	Weakness	Nightmares
Dizziness	Abdominal pain	Difficulty waking in morning
Slurred speech	Palpitations	Enuresis
Mydriasis	Poor concentration	
Visual disturbance		

al., 1989; Macfarlane *et al.*, 1989). Some symptoms such as abdominal pain occur only in children, and may be confused with the features of hyperglycemia and ketoacidosis. Altered behavior is particularly common in the young child and this may take the form of being naughty, having a temper-tantrum or appearing drowsy and apathetic. In toddlers, these features may be unrelated to hypoglycemia so that previous experience of the response of the individual child to hypoglycemia is essential; constant vigilance and suspicion of possible hypoglycemia has to be maintained by the carers of the young diabetic child.

It is extremely difficult to assess whether the symptoms and behavioral changes precipitated by hypoglycemia change during childhood or whether improved recognition occurs with increasing maturity and comprehension. About 50% of adult diabetic patients with diabetes of more than 20 years' duration will have some degree of altered awareness of hypoglycemia (Pramming *et al.*, 1991) but very little is known about the prevalence and nature of altered hypoglycemia awareness in diabetic children, if it occurs at all in this age group. The possible effects of strict glycemic control on the perception of hypoglycemia in diabetic children are not known at present.

25.4 FREQUENCY OF HYPOGLYCEMIA IN CHILDREN

A true estimate of the frequency of hypoglycemia in diabetic children is difficult to ascertain and varies considerably between studies. Factors contributing to this variation include differences in definition of mild and severe hypoglycemia, the population size and period of observation and whether the assessment was made retrospectively or prospectively. Goldstein *et al.* (1981) found that 3% or more of diabetic children experience recurrent episodes of severe hypoglycemia. Many studies determining the incidence of hypoglycemia are not therefore comparable, as frequency is sometimes expressed as the incidence (i.e., number of hypoglycemic episodes per 100 person-years), or is reported as the prevalence (i.e., the percentage of children who have suffered one or more hypoglycemic episodes). The principal studies which have reported the frequencies of both severe and mild to moderate hypoglycemia are summarized in Table 25.2.

25.5 CAUSAL FACTORS OF HYPOGLYCEMIA IN DIABETIC CHILDREN

25.5.1 PATIENT OR PARENTAL 'ERROR'

Many episodes of hypoglycemia result inadvertently from mistakes in the management of diabetes either by the individual patient or by the carer resulting in a mismatch between glucose availability and plasma insulin concentrations. Severe hypoglycemia in children has been attributed to patient or parental error to a varying degree, ranging from 33–85% of episodes, with the common causes being prolonged or additional exercise, delayed or insufficient food or errors in determining insulin dosage (Aman *et al.*, 1989; Bergada *et al.*, 1989; Daneman *et al.*, 1989; Bhatia & Wolfsdorf, 1991). Factitious hypoglycemia resulting from deliberate overdose of insulin, although uncommon, has been described and is usually surreptitious and associated with psychological disturbance (Dershewitz *et al.*, 1976; Mayefsky *et al.*, 1982; Grunberger *et al.*, 1988).

25.5.1.1 Exercise

Protracted physical activity predisposes to hypoglycemia although occasionally may not occur until several hours after the strenuous exercise (MacDonald, 1987). Factors such as the weather, season of the year, school

Table 25.2 The reported frequency of hypoglycemia in diabetic children.

Reference	Definition of severe hypoglycemia	Frequency of hypoglycemia		Study design	
		Severe	Mild	Type	Period of study
Goldstein *et al*. (1981)	Marked CNS depression, prolonged 'sympathetic' reaction	2.7%[a]	31.3%[a]	Prospective	18 months
Aman *et al*. (1989)	Help of adult required	44%[a]	97%[a]	Retrospective	1 year
Bergada *et al*. (1989)	Coma or convulsion	6.8%[a]	–	Prospective	1 year
Daneman *et al*. (1989)	Coma or convulsion	6.8%[a]	3.5%[a]	Retrospective	4.6 years
Macfarlane *et al*. (1989)	Not given	–	62%[a]	Prospective	14 weeks
Soltesz & Acsadi (1989)	Intravenous or intramuscular glucagon required	7.7%[a] 12.0[b]	–	Retrospective	5 years
Egger *et al*. (1991)	Coma + low blood glucose or response to glucagon	5.9[b]	–	Prospective	8 years
Bhatia & Wolfsdorf (1991)	Coma or convulsion	12.2[b]	–	Prospective	2 years
Limbert *et al*. (1993)	Need for assistance	44%[a] 77%[b]	– –	Prospective	1 year

[a] prevalence of hypoglycemia expressed as the percentage of children experiencing one or more episode.
[b] incidence of hypoglycemia expressed as the number of episodes of hypoglycemia per 100 patient-years.

holidays and the age and physical activities of the child will influence the intensity of physical exercise. Exercise in children varies greatly with respect to energy expenditure and can not always be anticipated. Appropriate ingestion of additional carbohydrate or adjustments to insulin treatment are often difficult to predict or achieve. The proportion of episodes of hypoglycemia attributable to exercise has been estimated between 25% and 71% (Bergada *et al.*, 1989; Daneman *et al.*, 1989; Macfarlane *et al.*, 1989; Bhatia & Wolfsdorf, 1991).

25.5.1.2 Delayed or insufficient food

A regular eating pattern is not always easy to maintain, particularly in young children in whom eating habits are erratic and refusal of food is common, so predisposing to hypoglycemia. One-third of all episodes of hypoglycemia have been attributed to delayed or insufficient ingestion of food (Daneman *et al.*, 1989; Macfarlane *et al.*, 1989; Bhatia & Wolfsdorf, 1991).

25.5.1.3 Deviation from usual insulin dosage

It has been estimated that up to a quarter of episodes of severe hypoglycemia result from errors of insulin administration which include mistakes in estimating dosage, giving the wrong insulin formulation and unsatisfactory insulin injection technique (Daneman *et al.*, 1989; Bhatia & Wolfsdorf, 1991). Inadvertent intramuscular (instead of subcutaneous) injection, the effect of localized lipohypertrophy at injection sites, changes in the anatomical site of injection and exercise after injecting into the lower limb can all influence the rate of insulin absorption and may induce hypoglycemia.

25.5.2 GLYCEMIC CONTROL AND MODE OF INSULIN DELIVERY

25.5.2.1 Glycemic control

Glycated hemoglobin concentrations have almost invariably been found to be lower in diabetic children and adults who have experienced recurrent severe hypoglycemia (Goldstein *et al.*, 1981; Casparie & Elving, 1985; Aman *et al.*, 1989; Daneman *et al.*, 1989; Egger *et al.*, 1989; The DCCT Research Group, 1993). The relationship between glycated hemoglobin and the frequency of episodes of mild symptomatic hypoglycemia is less certain. Some studies have shown no relationship (Goldstein *et al.*, 1981; Aman *et al.*, 1989; Daneman *et al.*, 1989) but Macfarlane *et al.* (1989) observed that children with the lowest glycated hemoglobin concentrations recorded more episodes of symptomatic hypoglycemia.

25.5.2.2 Insulin dosage

Most studies have shown no association between the daily dose of insulin and the frequency of hypoglycemia in children (Goldstein *et al.*, 1981; Aman *et al.*, 1989; Daneman *et al.*, 1989) with the exception of a prospective study of 350 children with Type 1 diabetes (Bergada *et al.*, 1989) in which the daily insulin dose (in units/kg body weight) of the children reporting severe hypoglycemia was shown to be significantly higher at the time of the episode.

25.5.2.3 Frequency of insulin injections

In a group of 92 diabetic children, Aman *et al.* (1989) found no relationship between the frequency of hypoglycemia and the number of injections of insulin per day. In other studies, children receiving more than one injection of insulin per day experienced more severe hypoglycemia, although these children also had lower glycated hemoglobin concentrations, and may have had a greater susceptibility to hypoglycemia because of strict glycemic control (Whincup & Milner, 1987; Daneman *et al.*, 1989; Egger *et al.*, 1991). In a small study of six preschool diabetic children who had pronounced metabolic instability characterized by chronic hyperglycemia and recurrent severe hypoglycemia, the introduction of continuous subcutaneous insulin infusion (CSII) produced more stable glycemic control and fewer episodes of hypoglycemia (Brambilla *et al.*, 1987) and these findings have been confirmed by others (Bougneres *et al.*, 1984). Schiffrin *et al.* (1984) utilized a similar method of insulin delivery in adolescents with Type 1 diabetes, and although metabolic control was improved the frequency of hypoglycemia was not reduced. This observation is consistent with a study in young adults with insulin dependent diabetes (Arias *et al.*, 1985). CSII has not been adopted widely for diabetic management and the practical importance of these findings is of greater relevance to the increasing use of basal-bolus insulin regimens many of which employ pen devices for insulin delivery. In a study of diabetic adolescents, multiple injection insulin therapy was found to improve glycemic control without increasing the incidence of severe hypoglycemia (Bougneres *et al.*, 1993). Initial trials of implantable insulin pumps have also shown an encouraging decrease in the risk of severe hypoglycemia produced by CSII (Selam *et al.*, 1992).

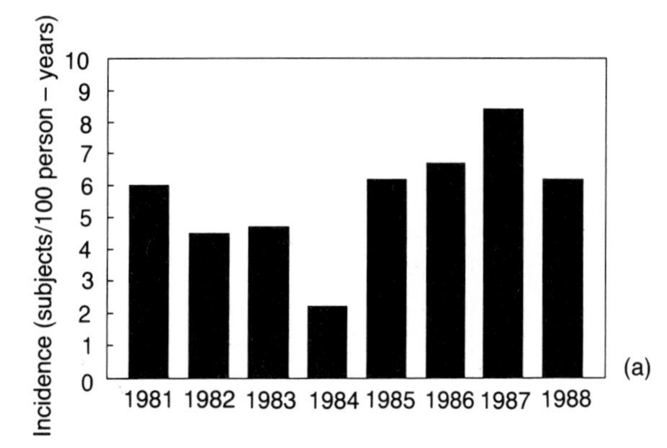

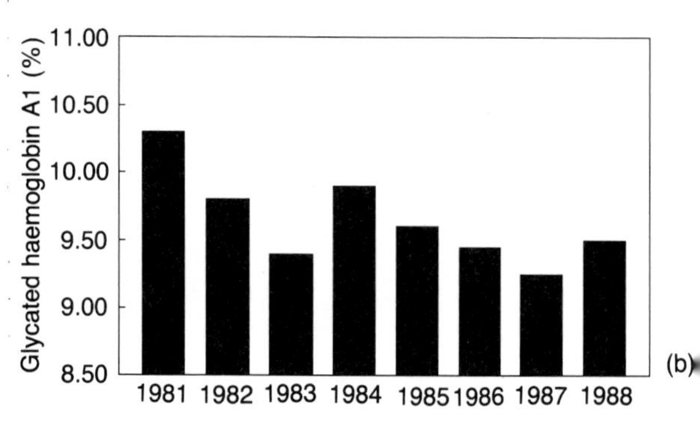

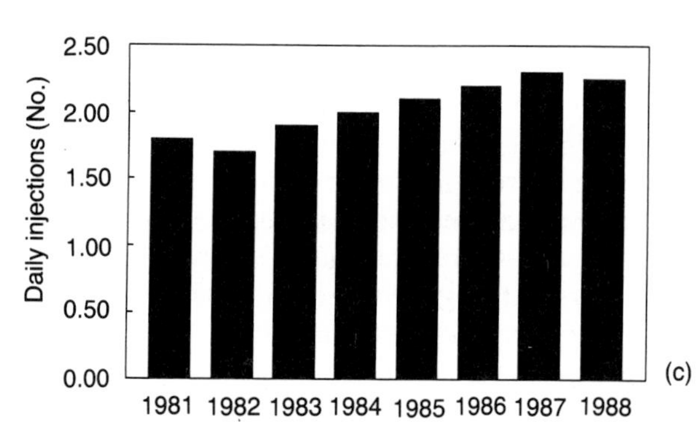

Figure 25.1 Data are provided on 155 Type 1 diabetic children collected between 1981 and 1988: (a) incidence of hypoglycemic coma, (b) mean glycated hemoglobin concentrations, (c) frequency of daily injections of insulin (accepted with permission from Egger, M. *et al. Diabetes Care*, **14**, 1001–1005, 1991. Copyright © 1991 by American Diabetes Association, Inc.).

25.5.2.4 Insulin species

Insulin species has not been shown to be a relevant predisposing factor in the causation of hypoglycemia in diabetic children (Bhatia & Wolfsdorf, 1991; Egger *et al.*, 1991). A detailed review of the effect of insulin species in adults can be found elsewhere (Fisher & Frier, 1993).

25.5.3 AGE AND DURATION OF DIABETES

Neither the age of the child nor the duration of diabetes appear to predispose to isolated episodes of severe hypoglycemia (Goldstein *et al.*, 1981; Aman *et al.*, 1989), although one study did suggest that hypoglycemia may be more frequent during the first year after diagnosis, possibly as a result of inexperience with the management of diabetes within the family group (Bergada *et al.*, 1989). Children who had experienced recurrent episodes of severe hypoglycemia had diabetes of longer duration and were younger at the time of the first episode (Daneman *et al.*, 1989; Egger *et al.*, 1991), although a case-control analysis showed that much of the increase in frequency could be attributed to improved glycemic control (Egger *et al.*, 1991) (Figure 25.1). The same study also showed that complete absence of pancreatic β cell function, estimated by plasma C-peptide concentration, was an important risk factor for hypoglycemic coma.

25.5.4 TIMING OF HYPOGLYCEMIA

A seasonal variation in the frequency of hypoglycemia in children is recognized, with more episodes occurring during the spring and summer months probably as a result of more frequent exercise (Daneman *et al.*, 1989). Severe hypoglycemia is more common during sleep immediately before awakening and also during waking hours before midday (Aman *et al.*, 1989; Bergada *et al.*, 1989; Macfarlane *et al.*, 1989). Although mild episodes of hypoglycemia have been reported to occur more frequently during waking hours and during play (Aman *et al.*, 1989), similar episodes during sleep are much less likely to waken the patient or cause restlessness. They are therefore less likely to be identified during sleep and the frequency of mild nocturnal hypoglycemia is probably underestimated.

25.5.5 DEFECTIVE GLUCOSE COUNTER-REGULATION

In adult diabetic patients treated with insulin, a history of previous severe hypoglycemia is an important risk factor for recurrent severe hypoglycemia (DCCT Research Group, 1991). Goldstein *et al.* (1981) noted that 3% of diabetic children had recurrent severe hypoglycemia and other studies have reported a similar percentage of children who are vulnerable to recurrent severe episodes (Eeg-Olofsson & Petersen, 1966; Bergada *et al.*, 1989; Soltesz & Acsadi, 1989). It is possible that in some children these observations of recurrent severe hypoglycemia are associated with deficient counter-regulatory hormonal responses to hypoglycemia.

25.6 METABOLIC AND HORMONAL RESPONSES TO HYPOGLYCEMIA IN CHILDREN

25.6.1 FASTING

Fundamental differences in blood glucose homeostasis exist between nondiabetic adults and children. Children have a lower tolerance to fasting and are much less resistant to the development of hypoglycemia than adults (Haymond *et al.*, 1974; Thomas, 1974; Kelnar, 1976; Haymond *et al.*, 1982). In addition, children in the fasted state are much more susceptible to ketosis than adults (Senior, 1973; Haymond *et al.*, 1974 & 1982). This may represent a protective mechanism for the child's brain, the weight of which is proportionately greater and requires a greater proportion of energy expenditure. Although endogenous glucose production is directly proportional to the weight of the brain in nondiabetic children (Bier *et al.*, 1977), ketones may provide an additional alternative source of fuel to help avoid the development of severe neuroglycopenia. Ketogenesis in children may be enhanced because of the lower availability of gluconeogenic amino-acids in children as a result of either decreased mobilization or increased glucose utilization (Haymond *et al.*, 1974 & 1982). The skeletal muscle mass is proportionately smaller in children; it is a major source of gluconeogenic substrates such as alanine and lactate and the availability of these substrates is greater in adult males than in women and children. The secretion of cortisol and growth hormone is much higher in fasting nondiabetic children than adults, which further potentiates free fatty acid release.

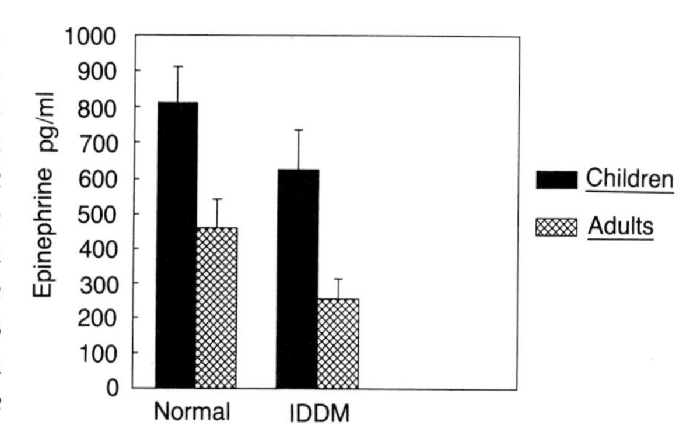

Figure 25.2 The peak epinephrine responses to acute hypoglycemia (2.8 mmol/l) in 49 nondiabetic and insulin-dependent adults and children (adapted from Amiel *et al.*, 1987b, with permission of *Journal of Pediatrics*).

25.6.2 HYPOGLYCEMIA

In response to acute insulin-induced hypoglycemia in humans, several counter-regulatory hormones provide the principal homeostatic mechanism to restore blood glucose to normal. The most potent hormones which cause a rise in blood glucose are glucagon and epinephrine, and a hierarchy of hormonal efficacy has been described (Gerich *et al.*, 1980). These counter-regulatory responses are similar in children although the magnitude of the hormonal secretion may differ. Using a hyperinsulinemic stepped glucose clamp technique, Jones *et al.* (1991) showed that the sustained epinephrine and symptom responses to hypoglycemia were greater and commenced at a higher blood glucose concentration in nondiabetic children than in adults. Furthermore, the threshold for sustained release of epinephrine in diabetic children occurred at a higher blood glucose than in normal children. Poorer glycemic control was also found to shift the threshold for epinephrine secretion to a higher blood glucose value which is consistent with observations in diabetic adults (Boyle *et al.*, 1988). Amiel *et al.* (1987b) extended their earlier glucose clamp studies in diabetic adults (Amiel *et al.*, 1987a), to compare the counter-regulatory hormonal responses between normal and diabetic children. The responses of norepinephrine and epinephrine were exaggerated in diabetic children when compared with diabetic adults (Figure 25.2). Diabetic children and adults failed to demonstrate a glucagon response, while neither growth hormone nor cortisol responses were affected by childhood and diabetes, and puberty did not appear to influence these hormonal responses. Hoffman *et al.* (1991) have also shown that the catecholamine responses to hypoglycemia were lower in diabetic children than those in age-matched nondiabetic controls, although the responses were still greater than in adults. Intensive insulin treatment further suppressed these responses. It appears therefore, that catecholamine-mediated counter-regulation is impaired in diabetic children, as it is in diabetic adults (Bolli *et al.*, 1983). However, diabetic children still exhibit an exaggerated rise in catecholamines, and the threshold for initiation of this response occurs at higher blood glucose concentrations than in diabetic adults. This may result in wide excursions of blood glucose in diabetic children, even after mild hypoglycemia, particularly if excessive carbohydrate is consumed to treat the low blood glucose.

In adult diabetic patients the glucagon response to hypoglycemia is lower than in healthy nondiabetic adults and becomes deficient in patients who have diabetes of greater than five years' duration (Bolli *et al.*, 1983; Amiel *et al.*, 1987a). Impaired glucagon responses have also been demonstrated in diabetic children (Brambilla *et al.*, 1987; Amiel *et al.*, 1987b; Aman & Wranne, 1988a; Singer-Granick *et al.*, 1988) and particularly in diabetic children who are C-peptide negative. Both in nondiabetic and insulin-dependent diabetic adults, hyperinsulinemia suppresses the epinephrine and growth hormone responses to hypoglycemia (Diamond *et al.*, 1991; Liu *et al.*, 1992) and it is possible that suppression may occur in diabetic children which would further reduce their counter-regulatory hormonal responses.

Ketone infusion appears to protect the brain from some of the effects of hypoglycemia (Amiel *et al.*, 1991) and as insulin suppresses ketogenesis, diabetic children with hyperinsulinemia may be more susceptible to cerebral damage from hypoglycemia.

25.7 NOCTURNAL HYPOGLYCEMIA

All diabetic patients are more vulnerable to hypoglycemia during sleep, which is a recognized risk factor for severe hypoglycemia (DCCT Research Group, 1991). The risk of nocturnal hypoglycemia is a constant source of worry to children with diabetes and their parents as hypoglycemia during sleep is often asymptomatic, and retrospective studies undoubtedly underestimate the incidence of nocturnal episodes. Winter (1981) studied children with diabetes in hospital and observed that 18% of the children had a blood glucose of less than 3.6 mmol/l during the night, which was confirmed by Baumer *et al.* (1982) who reported that 19% of children had blood glucose values of less than 3.0 mmol/l recorded during the night. In a larger study of 135 diabetic children, Shalwitz *et al.* (1990) found that 14.4% had a blood glucose of less than 3.3 mmol/l at 02.00 hours, 7% fell to below 2.8 mmol/l and 2% had a blood glucose lower than 2.2 mmol/l. Unfortunately the number of symptomatic episodes which wakened the patients was not documented. Nocturnal hypoglycemia has been observed to occur more frequently in children who are taking twice-daily insulin compared with once-daily administration, probably because they have a better quality of glycemic control (Whincup & Milner, 1987)

The blood glucose value at 22.00 hours has been shown to be an important predictor of the development of hypoglycemia during the night. Whincup & Milner (1987) studied two groups of diabetic children; if the blood glucose at bedtime was less than 7.0 mmol/l, it declined to below 3.0 mmol/l during the night in 13 of 14 diabetic children. A snack was given to the second group to children at bedtime if blood glucose was less than 7.0 mmol/l and this prevented nocturnal hypoglycemia in 12 of 15 children. In a similar study of 135 diabetic children Shalwitz *et al.* (1990) found that in 65 (48%) who had blood glucose values below 5.6 mmol/l at bedtime, the blood glucose declined to less than 3.3 mmol/l at 02.00 hours and had declined to below 2.8 mmol/l in 33 (24%) of patients. Both of these studies also showed that the fasting blood glucose concentrations in the morning did not provide an accurate indicator of whether hypoglycemia had occurred during the preceding night.

Fasting hyperglycemia appears to be very uncommon after nocturnal hypoglycemia, although Winter (1981) has demonstrated a significant rise in plasma growth hormone associated with nocturnal hypoglycemia and with fasting (morning) hyperglycemia of over 17.0 mmol/l. Studies in diabetic adults have failed to provide convincing evidence for the existence of post-hypoglycemic hyperglycemia, or the so-called 'Somogyi' phenomenon (Somogyi, 1959), and allege that it has no great clinical significance (Gale *et al.*, 1980; Tordjman *et al.*, 1987; Lerman & Wolfsdorf, 1988; Havlin & Cryer, 1987; Hirsch *et al.*, 1990). It is more likely that the ingestion of excessive quantities of refined carbohydrate to treat or prevent nocturnal hypoglycemia contributes to the subsequent fasting hyperglycemia observed on the following morning.

25.8 THE EFFECT OF HYPOGLYCEMIA ON THE BRAIN

25.8.1 NEONATAL HYPOGLYCEMIA

In human neonates, untreated severe hypoglycemia in the first week of life can result in extensive neuronal degeneration throughout the nervous system (Anderson *et al.*, 1967). Treatment of severe neonatal hypoglycemia has been shown to reduce the severity of abnormalities observed at necropsy. Banker (1967) described microcephaly caused by hypoglycemia in three human infants who had been exposed to severe hypoglycemia, and although gross pathological changes were demonstrable, Griffiths and Laurence (1974) claimed that hypoxia was a more important factor causing this cerebral damage. Several reports have suggested that neonatal hypoglycemia can cause permanent behavioral, EEG and cognitive changes (Hawarth & Coodin, 1960; Hawarth & McRae, 1965; Pildes *et al.*, 1974; Lucas *et al.*, 1988). In the absence of overt pathological lesions it is likely that subtle functional changes can occur after recurrent hypoglycemia, which result in a more insidious deterioration in neuropsychological function.

25.8.2 NEUROLOGICAL ABNORMALITIES

Anecdotal case reports of cerebral dysfunction in children occurring during acute hypoglycemia have been published. Transient hemiplegia, possibly following hypoglycemia, has been described in diabetic children (Wayne *et al.*, 1990; Stirling *et al.*, 1992) although this is reputed to be uncommon (Whincup & Milner, 1987). Cortical blindness has also been observed during documented hypoglycemia in a 3-year-old nondiabetic child with glycogen storage disease (Mukamel *et al.*, 1981).

25.8.3 NEUROPSYCHOLOGICAL AND COGNITIVE EFFECTS

The neurobehavioral complications of Type 1 diabetes are probably of multifactorial etiology (Ryan, 1988), but many anecdotal reports have alleged that diabetic children who had been exposed to recurrent hypoglycemic episodes, developed permanent cerebral damage (Murphy & Purtell, 1943; Fischer & Dolger, 1946). The IQs of diabetic children have been found to be significantly lower than age-matched nondiabetic controls with a similar educational background, and, in diabetic children, the deficit in IQ appeared to be associated with the number of preceding episodes of severe hypoglycemia (Ack *et al.*, 1961).

Eeg-Olofsson and Petersen (1966) noted that although EEG abnormalities were more prevalent in all diabetic children, those who had a history of recurrent severe hypoglycemia were most likely to have permanent EEG abnormalities and confirmed these findings in a subsequent study (Eeg-Olofsson, 1977). Fallstrom (1974) showed that 59 diabetic children had more problems with perceptual disturbance and behavior, and had increased anxiety when compared with healthy nondiabetic children of the same age. In addition, the severity of these abnormalities appeared to correlate with the frequency of previous severe hypoglycemia causing convulsions. Other studies have demonstrated abnormal EEGs in 80% of children who had suffered more than five episodes of severe hypoglycemia (Haumont *et al.*, 1979; Soltesz & Acsadi, 1989). Abnormalities of visual evoked potentials are more frequent in diabetic children compared with normal subjects (Cirillo *et al.*, 1984) although it is not known if this is related to hypoglycemia.

Several studies of cognitive and neurophysiologic function in diabetic children and adolescents have shown evidence of dysfunction and abnormality, in which the exposure to severe hypoglycemia could be implicated as a possible causal or contributory factor. Ryan *et al.* (1984, 1985) demonstrated poorer cognitive function in adolescent diabetic patients compared with matched nondiabetic controls and found that the poorest performance occurred in those children who had developed diabetes before the age of 5 years. Multiple regression analysis showed that verbal and learned skills were poorer when associated with a long duration of diabetes, whereas early age of onset particularly affected the tests which measured the ability to process new information. Children with diabetes also appear to have poorer reading ability (Gath *et al.*, 1980). None of these studies examined any possible association with the frequency of previous hypoglycemia but subsequent studies have shown that the diabetic children who performed poorly on cognitive function testing had a history of hypoglycemic convulsions (Rovet *et al.*, 1987; Golden *et al.*, 1989). Frequent episodes of mild or asymptomatic hypoglycemia were also related to poorer performance by diabetic children on cognitive function testing (Golden *et al.*, 1989). In a 3-year prospective study of 63 diabetic children, no major decline in cognitive function was observed (Rovet *et al.*, 1991). However, those children with onset of diabetes before 5 years of age experienced more asymptomatic episodes of hypoglycemia and had poorer spatial ability, while those with onset of diabetes after 5 years of age were more likely to have experienced frequent symptomatic mild and moderate episodes of hypoglycemia and had poorer verbal skills. These results are in accordance with the results of some studies in adult insulin-treated diabetic subjects in which a deficit in IQ correlated with the frequency of previous exposure to severe hypoglycemia (Wredling *et al.*, 1990; Langan *et al.*, 1991; Deary *et al.*, 1993). The neuropsychological changes may be more profound in diabetic children because the developing brain may be more vulnerable to hypoglycemia.

It is difficult to study the effects of acute hypoglycemia in children or adolescents because of ethical considerations and the inability of young children to cooperate. Cognitive assessments in adolescent diabetic children who are able to cooperate with formal testing, have demonstrated deterioration of fine motor coordination, memory, and concentrating ability at a range of venous blood glucose from 2.9–3.6 mmol/l (Flender & Lifshitz, 1976). By using the hyperinsulinemic glucose clamp technique to induce controlled hypoglycemia in a group of children with Type 1 diabetes, Ryan *et al.* (1990) have shown impairment of mental flexibility, planning and decision-making, attention to detail and reaction times at arterialized plasma glucose concentrations of 3.3–3.6 mmol/l. Abnormal auditory and somatosensory-evoked potentials have been recorded in nondiabetic children in whom the blood glucose fell below 2.6 mmol/l following prolonged fasting or during an insulin tolerance test (Koh *et al.*, 1988b). Recovery of function was also noted to be delayed following the restoration of normoglycemia with marked inter-subject variability in the degree of neurophysiologic and cognitive impairment, as has been demonstrated in adult diabetic subjects (Herold *et al.*, 1985; Hoffman *et al.*, 1989). At a diabetic summer camp, 24 diabetic children underwent cognitive testing after the resolution of a hypoglycemic episode in which the blood glucose was documented to be less than 3.3 mmol/l (Puczynski *et al.*, 1990). The results showed that an impairment of cognitive function persisted after the blood glucose had returned to normal and the children no longer had symptoms of hypoglycemia, when compared with diabetic children who were documented to be normoglycemic before cognitive testing. This suggests that there is a dissociation in the rate of resolution of physical symptoms and the rate of recovery of cognitive function in the diabetic child following relatively mild hypoglycemia. This is of relevance to performance at school and during examinations, although no studies have addressed this issue specifically.

In conclusion, both acute and recurrent hypoglycemia cause changes in cognitive function in diabetic children which may result in impaired learning ability and cause suboptimal school performance. It has been suggested that diabetic children with early onset of the disease should be considered for neuropsychological testing if they have a history of recurrent hypoglycemia (Puczynski *et al.*, 1992).

25.9 MANAGEMENT OF HYPOGLYCEMIA IN CHILDREN

Mild hypoglycemia which is recognized either by the child or by the carers may be treated satisfactorily by oral administration of 20–25 g of carbohydrate in the form of glucose drinks and tablets or high carbohydrate foods, e.g., chocolate bars. If no obvious improvement or recovery occurs after 10 minutes, the dose should be repeated. If the child is unable to take oral carbohydrate, jam or 'Hypostop' may be applied to the buccal mucosa but 'force-feeding' should be avoided as aspiration might occur, particularly if the child is semi-conscious or convulsing.

Physiologic glucagon secretion is suppressed in children with Type 1 diabetes, especially those undergoing intensive insulin therapy (Soltesz *et al.*, 1988; Aman & Wranne, 1988a) and administration of subcutaneous or intramuscular glucagon is usually effective to treat severe hypoglycemia (Aman & Wranne, 1988b). All parents should be instructed in the administration of glucagon; a dose of 10–20 μg/kg body weight produces supraphysiologic plasma concentrations so that the contents of half a 1 mg vial should suffice in small children while a whole 1 mg vial should be given to older children. Some children develop nausea and abdominal pain after glucagon, which is probably dose-related and these symptoms may be confused with the manifestations of hypoglycemia.

If hypoglycemia does not respond to the above measures after ten minutes then emergency medical help should be obtained, and the patient treated in hospital if necessary. Intravenous glucose (0.2 g/kg) should be given at a rate of 4–6 mg/kg/min. Rarely, sudden death has been associated with the administration of excessive quantitites of intravenous glucose for resuscitation following hypoglycemia during an insulin tolerance test (Shah *et al.*, 1992) and the rapid intravenous infusion of hyperosmolar solutions of dextrose should be avoided. Delayed recovery following hypoglycemia may be associated with the serious and potentially lethal complication of cerebral edema which requires specific therapy such as mannitol, and intensive care should be instituted.

25.10 PREVENTION OF HYPOGLYCEMIA IN CHILDREN

Diabetic children and adults treated with insulin are routinely taught blood glucose monitoring. This has been shown to provide a practical basis for the improvement of glycemic control and provides reassurance that hypoglycemia is not imminent (Baumer *et al.*, 1982). Children and their parents should be taught how to adjust insulin doses according to blood glucose results and to modify the diet to match planned physical activity. Extra carbohydrate should be available and given if the child has taken the usual insulin dose and is then involved in extra physical activity. Insulin doses may need to be reduced in the summer months. To avoid nocturnal hypoglycemia extra bedtime snacks should be given if blood glucose concentrations at bedtime are less than 7.0 mmol/l (section 25.7) or if the child has been undertaking more vigorous physical activity than usual during the day. Delayed food intake should be avoided if possible and the parents and the diabetic child should both carry an emergency supply of carbohydrate with them at all times. It has been shown that application of the above measures can enable an improvement in glycemic control with a simultaneous reduction in the frequency of hypoglycemia (Golden *et al.*, 1985).

25.11 CONCLUSIONS

Hypoglycemia is a common and potentially dangerous side effect of insulin treatment in diabetic children and has a substantial morbidity. Although it may be impossible to avoid completely, appropriate education, with regular reinforcement, of both diabetic children and their carers should reduce the incidence of severe episodes. It is also important for the physician to address the therapeutic dilemma which is emerging in the modern management of diabetes: should diabetic patients have to risk sacrificing intellectual capacity, as a result of exposure to recurrent severe hypoglycemia associated with the maintenance of excessively strict glycemic control, to try and avoid the long-term microvascular complications of diabetes? This is of particular relevance to the management of very young diabetic children, in whom recurrent severe hypoglycemia may have a profound, deleterious and permanent effect on cerebral and intellectual development. The damage to intellectual function in all diabetic children will limit their potential for achievement in adult life, and must therefore be strenuously avoided.

REFERENCES

Ack, M., Miller, I. and Weil, W.B. (1961) Intelligence of chidren with diabetes mellitus. *Pediatrics*, **28**, 764–70.

Aman, J. and Wranne, L. (1988a) Hypoglycaemia in childhood diabetes. I. Clinical signs and hormonal counterregulation. *Acta Paed. Scand.*, **77**, 542–47.

Aman, J. and Wranne, L. (1988b) Hypoglycaemia in childhood diabetes. II. Effects of subcutaneous or intramuscular injection of different doses of glucagon. *Acta Paed. Scand.*, **77**, 548–53.

Aman, J., Karlsson, I. and Wranne, L. (1989) Symptomatic hypoglycaemia in childhood diabetes: a population-based questionnaire study. *Diabetic Med.*, **6**, 257–61.

Amiel, S.A., Tamborlane, W.V., Simonson, D.C. *et al.* (1987a) Defective glucose counterregulation after strict glycemic control of insulin-dependent diabetes mellitus. *N. Eng. J. Med.*, **316**, 1376–83.

Amiel, S.A., Simonson, D.C., Sherwin, R.S. *et al.* (1987b) Exaggerated epinephrine responses to hypoglycemia in normal and insulin-dependent diabetic children. *J. Pediatr.*, **110**, 832–37.

Amiel, S.A., Archibald, H.R., Chusney, G. *et al.* (1991) Ketone infusion lowers hormonal responses to hypoglycaemia: evidence for acute cerebral utilization of a non-glucose fuel. *Clinical Science*, **81**, 189–94.

Anderson, J.M., Milner, R.D.G. and Strich, S.J. (1967) Effects of neonatal hypoglycaemia on the nervous system. *J. Neurology, Neurosurgery and Psychiatry*, **30**, 295–310.

Arias, P., Kerner, W., Zier, H. *et al.* (1985) Incidence of hypoglycemic episodes in diabetic patients under continuous subcutaneous insulin infusion and intensified conventional insulin treatment: assessment by means of semiambulatory 24-hour monitoring of blood glucose. *Diabetes Care*, **8**, 134–40.

Aynsley-Green, A. (1991) Glucose: a fuel for thought! *J. Paediatr. and Child Health*, **27**, 21–30.

Banker, B.Q. (1967) The neuropathological effects of anoxia and hypoglycaemia in the newborn. *Devel. Med. and Child Neurology*, **9**, 544–50.

Baumer, J.H., Edelstein, A.D., Howlett, B.C. *et al.* (1982) Impact of home blood glucose monitoring on childhood diabetes. *Arch. Dis. Child.*, **57**, 195–99.

Bergada, I., Suissa, S., Dufresne, J. *et al.* (1989) Severe hypoglycemia in IDDM children. *Diabetes Care*, **12**, 239–44.

Bhatia, V. and Wolfsdorf, J.I. (1991) Severe hypoglycemia in youth with insulin-dependent diabetes mellitus: frequency and causative factors. *Pediatrics*, **88**, 1187–93.

Bier, D.M., Leake, R.D., Haymond, M.W. *et al.* (1977) Measurement of 'true' glucose production rates in infancy and childhood with 6,6-dideuteroglucose. *Diabetes*, **26**, 1016–23.

Bolli, G., De Feo, P., Compagnucci, P. *et al.* (1983) Abnormal glucose counterregulation in insulin-dependent diabetes mellitus. Interaction of anti-insulin antibodies and impaired glucagon and epinephrine secretion. *Diabetes*, **32**, 134–41.

Bougneres, P.F., Landier, F., Lemmel, C. *et al.* (1984) Insulin pump therapy in children with type 1 diabetes. *J. Pediatr.*, **105**, 212–17.

Bougneres, P.F., Landais, P., Mairesse, A.M. *et al.* (1993) Improvement in diabetic control and acceptibility of a three-injection insulin regimen in diabetic adolescents. *Diabetes Care*, **16**, 94–102.

Boyle, P.J., Schwartz, N.S., Shah, S.D. *et al.* (1988) Plasma glucose concentrations at the onset of hypoglycemic symptoms in patients with poorly controlled diabetes and in non-diabetics. *N. Eng. J. Med.*, **318**, 1487–92.

Brambilla, P., Bougneres, P.F., Santiago, J.V. *et al.* (1987) Glucose counterregulation in pre-school-age diabetic children with recurrent hypoglycemia during conventional treatment. *Diabetes*, **36**, 300–304.

Casparie, A.F. and Elving, L.D. (1985) Severe hypoglycemia in diabetic patients: frequency, causes, prevention. *Diabetes Care*, **8**, 141–45.

Cirillo, D., Gonfiantini, E., De Grandis, D. *et al.* (1984) Visual evoked potentials in diabetic children and adolescents. *Diabetes Care*, **7**, 273–75.

Daneman, D., Frank, M., Perlman, K. *et al.* (1989) Severe hypoglycemia in children with insulin-dependent diabetes mellitus: frequency and predisposing factors. *J. Pediatr.*, **115**, 681–85.

The DCCT Research Group. (1991) Epidemiology of severe hypoglycemia in the diabetes control and complications trial. *Am. J. Med.*, **90**, 450–59.

The DCCT Research Group. (1993) The effect of intensive treatment of diabetes on the development and progression of long-term complications in insulin-dependent diabetes mellitus. *New Eng. J. Med.*, **329**, 977–86.

Deary, I.J., Crawford, J.R., Hepburn, D.A. *et al.* (1993) Severe hypoglycemia and intelligence in adult patients with insulin-treated diabetes. *Diabetes*, **42**, 341–44.

Dershewitz, R., Vestal, B., Maclaren, N.K. *et al.* (1976) Transient hepatomegaly and hypoglycemia. *Am. J. Dis. Child.*, **130**, 998–99.

Diamond, M.P., Hallarman, L., Starick-Zych, K. *et al.* (1991) Suppression of counterregulatory hormone response to hypoglycemia by insulin *per se*. *J. Clin. Endocrinol. Metab.*, **72**, 1388–90.

Eeg-Olofsson, O. (1977) Hypoglycaemia and neurological disturbances in children with diabetes mellitus. *Acta Paed. Scand.*, **270** (suppl. 1), 91–96.

Eeg-Olofsson, O. and Petersen, I. (1966) Childhood diabetic neuropathy. A clinical and neurophysiological study. *Acta Paed. Scand.*, **55**, 163–76.

Egger, M., Gschwend, S., Davey Smith, G. *et al.* (1991) Increasing incidence of hypoglycemic coma in children with IDDM. *Diabetes Care*, **14**, 1001–1005.

Fallstrom, K. (1974) On the personality structure in diabetic school children aged 7–15 years. *Acta Paed. Scand.*, **251** (suppl.), 1–70.

Fischer, A.E. and Dolger, H. (1946) Behaviour and psychologic problems of young diabetic patients. *Arch. Int. Med.*, **78**, 711–32.

Fisher, B.M. and Frier, B.M. (1993) 'Hypoglycaemia and human insulin', in B.M. Frier and B.M. Fisher (eds). *Hypoglycaemia and diabetes. Clinical and physiological aspects*, pp. 314–27. Edward Arnold, London.

Flender, J. and Lifshitz, F. (1976) The effects of fluctuations of blood glucose levels on the psychological performance of juvenile diabetics. *Diabetes*, **25** (suppl. 1), 334A (abstract).

Gale, E.A.M., Kurtz, A.B. and Tattersall, R.B. (1980) In search of the Somogyi effect. *Lancet*, **ii**, 279–82.

Gath, A., Smith, M.A. and Baum, J.D. (1980) Emotional, behavioural, and educational disorders in diabetic children. *Arch. Dis. Child.*, **55**, 371–75.

Gerich, G., Cryer, P. and Rizza, R.A. (1980) Hormonal mechanisms in acute glucose counterregulation: the relative roles of glucagon, norepinephrine, growth hormone, and cortisol. *Metabolism*, **29**, 1164–72.

Golden, M.P., Russell, B.P., Ingersoll, G.M. *et al.* (1985) Management of diabetes mellitus in children younger than 5 years of age. *Am. J. Dis. Child.*, **139**, 448–52.

Golden, M.P., Ingersoll, G.M., Brack, C.J. *et al.* (1989) Longitudinal relationship of asymptomatic hypoglycemia to cognitive function in IDDM. *Diabetes Care*, **12**, 89–93.

Goldstein, D.E., England, J.D., Hess, R. *et al.*

(1981) A prospective study of symptomatic hypoglycemia in young diabetic patients. *Diabetes Care*, **4**, 601–605.
Griffiths, A.D. and Laurence, K.M. (1974) The effect of hypoxia and hypoglycaemia on the brain of the newborn infant. *Develop. Med. and Child Neurol.*, **16**, 308–319.
Grunberger, G., Weiner, J.L., Silverman, R. *et al.* (1988) Factitious hypoglycemia due to surreptitious administration of insulin. *Ann. Int. Med.*, **108**, 252–57.
Haumont, D., Dorchy, H. and Pelc, S. (1979) EEG abnormalities in diabetic children. Influence of hypoglycemia in children and adolescents with IDDM. *Clin. Pediatr.*, **18**, 750–53.
Havlin, C.E. and Cryer, P.E. (1987) Nocturnal hypoglycemia does not commonly result in major morning hyperglycemia in patients with diabetes mellitus. *Diabetes Care*, **10**, 141–47.
Hawarth, J. and Coodin, F.J. (1960) Idiopathic spontaneous hypoglycemia in children. Report of seven cases and review of the literature. *Pediatrics*, **25**, 748–65.
Hawarth, J.C. and McRae, K.N. (1965) The neurlogical and developmental effects of neonatal hypoglycemia. *Can. Med. Assoc. J.*, **92**, 861–65.
Haymond, M.W., Karl, I.E. and Pagliara, A.S. (1974) Ketotic hypoglycemia is an amino acid substrate limited disorder. *J. Clin. Endocrinol. and Metab.*, **38**, 521–30.
Haymond, M.W., Karl, I.E., Clarke, W.L. *et al.* (1982) Differences in circulating gluconeogenic substrates during short-term fasting in men, women and children. *Metabolism*, **31**, 33–42.
Hepburn, D.A., Deary, I.J., Frier, B.M. *et al.* (1991) Symptoms of acute hypoglycemia in humans with and without IDDM. Factor-analysis approach. *Diabetes Care*, **14**, 949–57.
Herold, K.C., Polonsky, K.S., Cohen, R.M. *et al.* (1985) Variable deterioration in cortical function during insulin induced hypoglycemia. *Diabetes*, **34**, 677–85.
Hirsch, I.B., Smith, I.J., Havlin, C.E. *et al.* (1990) Failure of nocturnal hypoglycemia to cause daytime hyperglycemia in patients with IDDM. *Diabetes Care*, **13**, 133–42.
Hoffman, R.G., Speelman, D.J., Hinnen, D.A. *et al.* (1989) Changes in cortical functioning with acute hypoglycemia and hyperglycemia in Type 1 diabetes. *Diabetes Care*, **12**, 193–97.
Hoffman, R.P., Singer-Granick, C., Drash, A.L. *et al.* (1991) Plasma catecholamine responses to hypoglycemia in children and adolescents with IDDM. *Diabetes Care*, **14**, 81–88.
Jones, T.W., Boulware, S.D., Kraemer, D.T. *et al.* (1991) Independent effects of youth and poor diabetes control on responses to hypoglycemia in children. *Diabetes*, **40**, 358–63.
Kelnar, C.J.H. (1976) Hypoglycaemia in children undergoing adenotonsillectomy. *Brit. Med. J.*, **1**, 751–52.
Koh, T.H.H.G., Eyre, J.A. and Aynsley-Green, A. (1988a) Neonatal hypoglycaemia – the controversy regarding definition. *Arch. Dis. Child.*, **63**, 1386–98.
Koh, T.H.H.G., Aynsley-Green, A., Tarbit, M. *et al.* (1988b) Neural dysfunction during hypoglycaemia. *Arch. Dis. Child.*, **63**, 1353–58.
Langan, S.J., Deary, I.J., Hepburn, D.A. *et al.* (1991) Cumulative cognitive impairment following recurrent severe hypoglycaemia in adult patients with insulin-treated diabetes mellitus. *Diabetologia*, **34**, 337–44.
Lerman, I.G. and Wolfsdorf, J.I. (1988) Relationship of nocturnal hypoglycemia to daytime glycemia in IDDM. *Diabetes Care*, **11**, 636–42.
Limbert, C., Schwingshandl, J., Haas, J. *et al.* (1993) Severe hypoglycemia in children and adolescents with IDDM: frequency and associated factors. *J. Diab. Comp.*, **7**, 216–20.
Liu, D., Adamson, U.C.K., Lins, P.-E.S. *et al.* (1992) Inhibitory effect of circulating insulin on glucagon secretion during hypoglycemia in type 1 diabetic patients. *Diabetes Care*, **15**, 59–65.
Lucas, A., Morley R. and Cole, T. (1988) Adverse outcome of moderate neonatal hypoglycaemia. *Brit. Med. J.*, **297**, 1304–1308.
MacDonald, M.J. (1987) Postexercise late-onset hypoglycemia in insulin-dependent diabetic patients. *Diabetes Care*, **10**, 584–88.
Macfarlane, P.I., Walters, M., Stutchfield, P. *et al.* (1989) A prospective study of symptomatic hypoglycaemia in childhood diabetes. *Diabetic Med.*, **6**, 627–30.
McCrimmon, R.J., Gold, A.E., Deary, I.J. *et al.* (1994) Symptoms of hypoglycaemia in children with insulin-dependent diabetes mellitus (IDDM). *Diabetalogia*, **37** (suppl. 1), A165.
Mayefsky, J.H., Sarnaik, A.P. and Postellon, D.C. (1982) Factitious hypoglycemia. *Pediatrics*, **69**, 804–805.
Mukamel, M., Weitz, R., Nissenkorn, I. *et al.*

(1981) Acute cortical blindness associated with hypoglycemia. *J. Pediatr.*, **98**, 583–84.

Murphy, F.D. and Purtell, J. (1943) Insulin reaction and the cerebral damage that may occur in diabetes. *Am. J. Digest. Dis.*, **10**, 103–107.

Pildes, R.S., Cornblath, M., Warren, I. *et al.* (1974) A prospective controlled study of neonatal hypoglycemia. *Pediatrics*, **54**, 5–14.

Pramming, S., Thorsteinsson, B., Bendtson, I. *et al.* (1991) Symptomatic hypoglycaemia in 411 type 1 diabetic patients. *Diabetic Med.*, **8**, 217–22.

Puczynski, M.S., Puczynski, S.S., Reich, J. *et al.* (1990) Mental efficiency and hypoglycemia. *Develop. and Behav. Pediatr.*, **11**, 170–74.

Puczynski. S.S., Puczynski, M.S. and Ryan, C.M. (1992) Hypoglycemia in children with insulin-dependent diabetes mellitus. *Diabetes Educator*, **18**, 151–53.

Rovet, J.F., Erhlich, R.M. and Hoppe, M. (1987) Intellectual deficits associated with early onset of insulin-dependent diabetes mellitus in children. *Diabetes Care*, **10**, 510–15.

Rovet, J.F., Czuchta, D. and Ehrlich, R.M. (1991) Neuropsychological sequelae of diabetes in childhood. A three year prospective study. *Diabetes*, **40** (suppl. 1), 430A (abstract).

Ryan, C. (1988) Neurobehavioural complications of Type 1 diabetes. *Diabetes Care*, **11**, 86–93.

Ryan, C., Vega, A., Longstreet, C. *et al.* (1984) Neuropsychological changes in adolescents with insulin-dependent diabetes. *J. Consult. and Clin. Psychol.*, **52**, 335–42.

Ryan, C., Vega, A. and Drash, A. (1985) Cognitive deficits in adolescents who developed diabetes early in life. *Pediatrics*, **75**, 921–27.

Ryan, C.M., Atchison, J., Puczynski, S.S. *et al.* (1990) Mild hypoglycemia associated with deterioration of mental efficiency in children with insulin-dependent diabetes mellitus. *J. Pediatr.*, **117**, 32–38.

Schiffrin, A.D., Derosiers, M., Aleyassine, H. *et al.* (1984) Intensified insulin therapy in the type 1 diabetic adolescent: a controlled trial. *Diabetes Care*, **7**, 107–113.

Selam, J.-L., Micossi, P., Dunn, F.L. *et al.* (1992) Clinical trial of programmable implantable insulin pump for type 1 diabetes. *Diabetes Care*, **15**, 877–85.

Senior, B. (1973) Ketotic hypoglycemia. A tale (tail) Gauss? *J. Pediatr.*, **82**, 555–56.

Shah, A., Stanhope, R. and Matthew, D. (1992) Hazards of pharmacological tests of growth hormone secretion in childhood. *Brit. Med. J.*, **304**, 173–74.

Shalwitz, R.A., Farkus-Hirsch, R., White, N.H. *et al.* (1990) Prevalence and consequences of nocturnal hypoglycemia among conventionally treated children with diabetes mellitus. *J. Pediatr.*, **116**, 685–89.

Singer-Granick, C., Hoffman, R.P., Kerensky, K. *et al.* (1988) Glucagon responses to hypoglycemia in children and adolescents with IDDM. *Diabetes Care*, **11**, 643–49.

Soltesz, G. and Acsadi, G. (1989) Association between diabetes, severe hypoglycaemia and electroencephalographic abnormalities. *Arch. Dis. Child.*, **64**, 992–96.

Soltesz, G., Molnar, D., Decsi, T. *et al.* (1988) The metabolic and hormonal effects of continuous subcutaneous insulin infusion therapy in diabetic children. *Diabetologia*, **31**, 30–34.

Somogyi, M. (1959) Exacerbation of diabetes by excess insulin action. *Am. J. Med.*, **26**, 169–91.

Stirling, H.F., Goh, D., Darling, J.A.B. *et al.* (1992) Significant hypoglycaemia? – Transient hemiparesis complicating nocturnal hypoglycaemia in pre-pubertal diabetic children. *Eur. J. Pediatr.*, **151**, 393 (abstract).

Thomas, D.K.M. (1974) Hypoglycaemia in children before operation: its incidence and prevention. *Brit. J. Anaesth.*, **46**, 66–68.

Tordjman, K.M., Havlin, C.E., Levandovski, L.A. *et al.* (1987) Failure of nocturnal hypoglycemia to cause fasting hyperglycemia in patients with insulin-dependent diabetes mellitus. *N. Eng. J. Med.*, **317**, 1552–59.

Wayne, E.A., Dean, H.J., Booth, F. *et al.* (1990) Focal neurological deficits associated with hypoglycemia in children with diabetes. *J. Pediatr.*, **117**, 575–77.

Whincup, G. and Milner, R.D.G. (1987) Prediction and management of nocturnal hypoglycaemia in diabetes. *Arch. Dis. Child.*, **62**, 333–37.

Winter, R.J. (1981) Profiles of metabolic control in diabetic children – frequency of asymptomatic hypoglycemia. *Metabolism*, **30**, 666–72.

Wredling, R., Levander, S., Adamson, U. *et al.* (1990) Permanent neuropsychological impairment after recurrent episodes of severe hypoglycaemia in man. *Diabetologia*, **33**, 152–57.

26

Diabetes in the adolescent

R.W. NEWTON and S.A. GREENE

26.1 INTRODUCTION

Adolescence is defined as the period of 'growing up' – changing from childhood to adulthood; the adolescent is an individual involved in this period. The expression 'adolescence' is unfortunate in that it is seen by 'teenagers' as almost a derogatory term, and indeed appears to be very official, a standing disliked by many teenagers. 'Teenager' may indeed appear to be a more appropriate term for the patient, although thirteen is not a magic number, with many children starting adolescence well before or well after this age. The period is synonomous with a time of great physiologic change (growth and development) as well as behavioral and emotional changes relating to sexuality, increasing independence from parents and the development of outside emotional relationships. It is a time of experimentation and rebellion. Add insulin dependent diabetes mellitus (IDDM) and it can become a time of chaos!

Diabetes may become a focus for conflict and argument within the family, a restriction on social activities making the fun of teenage life more difficult. This may, in turn, lead to a feeling of being less than normal. Against this background it is crucial that health care professionals acknowledge rebellious behavior as normal in relation to diabetes care and avoid adopting a judgmental and critical role. Sticking to the ground rules of diabetes self-care becomes a minefield of issues: teenage rejection of the disease, the feeling of being different, change in ambition and life goals and the real fear of a shortened lifespan as a result of diabetic complications.

This chapter discusses the aspects of IDDM that have specific features for teenagers, and suggests an approach of management based on our experience with teenagers with IDDM in Tayside, Scotland, and as part of a United Kingdom-wide project for teenagers with diabetes, the Youth Diabetes Focus Group.

26.2 INCIDENCE AND PREVALENCE

Diabetes is one of the most common diseases occurring during teenage life. Overall the prevalence in Scotland is currently 1.4 cases per 1000 under the age of twenty (Smail, 1993), with an incidence of 19.1/1000 (Metcalf & Baum, 1991). The most common time of presentation is between the ages of 10–15 years with a peak age of onset at 12 years. Over 95% of cases are classic IDDM, presenting with weight loss, polyuria and polydipsia. This pattern appears to have changed in the last ten years with very few subjects now presenting with severe diabetic

Childhood and Adolescent Diabetes
Published in 1994 by Chapman & Hall, London
ISBN 0 412 48610 5

ketoacidosis (DKA) and coma. The vast majority of new patients can be managed initially on an outpatient basis, and in our experience only 5% require hospitalization. Most large district general hospitals will have around 100–150 teenagers and children under their management. General practitioners, however, will usually have only a small number (between 0 and 5). With the emphasis on a team approach to the management of IDDM in the young, we would advocate all young people (under 25 years of age) to attend a hospital-based clinic service.

A significant number of children (25%) present with diabetes under the age of 5 years (Metcalf & Baum, 1991). Hence many teenagers will have had IDDM for several years as they approach this period of lifestyle change. Some older teenagers will develop IDDM at a time of tremendous changes in their physical environment (e.g., at the start of college, having just moved away from home, at the begining of their first relationship). Both scenarios present challenges to the diabetic team advising on the management of the condition.

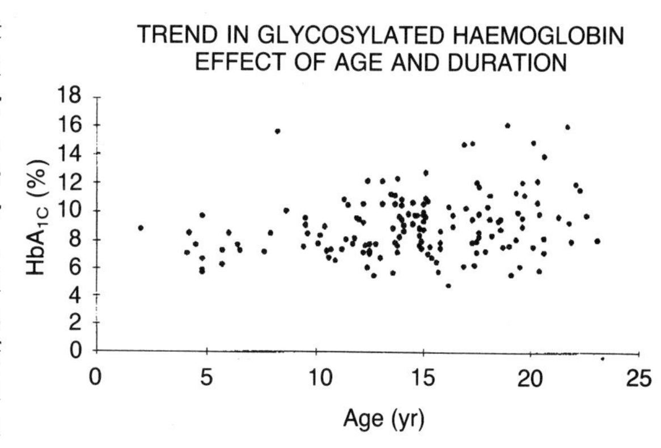

Figure 26.1 Trend in glycosylated hemoglobin effect of age and duration.

26.3 SPECIAL PROBLEMS

26.3.1 BLOOD GLUCOSE METABOLISM

There is an undoubted deterioration in blood glucose control during the teenage period (Figure 26.1). This is independent of duration of diabetes. This deterioration is far from universal in all teenagers, with the majority still able to keep excellent metabolic control. Some patients, however, deteriorate markedly during this period and give a 'bad name' to the diabetic teenager.

There are immense physiologic changes during this period. Insulin resistance develops with the onset of puberty (Hindmarsh *et al.*, 1988). Secondary to the hormonal changes associated with puberty and the lack of an integrated insulin release system, there are significant differences between diabetic and normal subjects in the circulating concentrations of insulin-like growth factor 1 (IGF1), IGF1 binding protein and growth hormone (Dunger *et al.*, 1993; Dunger & Cheetham, 1993). This abnormal hormonal milieu affects blood glucose control, particularly at night.

Attempting to overcome the insulin resistance by increasing the total daily dose of injected subcutaneous insulin, either by a conventional twice-daily regimen or by multiple injection regimen, fails to improve glycemic control over a sustained period (Mortensen *et al.*, 1988) and in our experience produces significant weight gain (Gregory *et al.*, 1992). In our view, increasing the total daily dose above 0.8–1.0 units per kg in prepuberty and 1.0–1.3 units during puberty is unlikely to improve glycemic control.

Other hormone therapies have been suggested in the past (e.g., somatostatin (Osei *et al.*, 1989)), but recent attention has been focused on the use of IGF1 therapy as an adjunct to insulin. In very preliminary observations, the addition of IGF1 injections in the evening improved glycemic control in the short term (Cheetham *et al.*, 1993). It remains to be seen if the addition of IGF1 to standard insulin regimens over a period of time will lead to a sustained improvement of control during this period. However, even if glycemic control does not improve 'normalization' of circulating IGF1, IGF1BP and growth hormone may be important, particularly for normal growth, both for height and weight, and also given the concern expressed about elevated growth hormone levels and the development of microvascular disease (Kohner, 1991).

While we have indicated the physiologic changes in puberty that give rise to the state of 'insulin resistance' we consider that for the majority of poorly controlled teenagers other, more practical and personal problems, are at the root of raised blood glucose concentrations. Correct these and the abnormal hormonal milieu will also correct itself.

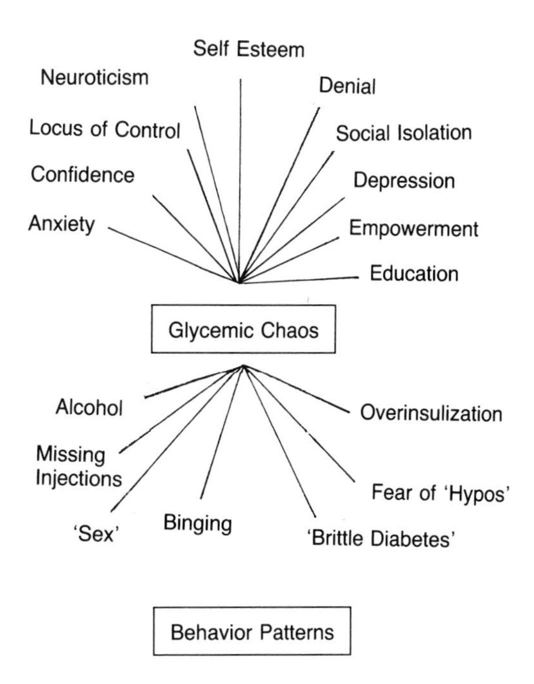

Figure 26.2 Relationships with poor glycemic control.

26.4 THE TOOLS TO ACHIEVE GOOD CONTROL

Education of the ground rules for self-management of IDDM has traditionally been the responsibility of the hospital-based team specializing in diabetes care. The problems that influence day-to-day management of diabetes, however, depend less on available information and more on learning to cope with diabetes and how it affects the family and environment. Contact with the hospital is necessarily sporadic and it is important to provide a support service for help and advice which is readily accessible.

The diabetes specialist nurse fulfils that role but the practice nurse may also be in a unique position to provide support as a friend and counsellor. Agreed policy on information to avoid confusion together with a philosophy of encouragement and avoidance of confrontation may foster an honest and open relationship over the problems of diabetic life.

The 'glycemic chaos' that occurs during the teenage period is influenced by many factors (Figure 26.2). While many of the psychological measures have been identified in teenagers and are responsible for the difficulties that occur in coping with diabetes, we feel that a more practical approach to investigating the specific difficulties that teenagers have expressed about IDDM is necessary (Davies & Newton, 1989).

26.4.1 EATING

Some kind of orderly pattern of eating whereby carbohydrate, reduced in 'free sugar' foods, is distributed over the day is fundamental to achieving diabetic control. It should not be restricted in calories and, for younger teenagers, should not differ greatly to that of the whole family. Problems with eating are the most commonly cited reason for poor diabetic control in insulin-dependent diabetics. There are a number of important aspects which contribute to this. Calorie intake typically increases during puberty and as parental influence subsides, unusual patterns of eating may develop, particularly when a proportion of eating may be out of the home. At least four out of five normal adolescents binge and the larger proportion consider themselves fat. Indeed obesity is a major association with insulin treatment particularly in the teenage girl and may be the result of handling bingeing episodes with ever-increasing doses of insulin to maintain diabetic control. Subsequent dieting to lose weight may be the forerunner of formal eating disorders of anorexia or bulimia which are especially common in diabetic girls (Steel *et al.*, 1989; Brook, 1993) (see Chapter 27).

26.4.2 INSULIN INJECTIONS

Insulin treatment during teenage years usually involves a twice-daily injection of soluble and isophane insulin before breakfast and the evening meal. A more acceptable alternative for many teenagers with erratic social commitments and irregular eating patterns is to use a more flexible multiple injection regimen whereby soluble insulin is given pre-meals from a 'pen' device and a longer-acting insulin administered at bedtime. Surprisingly, most teenagers are not uncomfortable with the need for multiple injections particularly when the bonus is greater flexibility, whereby the adolescent can engage in the fun and the 'unplanned' without concern about the consequences.

The other factor most consistently associated with a reduction of insulin requirement is the teenager who becomes physically fit as a result of regular sports activity. This raises an important but controversial question as to whether regular strenuous physical exercise should be recommended as part of the diabetes care regime (Chapter 19). 'Recommended' as opposed to 'prescribed' is perhaps acceptable!

26.4.3 TESTING

The 'way someone feels' is an extremely poor reflection of diabetic control; self-monitoring of blood glucose is an accurate and increasingly, convenient method of assessing glycemic control. However, success depends as much on the will to do regular tests as the know-how. Test results are primarily a means whereby the insulin-dependent diabetic can obtain the necessary information to make confident self-adjustments to the insulin dose. Tests are not done to satisfy nursing and medical staff, and the 'log book' of results should not become the point of confrontation at the diabetic clinic. A sympathetic approach acknowledging that many teenagers get fed up with blood testing is more likely to foster a sense of honesty and trust between doctor and patient. Gaining confidence in using blood tests is a gradual process which can be supported and prompted by everyone who works in diabetes care.

How often should the diabetic teenager test? Enough tests are needed to give the patient confidence about control and making appropriate insulin adjustments. When control is stable about 6–8 tests per week is as many as most will tolerate. Insistence on more tests inevitably leads to abandonment of testing and dishonesty in discussions about characteristics of control (Newton, 1987).

Many teenagers accept the 'deal' of having a test of glycated hemoglobin at a clinic visit, rather than 'badgering' with blood tests on a regular basis. Indeed 'on-line' capillary blood estimation of glycated hemoglobin, with the results available in the clinic, in our experience have proved invaluable in discussing problems of control with teenagers and are more relevant than diaries of blood tests. Teenagers invariably reject urine glucose testing although may still be happy to do some samples for urine ketone estimation, if this is appropriate at times of persistent glycemia or during illness.

There appear to be interrelationships between insulin injection regimens, testing and compliance with diet. Long intervals between insulin injection and eating, high numbers of daily eating occasions and high day-to-day variations in energy intake were associated with good metabolic control in Finnish teenagers past partial remission (Virtanen, 1992).

26.5 CHAOTIC DIABETIC CONTROL DURING TEENAGE LIFE

Normal adolescent behavior encompassing rebelliousness and experimentation will be reflected in many diabetic teenagers as chaotic blood glucose control. Open discussion with groups of teenagers with diabetes has had a dramatic role in elucidating these problems; much more so than complex scientific research designed to define complex metabolic explanations. It is crucial that we listen to these young people since it is clear that many explanations relating to poor diabetic control are attributable to psychosocial effects on the practical aspects of diabetic life (Davies & Newton, 1989).

When assessing reasons for poor control in individual patients it is worth considering the following:

- Binge eating, often of sugary foods, is perhaps the commonest cause of poor control. In some this may extend to a formal eating disorder with forced emesis or self-purgation.
- Missing insulin injections to achieve weight loss occurs, usually in teenage girls. Most teenagers experiment with missing insulin injections either 'to test the system' or alternatively as a 'denial' of diabetes. Deliberate stopping of insulin with resultant ketoacidosis is a common manipulative measure. Injection phobia is uncommon but may be difficult to treat. The use of devices such as the insuflon® reservoir system may help.
- Fear of hypoglycemia may lead to deliberate avoidance of blood glucose levels associated with symptoms of hypoglycemia. The net effect is chronic poor control. Concern about hypoglycemia may lead to teenagers administering insulin after meals rather than 20 minutes before.
- Failed 'crisis' management – it is clear that some teenagers relegate diabetes care to a low priority. They administer insulin only when they have symptomatic hyperglycemia. This leads to a chronic state of dramatically poor control. Failure to deal with the 'crisis' early enough results in accelerating diabetic ketoacidosis on occasion, leading to acceptance of the need for hospital assistance. This may be a common scenario!
- Over-insulinization may lead to dramatic swings in blood glucose. Hypoglycemia is inevitably followed by a period of hyperglycemia because of the need of sugar to counteract 'hypo' symptoms and the body's natural response to hypoglycemia. The net effect is a roller-coaster effect of wild swings between high and low blood glucose results. Such patients often gain weight.
- Alcohol excess has become an unhappy part of modern teenage life. Excess alcohol is the commonest cause of diabetic ketoacidosis in young males and a prominent cause of hypoglycemia. It appears to be the only recognizable factor in sudden unexplained nocturnal death in young people (Tattersall & Gill, 1991).
- 'Brittle diabetes' implies such extreme chaos of control as to disrupt the life of the teenager with recurrent episodes of DKA or hypoglycemia requiring hospitalization. Most of these patients are young females usually mildly obese and on a high insulin dose. Not uncommonly, episodes of

ketoacidosis are attributed to unsubstantiated urinary tract or viral infection. It seems likely that most episodes are self-manipulated and relate to a variety of psychosocial problems particularly in relation to the home environment and family pathology including sexual abuse. It is important to stress that these patients do not have any peculiar metabolic abnormality as compared to other insulin-dependent diabetics (Pickup & Williams, 1991).

It is clear that the teenager with diabetes has almost unique problems. He or she is expected to adhere to a strict regimen of self-care against a background of rebelliousness often seen by the health care professional as abnormal behaviour. Adolescence is a time when parents will be expected to let go of the responsibility for their child despite their great anxieties. It is important that we adopt an uncritical and encouraging role allowing the teenager the opportunity to take part in the fun of the teenage years and still adhere to many of the requirements of diabetic life. Most enlightened hospital services have realized the value of a special diabetes clinic for this age group involving both pediatrician and adult physician. The value of an informal environment where young diabetics can meet their own age group and discuss their problems should not be underestimated.

The practice nurse may be in an exclusive position able to offer friendship and support, and accessible advice during the transition of adult life.

26.6 DIABETIC COMPLICATIONS

26.6.1 MICROVASCULAR DISEASE

Teenagers who have had diabetes for a number of years may have a number of established complications. At this stage these are mostly asymptomatic and include excessive microalbumin excretion in the urine and a rise in blood pressure as markers of subsequent diabetic nephropathy, the development of retinopathy and measurable changes in peripheral nerve function (Greene, 1991). Complications practically never occur in prepubertal children but are generally associated with duration of the disease and it is not unusual to see 'malignant' rapidly progressive diabetic retinopathy or established raised blood pressure and proteinuria in the teenager. Retinal examination through dilated pupils, estimation of urinary microalbumin excretion and BP measurement should be undertaken at least annually as part of clinic routine. Despite this, it should be emphasized that the vast majority of youngsters with diabetes (well over 70%) will live a long and relatively healthy life. Furthermore, there is now compelling evidence from work in the United States that good diabetic control will prevent or delay diabetic complications. The results of the Diabetes Control and Complications Trial (DCCT) presented to the American Diabetes Association (Diabetes Control and Complication Trial Research Group, 1993) have shown that if blood glucose levels can be kept at near normal levels by intensive long-term therapy then the risks of diabetic eye disease, nephropathy and nerve damage are reduced by at least 50% respectively.

26.6.2 HYPOGLYCEMIA

Avoidance of long-term complications is only one factor in the battleground of achieving good control. The fear of hypoglycemia felt by many teenagers and their relatives should not be underestimated. The 'loss of face' following a hypoglycemic attack witnessed by friends, or the anxiety of the possibility of permanent damage due to unrecognized and prolonged nocturnal hypoglycemia in teenagers living alone, will naturally discourage many from accepting the risk of tight glycemic control.

Hypoglycemia is common in young people on insulin, the causes and clinical features have been described elsewhere (Frier, 1993) (see also Chapter 25). It is important to stress the frequency of 'late hypoglycemia' in the teenager often occurring up to 24 hours after a spell of sustained exercise or, for example, the inevitable association of spectacular hypoglycemia after alcohol in excess and the all-night 'rave party'!

Flavored dextrosol tablets (it is remarkable how many people dislike unflavored dextrosol) are useful immediate treatment for mild hypoglycemia. The availability of glucose gel (e.g., Hypostop) or glucagon for IM injection to be used by relatives can be a great source of reassurance in the event of severe hypoglycemia.

26.7 MANAGEMENT OF THE TEENAGER WITH DIABETES

We believe that with the problems outlined above, the diabetic teenager requires a specific service to help manage their diabetes. As for all age groups, a range of specialists should be available in the 'Diabetes Team' and individuals should be free to relate to whichever member of the team is most appropriate at the time, for the specific problem.

Sharing concerns and difficulties about the problems of an illness with fellow sufferers is invaluable and diabetic teenagers are no exception. Facilities should be available so that teenagers, if they wish, can meet up with each other either socially or as part of support groups.

While the above arrangements are to help the teenager overcome any problems he or she has in coping with their diabetes, it is vital that attention is paid also at this age to the concern of developing microvascular disease. Routine examination of the eyes, feet, blood pressure and urine for microalbumin levels we believe should start from the age of 14 and possibly earlier. The teenagers should be informed as to why these tests are being undertaken, the likelihood of problems and action if and when problems arise.

The teenager with long-standing diabetes will have usually come from a closely knit pediatric clinic, with a small number of team members who have known each other for several years. Transfer to the adult diabetes clinic, with its larger number of patients and staff and emphasis on the treatment of complications can be daunting for most young people. Many 'vote with their feet' and disappear from routine clinic visits for many years, with often disastrous consequences for the detection of microvascular disease. If transfer is required, moving to a completely different scene at 14 years seems to be the least best option; surely before puberty (if the facilities are appropiate) or around 18 years at the end of school are better times.

26.7.1 NATIONAL ORGANIZATION: THE YOUTH DIABETES (YD) FOCUS GROUP

The Youth Diabetes Project began in the UK in 1983 as a result of collaboration of pediatricians and adult clinicians involved in diabetes care. Its aims have focused on the perceived special problems of the teenager with diabetes. Supported by the British Diabetic Association, this project has provided an opportunity for young people to meet at annual YD conferences, weekends and holiday courses to share experiences of diabetes. As such, the project has become an important source of opinion on the development of diabetes care services for this age group.

REFERENCES

Brook, C.D.G. (ed.). (1993) *The practice of medicine in adolescence.* Edward Arnold, London.

Cheetham, T.D., Watts, A., Clayton, K. *et al.* (1993) *Growth hormone levels and insulin require-*

ments in IDDM: Short and longer term effects of rh IGF-1 administration. British Society for Paediatric Endocrinology Autumn Meeting, Oxford.

Davies, R.R. and Newton, R.W. (1989) Progress in the Youth Diabetes Project. *Practical Diabetes*, **6**, 6.

Diabetes Control and Complication Trial Research Group. (1993) The effect of intensive treatment of diabetes on the development and progression of long term complications in insulin-dependent diabetes mellitus. *N. Eng. J. Med.*, **329**, 977–86.

Dunger, D.B. and Cheetham, T.D. (1993) The adolescent with diabetes. *Current Paediatr.*, **3**, 125–29.

Dunger, D.B., Cheetham, T.D., Holly, J.M.P. *et al.* (1993) Does recombinant insulin like growth factor (IGF1) have a role in the treatment of insulin-dependent diabetes mellitus during adolescence? *Acta Paed.*, **388** (Suppl.), 49–52.

Frier, B. (1993) Hypoglycemia in the diabetic adult. *Clin. Endocrinol. Metab.*, **7**, 757–77.

Greene, S.A. (1991) 'Diabetes mellitus in childhood and adolescence', in J. Pickup and G. Williams (eds). *Textbook of Diabetes*, pp. 866–83. Blackwell Scientific Publications, Oxford.

Gregory, J.W., Wilson, A.C. and Greene, S.A. (1992) Obesity among adolescents with diabetes. *Diabetic Med.*, **9**, 344–47.

Hindmarsh, P.C., Matthews, D.R., Silvio, L.D.I. *et al.* (1988) Relation between height velocity and fasting insulin concentrations. *Arch. Dis. Child.*, **63**, 665–66.

Kohner, E., Porta, M. and Hier, S. (1991) The pathogenesis of diabetic retinopathy and cataracts, in J. Pickup and G. Williams (eds). *Textbook of Diabetes*, pp. 564–74. Blackwell Scientific Publications, Oxford.

Metcalfe, M.A. and Baum, J.D. (1991) Incidence of insulin dependent diabetes in children aged under 15 years in the British Isles during 1988. *Brit. Med. J.*, **302**, 443–47.

Mortensen, H.B., Hartling, S.G. and Petersen, E.E. (The Danish Study Group of Diabetes in childhood). (1988) A nationwide cross-sectional study of glycosylated haemoglobin in Danish children with IDDM. *Diabetic Med.*, **5**, 871–76.

Newton, R.W. (1987) Testing time. *Nursing Times*, January.

Osei, K., O'Dorisio, T.M., Malarkey, W.B. *et al.* (1989) Metabolic effects of long-acting somatostatin analog (Sandostatin) in type 1 diabetic patients on conventional therapy. *Diabetes*, **38**, 704–709.

Pickup, J. and Williams, G. (1991) 'Brittle diabetes', in J. Pickup and G. Williams (eds). *Textbook of Diabetes*, pp. 884–96. Blackwell Scientific Publications, Oxford.

Smail, P. (1993) Presentation at the Scottish Study Group for the Care of the Young Diabetic, October.

Steel, J., Young, R.J., Lloyd, G.G. *et al.* (1989) Abnormal eating attitudes in young insulin dependent diabetics. *Brit. J. Psychiatry*, **155**, 515–21.

Tattersall, R. and Gill, G. (1991) Unexplained deaths of type 1 diabetic patients. *Diabetic Med.*, **8**, 49–58.

Virtanen, S.M. (1992) Metabolic control and diet in Finnish diabetic adolescents. *Acta Paed.*, **81**, 239–43.

27

Eating disorders

J.M. STEEL

27.1 CLINICAL FEATURES

During the 1870s, Sir William Gull in Britain and Lasegue in France described a condition in which young girls became extremely thin and emaciated in the absence of any physical disease (Gull, 1874). The essential features of this illness, which became known as anorexia nervosa, are a compulsion to be thin and a disturbed body image, resulting in patients insisting they are fat even when very underweight. Weight is lost by avoiding fattening food, often associated with bizarre secretive eating habits and usually accentuated by additional devices such as abuse of laxatives, induced vomiting and strenuous exercise. Patients develop amenorrhea.

Bulimia nervosa was described much more recently by Russell (1979). Patients with this condition are again usually girls or women; they have food binges, sometimes eating several thousand calories at a time, usually in secret and follow this by vomiting or use of laxatives or severe dietary restriction. These patients also have excessive concern with their body weight and shape.

The official diagnostic criteria for these eating disorders have changed over the years and may change again. Many feel that these illnesses represent extremes of a range of behavior and that cut-off points are artifical. For some purposes, however, it is important to have clear criteria and those of the Diagnostic and Statistical Manual of Mental Disorders, revised third edition (DSM IIIR) (American Psychiatric Association, 1987) are shown in Table 27.1.

Anorexia nervosa in its extreme form is immediately obvious because the patient is emaciated, but lesser degrees are not always recognized as the patients tend to wear large baggy clothes and sometimes even fill their pockets with heavy objects. Some present with amenorrhea. Patients with bulimia may be more difficult to diagnose as they may be of normal weight or even overweight. Clinical examination may be normal although some have erosion of their front teeth as a result of repeated vomiting and some have parotid swelling. Some also present with menstrual irregularities. There have been occasional reports of acute gastric dilatation. Patients with either illness can develop major electrolyte disturbances, especially profound hypokalmia due to vomiting and laxative abuse and this can be fatal. Anorexia and bulimia share many features and some patients may have both conditions.

27.2 RISK FACTORS FOR EATING DISORDERS

Over recent years, eating disorders have been increasingly recognized and there is

Childhood and Adolescent Diabetes
Published in 1994 by Chapman & Hall, London
ISBN 0 412 48610 5

Table 27.1a DSM IIIR anorexia nervosa diagnostic criteria.

1. Weight loss and maintenance of body weight 15% below that expected for age and height.
2. Disturbance in the way in which one's body weight, size or shape is experienced.
3. Intense fear of gaining weight or becoming fat, even though underweight.
4. Absence of >3 menses when otherwise expected to occur.

Table 27.1b DSM IIIR bulimia nervosa diagnostic criteria.

1. Recurrent episodes of binge eating.
2. A feeling of lack of control over eating behavior during the eating binge.
3. Regular self-induced vomiting, use of laxatives or diuretics, strict dieting or fasting or vigorous exercise to prevent weight gain.
4. ⩾2 binges/1 week for ⩾3 months.
5. Persistent overconcern with body shape and weight.

also evidence that they are becoming more common (Kendell *et al.*, 1976; Crisp *et al.*, 1976; Cooper & Fairburn, 1983). It is now fashionable to be thin. The vital statistics of 'Miss World' have become smaller and smaller over the last 20 years and there is a lot of pressure particularly from films and magazines on the girls and women of today to be thin. While the majority of cases are female the conditions can occur in men; they too are encouraged by the media to be thin.

Models and ballet dancers are particularly at risk. The illnesses are also more common in people from upper social economic classes, particularly girls living in boarding schools.

27.3 DIABETES AS A RISK FACTOR

27.3.1 CASE REPORTS

The first case report of a patient with co-existing diabetes and anorexia nervosa was by Bruch (1973). She was eating very little and reduced her insulin to lose weight. Fairburn and Steel (1980) reported three cases and suggested that there might be an association between eating disorders and diabetes. This was followed by several other series of cases (Roland & Bhanji, 1982; Powers *et al.*, 1983; Szmukler, 1984) suggesting the possibility that eating disorders occur more frequently in association with IDDM than would be expected by chance.

27.3.2 REVIEW OF RECORDS

Steel *et al.* (1987) found that 7% of 208 female IDDM patients aged 16–25 years had a clinically apparent eating disorder. In that study even the higher prevalence was probably an underestimate, particularly of bulimia, as only known cases were included and patients were not specifically questioned.

In a retrospective review of 242 consecutive cases of eating disorders that had been treated between 1960 and 1984 at the Psychiatric and Child Psychiatric Clinics at Rigshospitalet (Copenhagen), Nielsen *et al.* (1987) found IDDM was present in five cases: four had anorexia nervosa and one bulimia. They claimed that this was six times more than would be expected by chance.

27.3.3 SELF-REPORT QUESTIONNAIRE

Attempts were subsequently made to evaluate more scientifically the frequency of eating disorders in patients with IDDM. Difficulties arise finding valid screening tests, agreeing diagnostic criteria, obtaining large enough samples and in finding appropriate control groups (Rodin & Daneman, 1992). These problems probably explain why some observers suggest that diabetes is a risk factor for eating disorders while others have found no such relationship.

Several groups have used the Eating Attitudes Test (EAT) devised by Garner and Garfinkel (1979). The EAT 40 is an objective, reliable and well-validated self-report measure of eating disorders and has been used as a screening instrument for detecting cases of anorexia nervosa in groups at high risk for this disorder and for identifying abnormal eating patterns, for example, among college students (Garner & Garfinkel, 1980). It consists of 40 questions describing attitudes or behavior. The questions are grouped into three subscales: dietary, bulimia and oral control. Another questionnaire used in several studies is the Eating Disorder Inventory (EDI) also designed by Garner *et al.* (1983). Wing *et al.* (1986) found higher scores in diabetic patients using the unmodified EAT but pointed out that the results were difficult to interpret as the answers to some questions (e.g., Do you avoid foods with sugar in them?) are likely to be affected by diabetes *per se*. Rodin *et al.* (1985), applying the original EAT and EDI to 46 female diabetic patients, found an incidence of 19% for clinically significant disorders of eating and weight. Rosmark *et al.* (1986) removed diabetes-related questions and found that 41 female diabetic patients had higher mean EAT scores than either female nondiabetic controls or male diabetic subjects. Steel *et al.* (1989) compared cohorts of 152 young IDDM women and 131 IDDM men with age and sex-matched controls, using the EAT and EDI. After diabetes-related questions were excluded, female diabetic patients scored significantly higher than their controls whereas there was no difference between male diabetics and their nondiabetic controls.

These studies suggest that clinical and subclinical eating disorders are particularly common in young female diabetic patients. Stancin *et al.* (1989) used another self-report questionnaire, the bulimia screening form, and found that 12% of 59 IDDM women met the DSM IIIR criteria for bulimia and Rodin *et al.* (1991) using an amended version of the Diagnostic Survey for Eating Disorders, found 13% of 103 girls with diabetes had eating disorders based on DSM IIIR criteria.

27.3.4 CLINICAL INTERVIEWS

Clinical interviews are likely to provide greater reliability and validity than self-report questionnaires. Rodin *et al.* (1986) conducted clinical interviews and identified present or past history of eating disorders in 13.8% of 58 young diabetic women. Fairburn *et al.* (1991) interviewed 54 diabetic women aged 17–25 years and a control group, using the Eating Disorder Examination, a semi-structured diagnostic interview with established reliability and validity, for the assessment of the specific psychopathology of eating disorders based on DSM IIIR criteria. The diabetic women scored higher but the differences were not statistically significant. The same group (Peveler *et al.*, 1992) went on to look at a younger age group. They diagnosed a clinical eating disorder in 9% of 33 girls aged 11–18 years compared with 6% of a control group. Streigel-Moore *et al.* (1992) interviewed 46 diabetic girls between the ages of 8–18 years. None of these studies found a difference between diabetic and control group but two of them included very young girls and all dealt with very small numbers. Peveler *et al.* (1992) stated that a sample size 10-fold greater would have been necessary to show a two-fold difference.

From all the reported observations, it seems likely that diabetes is a risk factor for eating disorders. There is no doubt that the coexistence of the two conditions is a common clinical problem and it is also clear that eating disorders not sufficiently severe to fulfil the DSM IIIR criteria can have serious psychological and metabolic implications.

27.4 CLINICAL FEATURES OF EATING DISORDERS AND DIABETES

Patients with diabetes who also have an eating disorder may show the clinical features already discussed. There are, however, several important features which cause additional problems.

27.4.1 OMISSION OF INSULIN IN ORDER TO CONTROL WEIGHT

In addition to the usual ways of losing weight by calorie restriction, exercise, vomiting and abuse of laxatives, patients with IDDM can lose calories through glycosuria by reducing or omitting their insulin. This was described in Bruch (1973) and has been observed in a high proportion of patients in every reported series (Hudson *et al.*, 1983; Szmukler & Russell, 1983). Stancin *et al.* (1989) reported that 23 (39%) of 59 women with IDDM aged 18–30 years used omission or underdosing as a means of weight reduction. This behavior was more common in those with eating disorders but also occurred in those who did not fulfil the criteria for an eating disorder. This method of inducing weight loss is not included in the DSM IIIR criteria although for diabetic women it clearly should be and it has been proposed for inclusion in DSM IV.

27.4.2 METABOLIC CONTROL

The relationship between eating disorders and diabetic control is complex. Many patients described in the literature have been poorly controlled (Hudson *et al.*, 1983; Szmukler, 1983; Hillard & Hillard, 1984) and those with high EAT and EDI scores tend to have high glycosylated hemoglobin (HbA_1) levels (Rosmark *et al.*, 1986; Rodin *et al.*, 1986; 1991). Psychiatrists seeing patients referred to them by physicians because of an eating disorder stress that eating disorders cause poor control (Hillard & Hillard, 1984). There are undoubtedly cases, particularly of bulimia, where this appears to be so. On the other hand, diabetologists seeing patients in the context of lifelong diabetes suggest that eating disorders tend to occur more frequently in patients who are already poorly controlled (Steel *et al.*, 1987) and that the emergence of an eating disorder in such patients appears to be another facet of longstanding behavioral disturbance. Indeed, eating disorders are a feature of 'brittle' diabetes (Pickup & Williams, 1991).

Table 27.2 Clinical variants of eating disorders in patients with diabetes

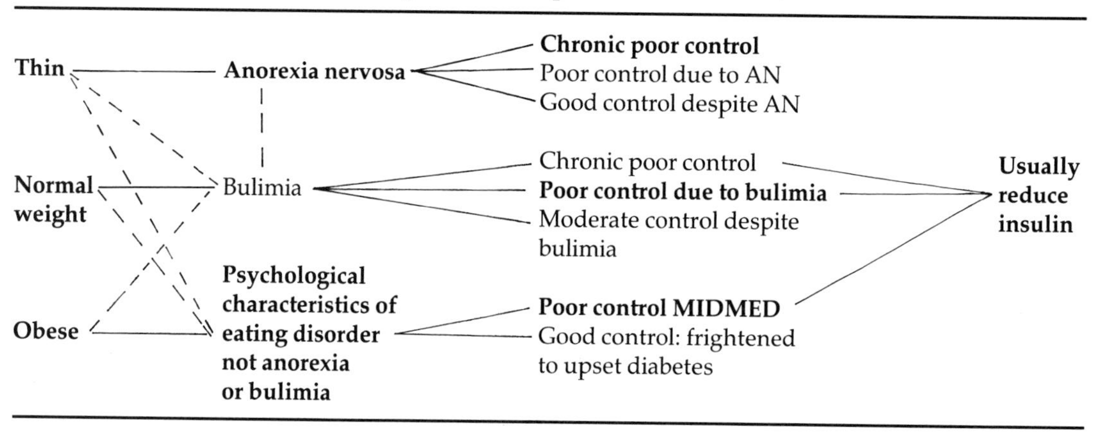

MIDMED: Manipulation of insulin as a manifestation of eating disorder.

There is also a third group of patients who manage to control their diabetes well despite suffering from an eating disorder. Some with anorexia nervosa manage to reduce their carbohydrate intake and insulin dose in parallel without developing either ketoacidosis or hypoglycemia. Some with bulimia increase their insulin in an attempt to compensate for a binge. This group is small; the majority of patients do have a high HbA_1. An eating disorder should always be considered in a patient who has a high HbA_1 for no obvious reason.

Their different clinical pictures are shown diagrammatically in Table 27.2. They are also illustrated by two pairs of female identical twins attending our clinic who are discordant for diabetes. In one pair, the diabetic twin has anorexia nervosa, and is extremely poorly controlled using heavy glycosuria to control her weight, whereas her twin is of normal weight and has a normal attitude towards food. In the other pair, the nondiabetic sibling has anorexia nervosa while the diabetic twin is obsessed by food and weight and has even more grossly abnormal attitudes to eating (measured by EAT) than her nondiabetic sister. However, she has never fulfilled the weight criteria for anorexia nervosa and says she has never dared cut down her food too much as she is concerned about maintaining good diabetic control at all times to prevent long-term complications.

27.4.3 SHORT AND MEDIUM-TERM COMPLICATIONS

Some patients reduce their insulin so much that they suffer from repeated episodes of ketoacidosis (Powers *et al.*, 1983; Hillard *et al.*, 1983). Other patients have been described who suffered from repeated episodes of hypoglycemia. One described by Gomez *et al.* (1980) died as a result of severe hypoglycemia. Growth retardation and pubertal delay may occur in girls who have not yet completed their pubertal growth spurt (Nielsen *et al.*, 1987). Occasionally growth failure and delayed sexual maturation are seen in the presence of a reasonably normal HbA_1. Prolonged amenorrhea is a classical feature of anorexia nervosa but may also occur in normal weight patients with bulimia.

27.4.4 LONG-TERM COMPLICATIONS

Several case reports have suggested a high incidence of early-onset microvascular complications in diabetic patients with eating disorders (Hillard *et al.*, 1983; Szmukler & Russell, 1983).

Steel *et al.* (1987) reported that 11 of 15 patients with eating disorders had a prolonged history of poor metabolic control. In this series there was a high incidence of early onset of diabetic complications. Eleven had retinopathy (six with proliferative changes); six had nephropathy, and six neuropathy. Four patients diagnosed with anorexia nervosa developed acute painful neuropathy with remission of the pain as weight gain was re-established. These symptoms were accompanied by abnormalities in peripheral nerve electrophysiology and autonomic nerve function and these measures improved as weight was regained.

Whether a direct relationship exists between the eating disorder and these complications or whether the latter are related purely to poor metabolic control remains speculative but it is possible that nutritional factors could be involved.

27.5 PSYCHOLOGICAL ASPECTS OF DIABETES RELATED TO EATING DISORDERS

It seems likely that there is more than a chance association between diabetes and eating disorders and there are several factors which may be at least partially responsible.

27.5.1 FOCUS ON DIET

Preoccupation with food is an inevitable problem in diabetic patients. Chronic dietary restraint, particularly the forbidding of sweet foods which they may enjoy and which children tend to be given for being 'good' can be very difficult for a diabetic child. A person with diabetes is often made to feel guilty if he or she cheats and after even a small binge may feel more guilty than someone who does not have diabetes.

27.5.2 FOCUS ON WEIGHT

Weight gain may trigger increased body dissatisfaction and a cycle of dieting and binging. Many diabetic adolescents, especially girls, rightly associate insulin with weight gain. Immediately after the start of treatment there is often a rapid weight gain as a result of rehydration and the anabolic effect of insulin. There may be a marked increase in weight over the first few months of treatment. Much of this may be regain of weight which was lost before the diagnosis of diabetes was made and they may not become overweight according to standard height-weight tables. However, many find this rapid change in their body image frightening (Steel *et al.*, 1990). Diabetic women tend to score highly on the 'drive for thinness' and 'body dissatisfaction' sub-scales of the EDI. Insulin-treated diabetic patients tend to be slightly heavier than their peers, probably partly because insulin delivered systemically, rather than into the portal circulation, overstimulates adipose tissue formation.

27.5.3 HYPOGLYCEMIA

Fear of hypoglycemia makes some people with diabetes overeat and so gain unwanted weight. In addition to this, hypoglycemia can precipitate a binge as it causes intense hunger. Many years ago, insulin was sometimes used as a treatment for anorexia nervosa on the grounds that it stimulated appetite.

27.5.4 SELF-ESTEEM

Diabetes, like other chronic illnesses, presents a severe challenge to an adolescent's self-esteem and to his or her positive body image. Low self-esteem is also correlated with the development of either anorexia nervosa or bulimia. Although IDDM is not often associated with overt psychological disturbances in adolescents and young adults, more subtle disturbances in ego development and self-image complexity have been found in young adults with diabetes compared with non-diabetic individuals (Hauser *et al.*, 1983). Diabetic girls score high in the EDI scores for 'introceptive awareness', feelings of 'ineffectiveness' and 'interpersonal distrust' reflecting problems commonly encountered in young diabetic women (Steel *et al.*, 1989).

27.5.5 CONFLICT BETWEEN DEPENDENCE AND INDEPENDENCE

The conflict between dependence and independence which occurs in adolescence is often more difficult for an adolescent with diabetes and for his or her parents. Difficulties in permitting age-appropriate autonomy in a child are risk factors for eating disorders. Minuchin *et al.* (1978) described several maladaptive characteristics in families of poorly controlled diabetic children: first, enmeshment, a term used to describe over-involvement of family members with each other so that changes in one family member or the relationship between two reverbate throughout the system; second, over-protectiveness, with family members hypersensitive to signs of distress in one another; third, distress in one another; fourth, rigidity and fifth, lack of family conflict resolution. These maladaptive characteristics are also common in families of patients with eating disorders.

27.6 TREATMENT

Milder cases can often be managed by an understanding physician who is able to see the patient frequently. Discussing the problem and explaining that others have similar difficulties is a great help and relief to many women.

27.6.1 DIABETIC MANAGEMENT

It is important to have a flexible approach to diabetic management while encouraging the patients to eat reasonably and regularly. The use of a pen device to give fast-acting insulin according to the amount of food to be eaten at each meal is the most appropriate way of delivering insulin in many cases. It is usually helpful to allow the patients to take some sweet foods in moderate amounts rather than banning them completely.

Patients should be encouraged to record in a diary the usual items such as date, dose of insulin, blood test results, hypoglycemic episodes, weight and HbA_1. In addition, they should record everything they eat and drink including binges and their feelings at the time of a binge or vomiting. Some people keep very full diaries and find it easier to write down their feelings than to talk about them. The book should be fully read and discussed at each interview and strategies to avoid future binges or other difficulties should be agreed either by thinking about the problem in a different way or by doing something which will avoid difficult situations arising again. For example, sometimes simple things like going to night school, to a sporting activity or to a social event in the evenings help patients who tend to sit alone and binge.

27.6.2 FAMILY INVOLVEMENT

In some cases, it is very helpful to involve members of the family in the treatment strategies. This can be particularly helpful in young patients where it may facilitate acceptance of the eating problem, identify the appropriate balance of autonomy permitted and help to moderate judgmental attitudes that some parents have regarding dietary lapses.

27.6.3 GROUP THERAPY

Discussion with other people with similar problems can be helpful to some. If a group is organized, it is essential that it should be led by someone with training and experience in group therapy. Drama and art therapy have occasionally been used.

27.6.4 PSYCHIATRIC TREATMENT

Severe cases are best treated by a psychiatrist. Some patients are extremely reluctant to be seen by a psychiatrist and it is sometimes possible for a physician to treat the patient in liaison with a psychiatrist.

The cognitive behavioral approach for the management of bulimia has been extensively studied by Fairburn (1981 & 1985). Peveler and Fairburn (1989) have reported the successful use of this technique in the treatment of diabetic women with anorexia nervosa and bulimia. This treatment attempts to modify self-defeating attitudes about diabetes management through a process of cognitive restructuring. They have suggested that diabetic women are sometimes more difficult to treat than their nondiabetic counterparts and in some cases they have also used interpersonal psychotherapy (Peveler & Fairburn, 1992).

27.6.5 DEPRESSION

A significant proportion of women with eating disorders also suffer from a depressive illness and this should be treated in its own right. The serotonin uptake inhibitors act as appetite suppressors in addition to their action as antidepressants. Their use may be preferable to the use of tricyclic antidepressants which have an appetite-stimulating effect in patients with bulimia whereas tricyclic antidepressants may be more suitable for those with anorexia.

27.6.6 DRUGS

Some workers have used drugs in patients with bulimia who are not depressed. Serotonin is one of several appetite-inhibitory peptides antagonizing norepinephrine-stimulated feeding at the level of the paraventricular nucleus. Injection of serotonin into the hypothalamus of hungry rats inhibits feeding. Serotonin re-uptake inhibitors such as fluoxetine and dexfenfluramine have been shown to reduce food intake in both experimental animals and in humans. They have have been used with limited success in the treatment of bulimia (Freeman, 1991; Walsh, 1991). So far there have been very few reports of the use of these drugs in diabetic patients with eating disorders (Ramirez *et al.*, 1990).

27.6.7 HOSPITALIZATION

Most patients can be managed on an out-patient basis but occasionally hospitalization is necessary if the patient's life is at risk, either from severe metabolic disturbance or from suicide.

27.7 PREVENTION

Prevalence studies are difficult enough but prevention studies would be even more so. However, with the present stage of knowledge, it seems sensible to discuss feelings about diet and weight with young girls, to make the diet reasonably flexible, include some sweet foods, explain the cause of initial weight gain and be prepared to reduce the diet at an early stage. It is very important to have a high index of suspicion so that any eating disorder can be recognized and treated at an early stage.

REFERENCES

American Psychiatric Association. (1987) *Diagnostic and Statistical Manual of Mental Disorders*, 3rd edn, revised. Washington DC.

Bruch, H. (1973) *Eating disorders: Obesity, Anorexia and the Person Within*, p. 357. Basic Books, New York.

Cooper, P.J. and Fairburn, C.G. (1983) Binge Eating and Self-induced Vomiting in the Community. A Preliminary Study. *Brit. J. Psychiatr.*, **142**, 139–44.

Crisp, A.H., Palmer, R.L. and Kalvey, R.S. (1976) How common is Anorexia Nervosa? A Prevalence Study. *Brit. J. Psychiatr.*, **128**, 549–54.

Fairburn, C.G. (1981) A Cognitive-Behavioural Approach to the Management of Bulimia. *Psychol. Med.*, **11**, 707–711.

Fairburn, C.G. (1985) 'Cognitive-Behavioural Treatment for Bulimia', in D.M. Garner and P.E. Garfinkel (eds). *Handbook of Psychotherapy for Anorexia Nervosa and Bulimia*, pp. 160–92. Guildford Press, New York.

Fairburn, C.G. and Steel, J.M. (1980) Anorexia Nervosa in Diabetes Mellitus. *Brit. Med. J.*, **280**, 1167–68.

Fairburn, C.G., Peveler, R.C., Davies, B. *et al.* (1991) 'Eating Disorders in Young Adults, with Insulin Dependent Diabetes Mellitus: A Controlled Study'. *Brit. Med. J.*, **303**, 17–20.

Freeman, C.P.A. (1991) Practical Guide to the Treatment of Bulimia Nervosa. *J. Psychosom. Res.*, **35**, 33–40.

Garner, D.M. and Garfinkel, P.E. (1979) The Eating Attitude Test: An Index of the Symptoms of Anorexia Nervosa. *Psychol. Med.*, **9**, 273–79.

Garner, D.M. and Garfinkel, P.E. (1980) Sociocultural Factors in the Development of Anorexia Nervosa. *Psychol. Med.*, **10**, 647–56.

Garner, D.M., Olmstead, M.P. and Polevy, J. (1983) Development and Validation of a Multidimensional Eating Disorder Inventory for Anorexia Nervosa & Bulimia. *Int. J. of Eating Disorders*, **2**, 15–34.

Gomez, J., Dally, P. and Isaacs, A.J. (1980) Anorexia Nervosa in Diabetes Mellitus. *Brit.*

Med. J., **281**, 261–62.

Gull. W.W. (1874) Anorexia Nervosa (Apepsia Hysterica, Anorexia Hysterica), *Trans. Clin. Soc. Lond.*, **7**, 22.

Hauser, S.T., Jacobson, A.M., Noam, G. *et al.* (1983) Ego Development and Self-image Complexity in Early Adolescence: Longitudinal Studies of Psychiatric and Diabetic Patients. *Arch. Gen. Psychiatry*, **40**, 325–32.

Hillard, J.R., Lobo, M.C. and Keeling, R.P. (1983) Bulimia and Diabetes. A Potentially Life-Threatening Combination. *Psychosomatics*, **24**, 292–95.

Hillard, J.R. and Hillard, P.J.A. (1984) Bulimia, Anorexia Nervosa and Diabetes Deadly Combinations. *Psychiat. Clin. North Am.*, **7**, 367–79.

Hudson, J.I., Hudson, M.S. and Wentworth, S.M. (1983) Self Induced Glycosuria. A Novel Method of Purging in Bulimia. *J. Am. Med. Ass.*, **249**, 2501.

Kendall, R.E., Hall, D.J., Hailey, A. *et al.* (1976) Epidemiology of Anorexia Nervosa. *Psychol. Med.*, **3**, 200–203.

Minuchin, S., Rosman, B. and Baker, L. (1978) 'Psychosomatic Families', in *Anorexia Nervosa in Context*, p. 30. Harvard University Press, Cambridge, Massachusetts.

Nielsen, S., Borner, H. and Kabel, M. (1987) Anorexia Nervosa/Bulimia in Diabetes Mellitus. A Review and a Presentation of Five Cases. *Acta Psychiatr. Scand.*, **75**, 464–73.

Peveler, R.C. and Fairburn, C.G. (1989) Anorexia Nervosa in Association with Diabetes Mellitus. A Cognitive-behavioural Approach to Treatment. *Behav. Res. Ther.*, **27**, 95–99.

Peveler, R.C., Boller, I., Fairburn, C.G. *et al.* (1992) Eating Disorders in Adolescents with IDDM. *Diabetes Care*, 15, 1356–60.

Peveler, R.C. and Fairburn, C.G. (1992) The Treatment of Bulimia Nervosa in Patients with Diabetes Mellitus. *Int. J. Eating Disorders*, 711169, 45–53.

Pickup, J.C. and Williams, G. (1991) '"Brittle" Diabetes', in J.O. Pickup and G. Williams (eds). *Textbook of Diabetes*, Vol. 2, p. 891. Blackwell Scientific Publications.

Powers, P.S., Malone, J.E. and Duncan, J. (1983) Anorexia Nervosa and Diabetes Mellitus. *J. Clin. Psychiatr.*, **44**, 133–35.

Ramirez, L.C., Rosenstock, J., Stowig, S. *et al.* (1990) Effective Treatment of Bulimia with Fluoxetine. A Serotonin Reuptake Inhibitor, in a Patient with Type 1 Diabetes Mellitus. *Am. J. Med.*, **88**, 540–41.

Rodin, G.M., Daneman, D., Johnson, L.E. *et al.* (1985) Anorexia Nervosa and Bulimia in Female Adolescents with Insulin Dependent Diabetes Mellitus. A Systematic Study. *J. Psychiatr. Res.*, **19**, 381–84.

Rodin, G.M., Johnson, L.E., Garfinkel, P.E. *et al.* (1986) Eating Disorders in Female Adolescents with Insulin Dependent Diabetes Mellitus. *Int. J. Psychiatry Med.*, **16**, 49–57.

Rodin, G.M., Craven, J., Littlefield, C. *et al.* (1991) Eating Disorders and Intentional Insulin Undertreatment in Adolescent Females with Diabetes. *Psychosomatics*, **32**, 171–76.

Rodin, G.M. and Daneman, D. (1992) Eating disorders and IDDM. *Diabetes Care*, **15**, 1402–1412.

Roland, O.M. and Bhanji, S. (1982) Anorexia Nervosa Occurring in Patients with Diabetes Mellitus. *Postgrad. Med. J.*, **58**, 354–56.

Rosmark, B., Berne, C., Holmgren, L. *et al.* (1986) Eating Disorders in Patients with Insulin Dependent Diabetes Mellitus. *J. Clin. Psychiatr.*, **47**, 547–50.

Russell, G.F.M. (1979) Bulimia Nervosa an Ominous Variant of Anorexia Nervosa. *Psychol. Med.*, **6**, 429–48.

Stancin, T., Link, D.L. and Reuter, J.M. (1989) Binge Eating and Purging in Young Women with IDDM. *Diabetes Care*, **12**, 601–603.

Steel, J.M., Young, R.J., Lloyd, G.G. *et al.* (1987) Clinically Apparent Eating Disorders in Young Diabetic Women Associated with Painful Neuropathy and Other Complications. *Brit. Med. J.* **294**, 859–62.

Steel, J.M., Young, R.J., Lloyd, G.G. *et al.* (1989) Abnormal Eating Attitudes in Young Insulin Dependent Diabetics. *Brit. J. Psychiatr.*, 7115569, 515–21.

Steel, J.M., Lloyd, G.G., Young, R.J. *et al.* (1990) Changes in Eating Attitudes During the First year of Treatment of Diabetes. *J. Psychosom. Res.*, **34**, 313–18.

Striegel-Moore, R.H., Nicholson, T.J. and Tamborlane, W.V. (1992) Prevalence of Eating Disorder Symptoms in Pre-Adolescent and Adolescent Girls with IDDM. *Diabetes Care*, **15**, 1361–68.

Szmukler, G.I. (1984) Anorexia and Bulimia in Diabetics. *J. Psychosom. Res.*, **28**, 365–69.
Szmukler, G.I. and Russell, G.F.M. (1983) Diabetes Mellitus, Anorexia Nervosa and Bulimia. *Brit. J. Psychiatry.*, **142**, 305–308.
Walsh, B.T. (1991) Fluoxetine treatment of bulimia nervosa. *J. Psychosom. Res.*, **351**, 33–40.
Wing, R.A., Nowalk, M.P., Marcus, M.D. *et al.* (1986) Subclinical Eating Disorders and Glycaemic Control in Adolescents with Type 1 Diabetes. *Diabetes Care*, **9**, 162–67.

28

Childhood diabetes and other endocrine/autoimmune diseases

A.C. MacCUISH

28.1 INTRODUCTION

The concept of insulin-dependent diabetes mellitus (IDDM) as an autoimmune disease (in the majority of cases) has been accepted since 1974, when antibodies reactive with cytoplasmic components of the pancreatic islet cells were first described (MacCuish, 1974). Over the past 20 years, a mass of further research in immunology, genetics and molecular biology has refined and extended our knowledge of etiopathogenesis to reach the present stage (Eisenbarth, 1986; Bottazzo, 1993), when intervention by immunotherapy or immunomodulation can be seriously considered to prevent or cure the disease.

Thus it has been natural to compare IDDM with the other classical autoimmune diseases which affect the endocrine system. By so doing, it can readily be appreciated that diabetes in juveniles is inextricably linked with other endocrine diseases; that clinical observations of an association between IDDM and other endocrinopathies have been established for well over a century, i.e., long before the concept of autoimmunity was introduced, and that a knowledge of such associations is highly relevant when considering the treatment of IDDM in childhood.

Childhood and Adolescent Diabetes
Published in 1994 by Chapman & Hall, London
ISBN 0 412 48610 5

28.2 THE POLYENDOCRINE SYNDROMES

IDDM has been associated with about 20 different genetic disorders but most are exceedingly rare. However the polyglandular autoimmune (PGA) syndromes are of extreme interest: each syndrome represents a group of endocrine and non-endocrine disorders, frequently coexistent in one individual or characterized by clustering in the same family. There are obvious similarities in the genetics and etiology of each disease and this is potentially important when considering prophylaxis as well as therapy for organ-specific autoimmunity.

The modern classification of polyglandular autoimmunity was devised and refined in 1980 (Neufeld *et al.*, 1980 & 1981), based primarily upon disorders which had been observed to coexist in patients with autoimmune Addison's disease (Spinner *et al.*, 1968; Irvine & Barnes, 1975). Types I and II PGA are the best characterized syndromes and are summarized in Table 28.1. A knowledge of both types is potentially important in the context of pediatric practice: it will be seen at once that IDDM is much more common in Type II PGA, affecting about half of all patients, but the onset of overt diabetes actually

Table 28.1 Types I and II polyglandular autoimmune (PGA) syndromes. Figures in brackets indicate the prevalence of individual disorders in the respective syndrome. (Modified from data of Neufeld *et al.* (1981).)

Type I PGA		Type II PGA	
Addison's disease	(100%)	Addison's disease	(100%)
Hypoparathyroidism	(80%)	Hyperthyroidism	(69%)
Mucocutaneous candidiasis	(73%)	Hypothyroidism	(69%)
Type 1 diabetes (IDDM)	(4%)	Type 1 diabetes (IDDM)	(52%)
Hypogonadism	(17%)	Hypogonadism	(4%)
B12 deficiency anemia	(13%)	B12 deficiency anemia	(0.5%)

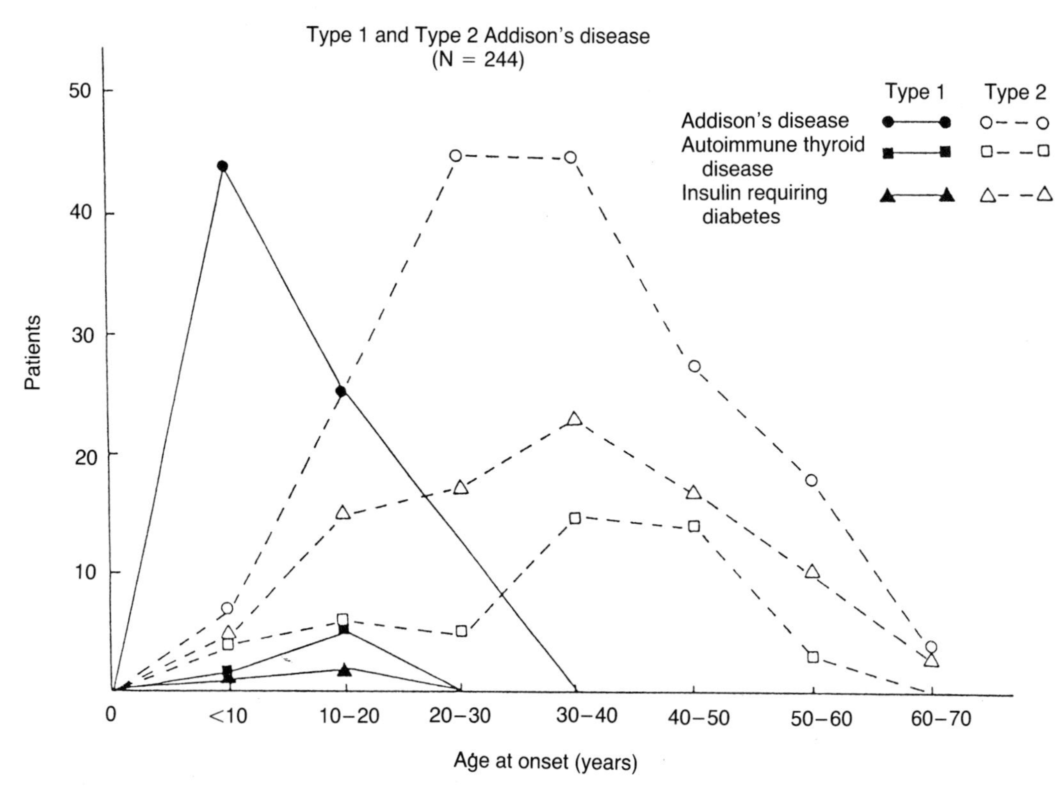

Figure 28.1 Type I and Type II Addison's disease (N = 244).

Respective ages of onset of Addison's disease, IDDM and autoimmune thyroid disease in Type I and Type II PGA syndromes. Addison's disease occurs before aged 10 years in most patients with Type I PGA but is rarely associated with IDDM: adrenal failure occurs later in Type II PGA but more than half the patients also develop IDDM (reproduced by kind permission of the editor of *Medicine* from Neufeld *et al.*, 1981. Two types of autoimmune Addison's disease associated with different polyglandular autoimmune (PGA) syndromes. *Medicine*, **60**(5), 355–62).

occurs before the age of 20 years in only about 20% of cases (Figure 28.1). By contrast, almost all cases of IDDM appear in childhood in the Type I PGA syndrome but only a small minority of children – less than 5% – ever become diabetic.

The major differences in etiology between Types I and II PGA may be summarized as follows. Type I PGA has no association with any HLA (MHC) gene, occurs in both sporadic and familial forms and seems to be inherited as an autosomal recessive trait, since families are described with multiple affected siblings but unaffected parents. The syndrome is probably due to underlying defects in cell-mediated immunity and thymus function (Arulanatham *et al.*, 1979), occurs mainly in early childhood and is manifest most commonly as a triad of mucocutaneous candidiasis and hypoparathyroidism (with clinical onset before age 5 years) and Addison's disease (mean age of onset 11 years). As noted, IDDM is comparatively rare and almost certainly different in pathogenesis from the majority of cases of the disease.

By contrast, Type II PGA is strongly associated with the Class II HLA alleles (DR3, DR4), which typify IDDM, and by linkage disequilibrium with Class I alleles (HLA-B8). The syndrome is characterized by excessive or aberrant Class II antigen expression on target tissues (β cell, thyroid, etc.) and most commonly inherited as an autosomal dominant trait. IDDM occurs in about 50% of patients and appears before age 25 years in up to two-thirds of cases (Papadopoulos & Hallengren, 1990), preceding adrenal failure in the majority of cases. After Addison's disease, autoimmune thyroid disease is the most common endocrinopathy but has no special temporal relationship to the other diseases and may appear at any age.

All these observations carry the strong implication that the presence of a coexisting adrenal or thyroid endocrinopathy in a child with IDDM reflects the presence of a Type II PGA syndrome. However, such is not always the case and it is appropriate now to consider what is known about each individual endocrine disease in the diabetic child and what impact such concurrent pathology may have upon the diabetic state.

28.3 ADDISON'S DISEASE

The first clinical account of coexisting diabetes mellitus and adrenal insufficiency (Ogle, 1886) appeared barely 11 years after Addison's classic description of the disease that bears his name and a wealth of subsequent reports (Beaven *et al.*, 1959; Solomon *et al.*, 1965; Nerup, 1974; MacCuish & Irvine, 1975) confirmed the association well before a comprehensive knowledge of autoimmune processes was acquired or the polyglandular syndromes were defined. Addison's disease is rare in the general population, the prevalence being estimated at 0.0039–0.0060% and although the condition is at least five times more common in the diabetic population (MacCuish & Irvine, 1975), even a large pediatric diabetic clinic will only contain a handful of such cases.

Idiopathic Addison's disease is accepted as an autoimmune disorder and has many features in common with IDDM. About half of all such patients develop adrenal failure as part of the Type II PGA syndrome (Papadopoulos & Hallengren, 1990) and in turn, 50% of patients with Type II PGA will develop diabetes mellitus. In other words, IDDM will eventually coexist with adrenal failure in around 25% of all patients with autoimmune Addison's disease, diabetes will frequently precede the development of Addison's disease and the majority of such cases will present at a young age.

Which diabetic children are particularly at risk of developing adrenal failure? From consideration of all available data, the following risk profile could be drawn. The vulnerable patient will be in the middle teenage years and will probably have developed IDDM when aged under 10 years. He or she will come from a family where there is already an established history of autoimmune endocrinopathy, usually adrenal or thyroid disease. (The biglandular association of Addison's disease with thyroiditis is known as Schmidt's syndrome (Schmidt, 1926) and is a particularly common manifestation (Carpenter *et al.*, 1964) of Type II PGA in young diabetics.) The diagnosis of adrenal insufficiency may be suspected when normal growth velocity tails off in a patient from such a family background – or more commonly, when the patient develops a strikingly increased sensitivity to insulin, with frequent and severe hypoglycemic reactions despite a marked decline in insulin requirements. Of course these phenomena primarily reflect the reduction in gluconeogenesis which is secondary to glucocorticoid deficiency but the onset of hypoglycemia during the years of growth is such an extraordinary phenomenon – except in young diabetic women who develop an eating disorder (see Chapter 27) – that it always merits most careful investigation.

In young diabetics with Addison's disease, the onset of insulin sensitivity invariably precedes the classical markers of adrenal insufficiency such as buccal pigmentation, hypotension or plasma electrolyte derangements. If the diagnosis is missed or delayed until these signs develop, the patient is likely to present with profound and intractable hypoglycemia. Before that stage is reached, the diagnosis should be readily confirmed by immunoassay of plasma ACTH and the usual dynamic adrenal function tests with synacthen. Serological demonstration of anti-adrenal antibodies (present in 60–70% of cases) and cytoplasmic pancreatic islet cell antibodies (ICA) often persisting for years after the original diagnosis of IDDM, clinches and refines the diagnostic process. Treatment with glucocorticoid replacement will effect a prompt return of insulin sensitivity to normal, hypoglycemic attacks will occur with no more than the expected frequency in young diabetics and insulin requirements will return to normal. Thus treatment is always gratifying for a condition in which successful diagnosis must depend upon a high index of suspicion, prompted by the family history. However, the careful clinician will not be content until the possibility of other, occult and coexistent endocrine disease has been excluded. It is particularly important to check for the presence of thyrogastric antibodies, although these are not highly predictive of future disease, and steroid cell antibodies, which certainly indicate a high risk of future premature gonadal failure.

Finally, and as anticipated from the commonest mode of inheritance of Type II PGA syndrome, it should always be remembered that autoimmune endocrinopathies are found in the close relatives of around 50% of all patients with Schmidt's syndrome. Hashimoto thyroiditis or IDDM without Addison's disease are the disorders most commonly present and the family members of any young person with Type II PGA syndrome should be screened accordingly.

28.4 THYROID AUTOIMMUNITY

Autoimmune thyroid disease is the most common form of autoimmune disease occurring in families with IDDM (Betterle *et al.*, 1984; Gorsuch *et al.*, 1980). The association of IDDM with thyroid autoimmune diseases has also been recognized for many years and of course thyroid disorders are much more common than adrenal insufficiency in the general population. It will be apparent from Table 28.1 that two of every three patients with PGA Type II syndrome will develop a thyroid disorder, either thyrotoxicosis (Graves' disease) or lymphocytic thyroiditis (juvenile Hashimoto's disease or juvenile hypothyroidism). About half of all those patients have IDDM and long before the stage

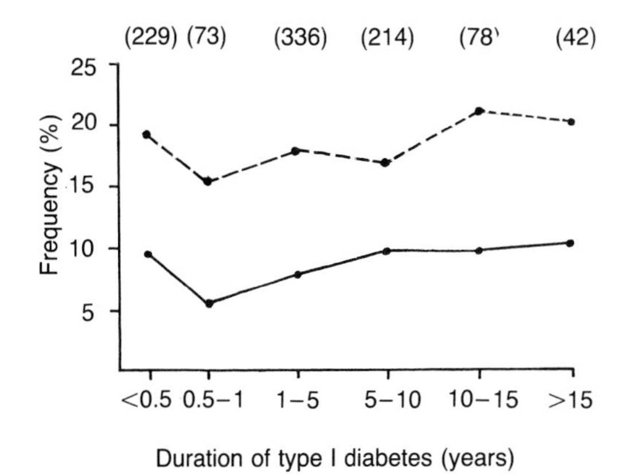

Figure 28.2 Prevalence of thyroid microsomal (------) and gastric parietal cell autoantibodies (——) in 972 patients (mean age 12.8 years) with IDDM, grouped by duration of disease. Figures in parenthesis represent the number of patients in each duration group (reproduced from Riley *et al.*, 1983 by kind permission of the editor of *Diabetologia*).

of clinically overt thyroid disease is reached, evidence of an autoimmune thyroid process can be inferred by the detection of circulating thyroid antibodies in the serum samples. The serological association was first established in 1961, when Pettit *et al.* described thyroid microsomal antibodies in 22% of diabetic children aged under 16 years and numerous subsequent studies have confirmed the observation in literally hundreds of subjects (Pettit *et al.*, 1961; MacCuish & Irvine, 1975; Christy *et al.*, 1977; Riley *et al.*, 1981; Bright *et al.*, 1982).

The results of a typical modern series (Riley *et al.*, 1983) are depicted in Figure 28.2. These authors searched for thyroid microsomal and gastric parietal cell autoantibodies in 972 young patients (mean age 12.8 years) with IDDM (mean age of onset 8.5 years) and detected thyroid antibodies in about 20% of patients. Of great interest was the fact that the frequencies of these antibodies did not change significantly over the ensuing 20 years following the diagnosis of diabetes, suggesting that the onset of autoimmune processes affecting the thyroid, gastric mucosa and pancreatic islets is simultaneous in a large subset – perhaps one quarter – of young persons who develop overt IDDM. Of course this is precisely what would be anticipated in a cluster of diseases with common etiology and immunopathology. Thyroid microsomal antibodies are by far the most common antibody detected, antibodies to thyroglobulin being comparatively rare, and very similar figures for thyroid antibody prevalence (15–25%) are found among first-degree relatives of patients with IDDM (Betterle *et al.*, 1984; Fialkow *et al.*, 1975). Indeed, sensitive enzyme-linked immuno-sorbent assay (ELISA) techniques for antibody measurement may yield even higher prevalence rates (Roman *et al.*, 1986).

The presence of circulating thyroid antibodies does not in any sense presage the imminent onset of clinical thyroid disease in IDDM but is a relatively simple method of screening young diabetics for susceptibility to thyroid disease. Since thyrogastric autoantibodies are found so commonly in juvenile diabetic sera, and tests for their detection are universally available, it seems sensible to undertake routine serological screening of all children when overt IDDM first appears. Such a screening procedure will also detect all patients with Type II PGA syndromes and allow the easiest possible detection of persons who are at risk for eventual development of clinical thyroid or gastric parietal-cell disease.

28.5 CHRONIC THYROIDITIS AND HYPOTHYROIDISM

The clinical features of chronic lymphocytic thyroiditis (juvenile Hashimoto's disease) are now well-known. The disease has an age-related spectrum of clinical characteristics and Hashimoto's original paper describes the variant seen in mainly elderly women, where the gland is invariably hard from extensive fibrosis. In diabetic children with the same disease, the thyroid gland is only moderately enlarged, with varying degrees of firmness in keeping with the degree of underlying lymphocytic infiltration. The vast majority of patients are clinically and biochemically euthyroid when first diagnosed and, as with Addison's disease, diagnosis itself depends upon a high suspicion index. Beware the teenage girl with IDDM and a slight fullness in the neck: irrespective of the gland's consistency on palpation, she may well have early chronic thyroiditis rather than a goiter of puberty. Such patients invariably possess moderate to high titers of thyroid microsomal antibodies but unlike the disease in middle-aged women, thyroglobulin antibodies are hardly ever detected.

The diagnosis is usually clinched by an assay of thyroid autoantibodies; radioisotope scan of the thyroid is rarely helpful, and needle biopsy of the gland is hardly ever necessary. Treatment with L-thyroxine should await biochemical evidence of evolving hypothyroidism, i.e., low free T4 and elevated TSH levels, except in patients (usually girls in the middle-teens) whose goiters are particularly large and therefore cosmetically unacceptable. In short, the diagnosis of Hashimoto thyroiditis *per se* is not an indication for immediate recourse to what may be lifelong hormone replacement therapy, this cautious approach being justified by the facts that only about half of all such children actually become hypothyroid through time, whilst shrinkage of the goiter itself is often capricious and disappointingly slow. In a group of predominantly euthyroid individuals with chronic thyroiditis, it is to be anticipated that the condition will exert virtually no effect on carbohydrate metabolism. Insulin dose will decline if the disease is missed and hypothyroidism develops, but, in my own experience, any required reduction in insulin is modest and cannot be compared with the dramatic insulin sensitivity observed in untreated Addison's disease.

28.6 THYROTOXICOSIS

Thyroid autoimmunity manifesting as Graves' disease is very much less common than either hypothyroidism or thyroiditis in IDDM juveniles (Riley *et al.*, 1981; Kontiainen *et al.*, 1990). The reason for this is unclear and considering the strong underlying autoimmune associations, the observation is surprising. The onset of thyrotoxicosis should have major adverse effects on carbohydrate tolerance, being associated with increased absorption of glucose from the gut, enhanced hepatic glucose production and increased sympathetic activity (Holdsworth & Besser, 1968; Karlander *et al.*, 1989).

In clinical practice, the consequences are not nearly so dramatic as might be expected on theoretical grounds. The child or teenager with diabetes may lose a little weight or growth velocity may falter; ambient glycemic levels and glycated hemoglobin values will rise modestly; there may be a mysterious, apparently inexplicable increase in insulin requirements and episodes of unexpected metabolic decompensation may become more frequent. The clinician with experience of childhood diabetes will immediately appreciate the non-specific nature of all these phenomena, which could quite easily be accepted as the standard pattern of poorly-controlled IDDM in teenagers who are disenchanted with or temporarily estranged from their disorder. Add to that the fact that thyroid ophthalmopathy (lid retraction, lid lag or any degree of exophthalmos) is uncommon in children with Graves' disease (Hayles *et al.*, 1959) and the diagnostic difficulties will be readily apparent. As with the other autoimmune endocrinopathies of childhood diabetes, successful diagnosis depends upon the clinical suspicion index and equally importantly, a knowledge of the individual diabetic patient which is sufficiently detailed to draw a distinction between the consequences of adolescent rejection of diabetes and the presence of an underlying metabolic disorder.

Once thyrotoxicosis comes to mind, the condition is readily proved or disproved by simple radioimmunoassay of serum TSH and free T4 levels, dynamic tests of thyroid function or autonomy being hardly ever necessary. Serological screening for thyrogastric antibodies should be performed as routine and treatment with Carbimazole – for a minimum of 18 months to 2 years – is usually satisfactory. The regaining of clinical and biochemical euthyroidism will be marked by a return to normal insulin sensitivity and a resumption of interrupted growth velocity.

In summary, thyroid autoimmunity is a remarkably frequent concomitant of IDDM in childhood (Dahlquist *et al.*, 1989). Just under half of the cases will be familial and associated with Type II PGA syndrome (very rarely Type I PGA), the remainder being sporadic. Serological abnormality, i.e., the presence of circulating antithyroid antibodies, especially microsomal, is the commonest and frequently the sole manifestation of thyroid autoimmunity. Thyroid antibodies are found in approximately 20% of diabetic children; in antibody-positive subjects, about 8% will have chronic thyroiditis with clinical and biochemical euthyroidism, approximately 7% will be hypothyroid and about 1% will suffer from Graves' disease. Thus the figures for clinical disease are small but by no means insignificant. Any group of patients where 20% carry a marker for potential chronic endocrine disease should be taken seriously as potential subjects for screening; diabetes in childhood is still sufficiently uncommon for us to encourage the adoption of serological testing as a routine and valuable practice in all patients.

28.7 GASTRIC AUTOIMMUNITY

Evidence of gastric autoimmunity is encountered with remarkable frequency in young persons with IDDM. As anticipated in diseases which share a common etiopathogenesis, there are strong parallels with the thyroid autoimmunity and evidence of both pathologies may exist in the same patient. The commonest manifestation of gastric autoimmunity is the presence of parietal cell antibodies (PCA) in sera from juvenile IDDM and a figure of 10% prevalence in childhood (Riley *et al.*, 1983) is typical (Figure 28.2). Others have recorded very similar figures: thus 15% of a group of 77 Italian diabetic children were PCA-positive (DeLuca *et al.*, 1985). As discussed earlier, the serological evidence suggests that the onset of thyrogastric and pancreatic autoimmunity is effectively simultaneous in such patients and once autoantibody production has been stimulatd, the antibodies will persist until or unless the target organ is destroyed. Antibody prevalence does not change significantly with the passage of time; in diabetic childhood, it equals the prevalence found in a nondiabetic population above 60 years of age and a consistent frequency of around 16–17% is recorded in middle-aged diabetics (MacCuish & Irvine, 1975).

However, gastric autoimmunity differs markedly from thyroid autoimmunity in diabetic children by the rarity with which serological abnormalities progress to any clinical disease. It is accepted that the appearance of parietal cell antibodies will be paralleled by varying degrees of lymphocytic infiltration of the gastric mucosa; but the classical pathological sequence which should then follow – mucosal atrophy, loss of gastric parietal cells, achlorhydria, elevation of plasma gastrin levels, iron deficiency anemia and ultimately B12 deficiency – either never occurs or is not completed until middle life. It has been estimated that no more than 3% per annum of PCA-positive patients will progress to pernicious anemia (Maclaren & Riley, 1982) and although it is prudent to check serum B12 levels from time to time, the assay need not be performed more than once every five years until the age of 40 has been passed. However, assay of serum ferritin concentration should be performed on a much more regular basis since achlorhydria is not uncommon in PCA-positive diabetic children and of course causes problems with absorption of oral iron.

Table 28.1 serves as a caveat that true B12 deficiency anemia is much more frequent (around 13% of cases) in teenagers with PGA Type I syndrome but of course IDDM itself is comparatively rare in this condition.

28.8 OTHER AUTOIMMUNE ASSOCIATIONS WITH IDDM

Antibodies to the adrenal medulla have been described in 7–16% of children with IDDM (Schopfer *et al.*, 1984; Scherbaum *et al.*, 1988), the higher prevalence figure being detected in recently-diagnosed cases, and a chronic lymphocytic infiltrate of the adrenal medulla ('adrenal medullitis'), with or without fibrosis, has been identified by a monoclonal antibody technique in pathological archive material from 20% of patients with IDDM (Brown *et al.*, 1990). These findings are an interesting parallel with the end-organ pathological changes seen in Hashimoto thyroiditis, Addison's disease and IDDM itself but there is no serious suggestion that they are of clinical significance.

Steroid cell autoantibodies are found uncommonly in patients with polyglandular autoimmune syndromes of which Addison's disease is one component. They cross-react widely with components of reproductive tissue and are implicated in the pathogenesis of, or are markers for, premature ovarian failure and hypergonadotrophic hypogonadism due to chronic lymphocytic gonaditis. It should be said that these phenomena are extremely rare in PGA Type II syndrome and almost unknown in childhood. They are comparatively common in the Type I PGA syndrome (Table 28.1) but very rarely associated with IDDM.

Autoantibodies which react with most cell types in the anterior pituitary gland were described (by an indirect immunofluorescence technique) about a decade ago in sera from 17% of young patients with recent-onset IDDM and an even higher proportion of their first-degree relatives (Mirakian *et al.*, 1982). Such a finding may occasionally be of clinical significance, i.e., it may precede the development of an autoimmune lymphocytic hypophysitis and there are sporadic reports of such cases, or of apparently spontaneous hypopituitarism (the 'empty sella') in the diabetic literature. However an autoimmune hypopituitarism is not a feature of childhood diabetes, even in patients with a strong autoimmune familial background and serological testing of children for this particular autoantibody group is unrewarding and unnecessary.

The rare hereditary neuromuscular disorder known as Wolfram's or DIDMOAD syndrome (diabetes insipidus, diabetes mellitus, optic atrophy, deafness) is sometimes erroneously assumed to be an autoimmune disorder since IDDM usually presents in childhood and is followed later by the insidious development of diabetes insipidus after the first two decades of life (Page *et al.*, 1976). In fact, the condition is inherited as an autosomal recessive trait that has no connection with autoimmunity, being marked neither by any particular HLA type or even serological evidence of autoimmunity (Scherbaum *et al.*, 1986) (see also Chapter 29).

Two chromosomal disorders merit inclusion when considering the association of IDDM with other autoimmune disorders. Down syndrome, due to trisomy or translocation of chromosome 21, carries a prevalence of diabetes which is estimated at 21 per thousand for children aged up to 14 years (Jeremiah *et al.*, 1973), i.e., grossly in excess of expected diabetic prevalence in an age-matched normal population and overwhelmingly IDDM in metabolic type (Milunsky & Neurath, 1968). In diabetic children with Down syndrome, an association with autoimmune thyroid disease has been reported with increasing frequency (Daniels & Simon, 1968; Shaheed & Rosenbloom, 1973; Ong & Schneider, 1976) and it now seems sensible to advise routine screening of such patients for evidence of thyroid autoimmunity. Turner syndrome (gonadal dysgenesis 45, XO karyotype or mosaic) is associated with carbohydrate intolerance in about 15% of prepubertal subjects (Polychronakos *et al.*, 1980; Wilson *et al.*, 1987) and nearly two-thirds of young adults with the syndrome are frankly diabetic (Nielson *et al.*, 1969) although only a minority are insulin-dependent. Thyroid autoimmunity is also remarkably common in gonadal dysgenesis (Williams *et al.*, 1964) and again it is appropriate to recommend routine screening for autoimmune disorders in patients with this syndrome.

28.9 CONCLUSIONS

IDDM in childhood and adolescence is frequently associated with autoimmune disorders of other endocrine glands. Multi-organ endocrinopathy reflects the common immunopathogenesis of autoimmune disease and may present either sporadically or as manifestation of an inherited polyglandular syndrome.

Comparatively few pediatric diabetic clinics currently undertake routine screening of all their patients for other autoimmune endocrine disorders. Those which do so will find serological evidence (especially thyrogastric antibodies) in around one-fifth of all subjects and will identify a smaller, but highly significant number of children with clinical disease. The impact of coexistent endocrinopathy upon the diabetic state is always harmful and ranges from the risk of gross hypoglycemia in Addison's disease to ketoacidosis with thyrotoxicosis and growth retardation with hypothyroidism.

Clinical signs of the autoimmune endocrinopathies may be subtle, especially in teenagers, and are easily mistaken for the metabolic problems of adolescent diabetes. To avoid such errors, always potentially harmful, it is difficult to escape the conclusion that formal serological screening for thyrogastric and adrenal autoimmunity should be undertaken as routine in all young patients with IDDM. Few exercises in clinical medicine offer such potential reward for the cost of a simple venepuncture.

REFERENCES

Arulanatham, K., Dwyer, J.M. and Genel, M. (1979) Evidence for defective immunoregulation in the syndrome of familial candidias endocrinopathy. *N. Eng. J. Med.*, **300**, 164–68.

Bearen, D.W., Nelson, D.H., Renold, A.E. *et al.* (1959) Diabetes mellitus and Addison's disease. A report on eight patients and a review of 55 cases in the literature. *N. Eng. J. Med.*, **261**, 443–54.

Betterle, C., Zanette, F., Pedini, B. *et al.* (1984) Clinical and subclinical organ-specific autoimmune manifestations in type 1 (insulin dependent) diabetic patients and their first-degree relatives. *Diabetologia*, **26**, 431–36.

Bottazzo, G.F. (1993) On the honey disease: a dialogue with Socrates. *Diabetes*, **42**, 778–800.

Bright, G.M., Blizzard, R.M., Kaiser D.L. *et al.* (1982) Organ-specific autoantibodies in children with common endocrine diseases. *J. Pediatr.*, **100**, 8–14.

Brown, F.M., Smith, A.M., Longway, S. *et al.* (1990) Adrenal medullitis in type 1 diabetes. *J. Clin. Endocrin. and Metab.*, **71**, 1491–95.

Carpenter, C.C.J., Solomon, N., Silverberg, S. *et al.* (1964) Schmidt's syndrome (thyroid and adrenal insufficiency): A review of the literature and a report of fifteen new cases including ten instances of coexistent diabetes mellitus. *Medicine*, **43**, 153–80.

Christy, M., Deckert, T. and Nerup, J. (1977) Immunity and autoimmunity in diabetes mellitus. *Clin. in Endocrin. and Metab.*, **6**, 305–32.

Dahlquist, G., Blom, L., Turemo, T. *et al.* (1989) The Swedish childhood diabetes study. Results from a nine year case register and a one year case-referent study indicating that type 1 (insulin-dependent) diabetes mellitus is associated with both type 2 (NIDDM) and autoimmune disorders. *Diabetologia*, **32**, 2–6.

Daniels, D.M. and Simon, J.L. (1968) Down's syndrome, hypothyroidism and diabetes. *J. Pediatr.*, **72**, 697–99.

DeLuca, F., Venelli, M., Magazzu, G. *et al.* (1985) Thyrogastric autoimmunity in a pediatric group of Type 1 diabetics. *Minerva Pediatrica*, **37**, 391–95.

Eisenbarth, G.S. (1986) Type 1 diabetes mellitus; a chronic autoimmune disease. *N. Eng. J. Med.*, **314**, 1360–68.

Fialkow, P.J., Zavala, C. and Nielsen, R. (1975) Thyroid autoimmunity: increased frequency in relatives of insulin-dependent diabetes patients. *Ann. Int. Med.*, **83**, 170–76.

Gorsuch, A.N., Dean, B.M., Bottazzo, G.F. *et al.* (1980) Evidence that type 1 diabetes and thyrogastric autoimmunity have different genetic determinants. *Brit. Med. J.*, **i**, 145–47.

Hayles, A.B., Kennedy, R.L.J., Beahrs, O.H. *et al.* (1959) Exophthalmic goitre in children. *J. Clin. Endocrin. and Metab.*, **19**, 138–42.

Holdsworth, C.D. and Besser, G.M. (1968) Influence of gastric emptying rate and of insulin response on oral glucose tolerance in thyroid disease. *Lancet*, **ii**, 700–703.

Irvine, W.M. and Barnes, E.W. (1975) 'Addison's disease and associated conditions: with particular reference to premature ovarian failure, diabetes mellitus and hypoparathyroidism', in P.G.H. Gell, R.R.A. Coombs and P.J. Lachmann (eds). *Clinical Aspects of Immunology*, pp. 1301–54, Blackwell, Oxford.

Jeremiah, D.E., Leyshon, G.E., Rose, T. *et al.* (1973) Down's syndrome and diabetes. *Psychological Med.*, **3**, 455–57.

Karlander, S.G., Kahn, A., Wajngot, A. *et al.* (1989) Glucose turnover in hyperthyroid patients with normal glucose tolerance. *J. Clin. Endocrin. and Metab.*, **68**, 780–86.

Kontiainen, S., Schlenzka, A., Koskimies, S. *et al.* (1990) Autoantibodies and autoimmune disease in young diabetics. *Diabetes Res.*, **13**, 151–56.

MacCuish, A.C. (1974) Editorial: Autoimmune diabetes mellitus. *Lancet*, **ii**, 1547–51.

MacCuish, A.C. and Irvine, W.J. (1975) Autoimmunological aspects of diabetes mellitus. *Clin. in Endocrin. and Metab.*, **4**, 435–71.

Maclaren, N.K. and Riley, W.J. (1982) Autoimmune endocrine diseases and the pediatrician. *Pediatr. Ann.*, **11**, 333–46.

Milunsky, A. and Neurath, P.W. (1968) Diabetes in Down's syndrome. *Arch. of Environmental Health*, **17**, 372–76.

Mirakian, R., Cudworth, A.G., Bottazzo, G.F. *et al.* (1982) Autoimmunity to anterior pituitary cells and the pathogenesis of insulin-dependent diabetes mellitus. *Lancet*, **i**, 755–59.

Nerup, J. (1974) Addison's disease – clinical studies. A report of 108 cases. *Acta Endocrinologica*, **76**, 127.

Neufeld, M., Maclaren, N.K. and Blizzard, R.M. (1980) Autoimmune polyglandular syndrome. *Pediatr. Ann.*, **9**, 145–62.

Neufeld, M., Maclaren, N.K. and Blizzard, R.M. (1981) Two types of autoimmune Addison's disease associated with different polyglandular autoimmune (PGA) syndromes. *Medicine*, **60**, 355–62.

Nielson, J., Johansen, K. and Yde, H. (1969) Frequncy of diabetes mellitus in patients with Turner's syndrome and pure gonadal dysgenesis. *Acta Endocrinologica*, **62**, 251–69.

Ogle, J.W. (1886) On disease of the brain as a result of diabetes mellitus. *St. George's Hospital Report*, **1**, 157.

Ong, E.A. and Schneider, G. (1976) Down's syndrome, hypothyroidism and diabetes mellitus. *Am. J. Dis. in Child.*, **130**, 335–36.

Page, M.M.J., Asmal, A.C. and Edwards, C.R.W. (1976) Recessive inheritance of diabetes: the syndrome of diabetes insipidus, diabetes mellitus, optic atrophy and deafness. *Quart. J. Med.*, **45**, 505–20.

Papadopoulos, K.I. and Hallengren, B. (1990) Polyglandular autoimmune syndrome Type II in patients with idiopathic Addison's disease. *Acta Endocrinologica*, **122**, 472–78.

Pettit, M.D., Landing, B.H. and Guest, G.M. (1961) Antithyroid antibody in juvenile diabetics. *J. Clin. Endocrin. and Metab.*, **21**, 209–10.

Polychronakos, C., Letarte, J., Collu, R. *et al.* (1980) Carbohydrate intolerance in children and adolescents with Turner's syndrome. *J. Pediatr.*, **96**, 1009–1014.

Riley, W.J., Maclaren, N.K., Lezotte, D.C. *et al.* (1981) Autoimmune thyroid disease in insulin dependent diabetes. The case for routine screening. *J. Pediatr.*, **99**, 350–45.

Riley, W.J., Winer, A. and Goldstein, D. (1983) Coincident presence of thyrogastric autoimmunity at onset of type 1 (insulin-dependent) diabetes. *Diabetologia*, **24**, 418–21.

Roman, S.H., Davies, T.F., Witt, M.E. *et al.* (1986) Thyroid autoantibodies in HLA-genotyped type 1 diabetic families: Sex-limited DR5 association with thyroid microsomal antibody. *Clin. Endocrin.*, **25**, 23–33.

Scherbaum, W.A., Wass, J.A.H., Besser, G.M. *et al.* (1986) Autoimmune cranial diabetes insipidus: its association with other endocrine diseases and histiocytosis X. *Clin. Endocrin.*, **25**, 411–20.

Scherbaum, W.A., Mogel, M., Boehm, B.O. *et al.* (1988) Autoantibodies to adrenal medulla and thyroid calcintonin cells in type 1 diabetes mellitus: a prospective study. *J. Autoimmunity*, **1**, 219–30.

Schmidt, M.B. (1926) Eine biglandulare Erkrankung (Nebennieren und Schilddruse) bei Morbus Addisonii. *Verhandlungen der Deutsche Gesellschaft fur Pathologie*, **21**, 212–21.

Schopfer, K., Matter, L. and Tenschert, R. (1984) Anti-glucagon and anti-adrenal medullary cell antibodies in islet cell antibody positive diabetic children. *N. Eng. J. Med.*, **310**, 1536–37.

Shaheed, W.A. and Rosenbloom, L. (1973) Down's syndrome with diabetes mellitus and hypothyroidism. *Arch. Dis. Child.*, **48**, 917–18.

Solomon, C., Carpenter, C.C.J., Bennett, I.L. *et al.* (1965) Schmidt's syndrome (thyroid and adrenal insufficiency) and coexistent diabetes mellitus. *Diabetes*, **14**, 300–304.

Spinner, M.W., Blizzard, R.M. and Childs, B. (1968) Clinical and genetic heterogeneity in idiopathic Addison's disease and hypoparathyroidism. *J. Clin. Endocrin. and Metab.*, **28**, 795–804.

Williams, E.D., Engel, E. and Forbes, A.P. (1964) Thyroiditis and gonadonal dysgenesis. *N. Eng. J. Med.*, **270**, 805–810.

Wilson, D.M., Frane, J.W., Sherman, B. *et al.* (1987) Carbohydrate and lipid metabolism in Turner's syndrome: effect of therapy with growth hormone, oxandrolone, and a combination of both. *J. Pediatr.*, **112**, 210–17.

29

Unusual diabetes and diabetes in the context of other disorders

J.A. BATCH and G.A. WERTHER

Most patients with diabetes diagnosed in childhood or adolescence will prove to have type I or insulin-dependent diabetes mellitus (IDDM). However diabetes mellitus which does not require insulin also occurs in childhood and adolescence. In addition a number of genetic diseases, chromosomal disorders and specific syndromes occuring in childhood have an associated predisposition for diabetes. Most of these conditions are rare, but some such as cystic fibrosis are relatively common. In addition, improvements in survival of many of these conditions means that diabetes associated with genetic disorders and syndromes will be seen more often in the future. The purpose of this chapter is to discuss these less common forms of childhood and adolescent diabetes. Maturity Onset Diabetes of Youth (MODY) will be discussed first, followed by various forms of secondary diabetes in childhood. In many of these secondary forms of diabetes, the mechanisms resulting in diabetes are not yet defined; however, many of them are associated with insulin resistance. The disorders discussed in this chapter are listed below and are noted in bold type in Table 29.1.

Childhood and Adolescent Diabetes
Published in 1994 by Chapman & Hall, London
ISBN 0 412 48610 5

29.1 MATURITY ONSET DIABETES OF THE YOUNG (MODY)

29.1.1 HISTORY, DEFINITION AND PREVALENCE

Maturity onset diabetes of youth (MODY) is a heterogenous disorder with the following characteristics: (a) onset before 25 years of age (b) non insulin-dependent diabetes (c) absence of ketosis and (d) autosomal dominant inheritance. In 1960, Fajans & Conn (1960) reported mild non insulin dependent diabetes in children, adolescents and young adults and used the term 'maturity onset type diabetes of young people' emphasizing the strong familial association of diabetes in such patients (Fajans & Conn, 1965). Autosomal dominant inheritance for MODY was postulated in 1974, on the basis of studies in three large families (Tattersall, 1974). In 1975, the abbreviation MODY for the term 'maturity onset type diabetes of young people' was coined, and this type of diabetes was differentiated from juvenile onset Type I diabetes on the basis of a large prospective study (Tattersall, 1975). Non insulin-dependent diabetes mellitus in the young (NIDDY) is another term which has also been used to describe this type of diabetes (Keen, 1982). As well, this type of diabetes has been termed 'Mason-type diabetes' as this was the surname of one of three large kindreds reported in the United Kingdom (Pyke, 1979).

MODY has been reported worldwide, including the United Kingdom, Europe, the United States, South America, South Africa, southern India, Japan and Australia (Fajans, 1989). The true prevalence of MODY is unknown, and appears to vary among ethnic groups. A German study estimated the prevalence of MODY as 0.15% (Panzram & Adolph, 1981), while an estimate of 4.8% has been made in southern India (Mohan *et al.*, 1985). A high prevalence (10%) in Indians in South Africa has also been reported although the diagnostic criteria used varied from the previous studies (Asmal *et al.*, 1981). MODY has been reported to account for up to 10% of all cases of diabetes in black American youths residing in southeastern United States (Winter *et al.*, 1987). The prevalence of MODY is probably greatly underestimated as it varies considerably among ethnic groups, and is dependent on the care taken in obtaining family histories and on routine testing of asymptomatic family members.

29.1.2 CLINICAL PRESENTATION

MODY has a heterogenous clinical presentation. MODY should be suspected if Type II diabetes occurs in three generations. It is usually diagnosed before 25 years of age, and is often diagnosed in adolescence. In adolescence it is frequently asymptomatic, and is often diagnosed on the basis of plasma glucose testing of young members of a family where this disorder is suspected. However, unless there is a high index of suspicion, MODY may not be diagnosed until middle age or later, when most type II diabetes is diagnosed. There is a wide spectrum of plasma glucose abnormalities in MODY, ranging from impaired glucose tolerance to fasting hyperglycemia. By repeated testing, it has been demonstrated that there is a variable rate of progression of these abnormalities, even within the same kindred (Fajans *et al.*, 1978). Several large kindreds with MODY have been studied and have served to illustrate the varying expression and natural history of the condition. Patients with MODY are generally non-obese, particularly in the younger age group, although obesity has been documented in some kindreds (Tattersall, 1982).

29.1.3 GENETICS/LINKAGE STUDIES AND MOLECULAR PATHOLOGY OF MODY

Fajans (1981) has reported on the prevalence of diabetes among seven kindreds of three to five generations with MODY. The inheritance patterns were consistent with autosomal dominant inheritance in these and other studies (Fajans, 1987). Sporadic occurrence of type II diabetes with the characteristics of MODY has also been reported. Another type of type II diabetes distinct from MODY has also been described (O'Rahilly & Turner, 1988). No association has been found between specific HLA antigens and MODY in Caucasians. Several studies have been performed looking for linkage between the insulin gene and the inheritance of MODY. The most recent of these using multipoint linkage provided strong evidence against a role for mutations in the insulin gene in the causation of MODY in the three families studied (O'Rahilly *et al.*, 1992). Recent studies have demonstrated linkage of MODY to chromosome 20 in one kindred (Bowden *et al.*, 1992) but not in two others (Bowden *et al.*, 1992). The most recent linkage studies have demonstrated close linkage of the glucokinase locus on chromosome 7p to MODY in 16 French families (Froguel *et al.*, 1992). The same group were the first to demonstrate a nonsense mutation in the glucokinase gene in one of the 16 families previously studied (Vionnet *et al.*, 1992), and have recently reported 16 mutations in 18 of the 32 families with MODY studied (Froguel *et al.*, 1993). As glucokinase has a signal recognition function in coupling glucose concentration and insulin release (Lenzen & Panten,1988), an abnormality in the glucokinase gene would be expected to lead to a disruption in glucose homeostasis. The glucokinase mutation in MODY is the first mutation found in a gene involved in glucose metabolism, and has provided great interest in the research into the molecular basis of type II diabetes.

29.1.4 STUDIES OF INSULIN SECRETION AND INSULIN SENSITIVITY

In an attempt to elucidate the cause of this form of diabetes, studies have been performed looking at the type of insulin secreted in MODY. Three variant or mutant insulins have been found in families with type II diabetes including MODY (Given *et al.*, 1980; Shoelson *et al.*, 1983; Nanjo *et al.*, 1986). Many studies have been performed in MODY subjects with similar degrees of fasting hyperglycemia comparing their insulin response to administered glucose loads (Fajans, 1989). These responses have ranged from very high to very low. Fajans (1986) has compared the insulin secretion of members of three MODY families (including members with mild fasting hyperglycemia or impaired glucose tolerance) with insulin responses to glucose in 150 healthy control subjects. In the different kindreds, responses varied from delayed and subnormal response; response above normal; to delayed, but ultimately higher insulin response with respect to controls. Thus in some MODY patients, delayed and subnormal insulin response appears to be the major pathogenetic mechanism for abnormal blood glucose levels. In time, the glucose-stimulated insulin response may become so low that it resembles those of early type I diabetes (Fajans, 1987). In childhood, normal children have a lower insulin response to administered glucose than adolescents, suggesting that they have a greater insulin sensitivity. It is interesting to speculate that the emergence of MODY in adolescence may be due at least in part to an inability of individuals with MODY and blunted insulin responses to raise their insulin response to administered glucose as normal adolescents would. As well as heterogeneity in insulin response to glucose administration, there is also heterogeneity in insulin resistance in MODY. Fajans (1986) has found no *in vitro* or *in vivo* evidence of insulin resistance in many MODY patients and familes studied. However, insulin resistance has been demonstrated in one of a pair of twins with MODY who had overt diabetes (Beck-Nielsen *et al.*, 1988). Non-obese Indian MODY subjects were also found to have insulin resistance (Sharp *et al.*, 1987).

Growth hormone, glucagon and cortisol levels have generally been found to be normal in MODY patients, as have levels of cholesterol and triglycerides. A low renal threshhold for glucose was reported in some family studies in MODY, but is not always found in MODY. In summary, individuals with MODY may demonstrate a wide spectrum of both insulin secretion and insulin sensitivity, but have otherwise normal biochemical and hormonal parameters.

29.1.5 TREATMENT

The aims of treatment in MODY are the same as treatment of any other form of diabetes, i.e., attainment and maintenance of euglycemia and prevention of long-term complications of diabetes. Hyperglycemia in MODY, because of the young age of presentation, is of longer duration than in other patients with type II diabetes. Although once thought to be a mild condition without long-term complications, it is becoming increasingly apparent that MODY can be associated with all the micro and macrovascular complications seen in type II diabetes.

The principles of treatment in MODY are the same as for type II diabetes. Dietary therapy including weight reduction in obese MODY individuals has been shown to reverse fasting hyperglycemia, improve or normalize glucose tolerance, reverse hyperinsulinemia or improve hypoinsulinemia and decrease insulin resistance. In non-obese MODY subjects, a carbohydrate-controlled diet alone may be sufficient to normalize postprandial blood sugars and glycosylated hemoglobin. Sulfonylurea treatment may be useful in the treatment of MODY subjects even in adolescence and in those individuals who have been shown to have a low insulin response to glucose, supporting the concept that sulfonylureas have extrapancreatic effects. The usefulness of this type of therapy has been demonstrated in some patients for over 30 years (Fajans, 1987). It has also been shown in some subjects with MODY that after a prolonged successful treatment period with sulfonylureas that it has been necessary to commence insulin therapy. This has been in the context of decreasing insulin secretory responses to glucose (Fajans, 1987).

29.1.6 COMPLICATIONS

MODY was originally thought to be a mild form of diabetes, easy to control and relatively free of long-term complications (Tattersall, 1974 & 1975). Subsequently two MODY patients were reported who developed severe complications, including marked retinopathy and nephropathy (Tattersall, 1979). The presence or absence of vascular complications in MODY appears to vary from one kindred to the next and may in part be related to the degree and duration of hyperglycemia. Reports of MODY kindreds followed for many years and showing little in the way of complications have mainly been in the context of mild hyperglycemia (O'Rahilly & Turner, 1988; Barbosa *et al.*, 1978). Estimates of the frequency of complications vary widely from one ethnic group with MODY to another. In South Africa, 19% of Indian MODY patients were reported to have vascular complications including microangiopathy, proliferative and background retinopathy and nephropathy (Jialal *et al.*, 1982). Estimates of frequency of complications in other ethnic groups vary widely (Fajans, 1989). Fajans (1989) concludes that MODY is not an innocuous form of hyperglycemia, and that complications are present in MODY patients in approximately the same proportion as they are in type II diabetic patients in general. Diabetic neuropathy has also been reported in MODY. Durruty found neuropathy in 24% of his MODY patients (Durruty *et al.*, 1985). A greater frequency of neuropathy has been reported in Indian MODY patients (Mohan *et al.*, 1985). As with vascular complications of diabetes, the frequency of diabetic neuropathy appears to vary greatly between one kindred and the next. The true prevalence of this condition is confused by differences in diagnostic criteria and lack of precise information about duration of hyperglycemia.

29.2 SECONDARY DIABETES

Diabetes mellitus (Both type I and type II) has been reported in a large number of genetic conditions and syndromes diagnosed in childhood. These conditions are summarized in Table 29.1 (for further information on individual conditions see Jones, 1988; Bankier & Rogers, 1992). Many of these conditions affect multiple systems and there is considerable overlap in the arbitrary grouping of Table 29.1. In the majority of these conditions the mechanism of diabetes is either unknown or poorly understood. Where the mechanism

Table 29.1 Conditions associated with diabetes mellitus.

Pancreatic disease

Cystic fibrosis
Thalassemia
Cystinosis
Post-surgery for hyperinsulinism
Hemochromatosis
α1-antitrypsin deficiency
Trauma
Infections
Toxins
Neoplasms
Congenital absence of pancreas/islets of Langerhans
Hereditary relapsing pancreatitis

Drugs

Glucocorticoids
L-Asparaginase

Chromosomal Disorders

Down syndrome
Turner syndrome
Klinefelter syndrome
Chromosome 6, partial duplication 6q
Chromosome 18, partial deletion 18p

Endocrine Disorders

Polyglandular autoimmune syndromes
DIDMOAD (Diabetes Insipidus, Diabetes Mellitus, Optic Atrophy, Deafness)
Cushing disease
Growth hormone deficiency
Panhypopituitarism
Laron dwarfism
Pheochromocytoma
Glucagon secreting tumors
Gigantism (growth hormone excess)

Obesity

Prader Willi syndrome
Laurence Moon Biedl syndrome
Alstrom syndrome
Pseudohypoparathyroidism
Cohen syndrome
Carpenter syndrome

Table 29.1 Continued

Celiac Disease

Neurological/Neuromuscular syndromes

DIDMOAD (Diabetes Insipidus, Diabetes Mellitus, Optic Atrophy, Deafness)
Alstrom syndrome
Muscular dystrophy
Late onset proximal myopathy
Huntington's disease
Machedo syndrome
Herrman syndrome
Friedreich's ataxia
Pseudo Refsum
Edwards syndrome
Flynn-Aird syndrome
Kearn Sayre syndrome

Insulin Resistance

Type A
Type B
Lipoatrophy/Lipodystrophy
Leprechaunism/Congenital/Acquired

Inborn Errors of Metabolism

Acute intermittent porphyria
Alaninuria
Cystinosis
Mannosidosis
Glycogen storage disease (Type I)
Hyperlipidemias (Types II, IV and V)
Methylmalonic acidaemia

Cutaneous Syndromes

Buschke-Ollendorf syndrome
Ectodermal dysplasia and arthrogryposis
Gastrocutaneous syndrome
Rud syndrome
Scalp, ear and nipple syndrome

Progeria Syndromes

Cockaynes syndrome
Werner syndrome
Progeria
Mulvihill-Smith syndrome
Metageria

(continued)

Table 29.1 Continued

Miscellaneous
Bloom syndrome
Chadaverian-Kaplan syndrome
Borjeson-Forssman-Lehman syndrome
Fetal rubella syndrome
Intrauterine dwarfism and ataxia
Mental retardation and hypergonadotrophic hypogonadism (Fryns-Vogel-Berghe type)
Pseudomongolism
Renal dysplasia, asplenia, pancreatic and portal fibrosis
Retinitis pigmentosa, deafness, mental retardation and hypogonadism
Retino-hepato-endocrine syndrome
Short stature, cranial hyperostosis and hepatomegaly
X-linked skeletal dysplasia
Anemia, thrombocytopenia and deafness
Multiple epiphyseal dysplasia

Further details on these conditions are contained in Jones (1988), and Bankier and Rogers (1992). Conditions in this table in bold type are discussed in the text. The order of conditions in this table does not necessarily indicate frequency of occurrence.

is known it will be briefly discussed, and readers are directed to the appropriate reference for further details. Many of these conditions occur rarely, and only those conditions seen more commonly are discussed in subsequent sections.

29.3 DIABETES DUE TO PANCREATIC DAMAGE

Secondary diabetes due to pancreatic disease has long been recognized and is an important cause of diabetes worldwide. Whereas alcohol is a major cause of pancreatitis and pancreatic damage in adult life, the major causes of pancreatic damage with secondary diabetes in childhood include inherited disorders such as cystic fibrosis, thalassemia and cystinosis.

29.3.1 CYSTIC FIBROSIS

Cystic fibrosis (CF) is the most common lethal genetic defect in Caucasians, occurring in approximately 1 in 2500 live births. It has an autosomal recessive mode of inheritance and is due to a defect of the cystic fibrosis transmembrane conductance regulator gene (CFTR) on chromosome 7 (Rommens *et al.*, 1989). The condition is associated with an elevation of sodium and chloride in sweat, although the exact biochemical basis of the disorder is not completely understood. Chronic respiratory infection is the major cause of morbidity in childhood, and is associated with fat malabsorption due to exocrine pancreatic insufficiency in 90% of cases.

Diabetes mellitus (DM) in CF (DM/CF) is predominantly a disease of adolescents and young adults, although onset as young as 2 and 4 years of age has been reported (Rodman *et al.*, 1986; Shwachman *et al.*, 1955). The mean age of onset in several studies is 18–20 years of age and although there is a tendency for females to be affected more often than males, there is no difference in age of onset between the sexes (Rodman *et al.*, 1986; Reisman *et al.*, 1990). The prevalence of DM/CF has changed with time and improvement in survival. Twenty years ago, a 1.3% incidence was reported (Shwachman & Holsclaw, 1969), whereas the same clinic reported a 12% incidence of diabetes in CF in 1991 (Krueger *et al.*, 1991). The prevalence of DM/CF is estimated as 40–200-fold higher than that of the general pediatric and young adult population (Krueger *et al.*, 1991). Molecular analysis of mutations of the CFTR gene responsible for CF, have led to correlations of genotype and phenotype. DM/CF is almost exclusively a disease limited to alleles associated with pancreatic insufficiency (reviewed in Krueger *et al.*, 1991).

DM/CF is invariably associated with gross histological changes in the pancreas and occurs against a background of impaired pancreatic exocrine function (Dodge & Morrison, 1992). The pancreatic ductules are blocked by inspissated secretions with subsequent cyst formation and fibrosis and fatty replacement of the acinar tissue. The insulin-producing islets of Langerhans are spared from damage until late in the disease, but ultimately the configuration is altered so that they exist in clusters separated by broad bands of fibrous tissue. Within remaining islets, both α (glucagon producing) and β (insulin producing) cells are affected with loss of β cells occuring first and to a greater degree than α cells. Nesidioblastosis (clustering of β cells within the islets) has been noted in a number of studies, but is probably not a major determinant of the presence or absence of diabetes. It has also been suggested that the relative sparing of β cells in DM/CF compared to type I IDDM, in conjunction with a normal proportion of glucagon secreting cells may explain the lack of ketosis in DM/CF (Abdul-Karim *et al.*, 1986).

As suggested by genotype/phenotype correlations, CF subjects with exocrine pancreatic disease are more likely to develop DM. CF patients with exocrine pancreatic disease are not only more likely to develop DM, but have impairment of α, β and pancreatic polypeptide cell function in comparison with CF patients without pancreatic insufficiency. In contrast to type I diabetes, no HLA type has been indentified which is associated with susceptibility to DM in the CF patient. Islet cell antibodies (ICA) have been found in up to 15% of one CF series, rising to 25% with glucose intolerance. There was also an age-related increase with ICA being found in 37% of patients aged 11–23 years (Stutchfield *et al.*, 1988). It has been suggested however that the presence of ICA seems to be a manifestation of an immune response which occurs selectively in type I diabetes in the general population but randomly, and without genetic predisposition in CF (Wilken, 1987). Familial susceptibility does not appear to play a role in the coincident occurrence of CF and DM.

Pathophysiologically, reduced glucagon secretion in response to arginine infusion is seen even in non-diabetic CF subjects, which is in keeping with the pathological observation that β cells tend to disappear from islets before α cells. The reduction in α cell activity in DM/CF may explain the heightened insulin sensitivity and tendency to hypoglycemia observed in DM/CF. Glucose homeostasis is also influenced by gastrointestinal function. The uptake of glucose by enterocytes in the jejunum has also been shown to be enhanced in CF (Frase, 1985) both *in vivo* and *in vitro*, while the ability of the liver to deal with a glucose load may be impaired in patients with CF and liver disease. Peripheral utilization of glucose is modulated by the number and affinity of peripheral insulin receptors. An increase in receptor numbers on the monocytes of patients with CF has been observed and attributed to insulinopenia or perhaps to the relatively poor nutritional status of some CF patients. Improvements in CF nutrition (such as enteral feeding) have therefore sometimes been associated with exacerbation or onset of hyperglycemia. The affinity of insulin receptors in CF has been reported as low (Lippe *et al.*, 1980).

DM/CF has some features in common with both type I and type II diabetes. DM/CF requires exogenous insulin therapy but is usually non-ketotic. It has been suggested that the characteristics of DM/CF are sufficiently different from either type I or II diabetes to conclude that DM/CF is a distinct entity and does not share a common etiology with either type I or type II diabetes. The major features of DM/CF and type I and II diabetes are summarized in Table 29.2. Typical type I diabetes has also been reported to occur in association with CF (Rodman

Table 29.2 Features of different types of diabetes.

Feature	Type I	Type II	DM/CF
Age of onset	child	adult	late teens
Speed of onset	acute	gradual	variable
Nutritional status	thin	obese	thin
HLA markers	DR3/DR4	nil	nil
Islet cell Abs*	high	low	low
Anti-insulin Abs*	high	absent	absent
C-peptide	absent	normal	low
Insulin production	low/absent	normal	low
Glucagon production	high	high	normal/low
Insulin dose/day	high	–	low/moderate
Insulin sensitivity	sensitive	resistant	increased
Complications	ketoacidosis	hyperosmolar non-ketotic	no ketosis
Microangiopathy	frequent	frequent	infrequent

* Abs = antibodies.

et al., 1986). The presenting symptoms of DM/CF are polyuria, polydipsia and loss of weight and appetite. DM/CF may be precipitated by the institution of intensive nutritional therapy such as enteral feeding or steroid therapy during a respiratory exacerbation. As well, puberty is normally associated with a physiologic increase in insulin resistance which may be sufficient to compromise pre-existing impairment of glucose tolerance in a subject with CF.

Once DM occurs in CF subjects, its role in future deterioration of respiratory function and the subject's overall status is not clear. Some studies have suggested a deterioration in lung function studies in DM/CF compared with normal controls. DM is more likely to be found in those CF subjects who have severe pancreatic impairment and have more severe respiratory disease. Reisman *et al.* (1990) examined the effect of DM in CF and found no difference in the respiratory studies of their matched DM/CF and CF groups 5 years prior to diagnosis, at the time of diagnosis and 5 years post-diagnosis. They also suggested that DM alone had no adverse effect on long-term survival in their DM/CF group although only 25% of the DM/CF group reached 30 years of age compared with 60% of nondiabetic CF patients.

The effect of DM in CF longevity requires further study. Microangiopathy is a serious complication of DM/CF and generally occurs 5 years or longer after onset of DM which has been poorly controlled. In a study of 21 DM/CF subjects, 3 had evidence of multisystem disease (i.e., retinopathy, nephropathy and neuropathy). In addition, use of such agents as aminoglycoside antibiotics for respiratory exacerbations may adversely influence the course of nephropathy. As the lifespan of CF subjects increases, more long-term vascular complications of DM may well be seen. Because of the increased likelihood of subjects with CF developing DM, some authors recommend routine screening of older patients with CF, consisting of regular measurement of glycosylated hemoglobin, postprandial glucose estimation and urinalysis. As well, the diagnosis of DM should be suspected in the event of weight loss or unexplained respiratory deterioration in a CF subject in their teens or beyond.

The treatment of DM/CF consists of insulin therapy and dietary modification. A diet high in complex carbohydrates and fats for high-calorie intake is usually recommended, and is contrary to the usual recommendation of a low-fat diet in IDDM. Good control should be emphasized in order to avoid both acute complications such as hypoglycemia (DM/CF subjects appear to be particularly prone to hypoglycemia) and the long-term problem of microangiopathy, as well as preventing any adverse effect of DM on overall CF survival. Unfortunately, compliance with DM management in adolescence is often poor. As well, the added burden of a second chronic disease in CF subjects may be quite demoralizing and thus undermine compliance and therapeutic strategies in both conditions.

29.3.2 THALASSEMIA

Type I diabetes is frequently a complication of thalassemia major and has a significant impact on the quality of life of these individuals and may influence their long-term survival. An Italian study performed in 1983 (De Sanctis *et al.*, 1988) found that 29 (6%) of their 448 subjects were affected by diabetes. The insulin-dependent diabetes which complicates thalassemia is thought to be due to iron overload which directly damages pancreatic β cells. Familial factors may also contribute, as one study found, that 75% of thalassemics with a family history of diabetes had impaired glucose tolerance or type I diabetes (Saudek *et al.*, 1977). Islet cell antibodies (ICA) are reportedly negative (Vullo *et al.*, 1980). Chronic hepatitis is also thought to play a role in the development of diabetes in thalassemia (De Sanctis *et al.*, 1986). Hyperinsulinism has been observed by several groups studying thalassemic patients with iron overload and/or cirrhosis. In adolescence, insulin sensitivity is reduced and hyperinsulinism is often seen. In iron-overloaded thalassemic subjects, impaired β cells may be unable to increase their output to cope with the insulin resistance of puberty and hyperglycemia may result. Viral infection may also be a compounding feature, as it has been observed in one study that the onset of type I diabetes was preceded by acute hepatitis in 28% of subjects (De Sanctis *et al.*, 1988). As the lifespan of patients with thalassemia improves, it is likely that microangiopathic complications may occur. To date, few such complications have been reported, although elevated albumin excretion (an early marker for nephropathy) has been reported in 17 of 33 thalassemic patients with type I diabetes (Vullo *et al.*, 1990).

29.3.3 CYSTINOSIS

Nephropathic cystinosis is an autosomal recessive disorder of lysosomal cystine transport resulting in excessive intracellular accumulation of free cystine in many organs. Cystine accumulation in the kidney leads to progressive renal damage and renal failure. Functional impairment of endocrine glands due to accumulation of cystine is uncommon. Thyroid dysfunction is sometimes seen, and insulin-dependent diabetes mellitus has been reported usually as a late manifestation of cystinosis (Broyer *et al.*, 1980). Both endocrine and exocrine pancreatic insufficiency have been reported in cystinosis, before and after renal transplant (Fivush *et al.*, 1987 & 1988).

29.3.4 SURGICAL TREATMENT OF HYPERINSULINEMIC HYPOGLYCEMIA

Hyperinsulinism accounts for approximately 1% of all cases of hypoglycemia (Thomas *et al.*, 1977), but is the most common cause of persistent neonatal hypoglycemia and may result in brain damage if untreated. The pancreas shows diffuse β cell and islet cell hyperplasia that is associated with fetal type budding from the pancreatic ducts, so called 'nesidioblastosis' (Laidlaw, 1938; Yakovac *et al.*, 1971). Medical treatment consists of intravenous glucose administration, and the use of drugs such as diazoxide which inhibits the secretion of insulin (Aynsley-Green *et al.*, 1981). Somatostatin given subcutaneously has also been used in the short-term management of hyperinsulinemic infants. Patients not responding to optimal medical treatment may require early pancreatic surgery. A 95% sub-total pancreatectomy is the operation of choice (Spitz *et al.*, 1986), as the recurrence rate is unacceptably high when the resection is conservative (75–85% pancreatectomy). In a recent study of 21 patients who had a 95% pancreatectomy for persistent hyperinsulinism, Spitz *et al.* (1992) reported varying degrees of hyperglycemia in all patients post-operatively. In most infants it occurred within 24 hours of surgery and lasted only a few days. Prolonged hyperglycemia lasting up to 18 months was encountered in four patients and required treatment with insulin. One patient became permanently diabetic.

Many children with secondary diabetes after pancreatectomy run a reasonably stable course, and experience suggests that the diabetes is less 'brittle' than that of many children with IDDM of a similar age (Green *et al.*, 1984).

29.4 DRUGS

29.4.1 GLUCOCORTICOID

The glucocorticoid group of drugs is the most common cause of drug-induced glucose intolerance and hyperglycemia in both adult and pediatric populations. Glucocorticoids decrease hepatic and peripheral tissue sensitivity to insulin by acting at a post-receptor level, leading to an inappropriately raised hepatic glucose output and impaired uptake of glucose by muscle and fat (Rizza *et al.*, 1982). Excessive administration of inhaled or topically applied steroids has also been shown to cause glycosuria and hyperglycemia (Gomez & Frost, 1976). Studies in normal adults have shown that significant increases in fasting glucose and serum insulin concentrations occur when doses of prednisolone of 30 mg/day or more are given (Pagano *et al.*, 1983). Steroids are given to children for a variety of disorders such as severe asthma, nephrotic syndrome and chronic arthritis. They may also be given in combination with other agents, particularly in chemotherapeutic regimes for childhood malignancy (see below). Steroid treatment will also worsen hyperglycemia in children with IDDM, MODY or type II diabetes. Treatment of steroid-induced or exacerbated diabetes consists of regular monitoring of blood glucose and introduction or alteration of insulin therapy until the steroids can be ceased, and glucose homeostasis returns to normal.

29.4.2 L-ASPARAGINASE

L-asparaginase is a key agent used in both induction and maintenance phases of chemotherapy for acute lymphoblastic leukemia in childhood. L-asparaginase is an enzyme obtained from cultures of *E. coli*, and causes depletion of the amino acid L-asparagine by hydrolyzing it to L-aspartic acid and ammonia. Cells unable to produce their own supply of L-asparagine (e.g., some malignant lymphoblasts) suffer impairment of protein synthesis and are unable to survive. Organs such as the liver and pancreas may be adversely affected (Altman & Schwartz, 1983). Pancreatitis occurs in up to 16% of children receiving L-asparaginase (Weetman & Baehner, 1974). The pancreatitis may be dose-related and of delayed onset. Hyperglycemia develops in up to 10% of children with leukemia treated with asparaginase and prednisolone, particularly in the induction phase of therapy. This complication is more common in obese children greater than 10 years of age and in patients with Down syndrome (Pui *et al.*, 1981). Insulin therapy may be necessary in the short term, but most patients return to euglycemia when L-asparaginase is withdrawn.

29.5 DIABETES IN ASSOCIATION WITH CHROMOSOMAL ABNORMALITIES

Impaired glucose tolerance or overt diabetes may be associated with a number of chromosomal abnormalities in childhood (Table 29.1). The chromosomal abnormalities most commonly associated with diabetes mellitus are Turner syndrome, Klinefelter syndrome and Down syndrome.

29.5.1 DOWN SYNDROME

Down syndrome is due to trisomy of chromosome 21, or translocations of parts of this chromosome. The characteristic physical findings include short stature, a large fissured protruding tongue; hypotonia, brachycephaly, short neck; typical facies; clinodactyly and endocardial cushion defects. A degree of mental retardation is usually found in this condition.

The prevalence of diabetes among prepubertal children with Down syndrome has been estimated to be 21 per 1000, which is considerably higher than the expected figure of 0.6–1.3 per 1000 in an age-matched normal population (Jeremiah *et al.*, 1973). In a series of 88 patients with Down syndrome and diabetes, over one-half were under the age of 20 years; 74% were insulin treated, 12% were taking oral hypoglycemic agents, and 14% could be controlled on diet alone (Milunsky & Neurath, 1968). A triad of Down syndrome, primary hypothyroidism and IDDM (including a marked tendency to ketoacidosis) has been reported (Ong & Schneider, 1976).

29.5.2 TURNER SYNDROME

Turner syndrome includes a wide range of phenotypic abnormalities resulting from complete or partial monosomy of the short arm of the X-chromosome. The most common abnormality is complete absence of the second X chromosome (45XO karyotype), which occurs in approximately 1 in 10 000 live-born female infants. Cytogenetic studies suggest that up to 95% of 45XO fetuses spontaneously abort. Isochromosomes, translocations and deletions of portions of the X chromosome also form part of the Turner syndrome spectrum. The principal features include short stature, gonadal dysgenesis with streak gonads and primary amenorrhea. Other clinical features may include a short webbed neck, low posterior hairline, pigmented naevi, cubitus valgus, absence of secondary sexual characteristics, cardiovascular abnormalities (coarctation, bicuspid aortic valve and hypertension), urinary tract abnormalities and peripheral lymphedema in the first year of life. If a mosaic pattern exists that includes the presence of the Y chromosome, the gonads should be removed because of the risk of gonadal malignancy in later life. Turner mosaic subjects do not usually have all the clinical features commonly seen in classical 45XO Turner syndrome.

Up to 15% of prepubertal subjects with Turner syndrome have impaired glucose tolerance (Wilson *et al.*, 1987) and 60% of young adults have frankly diabetic oral glucose tolerance tests (Nielson *et al.*, 1969). As well, 50% of patients with Turner syndrome may have positive thyroid antibodies (Polychronakos *et al.*, 1980). In a study of islet cell cytoplasmic antibodies in diabetes and disorders of glucose tolerance, Marner *et al.* (1991) found that islet cell antibodies were absent in 21 patients with Turner syndrome. Despite the relatively high incidence of impaired glucose tolerance and diabetic oral glucose tolerance tests, symptomatic diabetes occurs infrequently and is usually non insulin-dependent (Chan, 1991).

29.5.3 KLINEFELTER SYNDROME

Klinefelter syndrome occurs in phenotypic males the majority of whom have a 47XXY karyotype. Up to 10% are mosaics with a 46XY/47XXY pattern. Clinical features include increased height with eunuchoid proportions; gynecomastia, small testes and azoopsermia due to hyalinization of seminiferous tubules. Subjects with Klinefelter syndrome demonstrate an increased incidence of diabetic oral glucose tolerance tests (26%), but symptomatic diabetes is less common (7%) and is usually non insulin-dependent (Nielson *et al.*, 1969). Abnormally rapid and prolonged insulin responses to oral glucose among patients with Klinefelter syndrome have been observed, suggesting some degree of insulin resistance, and abnormal insulin receptor binding has also been demonstrated (Breyer *et al.*, 1981).

29.6 DIABETES ASSOCIATED WITH OTHER ENDOCRINE DISORDERS

Diabetes can be associated with a range of endocrine disorders as shown in Table 29.1. Most of these conditions occur uncommonly in childhood.

29.6.1 POLYGLANDULAR AUTOIMMUNE SYNDROMES

Diabetes in association with polyglandular autoimmune (PGA) syndromes usually falls into one of two main groups. Type I diabetes and autoimmune thyroid disease are occasionally seen in the type I PGA syndrome, in which adrenal failure, hypoparathyroidism and mucocutaneous candidiasis are prominent. The type II PGA syndrome frequently includes type I diabetes in association with adrenal and thyroid failure. Autoimmune disorders associated with both syndromes include alopecia, vitiligo, juvenile-onset pernicious anemia, chronic active hepatitis and gonadal failure. Both autosomal recessive and sporadic occurence of both syndromes have been reported (see Chapter 28).

29.7 DIDMOAD (*D*IABETES *I*NSIPIDUS, *D*IABETES *M*ELLITUS, *O*PTIC *A*TROPHY AND *D*EAFNESS)

DIDMOAD is a rare autosomal recessive condition usually diagnosed on a background of Type I diabetes which has presented in childhood (Page *et al.*, 1976). Diabetes insipidus usually develops later with an insidious onset. Optic atrophy and nerve deafness are usually also present.

29.8 GENETIC DISORDERS ASSOCIATED WITH OBESITY AND/OR TYPE II DIABETES IN CHILDHOOD

Genetic syndromes may be associated with type II diabetes presenting in childhood. Type II diabetes is most often diagnosed in obese adults after the third decade with gradual onset of symptoms. A family history of this condition is very common and there is no association with any other organ specific autoimmune disease. Individuals with type II diabetes have normal or elevated insulin concentrations and are not prone to ketoacidosis. Treatment usually consists of weight loss, dietary modification and possibly oral hypoglycemic agents. The genetic syndromes which may be associated with type II diabetes in childhood and their salient clinical features are summarized in Table 29.3.

29.8.1 PRADER-LABHART-WILLI SYNDROME

Prader Willi Syndrome (PWS) is associated with obesity, hypogonadotrophic hypogonadism, hypotonia and mental retardation. A

Table 29.3 Genetic syndromes and onset of type II diabetes in childhood.

Syndrome	Clinical features
Prader Willi	Obesity, short stature, mental retardation, micropenis
Laurence-Moon-Bardet-Biedl	Retinitis pigmentosa, obesity, polydactyly, hypogonadism
Alstrom	Retinitis pigmentosa, deafness, obesity
Pseudo-Refsum	Retinitis pigmentosa, ataxia, muscle wasting
Werner	Premature senility, cataracts
Progressive cone dystrophy	Color blindness, liver disease, deafness, mental retardation

deletion or translocation of chromosome 15 has been found at the molecular level in 75% of patients with the syndrome. Interestingly, this aberrant chromosome is always paternally derived, suggesting that the two parental chromosomes are differently imprinted (Hall, 1990). The prevalence of diabetes in PWS has been estimated as 10%, however more recently a lower frequency has been estimated (Bray *et al.*, 1983). The diabetes is type II in nature, with mild insulin resistance and little tendency to ketoacidosis (Bray *et al.*, 1983). Diabetic retinopathy has been reported (Savir *et al.*, 1974). Dietary modification and weight loss are the cornerstones of treatment in this condition.

29.8.2 LAURENCE-MOON-BARDET-BIEDL SYNDROME

The basic genetic defect of this autosomal recessive condition is not known. The diagnosis of this condition is based on a pattern of typical clinical features including obesity, mental retardation, polydactyly, hypogonadism, retinitis pigmentosa and glomerular sclerosis. Diabetes is uncommon and has been reported to occur in 6% of subjects in one study (Goldstein & Fialkow, 1973).

29.8.3 ALSTROM SYNDROME

Alstrom syndrome is an autosomal recessive condition first described in 1959 (Alstrom *et al.*, 1959). The principal features of this condition are blindness in childhood due to retinitis pigmentosa, severe nerve deafness, obesity, diabetes mellitus and diabetes insipidus. Diabetes insipidus, diabetes mellitus and hypogonadism may partly be explained by tissue resistance to vasopressin, insulin and gonadotrophins. Ninety per cent of affected subjects develop impaired glucose tolerance or diabetes mellitus in the second decade of life. The diabetes resembles type II diabetes and is often associated with hyperinsulism and acanthosis nigricans. Treatment with oral hypoglycemic agents may be required.

29.9 DIABETES ASSOCIATED WITH CELIAC DISEASE

The incidence of diabetes may be higher than expected in patients with celiac disease, with both conditions sharing common HLA antigens HLA-B8 and DR3. Symptomatic celiac disease accompanies type I diabetes more often than can be accounted for by chance alone, with an early study of serum screening in type I diabetic children giving a prevalence of 2.3% for celiac disease (Maki *et al.*, 1984). A more recent study in children with type I diabetes gave a higher figure of 3.5% (Savilahti *et al.*, 1986). In an adult series, the incidence was 4.3% with most requiring insulin treatment and three subjects being managed on diet or oral hypoglycemic agents alone (Walsh *et al.*, 1978). Pediatric patients with both celiac disease and diabetes usually have type I diabetes and require insulin therapy. Reported complications of diabetes in association with celiac disease have included ketoacidosis, microangiopathy and macrovascular disease (Walsh *et al.*, 1978).

29.10 NEUROLOGICAL/ NEUROMUSCULAR CONDITIONS

29.10.1 DYSTROPHICA MYOTONICA

Dystrophica myotonica is an autosomal dominant condition caused by an expansion of a trinucleotide repeat (CTG) at the 3′ end of its gene located on the proximal long arm of chromosome 19 (reviewed in Shelbourne & Johnson, 1992). Physical stigmata of this condition include frontal baldness, cataracts, cardiomyopathy, muscle wasting and myotonia. Muscle weakness with poor feeding may be profound in the neonatal period. Impaired glucose tolerance is common affecting up to 30% of subjects with this condition.

29.11 DIABETES ASSOCIATED WITH INSULIN RESISTANCE

Insulin resistance may be accompanied by frank hyperglycemia, or if adequate compensation can be made with elevation of circulating insulin levels, impaired glucose tolerance only may be seen. Insulin resistance occurs when a normal amount of insulin produces a subnormal biological response. Insulin-resistant states can be classified on the basis of their genetic inheritance, immune basis or association with endocrine or metabolic conditions (Table 29.4). Several syndromes of insulin resistance have been defined in association with acanthosis nigricans (Kahn *et al.*, 1976). Acanthosis nigricans is a skin disorder characterized by papillomatosis, hyperkeratosis and hyperpigmentation in the epidermis, which is commonly found at the neck, axillae, antecubital fossae and over the knuckles. Almost all patients with acanthosis nigricans show some degree of insulin resistance. Insulin resistance with acanthosis nigricans is also estimated to occur in 20–50% of women with polycystic ovarian disease (PCOD), manifesting as a combination of hirsutism, obesity and menstrual abnormalities. The etiological factors surrounding this complex group of abnormalities remain unclear. The syndromes of insulin resistance have been subdivided into type A and type B syndromes and their variants. The type A syndrome appears to be due to genetic abnormalities in the insulin receptor, whereas the type B syndrome is associated with anti-insulin receptor autoantibodies. Variants of the type A syndrome with normal insulin receptors but postreceptor defects (Bar *et al.*, 1978), have occasionally been termed the type C syndrome.

Table 29.4 Insulin resistance and diabetes.

Type A Insulin Resistance	(e.g., Rabson-Mendenhall syndrome)	
Type B Insulin Resistance	(e.g., ataxia telangiectasia)	
Lipoatrophy/Lipodystrophy	Leprechaunism	
	Congenital	Dunnigan syndrome
		Seip-Berardinelli syndrome
	Acquired	Lawrence syndrome
		Progressive partial lipoatrophy

29.11.1 TYPE A INSULIN RESISTANCE

The type A syndrome is typically diagnosed in young, thin females before the fourth decade. It may manifest as early as adolescence. Severe insulin resistance is usually found with marked glucose intolerance, acanthosis nigricans and hyperandrogenism (Kahn *et al.*, 1976). Males can also be affected. Other clinical findings include accelerated growth during childhood, acral hypertrophy and recurrent muscle cramps (Flier *et al.*, 1980). Young women and adolescents commonly present with primary or secondary amenorrhea, in association with varying degrees of virilization, elevated testosterone and a range of polycystic ovarian pathology. The presence of hyperinsulinemia may also aggravate the ovarian hyperstimulation. The type A insulin resistance syndrome has been shown in some cases to be due to mutant insulin receptors (reviewed in O'Rahilly & Moller, 1992). Studies on subjects with the type A insulin resistance syndrome have demonstrated reduced insulin binding (due to either reduced receptor number or altered receptor affinity) in both freshly-isolated or cultured cells. Others have been shown to have defective receptor autophosphorylation or abnormal post-translational processing of the receptor precursor (Yoshimasa *et al.*, 1988). These abnormalities occur in the absence of anti-insulin receptor antibodies or other circulating inhibitors of receptor function.

The Rabson-Mendenhall syndrome was first described in three siblings with deformed early dentition, dry skin, thick nails, hirsutism, precocious puberty, pineal hyperplasia and diabetes (Rabson & Mendenhall, 1956; West & Leonard, 1980). Affected individuals have severe insulin resistance and may die at puberty in ketoacidosis. Recently two individuals with this syndrome have been shown to have insulin receptor mutations (reviewed in O'Rahilly & Moller, 1992). The syndrome is associated with autosomal recessive inheritance.

29.11.2 TYPE B INSULIN RESISTANCE

Type B insulin resistance occurs uncommonly in childhood or adolescence and typically presents in the fourth to sixth decade (Kahn *et al.*, 1976). Autoimmune phenomena are commonly associated with the type B insulin resistance syndrome. The condition is due to autoantibodies directed against the insulin receptor. Ataxia telangiectasia is a rare autosomal recessive condition characterized by progressive cerebellar ataxia, telangiectasia affecting the retina and skin, recurrent upper and lower respiratory tract infections and various immune abnormalities. About 60% of patients with this syndrome have glucose intolerance, hyperinsulinemia and decreased sensitivity to exogenous insulin. Their insulin receptors are normal, but anti-insulin receptor antibodies have been found in several cases (Bar *et al.*, 1978).

29.11.3 DIABETES ASSOCIATED WITH LIPOATROPHY/LIPODYSTROPHY

Lipoatrophic diabetes encompasses a heterogenous group of rare syndromes characterized by insulin-dependent diabetes mellitus and poor development of subcutaneous tissue. Several different forms are distinguished on the basis of inheritance patterns and degree of lipoatrophy. The different forms of lipoatrophy are summarized in Table 29.4. Studies of insulin binding and receptor phosphorylation in the cultured cells from lipoatrophic subjects has revealed a wide range of results. Recently an insulin receptor mutation has been described in a patient with lipoatrophy (Yokota *et al.*, 1990).

29.11.3.1 Leprechaunism

Leprechaunism is a rare congenital syndrome characterized by intrauterine growth retardation, dysmorphic facies, decreased subcutaneous fat, acanthosis nigricans and severe insulin resistance with a tendency to fasting hypoglycemia (Donahue & Uchida, 1954). Some affected female neonates have ovarian hyperandrogenism and clitoromegaly (D'Ercole *et al.*, 1979). Most affected individuals die in infancy. Abnormalities which have been demonstrated in cultured cells from several patients with leprechaunism include defects in insulin binding, receptor autophosphorylation and kinase activity, and insulin-stimulated biological activity. Insulin receptor mutations have been defined in three patients with leprechaunism (reviewed in O'Rahilly & Moller, 1992). These mutations have been shown to directly or indirectly reduce insulin binding to extremely low levels, thus leading to a fundamental impairment of insulin action manifested by the intrauterine growth retardation seen in this very severe form of insulin resistance.

29.11.3.2 Dunnigan syndrome

This dominantly inherited generalized lipoatrophy was first described in two Scottish families (Dunnigan *et al.*, 1974). The lipoatrophy was associated with acanthosis nigricans, insulin-resistant diabetes and tubero-eruptive xanthomata.

29.11.3.3 Seip-Berardinelli syndrome

This syndrome is more common than Dunnigan syndrome and is also inherited in an autosomal recessive manner (Seip, 1971; Berardinelli, 1954). Parental consanguinity is common. Lipoatrophy is usually noted in early infancy, including loss of perivisceral and buccal fat. Mammary fat tissue may be spared. Acanthosis nigricans is commonly seen in this syndrome. Malformations in the region of the third ventricle, mental retardation and psychiatric disturbances are associated with congenital lipoatrophy. Other features include accelerated growth and advanced bone age, muscular hypertrophy and acromegaloid features with skin thickening and large hands and feet. Massive hepatomegaly due to increased lipid and glycogen storage may be seen and may result in cirrhosis with portal hypertension. Marked hypertriglyceridemia may result in eruptive xanthomata and lipemia retinalis. The basal metabolic rate may be markedly elevated. Polycystic ovaries with secondary menstrual irregularity is common in females. Diabetes usually occurs in the second decade and can be associated with long-term microvascular complications. The etiology of this condition remains unknown and anti-insulin or anti-insulin receptor antibodies have not been documented as a cause for the insulin resistance.

29.11.3.4 Lawrence syndrome

Acquired generalized lipoatrophy was first described by Lawrence (1946). These subjects show a generalized absence of body fat, insulin-resistant diabetes without ketosis, an elevated basal metabolic rate and hyperlipidemia with hepatomegaly. This condition occurs sporadically. Females are affected twice as often as males with onset often in childhood or shortly after puberty. Overt diabetes follows after an average of 4 years. Cirrhosis may be a problem and accelerated atherosclerosis may cause early coronary artery disease.

29.11.3.5 Partial lipoatrophy

In progressive partial lipoatrophy, fat is most commonly lost from the face and trunk; fat deposition below the waist is often normal or even increased, although occasionally loss may affect only the lower half of the body. Females are predominantly affected. It has been suggested that partial lipoatrophy is not a distinct entity and may only be part of the spectrum of generalized lipoatrophy as families have been described in which both forms of the disease occur. Unlike congenital lipoatrophy, autoimmune disorders such as systemic lupus erythematosus have been described in association with acquired lipoatrophy (Ipp *et al.*, 1977).

29.12 DIABETES ASSOCIATED WITH METABOLIC DISORDERS

Several metabolic disorders can be associated with diabetes in childhood. All of these conditions are uncommon, and the mechanism of the diabetes is not clearly understood. Acute intermittent porphyria is one of the more frequently seen metabolic disorders associated with diabetes. Porphyria is an autosomal recessive condition expressed more frequently and severely in females. Porphyria is due to an abnormality in the haem biosynthetic pathway, and occurs with a gene frequency of between 1 in 10 000 to 1 in 50 000. Acute attacks of porphyria may be precipitated by infection, pregnancy or exposure to drugs including barbiturates, sulfonamides, oral contraceptives and sulfonylureas. Endocrine abnormalities associated with porphyria include inappropriate secretion of growth hormone and antidiuretic hormone (ADH), isolated adrenocorticotrophin (ACTH) deficiency and impaired glucose tolerance.

29.13 CONCLUSIONS

Although the vast majority of children and adolescents who develop diabetes have type I or insulin-dependent diabetes mellitus, this chapter discusses the many rare types of diabetes which may also occur in childhood. Despite the fact that these forms of diabetes occur uncommonly, it is important to be aware of the possible association between various disorders and diabetes. It is also appropriate to screen 'at risk' groups, such as adolescents with cystic fibrosis for the development of diabetes. Early detection and appropriate treatment will help maintain wellbeing, may limit deterioration of the underlying condition, and possibly prevent long-term complications of diabetes.

REFERENCES

Abdul-Karim, F., Dahms, B. and Velasco, M. (1986) Islets of Langerhans in adolescents and adults with cystic fibrosis. *Arch. Pathol. Lab. Med.*, **110**, 602–606.

Alstrom, C., Hallgren, B., Nilsson, L. *et al.* (1959) Retinal degeneration combined with obesity, diabetes and neurogenous deafness: a specific syndrome (not hitherto described) distinct from Laurence-Moon-Bardet-Biedl syndrome. *Acta Psychiatr. Neurol. Scand.*, **129** (Suppl.), 1–35.

Altman, A. and Schwartz, A. (1983) 'Cancer Chemotherapy', in *Malignant Diseases of Infancy, Childhood and Adolescence*, p. 86. W.B. Saunders, Philadelphia.

Asmal, A., Dayal, D., Jialal, I. *et al.* (1981) Non insulin dependent diabetes mellitus with early onset in Blacks and Indians. *S. Afr. Med. J.*, **60**, 93–96.

Bankier, A. and Rogers, J. (1992) *POSSUM: Pictures of Standard Syndromes and Undiagnosed Malformations. Ed 3.4.* Computer Power Group and The Murdoch Institute for Research into Birth Defects, Melbourne.

Bar, R., Levis, W. and Rechler, M. (1978) Extreme insulin resistance in ataxia telangiectasia. Defect in affinity of insulin receptors. *N. Engl. J. Med.*, **298**, 1164–71.

Bar, R., Muggeo, M. and Roth, J. (1978) Insulin resistance, acanthosis nigricans and normal insulin receptors in a young women: evidence of a post receptor defect. *J. Clin. Endocrinol. Metab.*, **47**, 620–25.

Barbosa, J., Ramsay, R. and Goetz, F. (1978) Plasma glucose, insulin, glucagon and growth hormone in kindreds with maturity-onset diabetes of the young. *Arch. Intern. Med.*, **141**, 791–92.

Beck-Nielsen, H., Nielsen, O., Pedersen, O. *et al.* (1988) Insulin action and insulin secretion in identical twins with MODY: Evidence for defects in both insulin action and secretion. *Diabetes*, **37**, 730–35.

Berardinelli, W. (1954) An undiagnosed endocrinometabolic syndrome: report of two cases. *J. Clin. Endocrinol.*, **14**, 193–204.

Bowden, D., Gravius, T., Akots, G. *et al.* (1992) Identification of genetic markers flanking the locus for maturity-onset diabetes of the young on human chromosome 20. *Diabetes*, **41**:1, 88–92.

Bowden, D., Akots, G., Rothschild, C. *et al.* (1992) Linkage analysis of maturity-onset diabetes of the young (MODY): Genetic heterogeneity and nonpenetrance. *Am. J. Hum. Genet.*, **50**, 607–18.

Bray, G., Dahms, W., Swerdloff, R. *et al.* (1983) The Prader-Willi syndrome: A study of 40 patients and review of the literature. *Medicine*, **63**, 59–80.

Breyer, D., Cvitkovic, P., Zdenko, S. *et al.* (1981) Decreased insulin binding to erythrocytes in subjects with Klinefelter's syndrome. *J. Clin. Endocrinol. Metab.*, **53**, 654–55.

Broyer, M., Guillot, M., Gubler, M. *et al.* (1980) La cystinose infantile, réévaluation des symptomes précoces et tardifs. *Act. Nephr. Hop. Neck.*, 127–41.

Chan, A. (1991) 'Genetic and other disorders associated with diabetes mellitus', in J. Pickup and G. Williams (eds). *Textbook of Diabetes*, pp. 291–99. Blackwell Scientific Publications, London.

D'Ercole, A., Underwood, L., Groelke, J. *et al.* (1979) Leprechaunism: Studies of the relationship among hyperinsulinism, insulin resistance and growth retardation. *J. Clin. Endocrinol. Metab.*, **48**, 495–502.

De Sanctis, V., D'Ascola, D. and Wonke B. (1986) The development of diabetes mellitus and chronic liver disease in long term chelated β thalassemic patients. *Postgrad. Med. J.*, **62**, 831–36.

De Sanctis, V., Zurlo, M., Senesi, E. *et al.* (1988) Insulin dependent diabetes in thalassemia. *Arch. Dis. Child.*, **63**, 58–62.

Dodge, J. and Morrison, G. (1992) Diabetes mellitus in cystic fibrosis: a review. *J. R. Soc. Med.*, **185** (suppl. 19), 25–28.

Donahue, W. and Uchida, I. (1954) Leprechaunism: Euphemism for a rare familial disorder. *J. Pediatr.*, **45**, 505–519.

Dunnigan, M., Cochrane, M. and Kelly, A. (1974) Familial lipoatrophic diabetes with dominant transmission. *Quart. J. Med.*, **43**, 33–48.

Durruty, P., Munooz, M. and Garcia de los Rios, M. (1985) Clinical characteristics, inheritance of diabetes mellitus (DM) and insulin secretion in the NIDDM subgroup called maturity-onset diabetes in the young (MODY), S146. XII Congress of the IDF, Spain.

Fajans, S. (1981) Etiologic aspects of types of diabetes. *Diabetes Care*, **4**, 69–75.

Fajans, S. (1986) Heterogeneity of insulin secretion. *Diab. Metab. Rev.*, **2**, 347–61.

Fajans, S. (1987) MODY – a model for understanding the pathogenesis and natural history of type II diabetes. *Horm. Metab. Res.*, **19**, 591–99.

Fajans, S. (1989) Maturity-onset diabetes of the young (MODY). *Diabetes/Metabolism Reviews*, **5**:7, 579–606.

Fajans, S., Cloutier, M. and Crowther, R. (1978) Clinical and etiologic heterogeneity of idiopathic diabetes mellitus. *Diabetes*, **27**, 1112–25.

Fajans, S. and Conn, J. (1960) Tolbutamide-induced improvement in carbohydrate tolerance of young people with mild diabetes mellitus. *Diabetes*, **9**, 83–88.

Fajans, S. and Conn, J. (1965) 'Prediabetes, subclinical diabetes, and latent clinical diabetes: Interpretation, diagnosis and treatment', in D. Leibel and G. Wrenshall (eds). *On the Nature and Treatment of Diabetes*, **84**, 641–56. Excerpta Medica, Amsterdam.

Fivush, B., Green, O., Porter, C. *et al.* (1987) Pancreatic Endocrine Insufficiency in Post-Transplant Cystinosis. *Am. J. Dis. Child.*, **141**, 1087–89.

Fivush, B., Flick, J. and Gahl W. (1988) Pancreatic exocrine insufficiency in a patient with nephropathic cystinosis. *J. Pediatr.*, **112**:1, 49–51.

Flier, J., Young, J. and Landsberg, L. (1980) Familial insulin resistance with acanthosis nigricans, acral hypertrophy and muscle cramps. *N. Engl. J. Med.*, **303**, 970–73.

Frase, L. (1985) Enhanced glucose absorption in the jejunum of patients with cystic fibrosis. *Gastroenterology*, **88**, 478–84.

Froguel, P., Vaxillaire, M., Sun, F. *et al.* (1992) Close linkage of glucokinase locus on chromosome 7p to early onset non-insulin dependent diabetes mellitus. *Nature*, **356**, 162–64.

Froguel, P., Zouali, H., Vionnet, N. *et al.* (1993) Familial hyperglycaemia due to mutations in glucokinase. Definition of a subtype of diabetes mellitus. *N. Engl. J. Med.*, **328**, 697–702.

Given, B., Mako, M., Tager, H. *et al.* (1980) Diabetes due to secretion of an abnormal insulin. *N. Engl. J. Med.*, **302**, 129–35.

Goldstein, J. and Fialkow, P. (1973) Alstrom syndrome. *Medicine*, **52**, 53–71.

Gomez, E. and Frost, P. (1976) Induction of glycosuria and hyperglycaemia by topical corticosteroid therapy. *Arch. Dermatol.*, **112**, 1559–62.

Gregory, C., Kirkilionis, A., Greenberg, C. *et al.* (1990) Detection of molecular rearrangements in Prader-Willi syndrome patients by using genomic probes recognising four loci within the PWCR. *Am. J. Med. Genet.*, **35**, 536–45.

Hall, J. (1990) Genomic imprinting: review and relevance to human diseases. *Am. J. Hum. Genet.*, **46**, 857–73.

Ipp, M., Minta, J. and Gelfand, S. (1977) Disorders of the complement system in lipodystrophy. *Clin. Immunol. Immunopathol.*, **7**, 281–87.

Jeremiah, D., Leyshon, G., Rose, T. *et al.* (1973) Down's syndrome and diabetes. *Psychol. Med.*, **3**, 455–57.

Jialal, I., Welsh, N., Joubert, S. *et al.* (1982) Vascular complications in non-insulin dependent diabetes in the young. *S. Afr. Med. J.*, 155–57.

Jones, K. (1988) *Smith's recognisable patterns of human malformation*, 4th edn. Saunders, Philadelphia.

Kahn, C., Flier, J. and Bar, R. (1976) The syndromes of insulin resistance and acanthosis nigricans: insulin-receptor disorders in man. *N. Engl. J. Med.*, **294**, 739–45.

Kahn, C., Flier, J. and Bar, R. (1976) The syndrome of insulin resistance and acanthosis nigricans. Insulin receptor disorders in man. *N. Engl. J. Med.*, **294**, 739–45.

Keen, H. (1982) 'Problems in the definition of diabetes mellitus and its subtypes', in J.R.T. Kobberling and R. Tattersall (eds). *The Genetics of Diabetes Mellitus: Serono Symposia*, **47**, 1–11. Academic Press, London. Serono Symposium.

Krueger, L., Lerner, A., Katz, S. *et al.* (1991) Cystic fibrosis and Diabetes Mellitus: Interactive or Idiopathic? *J. Pediatr. Gastroenter. Nutr.*, **13**, 209–19.

Laidlaw, G. (1938) Nesidioblastoma, the islet tumour of the pancreas. *Am. J. Pathol.*, **14**, 125–39.

Lawrence, R. (1946) Lipodystrophy and hepatomegaly with diabetes, lipaemia and other metabolic disturbances. A case throwing new light on the action of insulin. *Lancet*, **i**, 724–31.

Lenzen, S. and Panten, U. (1988) Signal recognition by pancreatic β-cells. *Biochem. Pharmacol.* **37**, 371–78.

Lippe, B., Kaplan, S. and Neufeld, N. (1980) Insulin receptors in cystic fibrosis: increased receptor number and altered affinity. *Pediatrics*, **65**, 1018–22.

Maki, M., Hallstrom, O. and Huupponen T. (1984) Increased prevalence of coeliac disease in diabetes. *Arch. Dis. Child.*, **59**, 739–42.

Marner, B., Bille, G., Christy, M. *et al.* (1991) Islet cell cytoplasmic antibodies (ICA) in diabetes and disorders of glucose tolerance. *Diabet. Med.*, **8**, 812–16.

Milunsky, A. and Neurath, P. (1968) Diabetes in Down's Syndrome. *Arch. Environ. Health*, **17**, 372–76.

Mohan, V., Ramachandran, A., Snehalatha, C. *et al.* (1985) *Diabetes Care*, **8**, 371–74.

Nanjo, K., Sanke, T., Miyano, M. *et al.* (1986) Diabetes due to secretion of a structurally abnormal insulin (insulin Wakayama): Clinical and functional characteristics of (LeuA3) insulin. *J. Clin. Invest.*, **77**, 514–19.

Nielson, J., Johansen, K. and Yde, H. (1969) The frequency of diabetes mellitus in patients with Turner's syndrome and pure gonadal dysgenesis. *Acta Endocrinol.*, **62**, 251–69.

Ong, E. and Schneider, G. (1976) Down's syndrome, hypothyroidism and diabetes mellitus. *Am. J. Dis. Child.*, **130**, 335–36.

O'Rahilly, S., Patel, P., Lehmann, O. *et al.* (1992) Multipoint linkage analysis of the short arm of chromosome 11 in non-insulin dependent diabetes including maturity onset diabetes of youth. *Hum. Genet.*, **89**:2, 207–212.

O'Rahilly, S. and Moller, D. (1992) Mutant insulin receptors in syndromes of insulin resistance. *Clin. Endocrinol.*, **36**, 121–32.

O'Rahilly, S. and Turner, R. (1988) Early-onset type 2 diabetes vs maturity-onset diabetes of youth: Evidence for the existence of two discrete diabetic syndromes. *Diabetic Med.*, **5**, 224–29.

Pagano, G., Caballo-Perin, P., Cassader, M. *et al.* (1983) An *in vivo* and *in vitro* study of the mechanism of prednisolone-induced insulin resistance in healthy subjects. *J. Clin. Invest.*, **72**, 1814–20.

Page, M., Asmal, A. and Edwards, C. (1976) Recessive inheritance of diabetes: the syndrome of diabetes insipidus, diabetes mellitus, optic atrophy and deafness. *Quart. J. Med.*, **45**, 505–20.

Panzram, G. and Adolph, W. (1981) Heterogeneity of maturity onset diabetes at young age (MODY). *Lancet*, **2**, 986.

Polychronakos, C., Letarte, J., Collu, R. *et al.* (1980) Carbohydrate intolerance in children and adolescents with Turner syndrome. *J. Pediatr.*, **96**, 1009–1014.

Pui, C., Burghen, G., Bowman, W. *et al.* (1981) Risk factors for hyperglycaemia in children with leukemia receiving L-asparaginase and prednisone. *J. Pediatr.*, **99**, 46–50.

Pyke, D. (1979) The genetic connections. *Diabetologia*, **17**, 33–43.

Rabson, S. and Mendenhall, E. (1956) Familial hypertrophy of pineal body, hyperplasia of adrenal cortex and diabetes mellitus. *Am. J. Clin. Pathol.*, **26**, 283–90.

Reisman, J., Corey, M., Canny, G. *et al.* (1990) Diabetes mellitus in Patients with Cystic Fibrosis: Effect on Survival. *Pediatrics*, **86**, 374–77.

Rizza, R., Mandarino, L. and Gerich, J. (1982) Cortisol-induced insulin resistance in man. Impaired suppression of glucose production and stimulation of glucose utilisation due to a post-receptor defect of insulin action. *J. Clin. Endocrinol. Metab.*, **54**, 131–38.

Rodman, H., Doershuk, C. and Roland, J. (1986) The interaction of the two diseases: Diabetes mellitus and cystic fibrosis. *Medicine*, **65**, 389–97.

Rommens, J., Iannuzzi, M. and Kerem, B.-S. (1989) Identification of the cystic fibrosis gene: chromosome walking and jumping. *Science*, **245**, 1059–65.

Saudek, C., Hemm, R. and Peterson C. (1977) Abnormal glucose tolerance in β-thalassemia major. *Metabolism*, **26**, 43–52.

Savilahti, E., Simell, O., Koskimies, S. *et al.* (1986) Celiac disease in insulin-dependent diabetes mellitus. *J. Pediatr.*, **108**:1, 690–93.

Savir, A., Dickerman, Z., Zarp, M. *et al.* (1974) Diabetic retinopathy in an adolescent with Prader-Labhardt-Willi syndrome. *Arch. Dis. Child.*, **49**, 963–64.

Seip, M. (1971) Generalised lipodystrophy. *Ergeb. Inn. Med. Kinderheilk*, **31**, 59–95.

Sharp, P., Mohan, V., Levy, J. *et al.*, (1987) Insulin resistance in patients of Asian, Indian and European origin with non-insulin dependent diabetes. *Horm. Metab. Res.*, **19**, 84–85.

Shelbourne, P. and Johnson, K. (1992) Myotonic Dystrophy: Another Case of Too Many Repeats. *Human Mutation*, **1**, 183–89.

Shoelson, S., Fickova, M., Haneda, M. *et al.* (1983) Identification of a mutant human insulin predicted to contain a serine for phenylalanine substition. *Proc. Natl. Acad. Sci.*, **80**, 7390–94.

Shwachman, H. and Holsclaw, D. (1969) Complications of cystic fibrosis. *N. Engl. J. Med.*, **281**, 500–501.

Shwachman, H. and Leubner, H. (1955) Mucoviscidosis. *Adv. Pediatr.*, **7**, 249–322.

Spitz, L., Buick, R. and Grant, D. (1986) Surgical treatment of nesidioblastosis. *Ped. Surg. Int.*, **1**, 26–29.

Spitz, L., Bhargava, R., Grant, D. *et al.* (1992) Surgical treatment of hyperinsulinaemic hypoglycaemia in infancy and childhood. *Arch. Dis. Child.*, **67**, 201–205.

Stutchfield, P., O'Halloran, S. and Smith, C. (1988) HLA type, islet cell antibodies and glucose intolerance in cystic fibrosis. *Arch. Dis. Child.*, **63**, 1234–39.

Tattersall, R. (1974) Mild familial diabetes with dominant inheritance. *Quart. J. Med.*, **43**, 339–57.

Tattersall, R. (1979) Maturity-onset type diabetes in young people: A reassessment. *Pediatr. Adolesc. Endocrinol.*, **7**, 339–46.

Tattersall, R. (1982) 'The present status of maturity-onset type diabetes of young people (MODY)', in J.R.T. Kobberling and R. Tattersall (eds). *The Genetics of Diabetes Mellitus: Serono Symposia*, **47**, 261–70. Academic Press, London. Serono Symposium.

Tattersall, R. and Fajans, S. (1975) A difference between the inheritance of classic juvenile-onset and maturity-onset type diabetes of young people. *Diabetes*, **24**, 44–53.

Thomas, C., Underwood, M. and Carney, C. (1977) Neonatal infantile hypoglycaemia due to insulin excess. *Ann. Surg.*, **185**, 505–507.

Vionnet, N., Stoffel, M., Takeda, J. *et al.* (1992) Nonsense mutation in the glucokinase gene causes early-onset non-insulin dependent diabetes mellitus. *Nature*, **356**, 721–22.

Vullo, C., De Sanctis, V., Atti, G. *et al.* (1980) Islet cell surface antibodies in subjects with β-thalassemia affected by diabetes mellitus. *Haematologica*, **65**, 827–30.

Vullo, C., De Sanctis, V., Katz, M. *et al.* (1990) Endocrine abnormalities in thalassemia. *Ann. N. Y. Aca. Sci.*, **612**, 293–310.

Walsh, C., Cooper, B., Wright, A. *et al.* (1978) Diabetes mellitus and coeliac disease: a clinical study. *Quart. J. Med.*, **47**, 89–100.

Weetman, R. and Baehner, R. (1974) Late onset of clinical pancreatitis in children receiving L-asparaginase therapy. *Cancer*, **37**, 780–84.

West, R. and Leonard, J. (1980) Familial insulin resistance with pineal hyperplasia: metabolic studies and effect of hypohysectomy. *Arch. Dis. Child.*, 619–21.

Wilken, T. (1987) Autoimmunity, diabetes and cystic fibrosis. *Lancet*, **ii**, 157.

Wilson, D., Frane, J., Sherman, B. *et al.* (1987) Carbohydrate and lipid metabolism in Turner's syndrome: Effect of therapy with growth hormone, oxandrolone and a combination of both. *J. Pediatr.*, **112**, 210–17.

Winter, W., MacLaren, N., Riley, W. *et al.* (1987) Maturity-onset diabetes of youth in black Americans. *N. Engl. J. Med.*, **316**, 285–91.

Yakovac, W., Baker, L. and Hummeler, K. (1971) Beta cell nesidioblastosis in idiopathic hypoglycaemia in infancy. *J. Pediatr.*, **79**, 226–31.

Yokota, A., Moller, D. and Flier, J. (1990) Homozygous mutation at position 485 of the insulin receptor alpha-subunit in a patient with lipodystrophy and severe insulin resistance. *Diabetes*, **39** (suppl. 1), 235A (abstract).

Yoshimasa, Y., Seino, S. and Whittaker, J. (1988) Insulin resistant diabetes due to a point mutation that prevents insulin proreceptor processing. *Science*, **240**, 784–87.

30

Neonatal diabetes

H.F. STIRLING and C.J.H. KELNAR

30.1 DEFINITION

Hyperglycemia in the newborn infant (defined as a blood glucose concentration >7 mmol/l after a four-hour fast) occurs much less frequently than hypoglycemia. Diabetes in the newborn period is rare but well recognized, and may be transient or permanent: although the two conditions are distinct, it is impossible to distinguish between them at the outset.

A one-year study is commencing in the UK during 1994 under the auspices of the British Paediatric Surveillance Unit to establish incidence rates for the transient and permanent forms and to allow comparison of their clinical, physiological and genetic characteristics.

30.2 TRANSIENT NEONATAL DIABETES

This condition was probably first reported in 1852 by Kitselle who described his own son. The child developed polyuria, polydypsia, glycosuria ('honeyed napkins'), and emaciation a few days after birth, and died of a urinary tract infection at six months of age. Since then there have been repeated reports of such cases.

This condition characteristically occurs in full term infants of less than six weeks of age, who are born small for gestational age (SGA). They present with marked dehydration, fever, vomiting without diarrhea, failure to thrive and rapid weight loss despite adequate feeding. They usually have an alert open-eyed appearance which is unusual for their degree of dehydration. Thirst and polyuria are present but are less obvious to the carers, and may be more difficult to detect in such young infants (Hutchison *et al.*, 1962; Willi & Muller, 1968; Gentz & Cornblath, 1969; Pagliara *et al.*, 1973).

A period of transient symptomatic hypoglycemia (itself not uncommon in infants who are SGA) is not unusual before the hyperglycemia develops (Gentz & Cornblath, 1969).

The degree of hyperglycemia is variable, but blood glucose levels may reach 100 mmol/l. In a review of 15 cases by Cornblath and Schwartz (1976) the range of blood glucose at presentation was 13–73 mmol/l.

Ketosis is usually mild (Gentz & Cornblath, 1969) and may be absent. There is a striking resemblance to the hyperglycemic hyperosmolar coma seen in elderly patients, though infants with transient neonatal diabetes do not usually become comatose. However, they are capable of producing ketosis. It may be missed if only acetoacetic acid (detected by Ketotest™ or Ketostix™) is measured

Childhood and Adolescent Diabetes
Published in 1994 by Chapman & Hall, London
ISBN 0 412 48610 5

rather than the more abundant reduced β-hydroxybutyric acid. In the newborn, ketone bodies can be reabsorbed from the renal tubules with sodium and the young baby reabsosrbs practically all the sodium in the presence of an anion. Excessive hyperglycemia itself may in fact be antiketogenic, as may severe dehydration. The paucity of ketone production in the newborn period may itself contribute to the marked hyperglycemia as in an animal model ketones themselves have been shown to have a direct stimulatory effect on β cells (Madison *et al.*, 1964). For all these reasons, ketosis may only be mild or even absent at presentation in the infant with transient neonatal diabetes, or may only become apparent during rehydration.

Some infants do not conform to this typical clinical picture. McGill and Robertson (1986) described two siblings, each of normal birth weight who presented with hyperglycemia and glycosuria at eleven weeks and fifteen days of age respectively. These infants thrived without treatment although the hyperglycemia and glycosuria persisted until five and nine months respectively. These infants were unusual in that they were asymptomatic, although like other more typical cases they did not have antibodies to either insulin or islet cells and inappropriately low insulin levels for glucose levels suggesting poor insulin secretion.

Diagnosis in infants with neonatal diabetes may be delayed as diabetes mellitus is considered unlikely in this age group. Presentation may mimic other neonatal problems, for example severe sepsis and salt-losing congenital adrenal hyperplasia. Delay in diagnosis can lead to severe dehydration, and even death – possibly due to the thrombotic effects of such severe dehydration.

Transient diabetes mellitus lasts only for a few weeks, but the differentiation from permanent diabetes can only be made by the clinical course of the infant and repeated dynamic evaluations of β cell function (Cavallo *et al.*, 1987). C-peptide levels are a useful marker of β cell function. The mean duration of insulin therapy in a series of 35 patients (Cornblath & Schwartz, 1976) was 69 days with a range of 0–540 days.

Infants with transient diabetes are typically SGA and fail to thrive postnatally unless adequately treated with insulin. Insulin-like growth factor 1 (IGF1) has been shown to be significantly reduced pre-treatment in a child with this condition, with subsequent restoration to normal levels during the phase of insulin treatment. Spontaneous resolution of the condition at 2.5 months of age was associated with maintenance of normal IGF1 levels (Blethen *et al.*, 1981). There is usually good catch-up growth during the period of insulin treatment, with the insulin acting as a growth promoter.

30.3 ETIOLOGY

The etiology of transient neonatal diabetes is largely unknown and mechanisms are speculative.

Autopsy reports of affected neonates show in some patients a small pancreas with decreased numbers of islet cells (Devine, 1938; Lewis & Eisenberg, 1935). However, other reports have described the pancreatic appearance as normal (Hickish, 1956) and there is even one report of a pancreas with an unusually large number of islets (Osborne, 1965).

The favored etiological hypothesis of transient neonatal diabetes is delayed maturation of the pancreatic β-cells (Milner *et al.*, 1971; Pagliara *et al.*, 1973) with poor insulin response to glucose loading.

Insulin is known to be present in the fetal pancreas as early as eight to ten weeks of gestation (Schiff *et al.*, 1972). Release of insulin in response to glucose and tolbutamide is poor in the fetus. At term, release of insulin occurs in response to hyperglycemia, glucagon and amino acids, but not tolbutamide. The factors responsible for the maturation of insulin-releasing mechanisms are unknown. Acceleration of maturation occurs in the hyperinsulinemic infants of diabetic mothers who release insulin to tolbutamide immediately after birth and show an exaggerated response to glucose stimulation. In addition, infants born to diabetic mothers treated with sulfonylurea agents (which cross the placenta) have high insulin levels and exaggerated insulin responses.

Inappropriately low levels of plasma insulin for the hyperglycemia, with absent rise in response to a glucose challenge confirm insulin deficiency in affected infants rather than insulin resistance (Milner *et al.*, 1971).

The cause of delayed β-cell maturation is speculative. Infection is unlikely to be the cause – concomitant sepsis is more likely to be a complication of the diabetic state. There has only been one reported case of mumps in the mother at the time of delivery (Limper & Miller, 1935) and the infant had signs of pancreatitis at autopsy.

Infants with transient neonatal diabetes are usually SGA and it is likely that placental function has been poor prior to delivery. The placenta is a major source of fetal steroids, which may play a role in the development of the fetal pancreas. β-cells of fetal rat pancreas only grow in culture if the tissue is incubated in the presence of fetal rat adrenal cells, or in a medium containing hydrocortisone. Precocious development of rabbit fetal exocrine and endocrine pancreas was noted when cortisone or ACTH was administered to pregnant rabbits. Thus abnormal placental production of steroids may be implicated in the delayed maturation of the pancreas in these children (Ferguson & Milner, 1970).

Pagliara *et al.* (1973) postulated that the underlying defect related to delayed maturation of the adenyl cyclase-cyclic adenosine monophosphate system, due to either a deficient pancreatic β cell adenyl cyclase or an increased activity of the nucleotide phosphodiesterase. Evidence for this came from a SGA female infant who presented with hyperglycemia and inappropriately low insulin levels on day five of life. Insulin was continued until day thirty. Glucose and tolbutamide-mediated insulin release was absent during the diabetic phase whereas caffeine resulted in a substantial increase in plasma insulin, implying that insulin was present in the pancreas and that the defect was in the failure of the β cell to respond to glucose and tolbutamide. Caffeine, a phosphodiesterase inhibitor resulted in insulin release, and thus the underlying defect must be related to delayed maturation of the adenyl cyclase-cyclic adenosine monophosphate system.

Gerrard and Chin (1962) described an infant with transient neonatal diabetes whose mother had persistently low blood glucose levels during the pregnancy. They postulated that the hypoinsulinism in the child was due to a delay in development of the endocrine pancreas consequent on the absence of fluctuations in maternal glucose levels. Possibly such fluctuations are necessary for full β cell development in the fetus.

McGill and Robertson (1986) have suggested that the abnormality may lie in an inappropriately high threshold for insulin release which subsequently falls with age.

Plasma insulin levels are inappropriately low for the degree of hyperglycemia in the majority of reported cases (Milner *et al.*, 1971). C-peptide levels (Halliday *et al.*, 1986) were shown to be low for the first five months of life (<0.06 mmol/l) in a male infant with transient neonatal diabetes, with a progressive normalization of C-peptide reserve. C-peptide levels can be used as a measure of β cell function during insulin therapy (Cavallo *et al.*, 1987), as can serial arginine stimulation tests.

Genetic factors may be important in transient neonatal diabetes although unlike insulin dependent diabetes mellitus (IDDM) presenting later in childhood there is no definite HLA association. Siblings have been affected (Ferguson & Milner, 1970) including twins

(Nielsen, 1989) implying that inheritance is autosomal recessive. The condition has also occurred in three half-siblings (each with the same father but different mothers) raising the possibility, at least in some families, that the condition is autosomal dominant (Coffey & Killelea, 1982).

30.4 MANAGEMENT

The sulfonylurea drugs stimulate insulin secretion by the pancreatic β cells, with chlorpropamide longer acting than tolbutamide. Thus theoretically they could be effective in transient neonatal diabetes if abnormalities of insulin release from the β cells are postulated.

Chlorpropamide (Kuna & Addy, 1979) has been used in the management of babies with transient neonatal diabetes – a SGA baby presenting with diabetes at 6 days of age was initially controlled with insulin. At 40 days chlorpropamide was gradually substituted for the insulin over a 24-day period, and chlorpropamide was continued until 13 weeks, after which he remained well off treatment. It is difficult to be certain of the beneficial effect for chlorpropamide in this situation, as the natural history of the condition is for spontaneous remission over a similar period of time. More detailed studies in larger numbers of infants would be needed to prove the benefit of such treatment.

There is usually a dramatic response to insulin therapy. Experience suggests that a dose of 1–3 units/kg body weight/day is appropriate (Cornblath & Schwartz, 1976), with larger doses producing unacceptable episodes of hypoglycemia. Many infants can be maintained on oral feeding without recourse to intravenous fluids. If intravenous fluids are required, dehydration must be corrected slowly so as to minimize the risk of cerebral edema.

Once insulin therapy is started the dehydration corrects, weight gain ensues and the clinical manifestations are reversed.

The monitoring of serial C-peptide levels is a useful marker of β-cell function. Halliday *et al.* (1986) showed a rise in C-peptide levels between three and five months after birth in an infant with typical transient neonatal diabetes. He was able to discontinue insulin therapy once C-peptide levels were rising although they did not reach normal adult fasting values for at least the first year of life.

When stopping insulin therapy in these infants it is important to decrease the dose gradually to diminish the risk of renewed hyperglycemia.

30.5 INCIDENCE OF IDDM IN LATER LIFE

There are increasing reports of infants who had transient diabetes in infancy and a recurrence of IDDM, mostly in the second decade of life.

The phenomenon was first described by Campbell *et al.* (1978). An 18-year-old girl presented with necrobiosis lipoidica diabeticorum which had been present for two years, and had an abnormal glucose tolerance test. She had a past history of transient neonatal diabetes treated with insulin till aged 17 days. She had no detectable islet cell antibodies and was HLA type A2, A9, B12 (i.e., not those usually associated with IDDM, see Chapters 10 and 11). She was successfully managed with insulin.

Weimerskirch and Klein (1993) described IDDM occurring in two patients with transient neonatal diabetes after more than five years without insulin therapy. The first child had an abnormal glucose tolerance test (GTT) at 7.5 years, and developed symptomatic diabetes at 10 years of age. No islet cell antibodies were detected. The second child had an abnormal GTT at 8 years of age, again without the presence of islet cell antibodies.

There are similar reports from Shield and Baum (1993) in which a 13-year-old who had had typical transient neonatal diabetes presented with IDDM and ketoacidosis, and from Coffey and Killelea (1982) in which one of three half-siblings with transient diabetes developed IDDM aged 15 years. A further case reported by Gottschalk *et al.* (1992) supports the hypothesis that permanent IDDM occurring a significant time after the resolution of transient neonatal diabetes is unrelated to autoimmunity.

All reports of recurrence of IDDM in a child who had transient neonatal diabetes suggest that the condition is not like 'classical' IDDM presenting in childhood as there are several unusual features:

1) Islet cell antibodies have not been detected (cf. 'classical' IDDM presenting in childhood where the incidence of such antibodies at presentation is approximately 80%).
2) Such children are not homozygous for the diabetes susceptibility alleles at the HLA locus. In fact one child had HLA/DR2 which is usually associated with relative resistance to diabetes.
3) They seem to have low insulin requirements and are relatively easily controlled, raising the possibility that there is only partial β-cell dysfunction.

The absence of islet all antibodies and of the typical HLA alleles suggest that they may have a distinct nonimmunologic form of diabetes, which may be associated with mild insulin deficiency.

In the case described by Briggs (1986), an infant with transient neonatal diabetes was treated with insulin until eight months of age. She remained well, although she had an impaired GTT at 5 years of age. Diabetes was diagnosed at 12 years, and was successfully managed with diet and chlorpropamide.

Shield and Baum (1993) have postulated that the association between transient neonatal diabetes and the development of subsequent IDDM may add strength to the hypothesis that relates abnormal islet cell function and lower mean birth weight to abnormal glucose tolerance in later life (Hales *et al.*, 1991).

30.6 CONGENITAL PERMANENT NEONATAL DIABETES

Permanent IDDM is rare in infants under the age of 6 months, and is less common than transient neonatal diabetes. Differentiation from transient neonatal diabetes is difficult at presentation, and it is only by following the infant's clinical course that the two can be separated. The youngest child reported is a boy who presented at 24 hours of age with glycosuria (Hoffman *et al.* 1980) and who remained permanently diabetic.

One cause of permanent neonatal diabetes is pancreatic agenesis. Previously this was considered fatal. However, Winter *et al.* (1986) described congenital pancreatic hypoplasia in two brothers who presented with neonatal diabetes and subsequently developed pancreatic exocrine insufficiency at ages 5 and 21 years. There are other reports of similar cases (Howard *et al.* 1980). Wright *et al.* (1993) described a SGA infant who was hyperglycemic from birth and had associated pancreatic exocrine insufficiency consistent with pancreatic hypoplasia. Exocrine function needs to be evaluated in any infant with neonatal diabetes who fails to thrive despite appropriate insulin therapy.

Not all infants with permanent neonatal diabetes have pancreatic hypoplasia. Congenital absence of islets with normal exocrine pancreatic tissue was described by Dodge and Lawrence (1977) in an infant who developed diabetes on the third day of life. Another male sibling had probably also been affected, raising the possibility that this was an autosomal or X-linked abnormality.

Permanent IDDM is more likely than transient neonatal diabetes to be associated with more typical HLA typing (Ivarsson *et al.*, 1988), and associations with other HLA-linked conditions have been documented. An association with celiac disease has been described (Hattevig *et al.*, 1982). The patient was born at term with normal birth weight. At eight days of age he presented with vomiting, diarrhea, dehydration, acidosis and hyperglycemia. He responded well to insulin therapy, but at four months of age again developed diarrhea shortly after gluten-containing foods were introduced into his diet. Jejunal biopsy confirmed celiac disease. His insulin requirements persisted, and investigation at three weeks and twelve months of age showed a total loss of β-cell function. There was a strong family history of IDDM. HLA typing of the family showed an increased incidence of B8 and B15, and the child himself was homozygous for B8. There is a well-recognized association between IDDM and celiac disease, again with HLA types B8 and A1 being over-represented in patients with the condition (see Chapter 29).

Ivarsson *et al.* (1988) described a sibship of two HLA-Dw3/4 positive boys who developed permanent diabetes within the first week of life. Islet cell antibodies were negative, but both boys exhibited the presence of a novel acinar non-islet autoantibody.

Widness *et al.* (1982) described permanent diabetes mellitus in an infant of a diabetic mother, who developed persistent hyperglycemia from the first few days of life, but did not require insulin treatment until the age of 13 months. His mother had herself had IDDM from the age of 12 weeks. The family had none of the common HLA alleles associated with IDDM, nor any detectable tissue antibodies, and may represent a unique cause for the condition.

Pancreatic α cell function may also be impaired in infants with permanent diabetes mellitus (Knip *et al.*, 1983). In the child they reported there was maturation and recovery of α-cell function during the first month of life. Although β cell function improved on biochemical testing on two occasions, this was temporary and the child remained insulin dependent.

Like infants with transient neonatal diabetes, babies with permanent diabetes are also often SGA (Greenwood & Traisman, 1971). Catch-up growth is seen after initiation of insulin treatment, supporting the concept of insulin playing a role in the regulation of fetal growth (Wright *et al.*, 1993).

These infants are managed with subcutaneous insulin analagously to those with transient neonatal diabetes. However there is no recovery of insulin-secretory ability and they remain insulin dependent for the rest of their lives.

30.7 DIFFERENTIAL DIAGNOSIS OF NEONATAL HYPERGLYCEMIA

Hyperglycemia is commonly seen in sick or immature neonates. The incidence of hyperglycemia depends on birth weight, degree of stress, and the amount of dextrose infused per unit time. The risk for hyperglycemia is 18 times greater in infants weighing less than 1000 gms than in those weighing 2000 gms or more (Louik *et al.*, 1985). Glucose levels are significantly negatively correlated with Apgar scores, gestational age and birth weight, and positively correlated with inspired oxygen concentrations and severity of respiratory distress.

Hyperglycemia may be a compounding factor for increased mortality and morbidity in these vulnerable infants – hyperglycemia causes increased plasma osmolality which may result in brain cell dehydration, capillary dilatation and intracranial hemorrhage – but is difficult to evaluate as an independent cause.

In addition to exogenous glucose infusions other factors play a role in the etiology of hyperglycemia in the sick or immature neonate. Drugs such as caffeine, aminophylline (by activation of hepatic glycogenolysis and inhibition of glycogen synthesis) and steroids (used in the treatment of bronchopulmonary dysplasia) may be implicated. The stress of respiratory distress syndrome, sepsis, hypoxia, surgical procedures and lipid infusions can produce elevation of plasma glucose levels. In very low birth-weight infants without other obvious predisposing factors, the hyperglycemia is thought to be caused by persistent hepatic glucose production despite significant elevations in plasma insulin, i.e., insulin insensitivity.

Management usually consists of decreasing the rate of parenteral glucose administered. However this can compromise the total calories delivered to the infant and adversely affect nutrition. Cautious insulin therapy may therefore be necessary to maintain nutrition.

Other diseases can mimic neonatal diabetes and lead to confusion at presentation. Galactosemia can produce an ill neonate with reducing substances in the urine – thus both determination of the blood glucose level as well as testing the urine specifically for glucose are important in making an accurate diagnosis. Salt-losing congenital adrenal hyperplasia produces a similar clinical picture of dehydration, weight loss and vomiting. Blood glucose is likely to be low. Sepsis, which may itself produce mild hyperglycemia, may mimic the clinical picture of neonatal diabetes. To avoid these diagnostic errors it is recommended that the investigation of any young infant (particularly one who is SGA or post-mature) who is failing to thrive, vomiting or rapidly becoming dehydrated should include a complete urinalysis and a laboratory measurement of blood glucose.

REFERENCES

Blethen, S.L., White, N.H., Santiago, J.V. *et al.* (1981) Plasma somatomedins, endogenous insulin secretion, and growth in transient neonatal diabetes. *J. Clin. Endocrinol. Metabol.*, **52,** 144–47.

Briggs, J.R. (1986) Permanent non-insulin dependent diabetes mellitus after congenital transient neonatal diabetes. *Scott. Med. J.*, **31**, 41–42.

Campbell, I.W., Fraser, D.M., Duncan, L.J.P. *et al.* (1978) Permanent insulin-dependent diabetes mellitus after congenital temporary diabetes mellitus. *Brit. Med. J.*, **2**, 174.

Cavallo, L., Mautone, A., Laforgia, N. *et al.* (1987) Neonatal diabetes mellitus: evaluation of pancreatic beta-cell function in two cases. *Helv. Paediatr. Acta.*, **42**, 437–43.

Coffey, J.D. Jr. and Killelea, D.E. (1982) Transient neonatal diabetes in half sisters. A sequel. *Am. J. Dis. Child.*, **136**, 626–27.

Cornblath, M. and Schwartz, R. (1976) 'Transient diabetes mellitus in early infancy', in M. Cornblath and R. Schwartz (eds). *Disorders of Carbohydrate Metabolism in Infancy*, 2nd edn, pp. 105–112. W.B. Saunders, Philadelphia.

Devine, J. (1938) A case of diabetes mellitus in a young infant. *Arch. Dis. Child.*, **13**, 189.

Dodge, J.A. and Laurence, K.M. (1977) Congenital absence of islets of Langerhans. *Arch. Dis. Child.*, **52**, 411–13.

Ferguson, A.W. and Milner, R.D. (1970) Transient neonatal diabetes mellitus in siblings. *Arch. Dis. Child.*, **45**, 80–83.

Gentz, J.C.H. and Cornblath, M. (1969) Transient diabetes of the newborn. *Advances in Pediatrics*, **16**, 345–63.

Gerrard, J.W. and Chin, W. (1962) The syndrome of transient diabetes. *J. Pediatr.*, **61**, 89.

Gottschalk, M.E., Schatz, D.A., Clare-Salzer, M. *et al.* (1992) Permanent diabetes without serological evidence of autoimmunity after transient neonatal diabetes. *Diabetes Care*, **15**, 1273–76.

Greenwood, R.D. and Traisman, H.S. (1971) Permanent diabetes mellitus in an infant. *J. Pediatr.*, **79**, 296–98.

Hales, C.N., Barker, D.J.P., Clark, P.M.S. *et al.* (1991) Fetal growth and impaired glucose tolerance at age 64. *Brit. Med. J.*, **303**, 1019–22.

Halliday, H.L., Reid, M.M. and Hadden, D.R. (1986) C-peptide levels in transient neonatal diabetes. *Diab Med.*, **3**, 80–81.

Hattevig, G., Kjellman, B. and Fallstrom, S.P. (1982) Congenital permanent diabetes mellitus and coeliac disease. *J. Pediatr.*, **101**, 955–57.

Hickish, G. (1956) Neonatal diabetes. *Brit. Med. J.*, **1**, 95.

Hoffman, W.H., Khoury, C. and Byrd, H.A. (1980) Prevalance of permanent congenital diabetes mellitus. *Diabetologia*, **19**, 487–88.

Howard, C.P., Go, V.L.W., Infante, A.J. *et al.*

(1980) Long-term survival in a case of functional pancreatic agenesis. *J. Pediatr.*, **97**, 786–89.

Hutchison, J.H., Keay, A.J. and Kerr, M.M. (1962) Congenital temporary diabetes mellitus. *Brit. Med. J.*, **2**, 436–40.

Ivarsson, S.A., Marner, B., Lernmark, A. *et al.* (1988) Nonislet pancreatic autoantibodies in sibship with permanent neonatal insulin-dependent diabetes mellitus. *Diabetes*, **37**, 347–50.

Kitselle, J.F. (1852) *Jb. Kinderheilt*, **18**, 313.

Knip, M., Koivisto, M., Kaar, M.L. *et al.* (1983) Pancreatic islet cell function and metabolic control in an infant with permanent neonatal diabetes. *Acta Paediatr. Scand.*, **72**, 303–307.

Kuna, P. and Addy, D.P. (1979) Transient neonatal diabetes mellitus. Treatment with chlorpropamide. *Am. J. Dis. Child.*, **133**, 65–66.

Lewis, E. and Eisenberg, H. (1935) Diabetes mellitus neonatorium. *Am. J. Dis. Child.*, **49**, 408.

Limper, M.A. and Miller, A.J. (1935) Diabetes mellitus with extensive gangrene in early infancy. *Am. J. Dis. Child.*, **50**, 1216.

Louik, C., Mitchell, A.A., Epstein, M.F. *et al.* (1985) Risk factors for neonatal hyperglycaemia associated with 10% dextrose infusion. *Am. J. Dis. Child.*, **139**, 783–86.

McGill, J.M. and Robertson, D.M. (1986) A new type of transient diabetes mellitus of infancy. *Arch. Dis. Child.*, **61**, 334–36.

Madison, L.L. *et al.* (1964) The hypoglycaemic action of ketones. II. Evidence for a stimulatory feedback of ketones on the pancreatis beta cells. *J. Clin. Invest.*, **43**, 408.

Milner, R.D.G., Ferguson, A.W. and Naidu, S.H. (1971) Aetiology of transient neonatal diabetes. *Arch. Dis. Child.*, **46**, 724–26.

Neilsen, F. (1989) Transient neonatal diabetes mellitus in a pair of twins. *Acta Paediatr. Scand.*, **78**, 469–72.

Osborne, G.R. (1965) Congenital diabetes. *Arch. Dis. Child.*, **40**, 332.

Pagliara, A.S., Karl, L.E. and Kipnis, D.B. (1973) Transient neonatal diabetes: delayed maturation of the pancreatic beta cell. *J. Pediatr.*, **82**, 97–101.

Schiff, D., Colle, E. and Stern, L. (1972) Metabolic and growth patterns in transient neonatal diabetes. *N. Eng. J. Med.*, **287**, 119–22.

Shield, J.P. and Baum, J.D. (1993) Is transient neonatal diabetes a risk factor for diabetes in later life. *Lancet*, **341**, 693.

Weimerskirch, D. and Klein, D.J. (1993) Recurrence of insulin-dependent diabetes mellitus after transient neonatal diabetes: a report of two cases. *J. Pediatr.*, **122**, 598–600.

Widness, J.A., Cowett, R.M., Zeller, W.P. *et al.* (1982) Permanent neonatal diabetes in an infant of an insulin-dependent mother. *J. Pediatr.*, **100**, 926–29.

Willi, H. and Muller, F. (1968) Uber den transitorischen Diabetes Mellitus des Neugeborenen. *Helv. Paediatr. Acta.*, **3**, 231–41.

Winter, W.E., MacLaren, N.K., Riley, W.J. *et al.* (1986) Congenital pancreatic hypoplasia: a syndrome of exocrine and endocrine pancreatic insufficiency. *J. Pediatr.*, **109**, 465–68.

Wright, N.M., Metzger, D.L., Borowitz, S.M. *et al.* (1993) Permanent neonatal diabetes mellitus and pancreatic exocrine insufficiency resulting from congenital pancreatic agensis. *Am. J. Dis. Child.*, **147**, 607–609.

31

Maternal diabetes and the fetus

D.A. HEPBURN and J.M. STEEL

31.1 INTRODUCTION

Before the advent of insulin the outlook for the diabetic mother and her child was very poor. In 1909, 66 cases were reported; 27% of the mothers died at the time of labor or shortly thereafter, a further 22% died in the next two years, and in those that reached term one-third of the babies were stillborn (Peel, 1972). In 1920, DeLee reported that abortion and premature labor occurred in one-third of pregnancies in diabetic women and in pregnancies which reached term the infant often died shortly after birth (DeLee, 1920). In this series the perinatal mortality rate was 65% and about one third of the mothers died mainly from diabetic keto-acidosis. With the advent of insulin therapy in the 1920s the outlook for the diabetic mother improved substantially to a maternal mortality rate around 2% (Figure 31.1a). The perinatal mortality rate on the other hand did not fall as dramatically and has declined only slowly over time (Figure 31.1b).

By the 1950s the perinatal mortality rate had fallen to about 25% as a result of early delivery at or before 38 weeks, more intensive antenatal care and long-term or frequent admissions to hospital. When home blood glucose monitoring became widely practiced it was no longer necessary to admit women to control their diabetes and diabetic control improved markedly. Since then methods have become available for assessing fetal growth by ultrasound, fetal monitoring has become available and neonatal intensive care units with expert pediatric staff have opened. The perinatal mortality rate in experienced large centers is around 2–5% at the present time (Figure 31.2). Some partially unresolved problems such as macrosomia, congenital malformations and growth retardation in infants of mothers with diabetic renal disease and hypertension remain.

31.2 METABOLISM DURING PREGNANCY AND THE FETOPLACENTAL UNIT

During normal pregnancy, maternal metabolism adjusts to provide nutrition for both the mother and for the fetoplacental unit. Maternal fasting blood glucose decreases during normal pregnancy reaching a nadir by 12 weeks of gestation and remains suppressed for the rest of pregnancy (Fisher *et al.*, 1974), and this is probably caused by increased peripheral glucose utilization. From this early phase of pregnancy glucose homeostasis changes, with β cell hyperplasia and an increased insulin response to a glucose load (Lind, 1975; Freinkel, 1980). However,

Childhood and Adolescent Diabetes
Published in 1994 by Chapman & Hall, London
ISBN 0 412 48610 5

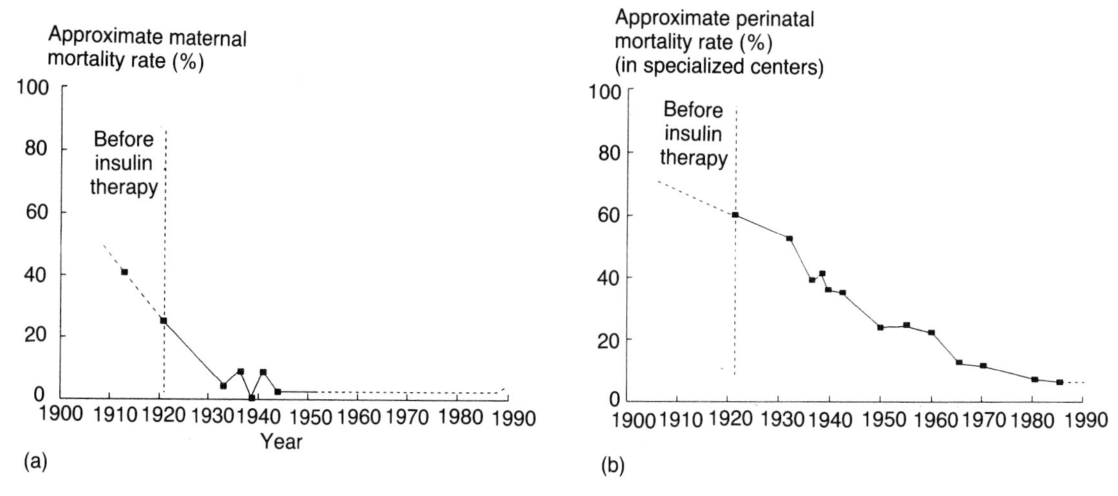

Figure 31.1 (a) Decrease in maternal mortality rate in diabetic pregnancies over time following the introduction of insulin for the therapy of diabetes. (b) Slower reduction in perinatal mortality rate in IDM after the introduction of insulin therapy. IDM = Infants of the diabetic mother.

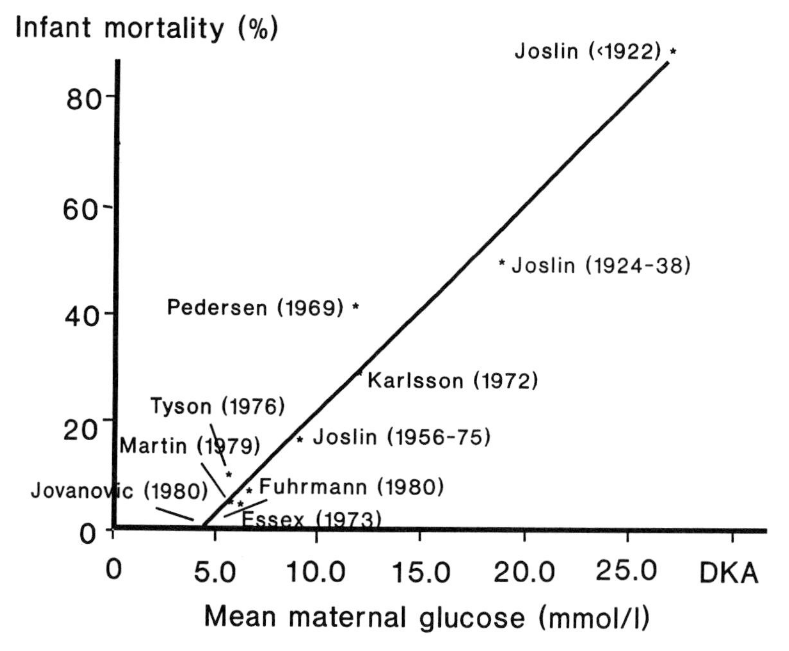

Figure 31.2 Graphical representation of the reduction in infant mortality in IDM with overall improvements in maternal blood glucose control.

despite the exaggerated insulin response blood glucose remains elevated for longer than in non-pregnant state. It has been shown that there is insulin resistance due to a post-receptor defect (Puavilai *et al.*, 1982; Gray *et al.*, 1984). Insulin disappearance is unaltered (Lind *et al.*, 1977). Other compensatory homeostatic mechanisms in the pregnant woman include increased protein catabolism, accelerated gluconeogenesis and therefore lower plasma amino acid concentrations. The early and mid-phases of pregnancy are periods of maternal anabolism with increased fat stores, promoted in part by the relative hyperinsulinism. Plasma glucagon concentrations are suppressed more following a meal than in the non-pregnant state, probably contributing to the more prolonged hyperglycemia and hyperinsulinemia after a meal (Freinkel *et al.*, 1974). Freinkel has called this 'facilitated anabolism'.

Many of the effects on maternal metabolism in the latter half of pregnancy are mediated via hormones, principally derived from the placenta. Human placental lactogen (hPL) and other hormones antagonistic to insulin, such as estrogen and progesterone, affect maternal glucose and amino acid utilization (Yen, 1973). In late pregnancy hPL stimulates maternal lipolysis, sparing glucose for use by the fetus. There is also decreased hepatic storage and enhanced mobilization of glycogen, maintaining glucose supplies to the fetus.

Not only does the fetoplacental unit secrete hormones that alter maternal metabolism, but it also controls transport and delivery of nutrients to the fetus. Glucose transport across the placenta is by carrier-mediated facilitated diffusion, so that the glucose concentration in the fetus is directly proportional to the maternal blood glucose concentration. The amount of glucose delivered to the fetus also depends on how much glucose is utilized by the placenta for its own function. Ketone bodies (β-hydroxybutyrate and actoacetate) diffuse freely across the placenta and may act as an alternative fuel for the fetus during periods of maternal starvation (Horton & Sadler, 1983). The placenta is impermeable to protein hormones such as insulin, glucagon and growth hormone. Maternal carbohydrate metabolism is homeostatically so well-regulated that fetal glucose concentrations are maintained within narrow limits. However, in the pregnant woman who has diabetes, periods of maternal hyperglycemia lead to fetal hyperglycemia, which can be detrimental in several ways.

31.3 PERINATAL MORBIDITY AND MORTALITY

31.3.1 FETAL DEATH

Although sudden fetal death occurred in 10–30% of diabetic pregnancies in the past, it is now rare in the intensively monitored and supervised pregnancy in a diabetic woman (Gabbe, 1980). Unfortunately, this event can still occur in pregnancies which do not receive optimal care or in whom this care is refused. Unexplained fetal death is seven times more common in diabetic women than nondiabetic women (Lang & Kunzel, 1989). Stillbirths have been associated with vascular disease, poor blood glucose control, hydramnios, fetal macrosomia or pregnancy-induced hypertension, and occur particularly after the 36th week of gestation. Previously it was thought that these fetal deaths could have been due to unnoticed hypoglycemia or asymptomatic undiagnosed diabetic ketoacidosis. However, episodes of severe maternal hypoglycemia have in general been associated with fetal survival and it is therefore unlikely that asymptomatic episodes of hypoglycemia would lead to *in utero* sudden fetal death. Conversely, diabetic ketoacidosis has been associated with perinatal mortality rates of between 50–90% (White, 1971;

Drury *et al.*, 1977). However, the precise cause of many unexpected fetal deaths remains unknown.

31.3.1.1 Fetal hypoxemia, intrauterine growth retardation and fetal death

Extramedullary hematopoeisis has been frequently observed at post-mortem in stillborn infants of diabetic mothers (IDMs), and this has suggested that chronic intrauterine hypoxia may have contributed to the fetal death (Landon & Gabbe, 1988). In studies, using fetal sheep, in which hyperinsulinemia is induced by direct infusion of glucose or insulin into the fetus, the high fetal insulin concentrations lead to increased glucose and oxygen uptake across the umbilical cord, hypoxia, acidosis and fetal death (Phillips *et al.*, 1982; Susa *et al.*, 1984). A similar phenomenon occurs in human pregnancies if large quantities of glucose are infused intravenously during labor, neonatal hypoxia and acidosis occur with increased frequency (Kenepp *et al.*, 1982; Lawrence *et al.*, 1982). There is also evidence of a relationship between reduced uteroplacental blood flow and poor maternal metabolic control (Nylund *et al.*, 1982), and the diabetic placenta has a decreased villous surface area (Bjork & Persson, 1982 & 1984). Cordocentesis has recently been used to demonstrate hypoxemia directly by measuring PO_2 in cord blood from a human diabetic pregnancy (Bradley *et al.*, 1988). Kirkinen and Jouppila (1983) using quantitative doppler measurements found low blood flow rates on the fetal side of the placenta in diabetic women with severe vascular complications and with evidence of intrauterine growth retardation. Studies using qualitative measurement of umbilical blood flow (doppler waveforms) have not found any differences between uncomplicated insulin-dependent diabetic pregnancies and nondiabetic pregnancies (Landon *et al.*, 1989; Johnstone *et al.*, 1991). Higher resistance doppler waveforms have been demonstrated in diabetic women with nephropathy, established hypertension and pregnancy-induced hypertension (Landon *et al.*, 1989; Kofinas *et al.*, 1990; Johnstone *et al.*, 1992), and these conditions are associated with intrauterine growth retardation and an increased risk of fetal death.

Ketoacidosis and pre-eclampsia have been reported to reduce uterine blood flow and Johnstone and Steel (1992) have demonstrated a relationship between blood glucose control, estimated by glycated hemoglobin concentrations, and uterine artery doppler waveforms. Poor metabolic control may also detrimentally affect placental function in addition to the effects on fetal oxygenation and growth. These data suggest that at least a proportion of unexpected fetal deaths may be caused by maternal hyperglycemia, leading to fetal hyperinsulinemia, an increase in fetal metabolic rate resulting in hypoxia and acidosis. This situation may be worsened by other factors which will also reduce utero-placental blood flow and explain the association between intrauterine death and pre-eclampsia and maternal vascular disease in diabetic pregnancies.

31.3.2 CONGENITAL ABNORMALITIES

In recent years, with the reduction in unexpected intrauterine deaths, birth injuries, and respiratory distress syndrome, congenital anomalies have become the most important cause of perinatal mortality. Congenital anomalies occur 2–5 times more frequently in the offspring of women who have diabetes and are currently the most frequent cause of perinatal mortality (Simpson *et al.*, 1983; Mills *et al.*, 1988). Whatever the insult to the developing fetus of the diabetic mother that causes malformations, it must occur before the seventh week of gestation (Mills *et al.*, 1979). There is a large diversity in the type of congenital anomalies reported in infants of diabetic mothers (IDMs) and analysis of data from many studies has revealed no specific anomaly purely reported in IDMs. The most frequent types of anomalies involve the central nervous system, cardiovascular, gastrointestinal, genito-urinary, and skeletal systems. Malformations of the central nervous system can involve any aspect of the neural axis, and neural tube defects are increased in IDMs compared to nondiabetic pregnancies (Pinter & Reece, 1988). There is also an increase in the rate of cardiac malformations in IDMs. Genitourinary anomalies may exist in isolation or in combination with other congenital abnormalities including duodenal atresia, Potter facies, and Meckel's diverticulum (Crooij *et al.*, 1982). Gastrointestinal abnormalities can occur throughout the gastrointestinal tract and may co-exist with other malformations. Skeletal abnormalities also occur and include sacral hypoplasia and agenesis, which is a rare condition which can occasionally occur in infants of nondiabetic mothers but is particularly increased in IDM (Mills *et al.*, 1979; Mills, 1982).

A number of different hypotheses have been raised in an attempt to explain the increased incidence of congenital anomalies in diabetic pregnancies. Unfortunately, the search for the precise teratogenic agent(s) causing diabetes-related congenital anomalies is hampered by the fact that diabetes is not a simple disorder of carbohydrate metabolism, but involves abnormalities in lipid and protein metabolism in addition. Among the hypotheses that have been proposed are: maternal hyperglycemia and poor metabolic control, maternal hypoglycemia, fetal hyperinsulinemia, uteroplacental vascular disease, and genetic factors. At the present time, the metabolic sequelae of maternal hyperglycemia occurring during early embryonic development are thought to be the primary teratogens.

31.3.2.1 Genetic factors

It is unlikely that a genetic predisposition is the primary cause of the increase in congenital malformations in IDMs, principally because there is no increase in the rate of malformations in infants of diabetic fathers and nondiabetic mothers, in contrast to the infants of diabetic mothers (Neave, 1984). However, it may be that a genetic predisposition could contribute if another teratogen is present.

31.3.2.2 Insulin

Insulin has also been proposed as a teratogen in the IDM, but fetal pancreatic β cells do not elaborate insulin until about 12 weeks of gestation, which is beyond the period of organogenesis, and maternal insulin does not cross the placenta in any substantial amount (Steinke & Driscoll, 1965; Kalhan *et al.*, 1975).

31.3.2.3 Vascular disease

Many years ago it was suggested that hypoxia caused by vascular disease may further augment the teratogenic effect of the altered metabolism, and that renal impairment may lead to delayed clearance of maternal toxins, both contributing to the teratogenic effect of hyperglycemia (Pedersen *et al.*, 1964). Pedersen (1977) found an increase in the rate of congenital abnormalities with increasing duration and severity of diabetes (according to White's classification (Table 31.1)), but others have not confirmed these findings. There is no relationship between duration of diabetes or microvascular disease and congenital abnormalities.

31.3.2.4 Hyperglycemia

Results from experimental and clinical studies support the current belief that disruption of developmental processes by metabolic perturbations, principally hyper-

Table 31.1 Simplified White's classification of insulin-dependent pregnant diabetic mothers.

White's classification	Age at onset of diabetes (yrs)		Duration of diabetes (yrs)	Complications
B	$\geqslant 20$	and	<10	Absent
C	10–19	or	10–19	Absent
D	<10	or	$\geqslant 20$	Background retinopathy
F				Nephropathy
R				Proliferative retinopathy

glycemia, cause the diabetes-related congenital anomalies seen in the IDM. Animal studies and whole embryo culture techniques have substantiated the teratogenic effects of elevated glucose concentrations. In pregnant rats who have had diabetes induced by streptozotocin on day six of gestation, a critical time for fusion of the neural tube, lumbar and sacral defects developed, but if diabetes was induced after day 6 or if blood glucose was reduced with insulin therapy there was no increase in the rate of malformations (Baker *et al.*, 1981). Rat embryos cultured in high concentrations of D-glucose exhibited neural tube defects (Cockroft & Coppola, 1977; Reece & Hobbins, 1986), and other studies have verified this effect and demonstrated growth retardation in addition to the teratogenesis (Goldman *et al.*, 1985; Pinter *et al.*, 1986).

A number of mechanisms have been suggested which may lead to the teratogenic effects related to maternal hyperglycemia. Inhibition of glycolysis has been suggested as one cause because D-mannose added to rat embryo cultures inhibited glycolysis and caused growth retardation and abnormal neural tube closure (Freinkel *et al.*, 1984). Goldman *et al.* (1985) have suggested that a functional deficiency of arachidonic acid may cause the increased incidence of anomalies in embryos cultured in hyperglycemic media. The addition of arachidonic acid to these rat and mouse embryo cultures prevents the anomalies induced by hyperglycemic culture media (Goldman *et al.*, 1985; Pinter *et al.*, 1986). Addition of prostaglandins, the products of the arachidonic acid cascade, can reverse the neural tube fusion defect in mouse embryos in hyperglycaemic culture media (Goldman *et al.*, 1989; Baker *et al.*, 1990; Goto *et al.*, 1992). Although hyperglycemia may be a major factor in the initiation of diabetic embryopathy, many studies suggest that other factors besides glucose *per se* are involved in the etiology of the diabetes-related congenital anomalies (Freinkel *et al.*, 1986; Sadler *et al.*, 1989). The concentrations of D-glucose required to produce anomalies in rodents in culture are much higher than in diabetic serum which has a similar effect to culture in artificial hyperglycemic media (Goldman *et al.*, 1985; Sadler *et al.*, 1989). β-hydroxybutyrate and somatomedin inhibitor, both of which are present in diabetic serum in elevated but subteratogenic levels, appear to act synergistically with D-glucose to result in a high incidence of anomalies and growth retardation in cultured rodent embryos (Freinkel *et al.*, 1986; Sadler *et al.*, 1989). The present data therefore suggest that a deficiency of prostaglandins as a result of inhibition of the arachidonic acid cascade may be the cause of hyperglycemia/diabetic serum-induced anomalies. One possible explanation of how hyperglycemia leads to a deficiency of prostaglandins is the involvement of *myo*-inositol as a primary defect in the mechanism. Glucose reduces *myo*-inositol uptake by cultured rat conceptuses in a dose-dependent fashion (Weigensberg *et al.*, 1990), and a deficiency of *myo*-inositol is reported in both animal and human diabetes. In rat embryos malformed by hyperglycemia, the tissue content of *myo*-inositol is reduced (Weigensberg *et al.*, 1990), and the anomalies are prevented by the addition of *myo*-inositol to the culture medium (Hod *et al.*, 1986; Baker *et al.*, 1990; Hashimoto *et al.*, 1990).

Clinical studies using glycated hemoglobin to assess recent blood glucose control have shown that a higher rate of anomalies occur in diabetic women who have higher glycated hemoglobin concentrations in the first trimester, indicating poorer glycemic control (Leslie *et al.*, 1978; Miller *et al.*, 1981). Miller *et al.* (1981) found that congenital anomalies correlated with the glycated hemoglobin concentration rather than with the White classification, in contrast to earlier studies (Pedersen *et al.*, 1964; Karlsson & Kjellmer, 1972).

If abnormalities are caused by hyperglycemia in early pregnancy it should be possible to prevent them by improved control. Table 31.2 shows the estimated time after ovulation at which congenital anomalies are thought to develop. The concept of pre-pregnancy care was first described by Steel *et al.* (1980) and elaborated in 1985 (Steel, 1985). The first study demonstrating a reduction in the incidence of congenital anomalies was that of Fuhrmann *et al.* (1983). Another study demonstrated that one group of insulin-dependent diabetic women in whom the insulin dose had been carefully adjusted preconceptually had no malformed offspring, while there was a malformation rate of 9.6% in a similar group of women who had not received the benefit of intensive insulin therapy (Goldman *et al.*, 1986). Attendance of diabetic women at a pre-pregnancy clinic, in an attempt to achieve tight control of blood glucose prior to conception, reduces the rate of congenital anomalies from 10.4% in those who did not attend pre-pregnancy counseling (mean HbA_1 10.5%) to 1.4% in those who attended pre-pregnancy counseling (mean HbA_1 8.4%) (Steel *et al.*, 1990; Kitzmiller *et al.*, 1991). In contrast, tight glycemic control started after the end of the first trimester improves other types of morbidity in the IDM but does not decrease the rate of congenital anomalies (Ballard *et al.*, 1984). These studies reinforce the importance of instituting optimal glycemic control in diabetic women prior to conception.

Table 31.2 Approximate timing of the initial development of congenital anomalies in IDDM.

Weeks after ovulation	Congenital anomaly
1	
2	
3	Caudal regression
4	Spina bifida
	Hydrocephalus
	Anencephalus
	Situs inversus
5	Transposition of great vessels
	Renal abnormalities
6	Ventricular septal defects
	Anal/rectal atresia

31.3.2.5 Hypoglycemia

Although the main cause of congenital abnormalities in the infant of the diabetic mother is thought to be hyperglycemia, there are some reports of congenital anomalies in rodent offspring following maternal hypoglycemia during the phase of organogenesis. The only reports of hypoglycemia as a possible cause of congenital anomalies originated from pregnancies in psychiatric patients who had been treated with insulin shock therapy for schizophrenia and depression (Sobel, 1960). In a review of the literature at that time Sobel (1960) reported 17 nondiabetic women who had been rendered comatose during insulin-induced hypoglycemia as part of their psychiatric therapy, six of whom suffered 'fetal damage'. Two of the six were spontaneous abortions, two were macerated fetuses with no evidence of congenital anomalies. The other two fetuses had congenital anomalies but one of the mothers did not receive insulin shock therapy until after the 14th week of gestation, leaving only one case in which an abnormality could possibly have been related to hypoglycemia.

Freinkel *et al.* (1983) has suggested that interference with the glycolytic process may result in congenital anomalies, and because of this it was suggested that hypoglycemia during early pregnancy could impair organ development by limiting the availability of glucose for obligate glycolysis at critical points in organogenesis (Freinkel *et al.*, 1985). In rats, maternal hypoglycemia led to fetal growth retardation and a small but significant incidence of gross developmental anomalies compared with the rat embryos from mothers kept euglycemic during the same level of insulin infusion, suggesting that the effect was due to hypoglycemia *per se* rather than insulin (Buchanan *et al.*, 1986). This finding was supported by work from Japan, in which rat embryos exposed to hypoglycemic serum manifested growth retardation and an increased frequency of neural tube defects (Akazawa *et al.*, 1987). The embryos exposed to hypoglycemia in this study (Akazawa *et al.*, 1987) demonstrated decreased glucose uptake and lactic acid formation, indicating decreased energy production via glycolysis, and this supports the suggestion that the defects might be mediated via metabolic interruption of embryogenesis. Continued work in this area using isolated rat embryo culture has demonstrated that the phase of organogenesis which is susceptible to the effects of hypoglycemia is equivalent to days 32–38 of development in human pregnancies (Buchanan & Sipos, 1989). Other studies from Japan have suggested that the effect of hypoglycemia on teratogenesis in the rat embryo may be enhanced by culture in hyperglycemic media (Akazawa *et al.*, 1989; Tanigawa *et al.*, 1991).

So far there have been no reports suggesting a relationship between hypoglycemia in early pregnancy and congenital anomalies in humans, and studies in rats may not be relevant in humans. In a detailed study of hypoglycemia in early pregnancy in eight insulin-dependent diabetic women, Bergman *et al.* (1986) found no abnormalities, and the Diabetes in Early Pregnancy prospective study of Mills *et al.* (1988) examined 347 insulin-dependent diabetic women over the period of organogenesis and found no relationship between the incidence of malformations and the frequency of hypoglycemia in the mothers. In a more recent study Kitzmiller *et al.* (1991) prospectively studied 84 diabetic women recruited prior to conception; 34 of these women reported mild symptomatic hypoglycemia and two had severe hypoglycemia but both delivered normal babies, while only one of the women who had experienced mild hypoglycemia delivered an abnormal child. These studies do not support the hypothesis that maternal hypoglycemia may cause congenital anomalies in human pregnancies. However, if the glycolytic dependency evident in rat embryos exists in early human pregnancy, human embryos, during a limited period of dependency on glycolysis (from 19–24 days post-ovulation), would also be susceptible to hypoglycemia. Although the studies discussed earlier have not disclosed a relationship between hypoglycemia and an increased incidence of congenital anomalies, these studies have not focused closely upon the susceptible period (i.e., under 3 weeks' gestation). In a prospective study of 88 IDDs from Edinburgh of maternal hypoglycemia occurring between 28–42 days of pregnancy (dated from first scan), which covers the time when rat conceptuses are susceptible to damage by hypoglycemia, 37 women had experienced hypoglycemia during this period. In 12 cases, the hypoglycemia was severe and none of these women delivered abnormal babies, and none of the four women who delivered babies with abnormalities had experienced hypoglycemia over the susceptible time period.

Current evidence therefore supports the hypothesis that congenital anomalies arising in IDMs principally occur as a result of maternal hyperglycemia, most likely due to effects on inhibition of glycolysis and functional deficiency of arachidonic acid. Hypoglycemia almost certainly does not cause fetal abnormalities but is of potential danger to the mother. It seems reasonable to individualize prescribed blood glucose targets, aiming at controlling the blood glucose in pregnant diabetic women as tightly as possible without causing a high risk of hypoglycemia.

31.3.3 MACROSOMIA

Fetal macrosomia, defined as a birth weight in excess of the 90th percentile when corrected for gestational age, occurs in approximately 30% of pregnancies in insulin-dependent women (Beard & Lowy, 1982), and may be associated with an increase in perinatal morbidity and mortality (Sack, 1969; Cowett & Schwartz, 1982; Stevenson *et al.*, 1982). If undetected before delivery, macrosomia may complicate vaginal delivery and lead to neonatal asphyxia and/or birth injuries, such as subdural hematoma, cephalhematoma, facial palsy, clavicular fracture, and brachial plexus injuries (Cowett & Schwartz, 1982). Diaphragmatic paralysis can result from damage to the phrenic nerve, and organomegaly may be associated with hemorrhage into the abdominal organs during delivery, particularly the liver and adrenal glands.

It has been suggested that maternal hyperglycemia in the third trimester of pregnancy allows abnormal quantities of glucose to cross the placenta by facilitated diffusion, thereby stimulating the fetal placenta to secrete insulin and render the fetus hyperinsulinemic. This forms the basis of the Pedersen hypothesis (Pedersen, 1954), which states that maternal hyperglycemia stimulates the fetal pancreas to secrete excess insulin, which produces adiposity and macrosomia (Figure 31.3). However, the mechanism by which insulin stimulates fetal growth is not yet clear. Insulin may produce its effect by altering metabolic substrate entry into cells, leading to anabolic processes such as lipogenesis, glycogenesis and protein synthesis. Conversely, insulin may exert its effects via other endocrine, paracrine, and autocrine systems, which then produce growth factors which stimulate growth. It has been postulated that insulin-like growth factors (IGFs) may play a role in the development of the macrosomic infant but recent evidence does not support this, with no elevation of IGF levels in macrosomic IDMs (Hill *et al.*, 1989). There is evidence now available which suggests that the Pedersen hypothesis should be modified to include additional metabolic fuels (e.g., amino acids and fatty acids) as causal agents for macrosomia (Kalkhoff *et al.*, 1988). It is of interest that the incidence of macrosomia is much reduced in IDMs whose mothers have vascular disease, hypertension and nephropathy, probably related to poor vascular supply and damage to the placental vascular

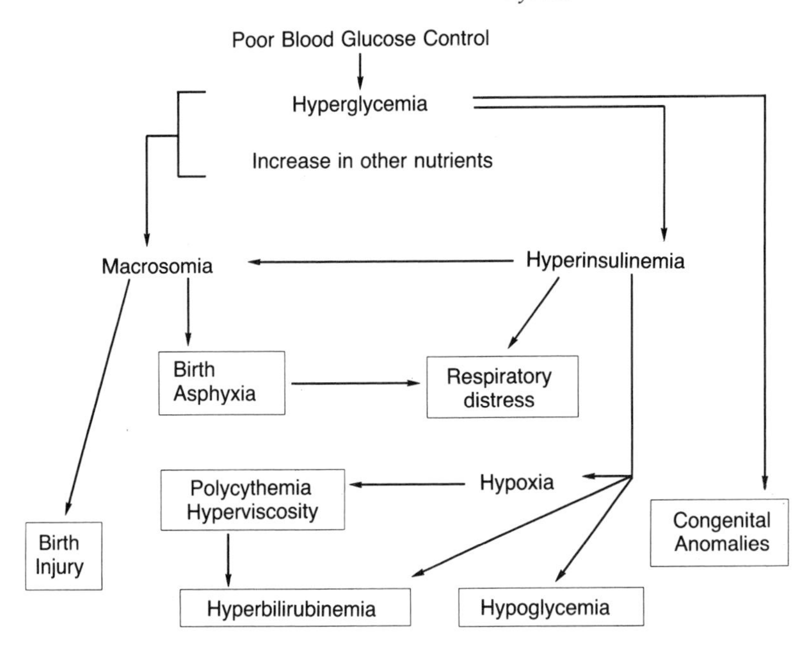

Figure 31.3 Schematic diagram of the causal factors and relationship between the major complications in IDM.

bed. In these cases the IDM is more likely to be growth retarded and poor maternal glycemic control in this situation does not encourage macrosomia.

It is generally thought that maintenance of good maternal blood glucose control exerts a favorable effect on macrosomia, preventing or slowing its further development. However, this remains controversial, with some studies reporting persistence of macrosomia despite apparent maternal 'normoglycemia' (Verhaaren *et al.*, 1984; Dandonna *et al.*, 1984; Visser *et al.*, 1984; Small *et al.*, 1987), while other studies report that meticulous efforts to achieve tight glycemic control can normalize birth weights in IDMs (Gabbe *et al.*, 1977; Coustan *et al.*, 1980; Jovanovic *et al.*, 1981). Although pregnant diabetic women may be attaining preprandial (fasting) blood glucose concentrations which are near normal, evidence is now available that postprandial (peak) blood glucose values are still elevated above those seen in nondiabetic women. These peak blood glucose levels are more predictive of the infant birth weight than preprandial measurements (Jovanic-Peterson *et al.*, 1991), a finding which is still consistent with the Pedersen hypothesis and continues to implicate glucose as a causal factor for macrosomia. This finding may in part explain the observation of macrosomia occurring in the IDMs of apparently 'normoglycemic' mothers whose preprandial blood glucose values are near normal, who may have higher undetected postprandial glucose peaks. However, other as yet unknown factors probably play a role because, although the swings in maternal blood glucose concentrations are less marked in mothers with gestational diabetes, there remains a relatively high incidence of macrosomia in their infants. Jovanovic-Peterson *et al.* (1991) also found evidence that maternal glycemic control in early and midgestation may influence the extent of fetal β cell hyperplasia and set the stage for the development of macrosomia in the context of continuing hyperglycemia in the third trimester. Although absolute blood glucose levels and swings are related to the development of macrosomia there must be other factors. Insulin antibodies have been suggested but infants of mothers treated with human insulin are no smaller than those treated with animal insulins.

31.3.4 RESPIRATORY DISTRESS SYNDROME

Respiratory distress, including the respiratory distress syndrome (RDS), used to be a frequent and potentially serious complication arising in the IDM. Lack of surfactant produced by Type II pneumocytes, which normally decreases surface tension at the air-to-alveolar interface, results in pulmonary atelectasis and thereby the cardinal signs of the disease. Respiratory distress syndrome develops because of lung immaturity and remains a major potential cause of mortality in the newborn, even though recently surfactant has become available for the treatment of this condition (Figure 31.3).

In a study of 934 pregnancies in diabetic women between 1940 and 1956 from the Joslin Clinic, 30.5% of viable infants developed respiratory distress clinically (Gellis & Hsia, 1959). In this cohort of patients, 95 of 104 infants who died were studied pathologically and 70% had evidence of hyaline membrane disease (RDS) (Driscoll *et al.*, 1960). Robert *et al.* (1976) compared 805 IDM with 10 512 infants of nondiabetic mothers, and found respiratory distress syndrome was nearly 24 times as likely in the IDM than in the infant of a nondiabetic mother. A major advance in the diagnosis and management of RDS was made by Gluck and Kulovich (1973) who recognized that lecithin/sphingomyelin (L/S) ratios in amniotic fluid were predictive of fetal lung maturation. However, there is delayed L/S maturation in patients with diabetes in White's classes A, B and C, whereas an accelerated maturation occurs in patients of classes D, E and F (Gluck & Kulovich, 1973). As a result, even when the L/S ratio equals 2.0, usually indicative of lung maturity, there may be an increased frequency of 'false positives' in all diabetic classes. An improvement in the diagnostic assessment of fetal lung maturity has been provided by estimation of phosphatidylglycerol (PG), one of the phospholipids in the lung which serves as an important role in maintaining alveolar stability. In the IDM, for unknown reasons, there is delayed maturation of PG synthesis so that the L/S ratio may be normal but with a lack of PG, with the potential for development of RDS. The best method of assessing the degree of fetal lung maturation is to analyze both the L/S ratio and PG levels. Even if the L/S ratio is 2.0 or greater the IDM should not be delivered until PG appears (Hallman & Teramo, 1979).

Over the last decade the L/S ratio has more rarely been measured as the risk of respiratory distress syndrome developing has fallen so dramatically with institution of optimal maternal glycemic control.

31.3.5 NEONATAL HYPOGLYCEMIA

Neonatal hypoglycemia is the most common metabolic complication experienced by the IDM and is diagnosed in term infants when the plasma glucose concentration is less than 1.8 mmol/l or less than 1.3 mmol/l in a preterm infant. The peak onset for hypoglycemia in IDMs is between 60–90 minutes after delivery and while many hypoglycemic IDMs may be asymptomatic, others manifest non-specific signs including jitteriness, tachypnea, apnea, twitching of the limbs, hypotonia, or even severe convulsions.

Hypoglycemia must be confirmed by determination of the plasma glucose concentration, initially performed at the cotside using a semiquantitative method, such as a glucose stick read by a glucose meter, and verified in the laboratory. Initially, all IDMs should have cotside glucose estimations performed hourly for the first six hours of life. Ideally, neonatal hypoglycemia should be prevented by early feeding, and initial treatment if this fails should be with oral glucose solutions. If it is not possible to correct it by oral glucose, neonatal hypoglycemia should be treated with an intravenous infusion of dextrose in a dose of 5–6 mg/kg/min. Bolus administration of hypertonic dextrose should be avoided because of the resulting stimulation of hyperinsulinemia and the risk of rebound hypoglycemia. In most instances, neonatal hypoglycemia in the IDM is transient but occasionally hypoglycemia may persist beyond the first three days of life and may require the use of other agents such as glucocorticoids.

A number of factors are known to contribute to neonatal hypoglycemia (Figure 31.3), the most important being fetal hyperinsulinemia at birth, caused by maternal hyperglycemia, leading to suppression of endogenous glucose production in the IDM (Kalhan *et al.*, 1977). Hence, prior maternal glucose homeostasis and maternal blood glucose control at and immediately prior to delivery are important (Cowett & Stern, 1987). Another possible contributory cause for neonatal hypoglycemia may be delayed maturation of glucose counterregulatory mechanisms (Cowett *et al.*, 1983). The prognosis for IDMs who develop hypoglycemia is usually favorable with no neurological sequelae, and it is unlikely that the occasional delay in motor development or psychological dysfunction observed after five years of life is related to neonatal hypoglycemia.

31.3.6 HYPOCALCEMIA, HYPOMAGNESEMIA AND HYPOKALEMIA

Hypocalcemia is another metabolic complication experienced by the IDM. The fetus usually has a higher concentration of calcium in the blood than the mother resulting in stimulation of calcitonin secretion. At birth, the combination of the relatively high calcitonin levels and the abrupt cessation of the supply of calcium from the mother leads to a fall in serum calcium. The reduction in neonatal serum calcium results in parathyroid hormone (PTH) and 1,25 dihydroxyvitamin D-induced calcium counterregulation thereby leading to restoration of serum calcium to normal. Approximately 50% of IDMs develop hypocalcemia within the first three days of life (Tsang *et al.*, 1979). This may be due to failure of PTH concentrations to rise appropriately in response to hypocalcemia, which has been observed in IDMs and is thought to be related to coexistent hypomagnesemia (Noguchi *et al.*, 1980). There may also more rarely be a fall in serum potassium in the fetus, caused by the effects of hyperinsulinemia and hypoglycemia, which could lead to cardiac arrhythmias (Jovanovic-Peterson & Peterson, 1992).

31.3.7 HYPERBILIRUBINEMIA, POLYCYTHEMIA AND HYPOXEMIA

Hyperbilirubinemia is another recognized complication in the IDM and was originally thought to occur because of prematurity. This is a factor but since jaundice is more common in IDMs than in age-matched normal infants, its exact pathogenesis remains uncertain. It has been suggested by Peevy *et al.* (1980) that only macrosomic IDMs are at risk of hyperbilirubinemia, with increased haem turnover a factor in its development. However, the main factor associated with hyperbilirubinemia in the IDM is likely to be polycythemia, diagnosed when venous hematocrit is greater than 65% (Figure 31.3). The incidence of polycythemia in IDMs used to be between 20% and 40%, and is sometimes associated with signs which include plethora, seizures, jitteriness, tachypnea, oliguria and priapism. Very rarely it may be necessary to initiate partial exchange transfusion, which will usually lead to a rapid resolution of signs. It has been demonsrated that fetal erythropoietin concentrations at delivery are related to antepartum maternal blood glucose control, assessed by glycated hemoglobin estimation (Widness *et al.*, 1990). Elevated fetal erythropoietin concentrations have been shown to be correlated with neonatal hyperinsulinemia (Widness *et al.*, 1981), which, as discussed earlier, is associated with poor maternal blood glucose control. Chronic hyperglycemia induced in fetal sheep by the constant infusion of glucose through an implanted catheter, results in increased oxygen consumption and a decrease in distal aortic arterial oxygen content (Carson *et al.*, 1980). This effect has been confirmed by Milley *et al.* (1984), who demonstrated that the hypoxemia produced by hyperinsulinemia was due to increased fetal extraction of available oxygen. In parallel studies, Philipps *et al.* (1982 & 1984) demonstrated the same phenomenon, and in some of the studies PO_2 fell to life-threatening levels in their fetal sheep so that the glucose infusion had to be discontinued. This phenomenon may explain anecdotal reports of decreased fetal movements in parallel with transient maternal hyperglycemia. It is therefore likely that poor maternal blood glucose control may lead to fetal hypoxemia resulting in increased erythropoietin secretion and thereby polycythemia (Figure 31.3). Polycythemia may be one factor in the increased incidence of the rare complication of renal vein thrombosis (Takeuchi & Benirschke, 1961) or other venous thromboses.

31.3.8 LONG-TERM OUTLOOK FOR THE IDM

The intrauterine environment imparts effects which are apparent at birth, and it has been suggested from anthropometric, neurologic and metabolic standpoints, that there are differences in IDMs from their peers (Freinkel, 1980).

31.3.8.1 Growth

Evidence suggests that the intrauterine environment can play a role in the development of heavy-for-height children. However, evidence from studies is conflicting with some studies reporting the children of women with diabetes being taller and heavier than standard charts (Breidahl, 1966; Adler *et al.*, 1977), although other studies have not reported any deviation from normal (Farquhar, 1959; Weitz & Laron, 1976; Farquhar, 1969). Hagbard *et al.* (1959) found that children of diabetic mothers were shorter and heavier than normals, while children of prediabetic women were no different from normals. Vohr *et al.* (1980) observed that macrosomic infants born to diabetic women were more likely to be obese in childhood and adolescence than normal birth weight infants. Evidence from Pima Indians, who have a high incidence of type 2 diabetes, suggests that the diabetic intrauterine environment is a causal factor of long-term obesity in IDMs (Pettitt *et al.*, 1987).

31.3.8.2 Glucose tolerance

Although the development of diabetes is multifactorial, there is a genetic component, and there are reports of high rates of diabetes in the offspring of people with diabetes. The effect of the diabetic intrauterine environment must therefore be considered in the context of the genetic background. In Pima Indians, diabetes occurred more commonly in offspring of women who developed diabetes before pregnancy than in offspring of women who developed diabetes after pregnancy or not at all (Pettitt, 1986). It is not clear if this operates in IDDM, in fact some studies suggest the opposite in that IDDM is commoner in offspring when the father is diabetic than when the mother is diabetic. One possible explanation for this observation is the mechanism of genetic imprinting with a gene from the mother being inactivated.

31.3.8.3 Neurologic outcome

There are a number of reasons why neurologic problems may occur in the children of diabetic women, including: more birth trauma and hypoxia, metabolic abnormalities *in utero* which may disturb neurologic development, neonatal hyperbilirubinemia leading to kernicterus, and neonatal hypoglycemia which may lead to permanent cognitive dysfunction. Two studies have observed an association between ketonuria during pregnancy and lower IQ in the offspring (Churchill *et al.*, 1969; Stehbens *et al.*, 1977), and in the study by Stehbens *et al.* (1977) low birth weight was also predictive of a lower IQ, but both studies have been criticized. However, in a recent study which excluded confounding variables, such as maternal obstetric complications and intrauterine growth retardation, the mental developmental index of the children studied correlated inversely with the mothers' plasma β-hydroxybutyrate levels (Rizzo *et al.*, 1991). This association between ketonemia in mothers with diabetes during pregnancy and altered neurologic scores in their children increases the importance of continued efforts to avoid ketoacidosis and accelerated starvation in all pregnant women. IDMs who experienced hypoglycemia in the neonatal period failed to show any relationship between neonatal hypoglycemia and any reduction in IQ (Persson & Gentz, 1984). There was also no association between severe hypoglycemia in the mother and IQ in the offspring (Churchill *et al.*, 1969). Several studies have failed to demonstrate any reduction in IQ in offspring of diabetic mothers who have received up-to-date medical and obstetric care, with meticulous blood glucose control throughout pregnancy (Cummins & Norrish, 1980; Persson & Gentz, 1984).

31.3.9 FUTURE DIRECTIONS

Rigorous control of diabetes during pregnancy and improved obstetric management have been shown to decrease infant mortality and morbidity. It is fairly clear that congenital anomalies can be reduced by preconception counselling and care. There is a need to target those women who are least likely to seek this type of care of their own volition. It will be necessary to develop new ways of treating diabetes before ideal diabetic control can be achieved before and throughout pregnancy which will prevent the fetus from recognizing that the mother has diabetes.

REFERENCES

Adler, P., Fett, K.D. and Bohåtka, L. (1977) The influence of maternal diabetes on dental development of the non-diabetic offspring in the stage of transitional dentition. *Acta Paediatr. Acad. Sci. Hung.*, **8**, 181–95.

Akazawa, S., Akazawa, M., Hashimoto, M. *et al.* (1987) Effects of hypoglycemia on early embryogenesis in rat embryo organ culture. *Diabetologia*, **30**, 791–96.

Akazawa, M., Akazawa, S., Hashimoto, M. *et al.* (1989) Effects of brief exposure to insulin-induced hypoglycemic serum during organogenesis in rat embryo culture. *Diabetes*, **38**, 1573–78.

Baker, L., Egler, J.M., Klein, S.H. *et al.* (1981) Meticulous control of diabetes during organogenesis prevents congenital lumbosacral defects in rats. *Diabetes*, **30**, 955–59.

Baker, L., Piddington, R., Goldman, A. *et al.*

(1990) *Myo*-inositol and prostaglandins reverse the glucose inhibition of neural-tube fusion in cultured mouse embryos. *Diabetologia*, **33**, 593–96.

Ballard, J.L., Holroyde, J., Tsang, R.C. *et al.* (1984) High malformation rates and decreased mortality in infants of diabetic mothers managed after the first trimester (1956–1978). *Am. J. Obstet. Gynecol.*, **155**, 111–18.

Beard, R.W. and Lowy, C. (1982) The British survey of diabetic pregnancies. *Br. J. Obstet. Gynaecol.*, **89**, 783–86.

Bergman, M., Seaton, T.B., Auerhahn, C.C. *et al.* (1986) The incidence of gestational hypoglycemia in insulin-dependent diabetic and non-insulin-dependent diabetic women. *New York State J. Med.*, **86**, 174–77.

Bjork, O. and Persson, B. (1982) Placental changes in relation to the degree of metabolic control in diabetes mellitus. *Placenta*, **3**, 367–78.

Bjork, O. and Persson, B. (1984) Villous structure in different parts of the cotyledon in placentas of insulin-dependent diabetic women. A morphometric study. *Am. J. Obstet. Gynecol.*, **121**, 789–94.

Bradley, R.J., Nicolaides, K.H., Brudenell, J.M. *et al.* (1988) Early diagnosis of chronic fetal hypoxia in a diabetic pregnancy. *Br. Med. J.*, **296**, 94–95.

Breidahl, H.D. (1966) The growth and development of children born to mothers with diabetes. *Med. J. Aust.*, **1**, 268–70.

Buchanan, T.A., Schemmer, J.K. and Freinkel, N. (1986) Embryotoxic effects of brief maternal insulin-hypoglycemia during organogenesis in the rat. *J. Clin. Invest.*, **78**, 643–49.

Buchanan, T.A. and Sipos, G.F. (1989) Lack of teratogenic effect of brief maternal insulin-induced hypoglycemia in rats during late neurulation. *Diabetes*, **38**, 1063–66.

Carson, B.S., Philipps, A.F., Simmons, M.A. *et al.* (1980) Effects of a sustained insulin infusion upon glucose uptake and oxygenation of the ovine fetus. *Pediatr. Res.*, **14**, 147–52.

Churchill, J.A., Berendes, H.W. and Nemore, J. (1969) Neuropsychological deficits in children of diabetic mothers. *Am. J. Obstet. Gynecol.*, **105**, 257–68.

Cockroft, D.L. and Coppola, P.T. (1977) Teratogenic effects of excess glucose on head-fold rat embryos in culture. *Teratology*, **16**, 141–46.

Coustan, D.R., Berkowitz, R.L. and Hobbins, J.C. (1980) Tight metabolic control of overt diabetes in pregnancy. *Am. J. Med.*, **68**, 845–52.

Cowett, R.M. and Schwartz, R. (1982) The infant of the diabetic mother. *Pediatr. Clin. North Am.*, **29**, 1213–31.

Cowett, R.M., Oh, W., Schwartz, J. *et al.* (1983) Persistent glucose production during infusion in the neonate. *J. Clin. Invest.*, **71**, 467–73.

Cowett, R.M. and Stern, L. (1987) 'Carbohydrate homeostasis in the fetus and newborn', in G. Avery (ed.). *Neonatology, Pathophysiology and Management of the Newborn*, pp. 691–709. Lippincott & Co, Philadelphia.

Crooij, M.G., Westhuis, M., Schoemaker, J. *et al.* (1982) Ultrasonographic measurement of the yolk sac. *Br. J. Obstet. Gynaecol.*, **89**, 931–34.

Cummins, M. and Norrish, M. (1980) Follow-up of children of diabetic mothers. *Arch. Dis. Child.*, **55**, 259–64.

Dandonna, P., Besterman, H.S., Freedman, D.B. *et al.* (1984) Macrosomia despite well-controlled diabetic pregnancy. *Lancet*, **i**, 737.

DeLee, J.B. (1920) *The principles and practice of obstetrics*, 3rd edn. W.B. Saunders, Philadelphia.

Driscoll, S.G., Benirschke, K. and Curtis, G.W. (1960) Neonatal deaths among infants of diabetic mothers. *Am. J. Dis. Child.*, **100**, 818–35.

Drury, M.I., Greene, A.T. and Stronge, J.M. (1977) Pregnancy complicated by clinical diabetes mellitus: a study of 600 pregnancies. *Obstet. Gynecol.*, **49**, 519–22.

Farquhar, J.W. (1959) The child of the diabetic woman. *Arch. Dis. Child.*, **34**, 76–96.

Farquhar, J.W. (1969) Prognosis for babies born to diabetic mothers in Edinburgh. *Arch. Dis. Child.*, **44**, 36–47.

Fisher, P.M., Hamilton, P.M., Sutherland, H.W. *et al.* (1974) The effect of pregnancy on intravenous glucose tolerance. *J. Obstet. Gynaecol. Br. Commonw.*, **81**, 285–90.

Freinkel, N. (1980) Banting lecture 1980. Of pregnancy and progeny. *Diabetes*, **29**, 1023–35.

Freinkel, N., Metzger, B.E., Nitzan, M. *et al.* (1974) 'Facilitated anabolism in late pregnancy: some novel maternal compensations for accelerated starvation', in W.J. Malaisse and J. Pirart (eds). *Diabetes*, p. 474. Excerpta Medica, Amsterdam.

Freinkel, N., Lewis, S., Akazawa, S. *et al.* (1983) The ' honey bee' syndrome, teratogenic effects of mannose during organogenesis in the rat embryo culture. *Trans. Assoc. Am. Physicians*, **96**, 44–55.

Freinkel, N., Lewis, N.J., Akazawa, S. *et al.* (1984) The honeybee syndrome: implications of the teratogenicity of mannose in rat-embryo culture. *N. Engl. J. Med.*, **310**, 223–30.

Freinkel, N., Dooley, S.L. and Metzger, B.E. (1985) Care of the pregnant woman with insulin-dependent diabetes mellitus. *N. Engl. J. Med.*, **313**, 96–101.

Freinkel, N., Cockroft, D.L., Lewis, N.J. *et al.* (1986) Fuel-mediated teratogenesis during early organogenesis: the effects of increased concentrations of glucose, ketones, or somatomedin inhibitor during rat embryo culture. *Am. J. Clin. Nutr.*, **44**, 986–95.

Fuhrmann, K., Reiher, H., Semmler, K. *et al.* (1983) Prevention of congenital malformations in infants of insulin-dependent diabetic mothers. *Diabetes Care*, **6**, 219–23.

Gabbe, S.G. (1980) 'Management of diabetes in pregnancy: six decades of experience', in R.M. Pitkin and F. Zlatkin (eds). *The Yearbook of Obstetrics and Gynecology*, pp. 112–121. Chicago, Yearbook Medical Publishers.

Gabbe, S.G., Mestman, J.H., Freeman, R.K. *et al.* (1977) Management and outcome of pregnancy in diabetes mellitus, classes B to R. *Am. J. Obstet. Gynecol.*, **129**, 723–32.

Gellis, S.S. and Hsia, D.Y.Y. (1959) The infant of the diabetic mother. *Am. J. Dis. Child.*, **97**, 1–41.

Gluck, L. and Kulovich, M.W. (1973) Lecithin/shingomyelin ratios in amniotic fluid in normal and abnormal pregnancy. *Am. J. Obstet. Gynecol.*, **115**, 539–46.

Goldman, A.S., Baker, L., Piddington, R. *et al.* (1985) Hyperglycemia-induced teratogenesis is mediated by a functional deficiency of arachidonic acid. *Proc. Natl. Acad. Sci. USA*, **82**, 8227–31.

Goldman, A.S., Kay, E.D. and Goto, M.P. (1989) Prevention of diabetic embryopathy by prostaglandins and lipokinin, a biological activator of phospholipase A_2. *Teratology*, **39**, 455–56 (abstract).

Goldman, J.A., Dicker, D., Felberg, D. *et al.* (1986) Pregnancy outcome in patients with insulin dependent diabetes mellitus with preconceptual diabetes control: a comparative study. *Am. J. Obstet. Gynecol.*, **155**, 293–97.

Goto, M.P., Goldman, A.S. and Uhing, M.R. (1992) PGE_2 prevents anomalies induced by hyperglycemia or diabetic serum in mouse embryos. *Diabetes*, **41**, 1644–50.

Gray, R.S., Cowan, P., Steel, J.M. *et al.* (1984) Insulin action and pharmacokinetics in insulin-treated diabetics during the third trimester of pregnancy. *Diabetic Med.*, **1**, 273–78.

Hagbard, L., Olow I. and Reinand T. (1959) A follow-up study of 514 children of diabetic mothers. *Acta Paediatr.*, **48**, 184–97.

Hallman, M. and Teramo, K. (1979) Amniotic fluid phospholipid profile as a predictor of fetal maturity in diabetic pregnancies. *Obstet. Gynecol.*, **54**, 703–707.

Hashimoto, M., Akazawa, S., Akazawa, M. *et al.* (1990) Effects of hyperglycaemia on sorbitol and *myo*-inositol contents of cultured embryos: treatment with aldose reductase inhibitor and *myo*-inositol supplementation. *Diabetologia*, **33**, 597–602.

Hill, W.C., Pelle-Day, G., Kitzmiller, J.L. *et al.* (1989) Insulin-like growth factors in fetal macrosomia with and without maternal diabetes. *Horm. Res.*, **32**, 178–82.

Hod, M., Star, S., Passonneau, J.V. *et al.* (1986) Effect of hyperglycaemia on sorbitol and *myo*-inositol content of cultured rat conceptus: failure of aldose reductase inhibitors to modify *myo*-inositol depletion and dysmorphogenesis. *Biochem. Biophys. Res. Comm.*, **140**, 974–80.

Horton, W.E. Jr. and Sadler, T.W. (1983) Effects of maternal diabetes on early embryogenesis: alterations in morphogenesis produced by the ketone body, beta-hydroxybutyrate. *Diabetes*, **32**, 610–16.

Johnstone, F.D., Steel, J.M., Haddad, N.G. *et al.* (1992) Doppler umbilical artery velocity waveforms in diabetic pregnancy. *Br. J. Obstet. Gynaecol.*, **99**, 135–40.

Johnstone, F.D. and Steel, J.M. (1992) 'The use of Doppler ultrasound in the management of diabetic pregnancy', in J.M. Pearce (ed.). *Doppler ultrasound in perinatal medicine*, pp. 178–88. Oxford University Press, New York.

Jovanovic, L., Druzin, M. and Peterson, C.M. (1981) The effect of euglycemia on the outcome of pregnancy in insulin-dependent diabetics as compared to normal controls. *Am. J. Med.*, **71**, 921–27.

Jovanovic-Peterson, L., Peterson, C.M., Reed,

G.F. *et al.* (1991) Maternal postprandial glucose levels and infant birth weight: the diabetes in early pregnancy study. *Am. J. Obstet. Gynecol.*, **164**, 103–111.

Jovanovic-Peterson, L. and Peterson C.M. (1992) Pregnancy in the diabetic woman. Guidelines for a successful outcome. *Endocrin. Metab. Clin. North Am.*, **21**, 433–56.

Kalhan, S., Schwartz, R. and Adam, P. (1975) Placental barrier to human insulin I^{125} in insulin-dependent diabetic mothers. *J. Clin. Endocrinol. Metab.*, **40**, 139–42.

Kalhan, S.C., Savin, S.M. and Adam, P.A.J. (1977) Attenuated glucose production rate in newborn infants of insulin dependent diabetic mothers. *N. Engl. J. Med.*, **296**, 375–76.

Kalkhoff, R.K., Kandaraki, E., Morrow, P.G. *et al.* (1988) Relationship between neonatal birth weight and maternal plasma amino acid in lean and obese nondiabetic women and in type 1 diabetic pregnant women. *Metabolism*, **37**, 234–39.

Karlsson, K. and Kjellmer, I. (1972) The outcome of diabetic pregnancies in relation to the mother's blood sugar level. *Am. J. Obstet. Gynecol.*, **112**, 213–20.

Kenepp, N.B., Shelley, W.C., Gabbe, S.G. *et al.* (1982) Fetal and neonatal hazards of maternal hydration with 5% dextrose before cesarean section. *Lancet*, **1**, 1150–52.

Kirkinen, P. and Jouppila, P. (1983) 'Ultrasonic measurements of human umbilical circulation in various pregnancy complications', in R.C. Sandes and M. Hill (eds). *Ultrasound Annual*, pp. 153–55. Raven Press, New York.

Kitzmiller, J.L., Gavin, L.A., Gin, G.D. *et al.* (1991) preconception care of diabetes. Glycemic control prevents congenital abnormalities. *J. Am. Med. Assoc.*, **265**, 731–36.

Kofinas, A.D., Penry, M. and Swain, M. (1990) Uteroplacental doppler flow velocity waveforms analysis correlates poorly with glycaemic control in diabetic pregnant women. *Society of Perinatal Obstetricians*, 10th Annual Meeting. Abstract no. 410, p. 427.

Landon, M.B. and Gabbe, S.G. (1988) Diabetes and pregnancy. *Med. Clin. N. Amer.*, **72**, 1493–1511.

Landon, M.B., Gabbe, S.G., Bruner, J.P. *et al.* (1989) Doppler umbilical artery velocimetry in pregnancy complicated by insulin-dependent diabetes mellitus. *Obstet. Gynecol.*, **73**, 961–65.

Lang, U. and Kunzel, W. (1989) Diabetes mellitus in pregnancy. Management and outcome of diabetic pregnancies in the state of Hesse, FRG; a five-year-survey. *Eur. J. Obstet. Gynaecol. Reprod. Biol.*, **33**, 115–29.

Lawrence, G.F., Brown, V.A., Parsons, R.J. *et al.* (1982) Feto-maternal consequences of high-dose glucose infusion during labour. *Br. J. Obstet. Gynaecol.*, **89**, 27–32.

Leslie, R.D.G., Pyke, D.A., John, P.N. and White, J.N. (1978) Haemoglobin A_1 in diabetic pregnancy. *Lancet*, **ii**, 958–59.

Lind, T. (1975) Changes in carbohydrate metabolism during pregnancy. *Clin. Obstet. Gynaecol.*, **2**, 395–405.

Lind, T., Bell, S., Gilmore, E. *et al.* (1977) Insulin disappearance rate in pregnant and non-pregnant women and in non-pregnant women given GHRIH. *Eur. J. Clin. Invest.*, **7**, 47–51.

Miller, E., Hare, J.W., Cloherty, J.P. *et al.* (1981) Elevated maternal hemoglobin A_{1c} in early pregnancy and major congenital anomalies in infants of diabetic mothers. *N. Engl. J. Med.*, **304**, 1331–34.

Milley, J.R., Rosenberg, A.A., Philipps, A.F. *et al.* (1984) The effect of insulin on ovine fetal oxygen extraction. *Am. J. Obstet. Gynecol.*, **149**, 673–78.

Mills, J.L. (1982) Malformations in infants of diabetic mothers. *Teratology*, **25**, 385–94.

Mills, J.L., Baker, L. and Goodman, A.S. (1979) Malformations in infants of diabetic mothers occur before the seventh gestational week. Implications for treatment. *Diabetes*, **28**, 292–93.

Mills, J.L., Knopp, R.H., Simpson, J.L. *et al.* (1988) Lack of relation of increased malformation rates in infants of diabetic mothers to glycemic control during organogenesis. *N. Engl. J. Med.*, **318**, 671–76.

Neave, C. (1984) Congenital malformation in offspring of diabetics. *Perspect. Pediatr. Pathol.*, **8**, 213–22.

Noguchi, A., Erin, M. and Tsang, R.C. (1980) Parathyroid hormone in hypocalcemic and normocalcemic infants of diabetic mothers. *J. Pediatr.*, **97**, 112–14.

Nylund, L., Lunell, N.-O., Lewander, R. *et al.* (1982) Uteroplacental blood flow in diabetic pregnancy: measurements with indium 113m and a computer-linked gamma camera. *Am. J. Obstet. Gynecol.*, **114**, 298–302.

Pedersen, J. (1954) Weight and length at birth of infants of diabetic mothers. *Acta Endocrinol.*, **16**, 330–42.

Pedersen, J. (1977) *The pregnant diabetic and her newborn*, 2nd edn, pp. 1–280. Munksgaard International Publishers Ltd., Copenhagen.

Pedersen, L.M., Tygstrups, I. and Pedersen, J. (1964) Congenital malformations in newborn infants of diabetic women: correlation with maternal diabetic vascular complications. *Lancet*, **i**, 1124–26.

Peel, J. (1972) A historical review of diabetes and pregnancy. *J. Obstet. Gynaecol. Br. Commonw.*, **79**, 385–95.

Peevy, K.J., Landaw, S.A. and Gross, S.A. (1980) Hyperbilirubinemia in infants of diabetic mothers. *Pediatrics*, **66**, 417–19.

Persson, B. and Gentz, J. (1984) Follow-up of children of insulin-dependent and gestational diabetic mothers. Neuropsychological outcome. *Acta Paediatr. Scand.*, **73**, 349–58.

Pettitt, D.J. (1986) The long-range impact of diabetes during pregnancy: the Pima Indian experience. *International Diabetes Federation Bull.*, **31**, 70–71.

Pettitt, D.J., Knowler, W.C., Bennett, P.H. *et al.* (1987) Obesity in offspring of diabetic Pima Indian women despite normal birth weight. *Diabetes Care*, **10**, 76–80.

Philipps, A.F., Dubin, J.W., Matty, P.J. and Raye, J.R. (1982) Arterial hypoxemia and hyperinsulinemia in the chronically hyperglycemic fetal lamb. *Pediatr. Res.*, **16**, 653–58.

Philipps, A.F., Porte, P.J., Stabinsky, S. *et al.* (1984) Effects of chronic fetal hyperglycemia upon oxygen consumption in the ovine uterus and conceptus. *J. Clin. Invest.*, **74**, 279–86.

Pinter, E., Reece, E.A., Leranth, C.Z. *et al.* (1986) Arachidonic acid prevents hyperglycemia-associated yolk sac damage and embryopathy. *Am. J. Obstet. Gynecol.*, **155**, 691–702.

Pinter, E. and Reece, E.A. (1988) 'Diabetes-associated congenital malformations: epidemiology, pathogenesis, and experimental methods of induction and prevention', in E.A. Reece and D.R. Coustan (eds). *Diabetes mellitus in pregnancy. Principles and practice*, pp. 205–245. Churchill Livingstone, Inc., New York.

Puavilai, G., Drobny, E.C., Domont, L.A. *et al.* (1982) Insulin receptors and insulin resistance in human pregnancy: evidence for a postreceptor defect in insulin action. *J. Clin. Endocrinol. Metab.*, **54**, 247–53.

Reece, E.A. and Hobbins, J.C. (1986) Diabetic embryopathy: pathogenesis, prenatal diagnosis and prevention. *Obstet. Gynecol. Surv.*, **41**, 325–35.

Rizzo, T., Metzger, B.E., Burns, W.J. *et al.* (1991) Correlations between antepartum maternal metabolism and intelligence of offspring. *N. Engl. J. Med.*, **325**, 911–16.

Robert, M.F., Neff, R.K., Hubbell, J.P. *et al.* (1976) Association between maternal diabetes and the respiratory distress syndrome in the newborn. *N. Engl. J. Med.*, **294**, 357–60.

Sack, R. (1969) The large infant. *Am. J. Obstet. Gynecol.*, **104**, 195–204.

Sadler, T.W., Hunter, E.S., Wynn, R.E. *et al.* (1989) Evidence for multifactorial origin of diabetes-induced embryopathies. *Diabetes*, **38**, 70–74.

Simpson, J.L., Elias, S. and Martin, A.O. (1983) Diabetes in pregnancy, Northwestern University Series (1977–1981). I. Prospective study of anomalies in offspring of mothers with diabetes mellitus. *Am. J. Obstet. Gynecol.*, **146**, 263–70.

Small, M., Cameron, A., Lunan, C.B. *et al.* (1987) Macrosomia in pregnancy complicated by insulin-dependent diabetes mellitus. *Diabetes Care*, **10**, 594–99.

Sobel, D.E. (1960) Fetal damage due to ECT, insulin coma, chlorpromazine and reserpine. *Arch. Gen. Psychiat.*, **2**, 606–611.

Steel, J.M. (1985) Pre-pregnancy counselling and contraception in the insulin dependent diabetic patient. *Clin. Obstet. Gynaecol.*, **28**, 553–66.

Steel, J.M., Parboosingh, J., Cole, R.A. *et al.* (1980) Pre-pregnancy counselling – a logical prelude to the management of the pregnant diabetic. *Diabetes Care*, **3**, 371–73.

Steel, J.M., Johnstone, F.D., Hepburn, D.A. *et al.* (1990) Can prepregnancy care of diabetic women reduce the risk of abnormal babies. *Br. Med. J.*, **301**, 1070–74.

Stehbens, J.A., Baker, G.L. and Kitchel, M. (1977) Outcome at ages 1, 3, and 5 years of children born to diabetic women. *Am. J. Obstet. Gynecol.*, **127**, 408–413.

Steinke, J. and Driscoll, S. (1965) The extractible insulin content of pancreas from fetuses and infants of diabetic and control mothers. *Diabetes*, **14**, 573–78.

Stevenson, D.K., Cohen, R.S. and Kerner, J.A. (1982) Macrosomia: causes and consequences. *J. Pediatr.*, **100**, 515–20.

Susa, J.B., Groppuso, P.A., Widness, J.A. *et al.* (1984) Chronic hyperinsulinemia in the fetal Rhesus monkey: effects of physiologic hyperinsulinemia on fetal substrates, hormones and hepatic enzymes. *Am. J. Obstet. Gynecol.*, **150**, 415–20.

Takeuchi, A. and Benirschke, K. (1961) Renal vein thrombosis of the newborn and its relation to maternal diabetes mellitus. *Biol. Neonate*, **3**, 237–56.

Tanigawa, K., Kawaguchi, M., Tanaka, O. *et al.* (1991) Skeletal malformations in rat offspring. Long-term effect of maternal insulin-induced hypoglycemia during organogenesis. *Diabetes*, **40**, 1115–21.

Tsang, R.C., Brown, D.R. and Steinchen, J.M. (1979) 'Diabetes and calcium disturbances in infants of diabetic mother', in I.R. Merkatz and P.A.J. Adam (eds). *The Diabetic Pregnancy. A Perinatal Perspective*, pp. 207–225. Grune & Stratton, New York.

Verhaaren, H.A., Craen, M., De Gomme, P. *et al.* (1984) Macrosomy despite well-controlled diabetic pregnancy. *Lancet*, **i**, 285.

Visser, G.H.A., van Ballegooie, J.P. and Sluiter, W.J. (1984) Macrosomy despite well-controlled diabetic pregnancy. *Lancet*, **i**, 284–85.

Vohr, B.R., Lipsitt, L.P. and Oh, W. (1980) Somatic growth of children of diabetic mothers with reference to birth size. *J. Pediatr.*, **97**, 196–99.

Weigensberg, M.J., Garcia-Palmer, F.J. and Freinkel, N. (1990) Uptake of *myo*-inositol by early-somite rat conceptus. Transport kinetics. *Diabetes*, **39**, 575–82.

Weitz, R. and Laron, Z. (1976) Height and weight of children born to mothers with diabetes mellitus. *Isr. J. Med. Sci.*, **12**, 195–98.

White, P. (1971) 'Pregnancy and diabetes', in A. Marble *et al.* (eds). *Joslin's Diabetes Mellitus*, 11th edn, p. 583. Lea & Febiger, Philadelphia.

Widness, J.A., Susa, J., Garcia, J.F. *et al.* (1981) Increased erythropoiesis and elevated erythropoietin in infants born to diabetic mothers and in hyperinsulinemic rhesus fetuses. *J. Clin. Invest.*, **67**, 637–42.

Widness, J.A., Teramo, K.A., Clemons, G.K. *et al.* (1990) Direct relationship of antepartum glucose control and fetal erythropoietin in human type 1 (insulin-dependent) diabetic pregnancy. *Diabetologia*, **33**, 378–83.

Yen, S.S.C. (1973) Endocrine regulation of metabolic homeostasis during pregnancy. *Clin. Obstet. Gynecol.*, **16**, 130–47.

PART FOUR

32

The diabetic child in context: the family

G.M. INGERSOLL and M.P. GOLDEN

32.1 INTRODUCTION

Descriptions of psychosocial aspects of insulin-dependent diabetes mellitus (IDDM) in children and adolescents routinely take note of the complexity of the self-care regimen. Management of IDDM requires unceasing, complex, and sometimes delicate, balancing of insulin administration, diet, exercise, and blood glucose monitoring. The treatment regimen is sufficiently difficult and intrusive that the responsibility for management of the disease rarely can rest solely on a child or adolescent; parents and other family members must assume varying degrees of responsibility for the diabetes management regimen. Thus, the presence of IDDM in a child may profoundly influence how a family functions.

At the same time, the normal pattern of family functioning has a major impact on the quality of the individual's and family's adjustment to the illness and on the quality of diabetes management. A premise taken here and elsewhere (Orr & Ingersoll, 1988; Ingersoll, 1992) is that children and adolescents with IDDM are first and foremost children and adolescents who need to master the same developmental tasks as children and adolescents without IDDM. How a child and family respond to the medical and psychosocial demands of IDDM management reflect and affect the ways in which they manage normal developmental tasks.

In the same fashion, the presence of IDDM does not operate as a monolithic stressor which, by itself, causes major disruption of family function. Rather, its presence magnifies normal patterns of family interaction and problem-solving. The child with diabetes resides in a family system whose functioning patterns exist independent of the presence or absence of IDDM (Hanson & Henggeler, 1984). In the context of family dysfunction, the presence of IDDM can both exacerbate and reflect a family's difficulties – such that the quality of diabetes management is a 'sensitive barometer of family function' (Wysocki & Wayne, 1992).

This chapter will review current thoughts regarding both how diabetes affects families and how families affect diabetes care. Further, how the special needs of a very young child are dealt with by families and how families and health care providers respond to a child's or adolescent's developing needs for autonomy are addressed in separate sections.

Childhood and Adolescent Diabetes
Published in 1994 by Chapman & Hall, London
ISBN 0 412 48610 5

32.2 IMPACT OF DIABETES ON FAMILY FUNCTIONING

The occurrence of diabetes (or any chronic illness) in a child may act as a profound stressor on family function (Hobbs *et al.*, 1985). Its presence forces parents and other family members to respond to cognitive, emotional, and behavioral challenges (Sargent, 1982). Family members must acquire a knowledge base about diabetes, its regimen, potential complications, and ways to respond to crises. They must cope with fears, anxieties, and frustrations that result from their interactions with the child with diabetes, and they must be able to modify family routines to accommodate the task demands of the illness. Concurrently, the family must deal with the financial demands caused by the illness. Thus, IDDM in a child forces the family to draw together its varied psychosocial resources to deal with the new problem. When these resources are inadequate, both individual family members and the family unit are adversely affected.

During the initial stages of disease onset, parents of children with diabetes feel guilt, resentment, and self-pity (Koski, 1969; Kovacs *et al.*, 1985 & 1990; Pond, 1979). Mothers appear more likely to respond to the presence of IDDM in their children with depression than fathers. As Wysocki and Wayne (1992) suggest, mothers' tendency to respond more negatively may be linked to the greater responsibility they assume for practical management of the diabetes.

Parental anxieties also reflect realistic worries about their child's future, including issues of growth, work, sex, marriage, and normal adult functioning, and while the structure and intensity of parents' worries shift over time, becoming less extreme as the child or adolescent matures (Vandagriff *et al.*, 1992), they do not totally dissipate. Parents of children with IDDM of greater or lesser longevity share common worries about risks of diabetes-related complications, their child's insurability, and that other of their children might develop the disease. On an affective dimension they worry that they worry too much (Vandagriff *et al.*, 1992). Further, parents' worries may be more intense than the children's or adolescents' (Ahlfield *et al.*, 1983).

In reflecting upon the impact of diabetes on family function it is worthwhile to recognize that the initial, acute reaction of parents and family members to the diagnosis of diabetes is generally more severe than their long-term, continued, adaptive responses. The initial response, however, is a significant predictor of parents' longer-term adjustment to the presence of diabetes in their child (Kovacs *et al.*, 1990; Newbrough *et al.*, 1985) and may be predictive of longer-term quality of regimen adherence (Hauser *et al.*, 1990; Koski, 1969).

Beyond the effects of the presence of diabetes (or another chronic illness) in a child and his or her parents, its presence may also have significant impact on health cognitions and behaviors of siblings (Eiser, 1985; Garrison & McQuiston, 1989). Bibace and Walsh (1981) speculate that children with direct, or indirect, experience of chronic conditions are likely to have impaired development of illness cognitions. Thus, even siblings of chronically-ill children might be expected to have less mature concepts of illness and health relative to children who do not have chronically-ill siblings. Siblings of children with diabetes, for example, have less cognitively mature conceptions of illness than siblings of other children (Carandang *et al.*, 1979).

There has been some speculation that siblings of chronically-ill or disabled children are prone to maladaptive behavior more than siblings of normal children (Breslau & Prabucki, 1987; Breslau *et al.*, 1981; Eiser, 1985; Lavigne & Ryan, 1979; Tritt & Esses, 1988) and self-report more medical problems than other children (Daniels *et al.*, 1986). There is a sense among such investigators, that siblings of chronically-ill children resent the excessive amount of attention their impaired sibling receives. In an attempt to gain their 'fair share' of parental attention, siblings of chronically-ill children may engage in 'acting out' behaviors. Additionally, there may be impairment to self-esteem among siblings of children with IDDM (Ferrari, 1987).

If it is evident that the presence of diabetes or a chronic illness can significantly affect other family members, converse evidence is particularly compelling that parental and family dynamics operate as important mediators of diabetic children's metabolic control.

32.3 IMPACT OF FAMILY FUNCTIONING ON DIABETES MANAGEMENT

The family environment establishes a salient context within which adaptation to and coping with the task demands of diabetes occur (Anderson & Auslander, 1980; Anderson *et al.*, 1981; Johnson, 1980). Quality of family organization and functioning relate directly to adolescents' abilities to adapt to stressors in their environment (Felner *et al.*, 1985; Hauser *et al.*, 1986).

It is clear that children and adolescents in extremely poor control, specifically those with recurrent hospitalizations for ketoacidosis, often come from markedly dysfunctional families. In these cases, a child's illness often serves to maintain a pre-existing unhealthy family structure (Golden *et al.*, 1985a; Minuchin *et al.*, 1978; Minuchin *et al.*, 1975; Swift *et al.*, 1967; White *et al.*, 1984). Similarly, even when children with better degrees of diabetes control are evaluated, positive family environments are correlated with better metabolic control and vice versa (Kronz *et al.*, 1989; Marteau *et al.*, 1987; Waller *et al.*, 1986). Treatment, therefore, should include work directed at restructuring the family system components that support illness management in the child (Orr *et al.*, 1983).

Coyne and Anderson (1988) have speculated that the relationship between family functioning and quality of diabetes management may sometimes reflect less a severe deficit in family structure and dynamics and more a well-intended, but poorly applied and inept, problem-solving system. This may be related to a lack of adequate education about diabetes management. There is ample evidence that children and adolescents with IDDM and their parents are poorly skilled in diabetes care (Johnson, 1980; LaGreca, 1988) and that what knowledge they do possess does not relate to effective diabetes care and metabolic control (Ingersoll *et al.*, 1986; Johnson, 1980; LaGreca, 1988). When a series of families initially seen with a child in poor diabetes control were given an educational intervention in which they learned aggressive insulin regulation and diabetes management skills, recurrent diabetic ketoacidosis was eliminated in one-third (Golden *et al.*, 1985a). Similar data were reported by Satin *et al.* (1989). When parents were provided with an opportunity to simulate living with IDDM, and thus managing it, the quality of metabolic control of their child's diabetes improved.

The ways in which parents respond to the normal, nondiabetes-related tasks of parenting reflect on their diabetes-related parenting. Diana Baumrind (1968) offers a differentiation between authoritative and authoritarian parenting styles that is noteworthy and relevant to this discussion. In Baumrind's view, both authoritative and authoritarian parents rate high in their use of structure and control. The difference lies in the context within which authority is exercised. Authoritarian parents use control in the absence of warmth and emotional support. Control is an end unto itself. The child is viewed as incompetent. The child is expected to obey without question and failure to comply with parental demands is met with harsh punitive reactions. Authoritative parents also use firm control, but their control is paired with high levels of emotional support. The parent assumes responsibility for decision-making but does so in a context of openness and caring. While decision-making authority rests with the parents, the child's views are valued.

As the child moves into the adolescent years, however, the balance between parents' authority and adolescents' need for autonomy must shift. A prime developmental task of adolescence includes relinquishing the secure, dependent role of child in favor of the independent role of adult (Ingersoll, 1989 & 1992). This transition, however, must be gradual and not precipitous. In the context of diabetes, parents must be encouraged initially to assume an authoritative stance linked to the developmental status of their child. During a child's early developmental stages parents must assume a central managerial role. They must maintain an active involvement in their child's diabetes regimen, gradually relinquishing control as the child or adolescent is developmentally capable of assuming self management activities. However, as will become evident, timing of the relinquishing of control might be less soon than thought.

32.4 YOUNG CHILDREN WITH IDDM

Early-onset IDDM, that is onset before age 5 years, presents parents and health care professionals with a complex, and psychologically stressful set of task demands. Management of IDDM in young children and infants is complicated by problems of administering and adjusting small doses of insulin, dietary inconsistency, and the inability of the very young child to detect and/or report symptoms of hypoglycemia. Combined with potential insulin sensitivity, young children with IDDM frequently experience severe hypoglycemia during insulin treatment (Golden *et al.*, 1985b; Grunt *et al.*, 1978; Sachsse, 1977). Further, the probability of ketoacidosis is higher among younger children with IDDM (Faich *et al.*, 1983; Glasgow & Altierri, 1984).

Because of their repeated exposure to elevated and diminished blood glucose levels, young children with IDDM appear to be at greater risk for development of abnormal neuropsychological sequelae and cognitive deficits than their nondiabetic peers and siblings and those who develop IDDM at a later age (Eeg-Olofsson, 1977; Golden *et al.*, 1989; Halonen *et al.*, 1983; Haumont *et al.*, 1979; Rovet *et al.*, 1987 & 1988; Ryan, 1988; Ryan *et al.*, 1985) (see also Chapter 25). Recent data (Golden *et al.*, 1989) suggest even repeated episodes of asymptomatic hypoglycemia may be problematic.

Since the toddler or infant is incapable of making decisions about or engaging in the behaviors needed for management of IDDM, the onus for management falls on the parent. With training, however, parents are quite capable of managing their child's diabetes (Golden *et al.*, 1985b). In the absence of training, parents seem to develop an attitude of learned helplessness with reference to their sense of competence to deal with the illness. Repeated episodes of 'lability' lead parents to feel the diabetes controls them and little they do makes any difference. They may feel their child's illness controls the family's life and limits the family's freedom. Mothers of preschoolers with IDDM report more family stress which they attribute to their child's diabetes (Wysocki *et al.*, 1989). The parents' role in maintaining continued metabolic control in the child with IDDM develops into a form of avoidance learning. They are admonished to maintain control in order to avoid hypoglycemia or ketoacidosis. Repeated failures to achieve good metabolic control (reflected in the child's lapses into seizures or coma) may result in lowered self-esteem, impaired feelings of self-efficacy, and feelings of being a pawn of the disease.

Both Golden *et al.* (1985a) and Kushion *et al.* (1991) emphasize the need for psychosocial support systems in combination with skill and knowledge training of parents of young children with IDDM. Skill training in combination with psychosocial support establishes an early sense of parental competence in dealing with their child's IDDM and thus their sense of efficacy and personal control. Improved parental self-efficacy leads to improved glycemic control in the children (Golden *et al.*, 1985b).

32.5 ISSUES OF AUTONOMY AND DIABETES SELF-MANAGEMENT

As individuals progress from childhood through adolescence to young adulthood, there is a normal expectation that they will assume greater self-reliance and autonomy from parents and adults. Indeed, the gradual establishment of emotional and psychosocial independence from parents is a hallmark of normal, healthy, psychological development (Greenberger, 1984; Ingersoll, 1989 & 1992; Steinberg & Silverberg, 1986). How does this shift toward greater autonomy take form in the context of diabetes self-management? Given the substantial needs for self-management of diabetes, at what point should the child or adolescent be expected to assume responsibility for simple and complex tasks?

Parents and professionals are not in accord on when children and adolescents are perceived as competent to engage in specific diabetes self-managerial behaviors (Wysocki *et al.*, 1992). On average, parents are more likely to see children as more capable than do health care professionals.

There are, however, risks of overestimation of capability and willingness of children and adolescents to assume self-management of their IDDM. In a study of adolescents with IDDM, Ingersoll (Ingersoll *et al.*, 1986) found that for children younger than age 15 years nearly all parents reported participating in insulin adjustment decisions. After age 15, very few reported participating in those decisions. Unfortunately, there was no evidence that the adolescents picked up the slack. Further, the prime predictor of adolescents' willingness to engage in diabetes self-managerial behaviors and thereby to maintain better metabolic control was level of cognitive maturity, independent of chronological age which by itself was a relatively poor predictor (Ingersoll *et al.*, 1986 & 1992).

As parents gradually relinquish authority over management of their child's or adolescent's diabetes they must help their child strike an appropriate balance between dependence and isolation. Just as excessive dependence on parents or others in authority during late adolescence would be viewed as unhealthy (Greenberger, 1984), too early expectations of autonomy could place the child or adolescent in jeopardy. Parents must temper their transfer of responsibility with reference to the developmental competence of their offspring which is not completely a function of age. Further, the ability of the child or adolescent to maintain self-management of IDDM may ebb and flow as the child addresses other, normal developmental tasks (Ingersoll, 1992).

32.6 CONCLUSIONS

How, then, should the health care provider treating children with diabetes address the needs of the family and of the child within the context of the family?

First, it is vital that all members of the family be included in the therapeutic relationship. To minimize potential negative effects following diagnosis of diabetes in a child or adolescent, family members should be encouraged to deal directly with strong emotions they may harbor. Those emotions may include anger, fear, and guilt. Physicians should help parents and siblings recognize that such feelings are normal. Additionally, parents (especially the mother) should be cautioned that in responding to the heightened demands that result from their child's diabetes, that they do not lose sight of their spouse's and other children's needs.

Secondly, family functioning should be considered part of the long-term treatment plan, particularly in view of the important role played by the family in determining metabolic control. Comprehensive diabetic education allows family members to feel in control of the illness and the child/adolescent patient to feel supported. Further, family crises such as illness, death and divorce can reasonably be expected to affect diabetes control, and added support and vigilance during these times can prevent metabolic deterioration.

Finally, it is important to encourage families to treat self-management of diabetes as they do other developmental tasks, with prolonged family supervision and support and gradual transfer of responsibility to the adolescent. With this approach, an adolescent can emerge into adulthood with confidence in his or her ability to care for their own illness and with a family which has successfully coped with the added difficulties imposed by raising a child with diabetes.

REFERENCES

Ahlfield, J.E., Soler, N.G. and Marcus, S.D. (1983) Adolescent diabetes mellitus: Parent/child perspectives of the effect of the disease on family and social interactions. *Diabetes Care*, **6**, 393–98.

Anderson, B.J. and Auslander, W.F. (1980) Research on diabetes management and the family: A critique. *Diabetes Care*, **3**, 696–702.

Anderson, B.J., Miller, J.P., Auslander, W.F. *et al.* (1981) Family characteristics of diabetic adolescents: Relationship to metabolic control. *Diabetes Care*, **4**, 586–94.

Baumrind, D. (1968) Authoritarian vs. authoritative control. *Adolescence*, **3**, 255–72.

Bibace, R. and Walsh, M.E. (1981) 'Children's conceptions of illness', in R. Bibace and M.E. Walsh (eds). *Children's Conceptions of Health, Illness, and Bodily Functions: New Directions in Child Development, Vol. 14*, pp. 31–48. Jossey-Bass, San Francisco.

Breslau, N. and Prabucki, K. (1987) Siblings of disabled children. *Arch. Gen. Psychia.*, **44**, 1040–46.

Breslau, N., Weitzman, M. and Messenger, K. (1981) Psychologic functioning of siblings of disabled children. *Pediatrics*, **67**, 344–53.

Carandang, M.L.A., Folkins, C.H., Hines, P.A. *et al.* (1979) The role of cognitive level and sibling illness in children's conceptualizations of illness. *Am. J. Orthopsychia.* **49**, 474–81.

Coyne, J.C. and Anderson, B.J. (1988) The 'Psychosomatic Family' reconsidered: Diabetes in context. *J. Marital and Family Therapy*, **14**, 113–23.

Daniels, D., Miller, J.J., Billings, A.G. *et al.* (1986) Psychosocial functioning of siblings of children with rheumatic disease. *J. Abn. Child Psychol.*, **15**, 295–308.

Eeg-Olofsson, O. (1977) Hypoglycemia and neurological disturbances in children with diabetes mellitus. *Acta Paed. Scand.*, **270** (Suppl.), 91–95.

Eiser, C. (1985) *The psychology of childhood illness*. Springer-Verlag, New York.

Faich, G.A., Fishbein, H.A. and Ellis, S.E. (1983) The epidemiology of diabetic acidosis: A population based study. *Am. J. Epidemiol.*, **117**, 551–58.

Felner, R., Aber, M., Primavera, J. *et al.* (1985) Adaptation and vulnerability in high-risk adolescents: An examination of environmental mediators. *Am. J. Comm. Psychol.*, **13**, 365–79.

Ferrari, M. (1987) The diabetic child and well sibling: Risk to the well child's self concept. *Children's Health Care*, **15**, 141–48.

Garrison, W.T. and McQuiston, S. (1989) *Chronic Illness during Childhood and Adolescence: Psychological Perspectives*. Sage, Newbury Park, CA.

Glasgow, A.M. and Altierri, M.F. (1984) Socioeconomic and demographic factors and readmissions at a children's hospital. *Diabetes*, **33** (suppl.

1), 195A.

Golden, M.P., Herrold, A.J. and Orr, D.P. (1985a) An approach to prevention of recurrent diabetic ketoacidosis in the pediatric population. *J. Pediatr.*, **107**, 195–200.

Golden, M.P., Ingersoll, G.M., Brack, C.J. *et al.* (1989) Longitudinal relationship of asymptomatic hypoglycemia to cognitive function in early onset insulin dependent diabetes mellitus. *Diabetes Care*, **12**, 89–93.

Golden, M.P., Russell, B.P., Ingersoll, G.M. *et al.* (1985b) Management of diabetes mellitus in children younger than 5 years of age. *Am. J. Dis. Child.*, **139**, 448–52.

Greenberger, E. (1984) 'Defining psychosocial maturity in adolescence', in P. Karoly and J.J. Steffen (eds). *Adolescent behavior disorders: Foundations and contemporary concerns*, pp. 3–38. Lexington Books, Lexington, MA.

Grunt, J.A., Banion, C.M., Ling, L. *et al.* (1978) Problems in the care of the infant diabetic patient. *Clin. Pediatr.*, **17**, 772–74.

Halonen, A., Hiekala, T. and Hakkinen, V.K. (1983) A follow-up EEG study in diabetic children. *Ann. Clin. Res.*, **15**, 167–72.

Hanson, C.L. and Henggeler, S.W. (1984) Metabolic control in adolescents with diabetes: An examination of systemic variables. *Family Systems Medicine*, **2**:1, 5–16.

Haumont, D., Dorchy, H. and Pelc, S. (1979) EEG abnormalities in diabetic children: Influence of hypoglycemia and vascular complications. *Clin. Paediatr.*, **18**, 750–53.

Hauser, S., Jacobson, A.M., Lavori, P. *et al.* (1990) Adherence among children and adolescents with IDDM over a four-year longitudinal follow-up: II. Immediate and long-term linkages with the family milieu. *J. Pediatr. Psychol.*, **15**, 527–42.

Hauser, S., Jacobson, A.M., Wertlieb, D. *et al.* (1986) Children with recently diagnosed diabetes: Interactions with their families. *Health Psychology*, **5**, 273–96.

Hobbs, N., Perrin, J.M. and Ireys, H.T. (1985) *Chronically Ill Children and their Families*. Jossey-Bass, San Francisco, CA.

Ingersoll, G.M. (1989) *Adolescents* (2nd edn), Prentice-Hall, Englewood Cliffs, NJ.

Ingersoll, G.M. (1992) 'Adolescent psychologic and social development', in E. McAnarney, C. Kriepe and D.P. Orr (eds). *Textbook on Adolescent Medicine*, pp. 91–98. W.B. Saunders, Philadelphia.

Ingersoll, G.M., Orr, D.P., Herrold, A.J. *et al.* (1986) Cognitive maturity and self-management among adolescents with insulin-dependent diabetes mellitus. *J. Pediatr.*, **108**, 620–23.

Ingersoll, G.M., Orr, D.P., Vance, M.D. *et al.* (1992) 'Cognitive maturity, stressful events, and metabolic control among diabetic adolescents', in E.J. Susman, L.V. Fegan, and W.J. Ray (eds). *Emotion, Cognition, Health, and Development in Children and Adolescents*, pp. 121–32. Lawrence Erlbaum, Hillsdale, NJ.

Johnson, S.B. (1980) Psychosocial factors in juvenile diabetes: A review. *J. Behav. Med.*, **3**, 95–115.

Koski, M.L. (1969) The coping processes in childhood diabetes. *Acta Paed. Scand.*, **198** (Suppl.), 1–56.

Kovacs, M., Finkelstein, R., Feinberg, T.L. *et al.* (1985) Initial psychologic reaction of parents to the diagnosis of insulin-dependent diabetes mellitus in their children. *Diabetes Care*, **8**, 586–95.

Kovacs, M., Iyengar, S., Goldston, D. *et al.* (1990) Psychological functioning among mothers of children with insulin dependent diabetes mellitus. *J. Consult. Clin. Psychol.*, **58**, 189–95.

Kronz, K.K., Marreros, D.G., Vandagriff, J.L. *et al.* (1989) *Parental involvement in care, self-esteem, perceived coping ability, and metabolic control in adolescents with IDDM*. Paper presented to the annual meeting of the American Association of Diabetes Educators, Seattle.

Kushion, W., Salisbury, P.J., Seitz, K.W. *et al.* (1991) Issues in the care of infants and toddlers with insulin-dependent diabetes mellitus. *The Diabetes Educator*, **17**, 107–10.

LaGreca, A.M. (1988) 'Children with diabetes and their families: Coping and disease management', in T. Field, R. McCabe, and N. Schnelderman (eds). *Stress and Coping Across Development*, pp. 139–59. Lawrence Erlbaum, Hillsdale, NJ.

Lavigne, J.V. and Ryan, M. (1979) Psychologic adjustment of siblings of children with a chronic illness. *Pediatrics*, **63**, 616–27.

Marteau, T.M., Bloch, S. and Baum, J.D. (1987) Family life and diabetic control. *J. Child Psychol. Psychia.*, **28**, 823–33.

Minuchin, S., Baker, L., Rosman, B.L. *et al.* (1975) A conceptual model of psychosomatic illness in children: Family organization and family therapy. *Arch. Gen. Psychia.*, **32**, 1031–38.
Minuchin, S., Rosman, B.L. and Baker, L. (1978) *Psychosomatic families: anorexia nervosa in context.* Harvard University Press, Cambridge, MA.
Newbrough, J.R., Simpkins, C.G. and Maurer, H. (1985) A family development approach to studying factors in the management and control of childhood diabetes. *Diabetes Care*, **8**, 83–92.
Orr, D.P. Golden, M.P., Myers, G. *et al.* (1983) Characteristics of adolescents with poorly controlled diabetes referred to a tertiary care center. *Diabetes Care*, **6**, 170–75.
Orr, D.P. and Ingersoll, G.M. (1988) Adolescent behavior and development: A biopsychosocial view. *Current Problems in Pediatrics*, **18**:8, 442–99.
Pond, H. (1979) Parental attitude toward children with a chronic medical disorder: special reference to diabetes mellitus. *Diabetes Care*, **2**, 425–31.
Rovet, J.F., Ehrlich, R.M. and Hoppe, M. (1987) Intellectual deficits associated with early onset of insulin-dependent diabetes mellitus in children. *Diabetes Care*, **10**, 510–55.
Rovet, J.F., Ehrlich, R.M. and Hoppe, M. (1988) Specific intellectual deficits in children with early onset diabetes mellitus. *Child Dev.*, **59**, 226–34.
Ryan, C.M. (1988) Neurobehavioral complications of Type I diabetes: Examination of possible risk factors. *Diabetes Care*, **11**, 86–93.
Ryan, C.M., Vega, A. and Drash, A. (1985) Cognitive deficits in adolescents who developed diabetes early in life. *Pediatrics*, **75**, 921–27.
Sachsse, R. (1977) Insulin treatment of the diabetic infant and small child. *Pediatr. Adol. Endocrinol.*, **2**, 129–31.
Sargent, J. (1982) 'Family systems theory and chronic childhood illness: Diabetes mellitus', in K. Flomenhaft and A.E. Christ (eds). *Psychosocial family interventions in chronic pediatric illness*, pp. 125–38. Plenum, New York.
Satin, W., LaGreca, A.M., Zigo, M.A. *et al.* (1989) Diabetes in adolescence: effects of multifamily group intervention and parent simulation of diabetes. *J. Pediatr. Psychol.*, **14**, 259–75.
Steinberg, L. and Silverberg, S. (1986) The vicissitudes of autonomy in early adolescence. *Child Dev.*, **57**, 841–51.
Swift, L.R., Seidman, F.L. and Stein, H. (1967) Adjustment problems in juvenile diabetes. *Psychosom. Med.*, **29**, 555–71.
Tritt, S.G. and Esses, L.M. (1988) Psychosocial adaptation of siblings of children with chronic medical illness. *Am. J. Orthopsychiatry*, **58**, 211–20.
Vandagriff, J.L., Marrero, D.G., Ingersoll, G.M. *et al.* (1992) Parents of children with diabetes: what are they worried about? *The Diabetes Educator*, **18**, 299–302.
Waller, D.A., Chipman, J.J., Hardy, B.T. *et al.* (1986) Measuring diabetes-specific family support and its relation to metabolic control: A preliminary report. *J. Am. Assoc. Child Psychia.*, **25**, 415–18.
White, K., Kolman, M.L., Wexler, P. *et al.* (1984) Unstable diabetes and unstable families: a psychosocial evaluation of diabetic children with recurrent ketoacidosis. *Pediatrics*, **73**, 749–55.
Wysocki, T. and Wayne, W. (1992) Childhood diabetes and the family. *Practical Diabetology*, **11**:2, 29–32.
Wysocki, T., Huxtable, K., Linscheid, T.R. *et al.* (1989) Adjustment to diabetes mellitus in preschoolers and their mothers. *Diabetes Care*, **12**, 524–29.
Wysocki, T., Meinhold, P.A., Abrams, K.C. *et al.* (1992) Parental and professional estimates of self-care independence of children and adolescents with IDDM. *Diabetes Care*, **15**, 43–52.

33

Childhood diabetes: the child at school

S. STRANG

33.1 INTRODUCTION

Despite the fact that the incidence of childhood diabetes appears to be rising (Metcalfe & Baum, 1991), it is still a relatively rare condition and therefore unlikely that there will be more than one child with diabetes in a primary school and probably only two or three in a secondary school. Of the 52 000 school children in Oxfordshire, approximately 160 have diabetes. Consequently, children can feel isolated and teachers may not previously have come into contact with pupils who have diabetes. Teachers are *in loco parentis* for up to seven hours a day for 39 weeks of the year, a considerable part of a child's life. In order that they can supply a secure environment and help the child to achieve his educational potential, they need to be provided with sufficient information and support. This may come from various sources – initially the child's parents with the back-up of the Clinic Team, and also the school medical officer and nurse. Ideally a pediatric diabetes specialist nurse (PDSN) should be the link person between the family, clinic and school, responsible for disseminating information, acting as a resource and providing overall support.

Childhood and Adolescent Diabetes
Published in 1994 by Chapman & Hall, London
ISBN 0 412 48610 5

The aim of this chapter is to give a comprehensive picture of children with diabetes in school and to address specific issues related to their care.

The terminology used relates to the UK education system – equivalent local concepts and usage will be readily apparent to other readers.

33.2 RETURNING TO SCHOOL AFTER DIAGNOSIS

Many children return to school within a relatively short time after diagnosis. This is because they are not unwell, and encouraging them to return to their normal routine helps to reinforce the view that diabetes is not an illness but a condition with which one can learn to live. At this stage, however, neither the children nor their parents have had a chance to master the practical aspects of diabetes or to come to terms with the condition. Children may worry that they will no longer be accepted by their peers, and that no one will know how to look after them – a fear shared by parents and teachers. Parents are apprehensive because it is difficult to hand over the care of your child to someone else when you are not yet confident yourself and they will need the help of the PDSN to explain in detail to the school staff the implications of having a pupil with diabetes. There is a fine balance between emphasizing the 'normality' of the child with diabetes while not underplaying the severity of the condition.

The PDSN should contact the school soon after diagnosis. It is useful if everyone can be addressed at a staff meeting but this is not always possible and the number of staff who are involved with a particular child will vary according to the age of the child and the size of the school. School secretaries, catering staff and playground assistants should also be included if possible. Information sheets from the British Diabetic Association School Pack (British Diabetic Association, 1994) can be left with the secretary and pinned on the staffroom notice board, where they can be brought to the attention of supply teachers. Sometimes it is necessary to be assertive as teachers may not always see the relevance of a visit from a PDSN, particularly if they have previously taught pupils with diabetes or have a relative with the condition, but it is important that every child is seen as an individual with differing needs dependent on age, personality and social and cultural background.

Teachers need to know how important it is for the child to have a regular intake of carbohydrate in order to keep the blood glucose stable. Snacks can usually be arranged to fit in with a break in lessons but children must have the confidence to know that they will not be told off if they have to eat in class. The effect of exercise, timing of meals and hypoglycemia should be addressed. Teachers also need to be aware of the symptoms of hyperglycemia and that if blood glucose levels are high, the child may need to pass urine frequently and should be allowed to leave the classroom when necessary. Children do not need to test their blood glucose levels routinely in school, but may do so during periods of erratic control. Blood glucose testing equipment may be kept by the school nurse for emergency use. Children are encouraged to wear some form of identification, though this is sometimes resented, and schools should allow necklaces and bracelets and not classify them as jewelry.

When a younger child returns to school the teacher may explain to the class why the child may need to eat in class and is not allowed sweets. The 'Althea' booklet is a useful aid (Braithwack, 1983). The child will be less embarrassed if permission is asked beforehand and will find classmates caring. Older children can be encouraged to tell their friends but may be reluctant for it to be widely known that they have diabetes. It may be helpful to speak to a teenager with a small group of school friends.

33.3 HYPOGLYCEMIA

Hypoglycemic episodes are one of the main concerns of children, parents and teachers. Their recognition, prevention and treatment should be discussed with reference to the individual child. Teachers need to know that if diabetic control is good, mild hypoglycemic episodes ('hypos') are to be expected but that these are easily treated and there is no need for parents to be contacted or for the child to be sent home. However, parents should be told if their child is having regular 'hypos'. It is encouraging for teachers to realize that knowing the child's personality and 'normal' behavior will help with the recognition of 'hypos', e.g., if the child becomes uncharacteristically quiet or disruptive. Likewise teachers may notice that the child lacks concentration during certain lessons at the same time of day or that handwriting has deteriorated. The child may appear to be all right but may be subclinically hypoglycemic.

Unless they are too young to carry glucose tablets, children are encouraged to treat their own 'hypos' in class at the first symptoms and only if these persist to go the medical room accompanied by another person. An emergency kit should be kept in a safe but accessible place, e.g., with the school secretary or in a classroom cupboard. This could contain spare glucose tablets, fun-size chocolate bars, some biscuits (cookies) and a sweet drink, such as a small carton of fruit juice. Severe hypoglycemic attacks are rare but the possibility should be discussed with the teachers who need to know the worst scenario, i.e., that the child could become unconscious and have a convulsion, but should be reassured that there is time to get medical help and that the child is not going to die. Parents, teachers and the PDSN should agree upon an action plan in the event of a severe 'hypo'. It is worth remembering that any 'hypo', severe or mild, could be embarrassing for children who may not be aware of what they have said or done.

33.4 SCHOOL MEALS

Lunchtime is a significant social occasion in the school day, and so as far as possible, children should continue with the same type of meal as before diagnosis, i.e., cooked or packed. If this is a cooked meal, photocopies of the menu can be obtained and the contents discussed with the dietitian or PDSN. Most schools are willing to provide fresh fruit or yogurt in place of dessert if artificial sweeteners are not used. Older children may have canteen-style meals to choose from, so they need to know how to make a suitable choice, although temptations will be greater. Teenagers sometimes leave school premises at lunchtime and buy lunch at the local 'take-out' to eat 'on the hoof'. This will need careful handling if teenagers are to change their eating habits without losing their peer group credibility. Larger schools sometimes have lunch in shifts which could mean that children have lunch at 12 noon one week and 1 p.m. the next. This presents no problems for children using an insulin 'pen' but other children may find that they have rather low blood glucose levels by 1 p.m. This can be resolved by either eating a small snack prior to lunch or by obtaining a pass to enable the child and a friend to eat regularly at an earlier shift. This pass could also allow the child to go to the front of the line if necessary.

33.5 EXERCISE

Children who have diabetes should be encouraged to participate in organized sport as it promotes physical fitness, peer bonding and possibly improved diabetes control (Greene, 1985). Extra carbohydrate may be required before gym class or sports activities but consideration should be given to the duration and intensity of the exercise and the time of day. Younger children will probably expend as much energy, if not more, kicking a football around the playground at break time as in an organized sports lesson, and this will be accounted for in their normal carbohydrate intake. However, an extra snack may be required before a match played after school.

At high school level, sports are more strenuous and of longer duration and most children will take some form of faster-acting carbohydrate before the activity, e.g., chocolate biscuit, fruit juice. This is also a welcome opportunity to eat sweet foods. Although large meals should not be eaten before swimming, some form of carbohydrate should be taken, as a hypoglycemic attack in the water is unpleasant and dangerous. Apparatus work in the gymnasium is another potentially hazardous situation. It is extremely important that physical education teachers are aware of children with diabetes in their classes and understand the connection between exercise, blood glucose and performance. There should be quick-acting carbohydrate at the playing field either in the child's pocket or with the teacher for safekeeping and if it is necessary for the child to return to base, he or she should be accompanied.

Children are usually required to remove jewelry during gym classes for their safety. This seems a reasonable precaution provided that teachers remember that the child has diabetes and that the identification is not lost.

33.6 BEHAVIOR AND BLOOD GLUCOSE

Children who have diabetes are primarily normal children going through the same stages as their peers and should be treated as such, with the same rules and discipline. Fluctuating blood glucose levels can affect behavior and both very high and very low levels may present with similar signs and symptoms which the children themselves can find confusing, e.g., headaches, aggression. Testing equipment can be left at school in order to ascertain blood glucose levels but written parental permission should be obtained. Sometimes children may display behavior which is unacceptable and it may be difficult to differentiate between cause and effect in these cases. Problems which alone could cause disturbed behavior may affect blood glucose levels, which in turn could provoke bad behavior. Often these problems are not easily resolved and need careful discussion between the family and the professionals. The help of a child psychiatrist or psychologist should be sought when necessary.

33.7 THE YOUNG CHILD

The fact that a very young child has diabetes will inevitably mean a close interdependency between mother and child and this may cause problems as the child moves towards independence and starts school. Sessions at toddler group, playgroup, day care or nursery school help the child to integrate and give the mother a chance to distance herself from the immediate care of her child. The carers in pre-school groups are usually very willing to take on a child with diabetes. They are used to looking after dependent children, the adult: child ratio is high and the child is only in their care for a few hours. Carers probably do not need a detailed explanation of diabetes but the timing of the snack and the type of biscuit offered to the child needs to be discussed as well as 'hypo' symptoms and treatment, with a caution to watch out for the child 'falling asleep' during the end of the morning story!

When a child first starts school it is an emotional time for all parents and this is heightened if the child has diabetes. Parents worry that a busy teacher may not notice if their child is unwell and that the child, even though he or she may recognize 'hypo' symptoms, may be too shy to tell the teacher, or ask for something to eat. The child will probably need reminding to eat a snack especially if there is not a convenient break. Children may need supervision to make sure they have eaten a snack before hurrying to join friends in the playground. Some schools have classroom assistants who take on this role. Older siblings attending the same school may be expected to look after a younger child during playtime and are sometimes called upon by teachers if there is a problem in class. It is important not to overburden children with this responsibility which may create resentment.

33.8 THE TRANSITION TO SECONDARY SCHOOL

The transfer to secondary school at the age of 11–13 years coincides with increasing independence and identification with the peer group. Children now function at a higher cognitive level and this is an ideal time for the Clinic Team to revise the children's diabetes knowledge so that they are able to deal with the increased physical exercise and canteen-style meals. A multiple injection regimen using an insulin 'pen' will give greater flexibility if no better control. The sheer size of a secondary school and numbers of pupils and staff will inevitably mean that not all staff are aware of pupils with diabetes, though hopefully they will know of any in their class. It is difficult for the PDSN to see everyone involved with a particular child, though the form teacher and physical education staff are important, and often information has to be passed on to other staff by the year tutor. The physical and emotional aspects of puberty exert extra pressure on adolescents who have diabetes, but sensitive teachers can help them come to terms with their condition both by gaining their confidence and by using lessons, e.g., biology and domestic science, to display the teenager's experiential knowledge.

33.9 BOARDING SCHOOL

Children may develop diabetes while already at boarding school or may have to board of necessity if parents live abroad. This can put quite a burden on a child who has diabetes, as sometimes even quite young children at boarding school are expected to take on responsibility for their own care which would not be expected at home. Boarding school staff will have 24-hour responsibility for children, with house parents and matrons having parochial care. It is important, however, that teachers are aware of their role in the care of the child. There is nearly always a trained nurse on the staff but she may not have had previous experience of a child with diabetes and will possibly need updating with the help of the local diabetes team. The child will probably sleep in a room with several other children who will need to know that their friend has diabetes. Food should be allowed at the bedside in order to treat night-time 'hypos'. Young non-medical house matrons may well be called if there is a severe hypoglycemic episode and should be aware of the signs and know how and when to get help. It is also important that kitchen staff are well-informed. The carbohydrate content of meals is not usually a problem but the fat content is often rather high. The provision of suitable snacks should also be discussed.

Several agencies may be involved with the diabetes care of a child at boarding school i.e., parents, school and home general practitioners (GPs) and the local diabetes team. It is therefore vital to have clear lines of communication so that the child is not isolated in the midst of poorly informed advisers. This is especially important if the parents live abroad.

33.10 SPECIAL SCHOOLS

Inevitably, some children with diabetes will have special educational requirements. Children with physical disabilities and those with learning and behavioral difficulties come into this category. These requirements may be met within special units in the mainstream school system or in special schools. Some children may have a multiprofessional assessment in order to identify their educational needs, however, this would be unusual in the case of a child who has only diabetes. When children have other problems it may be difficult to distinguish between diabetes-related symptoms and those related to the particular condition, e.g., the frustrations shown by deaf or dyslexic children may be mistaken for erratic blood glucoses (or vice versa). Although it may be more difficult to identify symptoms in children with special needs, the high staff: pupil ratio means that they are more closely observed.

33.11 PEN DEVICES AND PUMPS

Although 'pen' devices do not necessarily improve diabetic control, they do give teenagers the flexibility to have a lifestyle more in line with their peers and to cope with such things as haphazard meal times, more energetic sports and trips away from home. Introducing this regimen not only gives an opportunity for further diabetes education but also helps with the transfer of responsibility from parent to child. The school needs to know when a pupil is using a 'pen' at school, issues such as where it will be kept during school hours and where the injecting will take place should be addressed and also the procedure to follow should the 'pen' become lost.

Not many children are likely to be using insulin pumps. However, staff, especially the gym teachers, should be aware of the pump as it will need to be kept safe when it is removed and the child may require extra time in which to change and get reattached.

33.12 SCHOOL TRIPS

Most children will at some point have the opportunity to go on a school trip. This could be a day's outing, a week's outward-bound course or a long-distance day trip requiring a 4 a.m. start. Children gain independence and self-confidence from these trips and should be given every encouragement to participate. Trips should, however, be carefully planned and a meeting arranged between parents, child, teachers and PDSN to discuss various issues. Teachers may feel confident to take a child who has presented no problems in class, on a trip, but should be aware of the implications of having 24-hour care of a child with diabetes. The following list suggests some topics for discussion prior to a school field trip:

1. Travel: Departure time, method of travel, travel sickness pills, letters for Customs if crossing borders.
2. Program: Meal times, exercise.
3. Food: Provision of sufficient carbohydrates, snacks – especially bedtime. Discuss with field center beforehand.
4. Adjustment of insulin to account for increased exercise.
5. Supervision of injection, safety of kit.
6. Recognition and treatment of hypos.
7. Locate local general practitioner – inform him or her of diabetic in the party.
8. When to get medical help, i.e., severe hypo, vomiting.
9. Identification.
10. The importance of never omitting insulin.

33.13 EXAMINATIONS

Examinations can cause stress to all concerned. When the child has diabetes, this may manifest itself in a period of poor control which could affect performance. Some youngsters experience severe hypoglycemic attacks during the night prior to an examination and in cases such as this, a note from the clinic can be provided for use should there be an unexpected poor result. Notes may also be requested to allow food to be eaten in the examination room.

33.14 CAREERS GUIDANCE

Before they reach the stage of having to make a decision, children with diabetes need to be aware that there are some careers which are not open to them. These include the armed forces, police and fire services, and driving public service vehicles. Most other jobs are accessible and there is no reason why occupations which require shift work or using machinery should be barred, though careers officers sometimes have misconceptions about suitable jobs and may need some updating. It is important that supervisors of work experience placements and potential employers are aware of the diabetes. National diabetes associations produce information booklets related to applying for work.

33.15 PEER GROUP PERCEPTIONS

Young children will probably accept a classmate who has diabetes without question, and are likely to show more interest in why he or she is allowed to eat in class when they are not, and when given an explanation will be quite solicitous towards their friend. Their perception of the condition may be that the child has developed diabetes because he has done something wrong; they may even wonder if diabetes means that you will die, and need to be told that it is not catching.

It is another story in secondary schools. Conformity is important and if a child appears to be different (and feels different), peers can be unkind. Teenagers may be accused of taking drugs and be told that they will get AIDS because they are using syringes. It is understandable that teenagers are reluctant to let it be known that they have diabetes. Apart from all the usual pressures of puberty and adolescence, together with the influence of the peer group experimenting with smoking, alcohol and sex, teenagers with diabetes feel that they have to contend with parental and clinic attempts to constrain their lifestyle.

33.16 SCHOOL HEALTH SERVICE

Schools generally have a school nurse and medical officer allotted to them by the school medical service and sometimes employ their own nurse on the premises. They all need to be aware of children with diabetes in the school, but should have the support of the PDSN, and join in discussions about individual children. The school nurse is often someone to whom children can go as a counsellor and confidant. The nurse will understand about diabetes and the pressures of school and yet is removed from the authoritarian aspects of clinic staff and teachers. Children do not need to attend school medical examinations purely on account of diabetes especially if they are already attending a hospital clinic, as this only singles them out unnecessarily. They should have the same immunizations as their peers.

33.17 CONCLUSIONS

Since children between the ages of 5–16 years spend so much of their lives at school, it would be reasonable to expect that those who have responsibility for their care have, at least, a basic concept of how diabetes affects a child at school. Parents need to be confident in the knowledge that their child will be safe in the school environment and happily integrated with their peers. Research shows that this is not always the case. Bradbury and Smith (1983) showed a lack of knowledge of diabetes in schools in Liverpool, UK, and identified a need for more input from medical and nursing professionals. Yet in a study from Birmingham, UK, Warne (1988) showed that in spite of recorded visits from a PDSN many teachers denied knowledge of pupils with diabetes whom they taught. Others felt that there were inadequate sources of information. Parents too seem dissatisfied. In a study involving parents of newly diagnosed children, 50% of those interviewed were concerned about the lack of knowledge and understanding of diabetes by teachers (Lessing *et al.*, 1992). Even with a more common chronic condition, asthma, teachers appeared to have insufficient knowledge. Bevis and Taylor (1990) recommended that all primary school teachers should receive teaching about asthma during their training. It has been suggested that in-service training days could be used to give teachers insight into conditions such as diabetes (Brown *et al.*, 1990).

With the increasing incidence of diabetes in children under the age of 15 years (Metcalfe & Baum, 1991), there will be more children with diabetes in schools and teachers could also be in a position to observe the signs and symptoms of diabetes developing in a pupil. It is therefore important that they should at least have a background knowledge of the condition. School medical officers and nurses also need to keep up to date in order to supply practical support.

Hospital-based diabetes teams should continue to develop effective lines of communication with schools in order to ensure that children who have diabetes, not only achieve their educational potential but mature into healthy, well-adjusted members of society.

REFERENCES

Bevis, M. and Taylor, B. (1990) What do school teachers know about asthma? *Arch. Dis. Child.*, **65**, 622–25.

Bradbury, A.J. and Smith, C.S. (1983) An assessment of the diabetic knowledge of school teachers. *Arch. Dis. Child.*, **58**, 692–96.

Braithwack, A. (1983) *I Have Diabetes, by 'Althea'*. Dinosaur Publications, HarperCollins, London.

British Diabetic Association. (1994) *School Pack*. British Diabetic Association, London.

Brown, K., Chadwick, J. and North, J. (1990) Using 'Baker Days' for teacher education about diabetes. *Diabetes Update*, British Diabetic Association, London.

Greene, S.A. (1985) 'Exercise', in J.D. Baum and A.-L. Kinmonth (eds). *Care of the Child with Diabetes*, pp. 117–28. Churchill Livingstone, Edinburgh.

Lessing, D.N., Swift, P.G.F., Metcalfe, M.A. *et al.* (1992) Newly diagnosed diabetes: a study of parental satisfaction. *Arch. Dis. Child.*, **67**, 1011–13.

Metcalfe, M.A. and Baum, J.D. (1991) Incidence of insulin dependent diabetes in children aged under 15 years in the British Isles during 1988. *Brit. Med. J.*, **302**, 443–47.

Warne, J. (1988) Diabetes in school: a study of teachers' knowledge and information sources. *Practical Diabetes*, **5**, 210–15.

34

Liaison nursing – the diabetic home care team

A. McEVILLY

The child with diabetes should have a multidisciplinary team of health care professionals responsible for both day-to-day management and monitoring for future complications. The benefit of a team approach can be seen in the improved communications which develop between the different health care professionals, and this in turn leads to consistent advice for the child and family. Parents need to know that their child is seen as an individual and that the advice given is relevant to their particular needs. In order to develop this, a rapport needs to be established; this is best achieved by a diabetes nurse who can visit the family at home.

34.1 THE PEDIATRIC DIABETES SPECIALIST NURSE

The role of the pediatric diabetes specialist nurse (PDSN) differs in many ways from the role of the adult diabetes specialist nurse (DSN), not because of the diabetes, but more related to the client population. In the adult field the person with diabetes is usually the main carer, supported by their partner, whereas in childhood the ability of self-care alters as they grow and develop. This means that anyone responsible for the child must also be a carer and understand the possible problems which may arise. The education of the child and carers is the responsibility of the PDSN and the hospital-based Diabetes Team. Family-centered care enables the education to be adjusted to the individual child and family, adapting to their changing needs and leading to transfer of care (Figure 34.1). A member of the Diabetes Team should be available to help and support carers when needs arise, remembering that these will change as the child takes on new challenges.

In the UK, the problem of pediatric nursing support has been approached in many ways, with the result that nurses may be accommodated and financed by either the hospital or community, but wherever based they must be available to work in both areas. The Royal College of Nursing (RCN) Diabetes Forum Working Party, looking at the role of the diabetes nurse specialist, recognized that the nurse requires skills in nursing, teaching, counselling and in identifying special needs. Nurses also need to be flexible, available to visit either in hospital or the home (RCN, 1993a). A working party for the RCN Paediatric Diabetes Special Interest Group identified that the nurse responsible for children with diabetes should also have pediatric and com-

Childhood and Adolescent Diabetes
Published in 1994 by Chapman & Hall, London
ISBN 0 412 48610 5

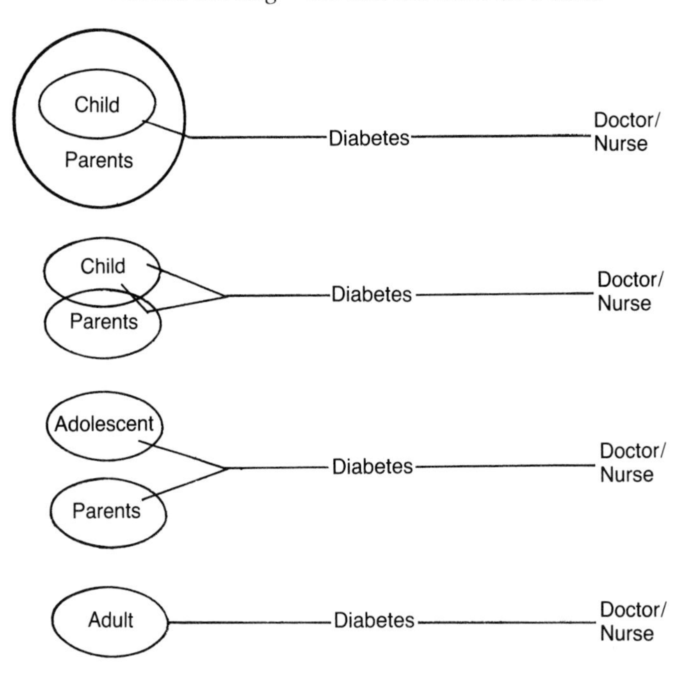

Figure 34.1 Adapting education to the changing needs of the child and family.

munity training (RCN, 1993b). Pediatric liaison posts have developed from many different backgrounds, with nurses taking on the responsibility for children with diabetes after working as adult DSNs, health visitors, district nurses, ward sisters or school nurses.

In England, since 1982 the basic diabetes nurse training has been provided by the English National Board 928 course, but more recently training has moved towards establishing courses to diploma or degree level. Newer courses will provide accreditation for accumulated learning, such as Continuous Accreditation and Transfer points. These courses still include only minimal training in pediatrics and management of children with diabetes. Currently the only training for nurses and dieticians in the management of childhood diabetes in the UK is held at the Children's Hospital, Birmingham.

Diabetes nurses have been in post in some areas since the 1950s, but recent years have seen a rapid increase in numbers, following the recognition of the need highlighted in the document *The Provision of Medical Care for Adult Diabetic Patients in the United Kingdom* produced by the Royal College of Physicians and the British Diabetic Association (BDA) in 1984. The recommendation of two clinical nurses in diabetes per health district of average size (200 000), does not make allowance for the time needed to educate and support children and their carers. Many nurses who have to combine the care of both adults and children, have found difficulty justifying the disproportionate time spent with their young patients, who often form such a small percentage of their case load. Recommendations produced by the RCN Paediatric Diabetes Special Interest Group suggest that the nurse: patient ratio in childhood diabetes should be one nurse whole time equivalent for every 100 children to enable development of total home management. This will vary depending upon the geographical spread, cultural background, socioeconomic status and other medical conditions of the case load (RCN, 1993b). The BDA also produced guidelines for parents identifying the service they should receive to support them in the care of their child with diabetes (BDA, 1991), and this has been further supported by the St Vincent Declaration (Krans *et al.*, 1992) (see Appendix A).

Pediatrics forms a very small part of the training of a registered general nurse (RGN) and therefore they have minimal understanding of the changing abilities, comprehension and learning skills of children in their care. The nurse needs to be aware of the psychological impact of a chronic condition on the child and family, and should have an understanding of the principles of the 1989 Children Act (Department of Health, 1991a) and the RCN pediatric nursing philosophy, enabling them to offer adequate support in the community. The National Association of Welfare for Children in Hospital (Department of Health, 1991b), identifies the need for children in hospital to be cared for by nurses with pediatric training and as more children are cared for in the home, this, along with community training, would be the ideal for their community care as well.

34.2 THE ROLE OF THE PEDIATRIC DIABETES SPECIALIST NURSE (PDSN)

The pediatric diabetes specialist nurse's role is multifaceted, involving both education and clinical care. Education is necessary to enable the transfer of management from parents as the child develops the skills needed for self-care. The nursing model most suited to this is Orem's self-care theory (Orem, 1971), because this acknowledges the changing and developing ability of the growing child, as well as the support needed by parents to allow independence.

Continuity of care and advice in the hospital and community is essential to give parents the confidence to manage difficult situations in the home. To ensure this, the PDSN must be involved in the education of hospital staff, community workers and the child and carers. This enables a smooth transition from hospital to home at the time of diagnosis and consistent support at other times.

A further aim of the PDSN must be to minimize the child's separation from parents and family, especially at the time of diagnosis. The newly diagnosed child who is not clinically ill may be cared for at home, if there is sufficient community support and the parents prefer home management. This would involve community visits from other team members. The final aim must be to offer support at times of crisis; to achieve this, the family must know how to obtain advice at any time of day or night.

The education now provided to the family, can increase their anxiety (Moyer, 1989). The expectation of good control is not always achieved and this can increase concern for the future as their awareness of the risk of complications is increased. Working closely with the family enables the nurse to become their friend and advocate, providing opportunities for them to express their concerns about the future and other difficulties.

34.3 THE DIABETIC TEAM

A pediatric diabetes specialist nurse cannot work in isolation and to be fully effective needs to be part of a multidisciplinary team providing shared care. The members of the team will vary depending on the number of children under their care, but there should be a minimum of senior pediatrician, middle grade pediatrician, pediatric dietician, ward sister and PDSN. Working in close proximity will aid good communications. Table 34.1

Table 34.1 The pediatric diabetes team.

Diabetes Team		Extended Diabetes Team
Pediatric Consultant	Hospital	OPD Sister
Secretary		A&E Sister
Registrar		Pharmacist
Pediatric Dietician		Senior House Officer
Ward Sister		
Pediatric diabetes specialist nurse	Community	Health Visitor
Psychologist		District Nurse
Psychiatrist		General Practitioner
Social Worker		Practice Nurse
Family Counsellor		School/Nursery Staff
		Local Pharmacist

shows the full pediatric diabetes team, including members of the extended team.

The team leader is usually the consultant, but all members play an equal part and their individual roles must be recognized, establishing each person as an integral member of the team. A nurse based in a diabetes center has more opportunity to interact with colleagues, reducing the feeling of isolation many experience, particularly in pediatrics. This interaction leads to team building as each member learns to appreciate the problems of the others.

Home support should be provided by all members of the team, whenever possible. Community visits by the medical members are particularly important at the time of diagnosis and help the family gain confidence. Dietetic home visits enable the dietician to assess the normal eating patterns of the family, so that the advice provided is relevant to that particular child. Joint visits by members of the team demonstrate to the family how each role is important in the care of their child. A visit from the dietician and nurse can highlight the importance of both aspects of care and may demonstrate how the two areas interact.

Teamwork helps in the development of care plans. Identifying each member's involvement in the care of a child with diabetes prevents misunderstandings within the team and leads to a greater understanding of each other's roles. To develop a care plan, the personal needs of the child should be identified and discussed during team meetings, so that the final plan reflects the needs of the individual child. Standards of care which are realistic, achievable and measurable should be set by the team, and protocols written so that each member knows the procedures to follow, in order to ensure that standards are maintained. Teamwork should ensure a consistent service, reducing the risk of conflicting advice to the child and family. Alwyn Moyer (1987) identified that parents wanted 'information that was individualized, readily available and timely'. Good teamwork should ensure this.

The role of the PDSN includes being the link between all the different team members (Figure 34.2). Principal carers will be the family, supported by the hospital team, but the extended community team should be aware of the recommendations being given to parents, to prevent conflicting advice. The

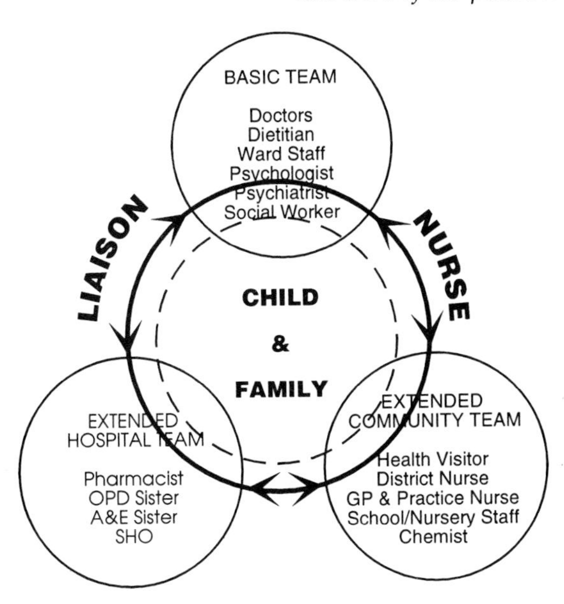

Figure 34.2 The pediatric diabetes specialist nurse link network.

family will contact their general practitioner for medication, and to enable continuity of care he and his team must have an understanding of the current management and should see the child at regular intervals. This should not be at a general practice diabetes mini clinic, where the young child may have to listen to adults discussing complications. The nurse should liaise with any other community team members involved with the family, when the need arises.

Nurses are ultimately responsible for their own decisions, and it is therefore essential that they keep accurate records of all patient contacts and teaching sessions with the children, their families or carers. Accurate record-keeping will also facilitate audit of the service and this in turn will help identify future needs. Protocols may need to be written and signed by the consultant responsible for the care of the children with diabetes. These should cover such points as the home management of illness and insulin adjustment.

34.4 THE WORK OF THE PEDIATRIC DIABETES SPECIALIST NURSE

34.4.1 CLINICAL

Establishing and maintaining easy access for the families to professional advice is a priority for the specialist nurse (Challen *et al.*, 1990). The newly diagnosed require a great deal of help and support, involving the nurse in frequent home visits for the first few days. This also offers the ideal environment for discussing questions of management and, whether in newly diagnosed or established patients, these should be followed up by telephone contact, until the problem is resolved. The home offers relaxed surroundings for the family to discuss their concerns and when there are other young children in the family, parents are relieved of the extra stress of finding a childminder while they visit the hospital. The home also provides the opportunity for the nurse to observe practical skills, which may help identify the reason for poor metabolic control. As the young person becomes adolescent, they may choose to discuss their diabetes away from home, in a situation where they know parents cannot listen.

The clinic offers an opportunity for the nurse to monitor growth and development, take blood for glycated hemoglobin or fructosamine and to check that annual reviews are completed. Any problems identified at clinic can be followed up by a home visit or telephone contact. A diabetes center can provide a 'drop-in' service, which some families find useful. However contact is maintained, it is essential the families are given guidelines on how and when to get advice, so that problems can be identified early and steps taken to maintain satisfactory glycemic control. Counseling skills may be used to help the child and family identify problems and then provide support as they come to terms with them.

In-patient care requires close liaison with the ward staff, and the multidisciplinary team should discuss policies and plan discharge to enable the development of the care plan. Hospital admission provides an opportunity for staff to assess the child's practical skills and identify their educational needs, which the liaison nurse can follow up after discharge. The admission of a newly diagnosed child offers the liaison nurse the chance to establish a rapport with the family and begin to assess their social needs before visiting them at home.

Liaison with other health care professionals and lay organizations is an important aspect of the nurse's role, as this ensures the continuity and consistency of care within the extended team.

34.4.2 EDUCATION

The planning, execution and evaluation of the education provided to the child and family at the time of diagnosis and during reassessment of their changing needs, is the responsibility of the liaison nurse. This involves the development of an educational program starting from the time of diagnosis and should include all aspects of diabetes and its management. The teaching needs to be evaluated a few weeks after diagnosis, to assess the family's comprehension of the information they have been given.

Ongoing education is required to cope with the changing ability of the child and this may include small group work or one-to-one sessions. Play makes learning more enjoyable and games, quizzes, and physical participation are essential elements of educational sessions for the children (Hatcher, 1990). Parents and carers also need the opportunity to develop their understanding of diabetes and this may be provided through educational sessions, which also offer the opportunity for them to meet other carers. Families in the UK should be introduced to the support and help available to them through the BDA.

To ensure the necessary continuity of advice for the child and family, the PDSN should be involved in the education of other health care professionals. This should include pre- and post-registration nurses, in the hospital and community, medical students and junior hospital medical staff. The nurse must be considered a resource to be used by other staff in the hospital and community, and education of carers should include anyone who may become involved with the child, for example, if going on holiday. With this support, the parents know their child is in the care of people with a knowledge and understanding of diabetes.

34.4.3 PROFESSIONAL

Depending on the size of the unit, the specialist nurse may be the manager of the service, with responsibility for the organization of the work and management of the budget. The nurse should keep up-to-date with research and developments in the care of childhood diabetes, ensuring that practice is research-based. In the UK, peer support can be obtained through the professional organizations, such as the BDA Education Section and the Royal College of Nursing Diabetes Forum and Paediatric Special Interest Group.

34.5 HOME MANAGEMENT PROBLEMS

34.5.1 ON DIAGNOSIS

The development of home stabilization and education has led to a decrease in hospital bed occupancy (Rayner, 1984). Support in the home enables the diabetes team to provide education at a rate to suit the individual child and family. All aspects of diabetes management, storage, care and disposal of equipment and when to get advice need to be explained gradually, so that the child and family can absorb the information they are given. The reaction of parents to the diagnosis varies, but most feel guilty and need reassurance that they have done nothing wrong. Diagnosis of any chronic condition can lead to feelings of loss, similar to those experienced at the time of death and the nurse's understanding of these emotions are essential to help parents through this difficult time.

An explanation of the different types of diabetes is needed at a very early stage because well-meaning friends often confuse parents by suggesting that their child will go on to tablets when they are older. Whenever possible, both parents should be involved in the management of their child's diabetes from diagnosis and educational sessions arranged at a time to include them both. Phobias about injections and blood tests may need to be overcome. Siblings often resent the attention given to their brother or sister; involving them in the education and management may overcome this and also allay their fears and confusion about what the diagnosis means. Introducing the family to others with diabetes may reduce the feelings of isolation and the nurse should be able to make a suitable introduction.

Other problems which the specialist nurse may experience may conveniently be divided into different age groups, but these are not exclusive to each group and may occur at any age.

34.5.2 THE PRE-SCHOOL CHILD

Parents are the prime carers for this group and their feelings of guilt experienced at diagnosis are increased as they have to cope with the traumas of injections and blood testing. They may find physically holding their child down for injections very traumatic, especially when the child responds with aggression towards them. Single parents have to be taught how to hold their child, to enable them to give an injection on their own and this reduces the sites available to them.

Dietary support is vital in this age group as all pre-school children have erratic eating patterns and the child with diabetes is no different. Inevitably, parents' anxiety increases once the insulin has been given and they know their child must eat. Children quickly sense this anxiety and may use it to manipulate parents, even at this early age. Hypoglycemia is a major concern in young children as they may not be capable of recognizing warning signs and therefore parents become reluctant to leave them in the care of others.

The nurse's responsibility is to support the parents in the education of carers and to try and alleviate their concerns. Young children will experience many intercurrent childhood illnesses, and support should be readily available to help parents as they learn to cope with these difficult situations. Parents need the opportunity to discuss their problems so that a strategy may be developed to help them cope. Regular home blood glucose monitoring, which is not excessive, should be encouraged and most young children will adapt to this provided the routine is maintained.

Starting school is a stressful time and the added problem of the diabetes increases parental anxiety. The support of the specialist nurse visiting the school helps the parents gain confidence.

34.5.3 PRIMARY SCHOOL

The child at junior school should be more involved in the management of diabetes, particularly the practical skills, which need to be assessed on a regular basis to ensure good techniques are maintained. This age group responds well to rewards and appreciates being presented with certificates identifying their achievements. Educational programs with rewards are entered with enthusiasm and parents begin to recognize the ability of their child in managing some aspects of their diabetes. Management may need to be adjusted as the school routine changes to prevent them feeling different because they have to eat at a different time. A problem which is not recognized may lead to manipulation of the diabetes and this can lead to erratic blood glucose control. This may be associated with emotional problems and the nurse's knowledge of the child and family can sometimes identify this in the early stages. Parents often need support to allow their child independence but must be encouraged to continue monitoring their skills to prevent bad habits developing.

34.5.4 ADOLESCENCE

It is hard to decide which is the most difficult age group to cope with, the pre-school child with erratic eating problems and temper tantrums or the teenager with erratic eating patterns and mood swings. Both offer a challenge to the PDSN. Management of diabetes is notoriously difficult in the teenage years, with the variable routine and the interaction of insulin and puberty hormones (see Chapters 5 and 26). The nurse must support the young person through these changes and be their advocate at times of major problems. Confrontation with their parents is common at this age and the nurse may become involved with persuading parents that this may be part of adolescence and not just because of the diabetes.

The first problems of adolescence may occur at the time of transfer to high school, when there is often a major change in routine, increased responsibility for their diabetes and feelings of isolation in a new and very different environment.

Education prior to this age would have been directed more towards the parents, but by the time the child moves to high school they should be able to comprehend more about their diabetes and therefore teaching should be organized to help them cope with the increased responsibility. The pubertal growth spurt may start even before they reach their teens and discussing the relationship between normal growth, development and blood glucose control may motivate a young person into trying to achieve better management of their diabetes.

Transition to adulthood is rarely easy and this is made harder by diabetes. A primary concern of the adolescent is to be the same as their peers, but this is not entirely possible if they have diabetes. The nurse must try and encourage teenagers to construct a routine which will fit into their lifestyle and at the same time give some thought to the management of their diabetes – not an easy combination! Parental pressure, a product of anxiety about their child's diabetes, may lead to greater confrontation and the nurse may become a mediator.

Diabetes has an impact on every aspect of the adolescent's life. They need to be aware of the implications for the future in such areas as complications, careers, smoking, driving, alcohol and starting a family. Girls should be aware of the need for pre-conceptual counselling (see Chapter 31) and why this is necessary. All these points need to be discussed at a time appropriate to the individual, and the specialist nurse must be sensitive to the needs of the young person, remembering that diabetes and its implications can distract from the spontaneous pleasure other young people experience.

The complications of diabetes cannot be ignored and the team must choose the right time to discuss these with the young person. Most parents are very aware of the risks and some use them as a threat when the adolescent is not compliant.

34.6 CONCLUSION

The PDSN must work with the diabetes team to achieve the best control possible for each individual child, taking into account their circumstances. The PDSN's role in education must encompass all carers, whether in the hospital or community; understanding the changing needs of the growing child should enable the specialist nurse to adapt teaching appropriately. Support in the home provides the opportunity for home stabilization and knowledge of the family dynamics is used by the team to devise individual care plans. The ultimate aim must be to see the child grow into a healthy, fit, stable and emotionally secure young adult.

APPENDIX: RESOURCE LIST

1. *School Pack*. (1994) British Diabetic Association, 10 Queen Anne St. London, W1M 0BD. Tel: 071 323 1531.
2. *I have diabetes*. (1983) Althea Braithwack. Dinosaur Publications. HarperCollins, London.
3. *Diabetes Employment Handbook*. (1988) British Diabetic Association, London.
4. *So your child has diabetes*. (1992) Bonnie Estridge and Jo Davies. Vermillion, London.
5. *Teenage Diabetes*. (1990) Judith North. Thorsons Publishing Group, London.
6. *If Your Child is Diabetic*. (1987) Joanne Elliott. Sheldon Press, London.
7. *Insulin Dependent Diabetes*. (1986) John Day. Thorsons Publishing Group and British Diabetic Association, London.
8. *Diabetes – A book for children and their families*. (1993) Boehringer Mannheim UK, London.
9. *Taming the Dragon*, Video. (1990) Novo Nordisk Pharmaceuticals Limited, London.

REFERENCES

British Diabetic Association. (1991) *What Professional Supervision Should Children with Diabetes and their Families Expect?* Leaflet, British Diabetic Association, London.

Challen, A.H., Davies, A.G., Williams, R.J.W. *et al*. (1990) Support for families with diabetic children: parents' views. *Practical Diabetes*, **7**:1, 26–31.

Department of Health. (1991a) *The Children Act 1989. An Introductory Guide for the NHS*. HMSO, London.

Department of Health. (1991b) *Welfare of Children in Hospital*. HMSO, London.

Hatcher, T. (1990) Learning is Fun. *Paediatric Nursing*, **2**:2, 10–12.

Krans, H.M.J., Posta, M. and Keen, H. (1992) *Diabetes Care and Research in Europe: The St Vincent Declaration Action Programme*. WHO Regional Office in Europe, Copenhagen.

Moyer, A. (1987) The specialist nurse and the child with diabetes. *Senior Nurse*, **7**:5, 31–4.

Moyer, A. (1989) Caring for a child with diabetes: the effect of specialist nurse care on parents' needs and concerns. *J. Adv. Nurs.*, **14**, 536–45.

Orem, D.E. (1971) *Nursing: Concepts of Practice*, 3rd edn. McGraw Hill, New York.

Rayner, P. (1984) A home care unit for diabetic children. *Practical Diabetes*, **1**:1, 5–6.

Royal College of Nursing, Diabetes Forum Working Party. (1993a) *The Role of the Diabetes Specialist Nurse*. RCN, London.

Royal College of Nursing, Paediatric Diabetes Special Interest Group. (1993b) *The role and qualifications of the nurse specialising in paediatric diabetes*. Eli Lilley Co. Ltd. and RCN, London.

Royal College of Physicians/British Diabetic Association. (1984) *The Provision of Medical Care for Adult Diabetic Patients in the U.K.* (Available from Royal College of Physicians, London).

35

Primary care and the community

C. WAINE and E.A. STAVELEY

35.1 INTRODUCTION

General practitioners' roles and responsibilities vary greatly from one country to another. This chapter is based on their position in the United Kingdom, which is more clearly defined. Over past decades there has been a tendency for the care of the child with diabetes to be taken over by hospital-based clinics. This is regrettable because it can exclude the potential contribution which the general practitioner and the primary care team can bring to the care of the child and family.

The general practitioner with an average list size will probably only have one child with diabetes – hardly enough to give him or her wide experience; but the child and family can reasonably expect their general practitioner and primary care team to be well-informed, competent and supportive. This has implications for those responsible for the training and continuing education of general practitioners and members of the primary care team (see Chapters 33 and 34).

Walford (1991) has deplored the old and prejudiced attitudes to general practitioner care for patients with diabetes, pointing out that general practitioners and diabetologists have been cooperating in diabetes care for several decades and arguing that the development of joint strategies can enhance diabetes care.

It is the policy of the Royal College of General Practitioners (RCGP, 1985) that much of the care of chronic disease should be via the general practitioner and primary care team working, when appropriate, in partnership with their specialist colleagues to form a team, united by the goal of enhancing patient care. Such a policy is based on solid foundations.

35.2 THE CASE FOR PRIMARY CARE

Four key principles affect health and the health services: the environment, prevention, accessibility and cost-effectiveness. For the child the environment is, quite simply, the home and the family. Prevention is assuming increasing importance in the work of the general practitioner and looking after children with diabetes is very much an exercise in prevention. General practice is certainly accessible and cost-effective and is the ideal place to unite therapeutic and preventive care (RCGP, 1983).

Chronic diseases, of which diabetes is a good example, are lingering and stubborn, more likely to be eased than cured and when they appear, often restrict their sufferer's

Childhood and Adolescent Diabetes
Published in 1994 by Chapman & Hall, London
ISBN 0 412 48610 5

choice and actions. This should be of great concern to family doctors (Waine, 1990).

The growing trend to start children on treatment at home logically demands the involvement of the general practitioner and primary care team. A diagnosis of diabetes in a child has an impact on the whole family, so involving those who look after that family in the management of the child is essential. The modern general practitioner is trained in both three-dimensional care – physical, social and psychological (Gray, 1991) – and in communication skills. These assets must be utilized.

The general practitioner is the doctor of first contact, who is specifically charged with the role of practising 'whole person' medicine and is the only doctor who works frequently with the whole family and invariably provides continuing care over many years (Gray, 1972).

Care by the general practitioner, as the doctor of first contact and continuing presence, can be considered as evolving through a number of consecutive stages: detection, assessment and referral, explanation and continuing care and support.

35.3 DIAGNOSIS

Table 35.1 details the presentation of 30 consecutive children. The triad of polyuria, polydipsia and weight loss were prominent presenting features and a urine test for glucose is mandatory for any child showing these symptoms. In only two instances was the parent a diabetic. The average age at presentation was 7.6 years, but four of the children were under 3 years of age.

All were seen and assessed at a pediatric unit, eleven were not admitted and 14 admitted for less than 24 hours, Only six had diabetic ketoacidosis, which suggests that the diagnosis was being made early. Only one was in hospital for more than two days.

The general practitioner is the most likely person to be consulted by the child and family so, while childhood diabetes may be uncommon, vigilance and a high level of suspicion are necessary at all times. Rapid early diagnosis will increase the confidence of the child and family in the general practitioner.

35.4 ASSESSMENT

Once the diagnosis has been made, the general practitioner must rapidly assess the child's condition so that appropriate decisions can be taken, the most important being whether or not the child's condition needs to be managed in hospital, or can be carried out at home.

If the child is not clinically dehydrated and not clinically ketoacidotic then, given the willingness of the family to cope, it is often possible to initiate treatment at home in collaboration with the pediatric diabetologist and diabetes specialist nurse.

The assessment should be predominantly clinical. For instance, one child with blood glucose 23.1 mmol/l was desperately ill and ketoacidotic, whereas another with blood glucose 62.2 mmol/l did not require admission (Table 35.1).

Nearly all children will have ketonuria at presentation: ketonuria without clinical dehydration and/or ketoacidosis does not necessarily require admission, but where ketonuria and vomiting co-exist, admission is mandatory.

Appropriate investigations should include blood glucose, urea and electrolytes and a urine test for ketones. Height and weight should be recorded. Other factors which need to be taken into consideration are the attitude of the parents and their willingness to cope at home, the availability of comprehensive support in the community by a diabetes specialist nurse, and the degree of expertise and willingness of the general practitioner and primary care team to be

Table 35.1 Children dealt with in the pediatric unit of North Derbyshire Royal Hospital NHS Trust.

Name & Age at Diagnosis	Diabetic Ketoacidosis (DKA)	Blood Glucose (mmol/l)	Urine Test (glucose/size ketones)	Diangosis made by	Presentation	Hospitalization
James 13 yrs	No	42.2	2%/large	GP	Polyuria, polydipsia, weight loss anorexia, lethargy – 2 weeks	Less 24 hours
Louise 5 yrs	No	30.6	2%/small	GP	Polyuria, polydipsia, weight loss, anorexia. Irritability – 2 weeks. Vomiting – 1 day	Less 24 hours
Mark 6 yrs	Yes	34.3	2%/large	GP	Weight loss, polyuria, polydipsia – 4 days	2 days
Laura 8 yrs	No	23.3	2%/moderate	GP	Polyuria, polydipsia. Weight loss – 2 weeks	No
Stephen 11 yrs	Yes	29.9	2%/large	Mother (tested urine)	Polyuria, polydipsia. Weight loss 2–3 weeks. Vomiting – 2 days	2 days
Shelley 12 yrs	No	18.0	2%/moderate	GP	Weight loss, polyuria, polydipsia. Tired – 2 months. Thrush – 1 month prior to diagnosis	No
Craig 8 yrs	Yes	33.7	2%/large	Hospital pediatric registrar	Polyuria, polydipsia, weight loss – 6–8 weeks. Abdominal pain and vomiting – 2 days	3 days
David 10 yrs	No	19.9	2%/moderate	GP	Polyuria, polydipsia. Anorexia – 3 weeks	No
Damien 8 yrs	No	29.9	2%/moderate	GP	Weight loss, polyuria, polydipsia – 3–4 weeks	Less 24 hours
Clare 12 yrs	No	15.9	2%/moderate	GP	Polyuria, polydipsia, weight loss – 2–3 weeks	Less 24 hours
Ryan 11 yrs	No	40.9	2%/moderate	GP	Weight loss, polyuria, polydipsia – 2 weeks. General malaise – 6 weeks	Less 24 hours
Peter 2 yrs	No	41.9	2%/large	GP	Polyuria, polydipsia – 2 weeks. Unwell since chicken pox 3 months previously	Less 24 hours
Alexandra 9 yrs	No	19.7	2%/no	GP	Polyuria, polydipsia, weight loss – 2 weeks	No
Jason 5 yrs	No	39.7	2%/small	GP	Polyuria, polydipsia, lethargy – 2 weeks	No
Laura 12 yrs	No	22.7	2%/strong	GP	Polyuria, polydipsia, weight loss	Less 24 hours
Samantha 5 yrs	No	28.0	2%/moderate	GP	Polyuria, polydipsia, tired, bed-wetting – 2–3 weeks. Vomiting – 1 day	Less 24 hours
Lee 15 yrs	No	30.7	2%/large	GP	Polyuria, polydipsia, weight loss – 2 weeks	No
Mark 15 yrs	No	29.3	2%/large	GP	Polyuria, polydipsia – 2–3 weeks. Down syndrome (deaf, unable to speak)	2 days

Table 35.1 *Continued*

Name & Age at Diagnosis	Diabetic Ketoacidosis (DKA)	Blood Glucose (mmol/l)	Urine Test (glucose/size ketones)	Diangosis made by	Presentation	Hospitalization
Suzanne 8 yrs	Yes	37.1	2%/large	GP	Polyuria, polydipsia, weight loss – 1 week. Vomiting – 3 days	Less 24 hours
Thomas 6 yrs	No	26.9	2%/moderate	Grandmother	Polyuria, polydipsia, lethargy, weight loss – 3–4 weeks	Less 24 hours
Andrew 4 yrs	No	62.0	2%/moderate	GP	Polyuria, polydipsia, lethargy, weight loss – 10 days	No
Rebecca 22 mths	No	17.6	2%/moderate	Mother (tested urine)	Polyuria, polydipsia – 2–3 weeks	Less 24 hours
Laura 2 yrs (twin of Rebecca above)	No	13.4	2%/no	Mother	Polyuria, polydipisa – 1 week	No
Helen 7 yrs	No	29.7	2%/moderate	GP	Weight loss, polyuria, polydipsia – 4 weeks. Mother insulin dependent diabetic	Less 24 hours
Kelly 1 yr	Yes	23.1	2%/large	Father	Several months unwell, weight loss, thrush, polyuria, polydipsia, several visits to GP. Father insulin dependent diabetic	2 days
Sarah 8 yrs	No	33.3	2%/moderate	Uncle checked blood glucose	Polyuria, polydipsia, weight loss – 3 months	No
Daniel 5 yrs	No	21.0	2%/moderate	GP	Polyuria, polydipsia, weight loss – 8–10 weeks	No
Georgina 4 yrs	No	29.6	2%/strong	GP	Weight loss, bed-wetting, polyuria, polydipsia, lethargy – 4–5 weeks	Less 24 hours
Richard 11 yrs	Yes	39.1	2%/large	GP	Lethargy, polyuria, polydipsia, weight loss – 2 weeks	Less 24 hours
Christopher 3 yrs	No	30.8	2%/moderate	GP	Polyuria, polydipsia, lethargy – 1 week	No

involved. Parents are only asked to take responsibility when they feel confident to do so.

Continuity of care and consistent advice are essential, so that soon after presentation clear lines of responsibility should be agreed between general practitioner, pediatrician and specialist nurse. In the early days after diagnosis the bulk of care, advice and support is usually given by the specialist nurse. Such nurses can provide the essential link between the specialist and the primary care team (see Chapter 34).

35.5 EXPLANATION

As their training includes communication skills and as he or she is likely to be known to child and family, it is appropriate that the general practitioner should play an integral part in explaining the condition to the child and family. In doing so, it is essential that there is close liaison with the hospital-based team so that both are giving the same message.

There is one absolute pre-requisite: the making of an adequate amount of time available to the child and family, time which allows the child and family to raise questions, reveal fears and problems and seek explanations. This is very difficult and demanding work which cannot be accomplished in a single session and is best achieved by a series of consultations paced by the child and the family.

Parents' reactions go through three stages (Gray, 1972). First, parents often experience a phase of surprise and shock, followed by the phase of emotion, shown outwardly as anger and resentment and inwardly, as guilt. Third, there is the phase of adjustment. Some, but by no means all, reach the stage of acceptance. Psychologists have compared these phases with the grief reaction.

35.6 CONTINUITY OF CARE AND SUPPORT

> Successful management of children with diabetes is nowadays recognised to depend on the effective transfer of skills and information to the diabetic child, his or her family, friends and community. (Young and Greenhouge, 1993)

The specialist and primary care teams' roles should complement and not duplicate each other; it is essential that information is shared and that effective lines of communication between the two are established at an early stage. Records held by parents can play a valuable role here.

Diabetes is a disease which has repercussions on the whole family and siblings, as well as the child with diabetes, have needs which must be met. Prophylactic counseling should be considered for all families (see also Chapter 32).

35.7 INTERCURRENT ILLNESS

The general practitioner has two roles in this area:

(a) Prevention by ensuring the child is fully up to date with all immunizations.
(b) Managing the child and family through the illness.

At times of illness, blood glucose monitoring should be increased and regular urine testing for ketones carried out. Doses of insulin may need to be increased and often extra doses given. Insulin should never be omitted because of anorexia. Children with diabetes are no more likely to get the usual childhood illnesses than other children but when they occur, the consequences of severe metabolic upset, such as diabetic ketoacidosis from a simple illness can be dramatic. Doctors should remember that children with diabetes should be protected each year by vaccination against influenza.

35.8 CLINICAL AUDIT

The general practitioner with an average list size may only have one child with diabetes, yet the child and family can reasonably expect their general practitioner and primary care team to be well informed, competent and supportive. Clinical audit can be one way of achieving this, because medical audit is a promising means to an essential end – improving the quality of medical care that the patient receives (Marinker, 1990).

The general practitioner and the primary care team must be creative in their search for good standards of practice and they must be their own sternest critics in searching for error.

Clinical audit can be looked at from three perspectives: contractual, managerial or educational. This section has been written solely from the educational perspective. Clinical audit is nothing less than an attempt to apply scientific methods to the quest for quality. In simple terms, it means looking critically at what you are doing to see if you can do it better.

Chronic conditions, of which diabetes is a prime example, are particularly suited to the practice of audit. Since children with diabetes can have their ability to work or play impaired, the question we must ask constantly is 'What can we do to help such patients live as fully as possible, given their circumstances?'

35.9 GETTING STARTED

The first need is to define therapeutic aims and construct or adopt guidelines for the management of a child with diabetes. The therapeutic aims might be:

1) To search for diabetes.
2) To maintain continuing communication with other patients with diabetes.
3) To achieve the degree of metabolic control likely to avoid complications.
4) To search for early indications of end organ damage.
5) To ensure that appropriate action is taken.

In the words of Kurtz (1985), 'The goals of therapy are set by doctors but have to be achieved by patients.' Measurements of performance can then be based on the following checks.

At each visit, the child and parents should be asked about problems since the last attendance, the results of blood and urine tests should be studied and the diet and dosage of tablets or insulin reviewed. The patient's height and weight should be measured and the feet inspected. Blood should be taken for random blood glucose and if 6–10 weeks have elapsed since the last visit, glycosylated hemoglobin. Urine should be checked for albumin and injection sites should be inspected.

Periodically, checks should be made on the technique of drawing up and injecting insulin and the technique for measuring blood glucose.

Once a year, there should be checks of creatinine and blood pressure; and a check of visual acuity and inspection of the optic fundus after preliminary dilatation of the pupils (after five years of diabetes). In addition, regular reviews of diet by the dietician are highly desirable (RCGP, 1993).

Because the number of children with diabetes in any one practice is likely to be small, there is much to be said for collaborative audit involving a whole health district, especially as all those concerned with diabetes care should be moving towards developing measures of outcome. This in turn, demands collaboration with the physicians responsible for the care of adults with diabetes, but as the general practitioner is the doctor of first contact and continuing presence, he or she is well placed to be a key participant in any form of district audit.

35.10 CONCLUSION

In the future, general practitioners and primary care teams are likely to have a greater part to play in the management of children with diabetes. This has major implications for their training and continuing education which must be addressed. Care by the general practitioner and primary care team occurs logically through consecutive stages: detection, assessment and referral, explanation and continuity of care and support.

The care of the child with diabetes must be integrated with the care of the whole family. A holistic approach is essential and the general practitioner and primary care team are trained to deliver this. The needs of children with diabetes and their families are best met when the general practitioner and primary care team share goals for their management with the hospital-based pediatric team. The needs of the family, as well as those of the child, must be acknowledged and appropriate steps taken to meet them.

REFERENCES

Gray, D.J. Periera. (1987) *The frontline of the health service*, RCGP Report from General Practice, 25. Royal College of General Practitioners, London.

Gray, D.J. Pereira. (1972) The care of the handicapped child in general practice. Huntarian Society Gold Medal Prize Essay.

Kurtz, A.B. (1985) quoted in Waine, C. (1988) *Why Not Care for your Diabetic Patients?*, 2nd edn, p. vii. Royal College of General Practitioners, London.

Marinker, M. (1990) *Medical Audit and General Practice*. British Medical Journal, for the MSD Foundation, London.

Royal College of General Practitioners. (1983) *Healthier Children – Thinking Prevention*. Report from General Practice No. 22. Royal College of General Practitioners, London.

Royal College of General Practitioners. (1985) *Quality in General Practice*, Policy Statement No. 2. Royal College of General Practitioners, London.

Royal College of General Practitioners. (1993) *Guidelines for the care of patients with diabetes*. Royal College of General Practitioners, London.

Waine, C. (1990) Audit of chronic disease, in M. Marinker (ed.). *Medical Audit and General Practice*, pp. 67–100. BMJ, London.

Waine, C. (1992) *Diabetes in General* Practice (3rd edn). Royal College of General Practitioners, London.

Walford, S. (1991) Editorial. *Diabetic Medicine*, **8**, 307–308.

Young, R.J. and Greenhouge, S. (1992) The new diabetic child. *Diabetes Care*, **1**, 2.

36

Camps for diabetic children and teenagers

C. THOMPSON, S.A. GREENE and R.W. NEWTON

36.1 INTRODUCTION

Prior to the discovery of insulin in 1922, the prospects for a nomal healthy outdoor life were negligible for the young person with insulin-dependent diabetes mellitus, and its therapeutic impact can be gauged by the advent of camping holidays for children with diabetes within only a few years of its clinical introduction. As early as 1925 a summer camp was held in Detroit, and the early success of this project led to the proliferation of camps throughout the United States, which were being offered in 43 states by 1988 (Delcher, 1991). Since 1936 the British Diabetic Association (BDA) has run holidays for children with diabetes; over 100 000 children and young adults in the UK have now enjoyed the challenge of diabetic holidays and in 1992 the BDA allocated £110 000 towards the cost of holidays, representing a subsidy of £220 per child (G. Hood, personal communication). Most holidays occur in the summer vacation, although winter skiing trips are also offered and the range of activities varies from leisurely pastimes to more physically demanding pursuits typified by the Eskdale Outward Bound Mountain Course (Hillson, 1984a) and the Firbush Course in Tayside (Newton *et al.*, 1985) as part of the Youth Diabetes Project. In this chapter we will review the general principles of camp aims and organization, with illustrative examples taken from the Firbush Project on Loch Tay in Scotland.

36.2 AIMS AND PHILOSOPHY

The original intention behind the early BDA camps was to offer healthy supervised holidays to children from underprivileged households, but throughout subsequent decades children from all social and geographical backgrounds have been represented. The most important aim of the camps is to provide an enjoyable holiday with a variety of exciting activities, properly supervised by experienced staff. A happy camp is an absolute prerequisite to create the conditions to develop the secondary goals: learning social skills, gaining the self-confidence to participate in unfamiliar physical activities, education in self-management of diabetes, and sharing the experience of coming to terms with diabetic life.

Development of social skills is an important part of diabetic camps (Delcher, 1991). Prior to camp many children have

Childhood and Adolescent Diabetes
Published in 1994 by Chapman & Hall, London
ISBN 0 412 48610 5

never had the opportunity to meet other youngsters with diabetes, particularly in a recreational setting with the time and encouragement to discuss thorny issues such as injections, diets and hypoglycemia. The relaxed, non-threatening environment of a camp facilitates discussion, with many youngsters prompted to talk for the first time about living with diabetes. The experience is almost uniformly positive, with most teenagers reporting improved self-confidence following diabetic holidays (McCraw & Travis, 1973), an assessment echoed by the parents of children attending camps (Vyas *et al.*, 1987).

> 'I had never met another young diabetic before – a totally new experience for me to be with other people who were having injections at the same time – to be able to talk about sticking to a diet.'

Many youngsters with diabetes avoid strenuous activities, principally because of the fear of hypoglycemia, and camps provide the ideal environment for instruction and coaching through the insulin and dietary adjustments necessary to cope with unfamiliar exercise. Almost all camps offer some form of physical activity. Some have incorporated a fitness program with a formal assessment of physical fitness index pre- and post-camp (Åkerblom *et al.*, 1980) while others have clearly defined physical objectives (Hillson, 1984a). Most provide the opportunity simply to enjoy sports and pursuits under the supervision of trained instructors and experienced medical staff. In this respect, one of the most important goals of camps is to convey the message that diabetes is entirely compatible with an active outdoor life, and that, with a little care and planning, most sports and pursuits can be easily attempted. In the US, development of camping skills is encouraged (Delcher, 1991) although in the more inclement weather of the UK, most 'camps' are actually held in dormitory-type accommodation and camping skills are therefore not an issue.

Education remains of paramount importance to the concept of the diabetic camp, a view stressed in a recent BDA report of the Young Persons Holiday Programme (G. Hood, personal communication), and the role of the medical team – doctors, nurses and dietitians – is not simply the provision of medical cover, but also to contribute educational input and encouragement. This is particularly important for younger children, up to 25% of whom may not be injecting their own insulin when they come to camp; less than 1% leave without the ability to do so (Delcher, 1991). Blood glucose monitoring may likewise be a technique not yet mastered, but amenable to education at camp. The educational value of camps for younger children was emphasized by a postal survey of the parents of children attending two educational camps; there were significant increases in children doing blood tests on their own, more confidence in the recognition of hypoglycemia and a sustained increase in independence with insulin injections (Vyas *et al.*, 1987). Older teenagers are almost universally independent in such respects (in some camps this is a prerequisite to attendance) and tend to seek advice on more adult topics such as alcohol, sport, exercise, complications and contraception. However, most older teenagers still report increased self-confidence in dealing with their diabetes, both technically and emotionally, after having attended an educational holiday camp.

The educational worth of a diabetic camp to the attending medical team should also not be underestimated. Most health professionals recognize the value of having personally attended an educational holiday (Walker & Sharland, 1987). The advantages come in several forms. First, it is usually their first experience of living in close quarters with diabetes over a prolonged period of time, with a more intense exposure to the practicalities of living with diabetes than it is possible to obtain from hospital wards or clinics.

> 'A doctor will say you have to do this or do that, but they aren't going through it. They don't know what it's like to be eighteen, with all your friends going off hiking, and you have to stand by and watch. Careful in case you go hypo. Or maybe you get invited to an all-night party – it's a long time since a lot of them were eighteen. They can sympathize, but they can't say like I can, don't worry I've managed it this way.'

Second, the relaxed setting of a holiday camp, where teenagers and staff are on first-name terms, often having shared a vigorous soaking in mountainside rain, provides an environment more conducive to frank talk and discussion than the oppressive, hierarchical setting of a hospital.

> 'It's very authoritarian. It's like you don't go to clinics for reassurance and advice, you go there for a row. They give you a lecture about how badly you have been doing.'

Young people are far more comfortable on holiday than in clinics and their honest and often forthright comments about their perspective of diabetes – and how it is managed by health care professionals – can be a sobering experience which gives pause for reflection on one's own practices. Finally, interactive discussion groups rarely fail to alert the health care professional to new methods of managing diabetes. It is highly unusual for a member of the medical team to leave a camp without modification to his or her attitudes towards teenage diabetes – so much so that it has been suggested that attending an educational holiday camp should be formally incorporated into the training structure of aspiring diabetes specialists.

The Firbush Outdoor Activity Centre provided the setting for a novel camp, begun in 1983, which, while embracing the aims and ideals noted above, also sought to harness the powerful benefits of association between teenagers with diabetes, in order to encourage those who are independent and well-adjusted to help those less able to cope with diabetic life (Newton *et al.*, 1985). As such, it became the forerunner and eventually the focal point of the Youth Diabetics Project, a nationwide network of active young people with diabetes, able to articulate the difficulties and needs of their age-groups. Although the original aims – to produce 'Young Diabetic Leaders' – have been perceived by some as elitist and threatening, the intended role of such 'leaders' was to be supportive and friendly. It was hoped that young people attending the Firbush camp might fulfil a reassuring and supportive role to newly-diagnosed teenagers in their home clinics or hospitals, form the nucleus of local Youth Diabetic groups throughout the country, and provide feedback to the medical profession, at both local and national level, on the structure and style of diabetes service they wished to see implemented.

> 'I feel a responsibility towards others. I have now found out that I have something I can give to another diabetic.'

Many clinics run local camps specifically for their own children, and in Dundee we have done so since 1987. We believe that the information gained from these camps is unobtainable in the normal clinic setting or even from home visits, and bonds between children and clinic staff develop in the camp setting which render subsequent clinic visits entirely different in character. As many of our children are leaving home with diabetes for the first time, we have adopted a weekend format, rather than the longer holidays favored by the BDA. Even in this short time period however, we have found these camps an ideal setting in which to get to know the children attending our local clinic, identify problems of diabetes management and adopt strategies to deal with them.

36.3 CAMP ORGANIZATION

36.3.1 SELECTION: TEENAGERS AND STAFF

One of the basic tenets of both the Firbush camp and the BDA education holidays is that they should be open to children from all ethnic, geographical and socioeconomic backgrounds, and that no unreasonable financial obstacle should discourage attendance. To this end the Firbush camp was free to participants until 1993, with course finance provided by Novo Nordisk UK and travel costs by the BDA; burgeoning costs have led to the introduction of a standard £100 contribution, though local clinics are encouraged to volunteer the money in needy cases. If no local funds are available, the costs are waived. The BDA operates a similar arrangement, with an average subsidy per child of £220 per holiday. It is common sense to age-stratify the camps so that the nature of the camps and their constituent pursuits are appropriate to emotional and physical development. It is also sensible to solicit an appraisal of the suitability of applicants from their local consultant; although one strives not to reject applicants, a history of manipulative ketoacidosis might be dangerous in an outward bound camp with prolonged periods away from medical care, and an inability to swim might preclude enjoyment of a water-sports holiday. The consultant's appraisal can also give valuable insight into personality traits, tendency to hypoglycemia and ability to socialize, so that potentially vulnerable campers can be identified early.

The exact number and composition of staff varies according to the nature of the holiday: the larger the number of youngsters, the larger the number of staff required; and the more specialized or potentially hazardous the sporting activities, the more expert instructors are required. In addition, some camps are used for training purposes for medical staff and may have a higher staff: teenager ratio. At the 1993 Firbush Project there were five doctors, two diabetes nurses and one dietitian, as well as three specialized instructors, for 28 young people. The high staff : youngster ratio reflects the simultaneous running of three or more sporting activities and the emphasis on small interactive discussion groups. A balance is attempted between 'old hands' and professionals who have never previously attended a camp; in this respect, the camp is viewed as fulfilling a training role and in the past interested medical students have joined the staff. The employment of expertly trained instructors is imperative to ensure the safety of outdoor activities (Hillson, 1987); although the conduct of sporting pursuits and the provision of suitable equipment is their area of responsibility, prior consultation with instructors is suggested to ensure that activities are timed to accommodate meals and insulin, and potential hazards, particularly involving hypoglycemia, identified and contingency plans drawn up.

For this reason a staff meeting prior to the arrival of the participants is recommended to establish the timetable of pursuits for the week and to allocate specific tasks such as banking, and care of the medical kit. The participants are discussed in the light of their consultants' letters and potential problems talked over. The activities can be planned with the help of the expert staff, pitfalls identified and solutions agreed upon. In addition, staff can get to know each other and areas of special expertise can be identified.

There should be an early contact between the dietitian and the caterers who will be providing and cooking food (Hillson, 1984b), preferably with a site visit to assess facilities. Guidelines for dietitians attending camps are available from the BDA, along with copies of BDA Dietary Recommendations, and recipe books for the center can be supplied by the BDA. An adequate intake of carbohydrate is crucial; one study of children aged 6–9 years found the average pre-camp carbohydrate prescription to be 44 g below minimal recommended values (Frost *et al.*, 1986) and some youngsters may require up to 100 g extra carbohydrate per day without loss of glycemic control (Hillson, 1984b). Although in general the principle of a high-carbohydrate, high-fiber, moderate-fat diet should be followed, palatability must be maintained; young people are notoriously fastidious and failure to provide a suitable diet may lead to mass hypoglycemia! However, camps are an ideal time to introduce the principles of a healthy diet.

36.3.2 TIMETABLE OF ACTIVITIES

An evening meeting of staff and campers on the evening of arrival is an ideal time for introductions, explanation of camp 'ground rules', advice about prevention of hypoglycemia and blisters, and an outline of the weekly activities; a timetable sample from Firbush is shown in Table 36.1.

Following breakfast, our practice is to divide the campers into groups of 4–6 people with one or two members of staff; they remain as a unit for small group discussion for the entire week. It is useful to start off with an exploration of expectations of the week, and towards the end of the holiday, discuss achievements and disappointments. Other popular topics include 'problems of diabetic life in the teenage years' and 'how should a hospital service provide care for teenagers with diabetes?'. The groups meet for about an hour, after which the daily activities begin.

It is a useful exercise for everyone to spend the first day together, and we have found that a long group hike facilitates bonding and familiarity, with its sense of shared achievement, and the camaraderie of swapping stories and comparing blisters back at camp. On subsequent days our practice is to divide the campers into three or four groups who rotate through the various activities provided, leaving the opportunity for two days at the end of the holiday to concentrate on a favored sport, and develop some expertise. Many teenagers trace lifelong hobbies to fumbled beginnings at camp.

Following the evening meal, there are large group educational sessions for an hour, in which the teenagers are encouraged to play a major role. Although some are obviously shy, for many the experience is highly important and may be tremendously cathartic. For example, an 18-year-old girl with a history of frequent and prolonged hospitalization for recurrent ketoacidosis attended camp and was intermittently bed-ridden with mild unexplained ketoacidosis. After intently following a lively large group discussion on 'missing insulin injections' during which the consensus was reached that 'we all do it', she gave an unsolicited and moving account of her years of insulin manipulation, concluding that she was until that moment unaware that anyone else shared or understood her problem, and had never felt sufficiently confident or relaxed to discuss it.

After the educational sessions have ended, the evenings are host to a variety of relaxing social events, such as dances, barbecues, and on the final evening, a cabaret show performed by staff and campers.

36.3.3 THE MEDICAL KIT

A multiplicity of physical injuries and illness can be sustained by a group of active young people participating in physically demanding activities and living in close proximity to each other, and although it is impossible to cover

Table 36.1 Timetable of activities at Firbush Outdoor Activity Camp.

	Friday	Saturday	Sunday	Monday	Tuesday	Wednesday	Thursday	Friday
0815				Advice if needed – Mini-Clinic Session				
0830				Breakfast				
0930				Small Group Discussion				
1030	Arrival	Hiking	Canoeing	Sailing/ Abseiling	Windsurfing	Two days spent in activity of choice		Home
1800				Evening Meal				
1930				Whole Group Education Session				
	Welcome Program. House Rules. Hypos & Blisters	Diabetes and Sport	Sex, Pregnancy and Contraception	The Diabetic Clinic	Free Time	'Good' Control. How to achieve it and pitfalls	Summing up	
2030				Social Activities				

Table 36.2 Contents of typical medical bag at diabetic camp.

Antibiotics	Phenoxymethylpenicillin Erythromicin Ampicillin Flucloxacillin Otosporin ear drops
Antihistamines	Chlorpheniramine (Oral and IV)
Analgesia	Aminocetophen Dihydrocodeine
Antiemetic	Metoclopramide (Oral and IV)
Antidiarrheals	Loperamide Kaolin & morphine mixture
Miscellaneous	Hydrocortisone IV Epinephrine 1:10 000 IV Diazepam IV & rectal solution Salbutamol inhaler Glucagon Insulin – soluble and isophane Syringes, needles, intravenous cannulae Stitch set and lignocaine 2% local anesthetic Bags of 0.9% sodium chloride and 10% dextrose for infusion Dextrose 25% (25 ml) for IV injection Airways Calamine lotion Mouthwash solution tablets Povidone – iodine antiseptic solution 10% Dry & gauze dressing, bandaids and cotton wool Sterets injection swabs

every eventuality, it is prudent to be prepared for the likelihood. Table 36.2 shows the contents of the medical kit which we take to Firbush, and although most items are self-explanatory, one or two contents are worthy of comment. A stock of soluble and isophane insulin, plus syringes, is obvious for those inevitable few who forget their own supply, but what cannot be sufficiently stressed is that an adequate amount of dextrose tablets, glucagon and IV dextrose should be taken as the incidence of hypoglycemia, usually mild, occasionally severe, will almost always exceed expectations. A supply of antibiotics to treat the commoner infections may obviate the need for tedious visits to the local general practitioner, and as gastroenteritis may very rapidly spread through a community of young people, antidiarrheals and antiemetics are often very useful. Because of the potential for ketoacidosis, either associated with illness such as gastroenteritis, or due to manipulation of insulin, we always take cannulae and intravenous fluids. It is always courteous to inform in advance local general practitioners and hospital staff of the sudden presence in their midst of a group of young diabetic campers. Supervision of the medical kit is usually delegated to one member of staff (traditionally a nurse), though each member of staff carries a 'hypo kit' at all times (Table 36.3).

Table 36.3 Contents of portable 'Hypo Kit' carried in watertight box by medical staff during all activities.

Autolet + BM 20-800 Glycemia Test Strips
Dextrosol
Hypostop
25 ml + 50 ml syringes
50% Dextrose for injection
Glucagon 1 mg for injection (×2)

36.3.4 TROUBLESHOOTING

The major worry for teenagers about to partake in heavy or unfamiliar exercise is hypoglycemia and despite the most meticulous precautions virtually everyone suffers mild early hypoglycemia. Frost *et al.* (1986) found an incidence of 85 clinical episodes of hypoglycemia in 38 children in the first week of two consecutive camps, and although most episodes are mild and rapidly treated, severe hypoglycemia is not rare, and fits have been reported (Swift & Waldron, 1990). Most camps instruct participants to reduce their total daily insulin dose by around 25% on day 1 and to monitor blood glucose frequently to allow further adjustment. Hypoglycemia occurs far more frequently when the insulin dose exceeds 0.7 u/kg body weight (Frost *et al.*, 1986), and staff should be alert to the strong possibility of hypoglycemia in children on large doses of insulin. Some individuals, often those who usually take a low dose of insulin, prefer to increase carbohydrate consumption rather than reduce insulin to prevent hypoglycemia and this should not be discouraged; it is, after all, what a nondiabetic child would do during periods of unusual exercise. During a winter skiing camp for teenage diabetics, a Finnish group found a mean decrease in daily insulin dose of 11.8% compared with pre-camp and an increase in caloric intake of 31% (Åkerblom *et al.*, 1980).

The increase in carbohydrate intake should be catered for not only at meal times, but at snack times (snack carbohydrate content should be doubled from day 1), and by a policy of each participant carrying readily absorbable carbohydrate in the form of dextrose tablets, cereal bars and chocolate bars at all times. Many participants cheerfully ignore or forget such exortations, however, and it is incumbent upon the staff to carry extra carbohydrate on day outings, particularly long days in the hills, which have the potential to be delayed past normal meal times by inclement weather or unfit participants. In this respect the confounding effect of cold should be mentioned. Hypoglycemia is far commoner in individuals who are cold, especially those who are cold and wet, and particular vigilance should be exercised during cold weather or when participating in water sports with regular dousing in cold lakes or rivers. In addition, hypoglycemia may precipitate hypothermia (Gale *et al.*, 1981), and it may be difficult to discern hypoglycemia in cold, frightened, shivering youngsters (Hillson, 1984b). If in any doubt, glucose is given. Because water sports particularly predispose towards hypoglycemia by reason of the cold and exceptional physical effort involved, and because the consequences of hypoglycemia in a canoe or on a windsurfer in the middle of a lake are potentially disastrous, we take particular care in such circumstances. At Firbush trained instructors in a motorized boat patrol the water with a large supply of chocolate and dextrose tablets at all times.

The question of alcohol consumption may arise at some of the camps for older teenagers and young adults. If the legal age for purchase of alcohol has been attained, it is difficult to be prescriptive, and it is probably undesirable to ban acohol totally anyway. From a practial point of view, however, the potential for hypoglycemia is considerably amplified by ingestion of large amounts of alcohol following prolonged vigorous exercise, and ketoacidosis may also occasionally be precipitated. In addition, full enjoyment of the subsequent day's activities is unlikely following a night of little sleep and excess alcohol. In Firbush we run a small bar on site for the sale of beer and wine, but participants are requested not to bring spirits purchased elsewhere to camp, and the bar closes early to discourage late-night parties. With the physical demands of an outdoor holiday, particularly in warm summer weather, there will be a considerable increase in fluid requirement, for which reason the camp should be well-stocked with a readily available supply of non-alcoholic low-calorie drinks.

Blistering can be a painfully frequent problem at a camp in which long hikes or mountain climbing are part of the schedule. At the camp meeting on the first night, participants are advised to wear two pairs of socks on all walking or climbing expeditions and are made aware of the presence of 'blister kits' among the medical staff, for treatment of painful blistering both on the hillside, and back in camp. This is a very important aspect of walking holidays as blistering is common, painful and a possible avenue for infection.

36.3.5 PROBLEMS DURING CAMP

The most common medical problem encountered during camps is hypoglycemia, which was addressed in detail in the previous section. Despite reduction of insulin dosage, increase in carbohydrate intake and frequent blood glucose monitoring, most participants become hypoglycemic at some stage during camp, though a high level of awareness of the problem and the ready availability of dextrose means that the overwhelming majority of cases are trivial.

Much less common, though potentially more serious is ketoacidosis. Warning signs may be derived from the report of the referring clinic doctor and include frequent hospital admissions, high HbA_1, low insulin dosage and dislike of injections. Many episodes are manipulative (Hillson, 1984b), usually as attention-seeking episodes, though during savagely inclement weather, mild ketoacidosis and 'tummy upset' tend to mysteriously occur in those physically or psychologically less robust! The importance of recognizing ketoacidosis is that it is dangerous to allow ketoacidotic youngsters to participate in strenuous exercise, which will increase the acidosis, and particularly for them to embark on long hikes or climbs remote from medical services. Death from cerebral edema complicating ketoacidosis has occurred at camp in the US (Delcher, 1991).

Because of the level of medical supervision at camps, most episodes of ketoacidosis are recognized early and can readily be treated at base with bed rest and frequent injections of soluble insulin. In more serious cases, however, it is sensible to admit early to local hospital facilities. One reasonably common medical precipitant of ketoacidosis is gastroenteritis, which can spread with some rapidity through the close confines of a camp. Bed, frequent fluids, antiemetics, antidiarrheals and frequent injections of soluble insulin are generally sufficient, though a liter of intravenous sodium chloride, with 40 mmol of added potassium chloride, given over six hours can expedite a return to wellbeing in those who find oral fluids difficult. Significant dehydration should be treated with hospitalization, and spread can be limited by close attention to hygiene.

Soft tissue injuries, sprains, bumps and bruises abound during camps and need little beyond simple analgesia and support with crepe or ace bandages or Tubigrip. We routinely stock medical equipment to manage simple sprains, abrasions and lacerations. Occasional fractures occur – bilateral fracture of the humerus during mountain biking, for instance – and require attention at local hospitals. Asthma is very common in teenagers and may be exacerbated by exercise, and it is worth keeping a close watch on those prone to bronchospasm. We routinely carry salbutamol and hydrocortisone, while others also recommend aminophylline (Hillson, 1984b). Homesickness is commoner in camps for younger children and best managed with sympathy and encouragement. Loneliness and homesickness are common fellow travellers and it is important to ensure that each camper is integrated into a group of friends.

Because of the potential for illness or accident at a diabetic camp it is advisable to be covered by an insurance policy. Most outward bound centers will be able to provide this as part of the hire agreement.

36.4 SUMMARY

Camps for children and teenagers with diabetes have been established for many decades now. The aim of camps is to provide a safe, enjoyable holiday which creates a friendly atmosphere in which social skills and self-esteem are developed, and provides a forum for education concerning self-management of diabetes. They are of proven short-term value in this respect, though the long-term impact of camp attendance has not been evaluated. The interactive nature of camps is also of immense educational value to doctors, nurses and dietitians who are members of staff.

> Discovering other people like yourself makes you think; if they've got it, it can't be that bad after all.

REFERENCES

Åkerblom, H.K., Koivukangas, T. and Ilkka, J. (1980) Experiences from a winter camp for teenage diabetics. *Acta Paed. Scand.*, **283** (Suppl.), 50–52.

Delcher, H.K. (1991) Camps for children with diabetes mellitus', in J.K. Davidson (ed.). *Clinical Diabetes Mellitus: a problem orientated approach*, pp. 767–69. Thieme Medical Publishers, New York.

Frost, G.F., Hodges, S. and Swift, P.G.F. (1986) Dietary carbohydrate deficits and hypoglycaemia in the young diabetic on holiday. *Diabetic Med.*, **3**, 250–52.

Gale, E., Bennett, T., Green, J.H. *et al.* (1981) Hypoglycaemia, hypothermia and shivering in man. *Clinical Science*, **61**, 463–69.

Hillson, R.M. (1984a) Diabetes Outward Bound Mountain Course, Eskdale, Cumbria. *Diabetic Med.*, **1**, 59–63.

Hillson, R.M. (1984b) Suggested supplies for Outdoor Diabetic Camps. *Practical Diabetes*, **1**, 43–45.

Hillson, R.M. (1987) British Diabetic Association activities for young people – safety while adventuring. *Practical Diabetes*, **4**, 233–34.

McGraw, R.K., and Travis, L.G. (1973) Psychological effects of a special summer camp on juvenile diabetics. *Diabetes*, **22**, 275–78.

Newton, R.W., Isles, T. and Farquhar, J.W. (1985) The Firbush Project – sharing a way of life. *Diabetic Med.*, **2**, 217–24.

Swift, P.G.F. and Waldron, S. (1990) Have diabetes – will travel. *Practical Diabetes*, **7**, 101–104.

Vyas, S., Mullee, M.A. and Kinmonth, A.-L. (1987) British Diabetic Association holidays – what are they worth? *Diabetic Med.*, **5**, 89–92.

Walker, R. and Sharland, V. (1987) Benefits of BDA educational holidays – chance or design? *Practical Diabetes*, **4**, 163–65.

37

Self-help in childhood diabetes

P.G.F. SWIFT, J. NORTH and S. REDMOND

37.1 INTRODUCTION

The management of diabetes in children is both complex and intrusive. Many new skills must be acquired and family lifestyles modified. Education in diabetes should be concerned therefore not only with providing factual information but sharing confidences and feelings. Effective education helps parents and children to understand their situation more clearly and in this way take control of their own management. Such a patient-centered approach can only succeed on the basis of a trusted partnership between the family and professionals.

Even when such a partnership exists, the medical care team cannot, and should not, expect to be able to provide totally comprehensive personal and social support for the child and family. There is a universal need for external support mechanisms to enhance medical care. Thus parents seek help from friends, relatives, the church, social acquaintances and other parents of children with diabetes. It is from these contacts that self-help groups, networks and organizations evolve.

37.2 THE MEDICAL APPROACH

There has developed in recent years a misguided perception that modern medicine is infallible. When this perception is found to be false, the medical establishment finds itself heavily criticized to the extent that, far from providing comprehensive care, it may be accused of endangering health. Doctors are said to be over-dependent upon modern technology, lack empathy with patients and even to 'expropriate the individuals's power to shape his own environment' (Illich, 1975).

Some support for these concerns can be found in studies showing that in many consultations patients are not encouraged to ask questions and close interaction is inhibited. A survey of British Diabetic Association adult members reported that 60% found it easier to talk to another diabetic person than doctors or nurses (Kelleher, 1991) and a research study showed that in 70% of consultations the doctor interrupted the patient within 18 seconds of the patient beginning to speak (Beckman & Franhel, 1984). In contrast, other studies indicate that when patients do ask questions, higher levels of satisfaction result (Blau, 1989) and there may even be physiologic improvements when patients feel in control – lower blood glucose levels have been documented when consultations are structured to encourage patients to interrupt and ask questions (Kaplan *et al.*, 1989). Team-based education programs using non-authoritarian, interactive approaches giving real responsibility to the patient are more

Childhood and Adolescent Diabetes
Published in 1994 by Chapman & Hall, London
ISBN 0 412 48610 5

effective than didactic teaching methods (Sulway *et al.*, 1980). Therefore it has become scientifically respectable for medical personnel to attempt to influence the outcome of the disorder by encouraging patients to express their feelings about diabetes and their ability to control its impact on their lives (Coles, 1990).

37.3 SELF-MANAGEMENT

Diabetes has been in the vanguard of promoting patient-centered education and self-management strategies, which are particularly appropriate in childhood diabetes. Parents and children who are enabled to feel in control from an early stage, particularly on a domiciliary basis, are likely to show greater self-confidence and independence (Walker, 1953; Swift *et al.*, 1993). Other aspects of education which foster self-management have been discussed in detail elsewhere (Day, 1991) but the idea of sending regular written information to children and parents exemplifies the recent attempts at improving communication (Tattersall, 1990; Savage, 1991). The concept of self-management is not new. Dr Robin Lawrence, whose first edition of *The Diabetic Life* was published in 1925, highlighted the importance of education, emphasizing that 'every diabetic must realize that his health lies mainly in his own hands . . . and depends on the thorough understanding of the care . . . and persistence with which he carries it out' (Lawrence, 1925, p. 187). It was with his persistence and enthusiasm that one of his famous patients (the author H.G. Wells) helped to form the world's first patient-initiated and patient-orientated association of people suffering from a particular disorder. Thus in 1934 the Diabetic Association was founded, becoming the British Diabetic Association (BDA) in 1954. Other associations such as the 'Portuguese Association for the Protection of Poor Diabetics' (1926) and the American Diabetes Association (ADA, 1940) were initiated by physicians and scientists and only later considered patient or lay involvement.

In a later description of the BDA, Lawrence wrote of a 'self-help' group, to develop 'something good and important for the lives of diabetics . . . the progress of knowledge . . . and to raise money for research' (Lawrence, 1952, pp. 420–21).

It is interesting to speculate whether the success of self-management spawns a greater search for self-help organizations. It might be argued that good self-management might obviate the need for self-help groups but in the UK the increasing emphasis on patient-centered education in the past two decades has been accompanied by a major expansion of self-help groups.

37.4 SELF-HELP ORGANIZATIONS AND ACTIVITIES

Organized groups such as diabetic associations have a number of fundamental and important characteristics (Robinson, 1985). These characteristics are readily recognized by parents and children when discussing the benefits derived from group activities (Table 37.1). It is important to analyse and understand the potential value and rationale of self-help organizations because some professionals feel threatened by their existence and criticize their activities. The characteristics described in Table 37.1 and the mechanisms by which participants may benefit from joining groups (Table 37.2) help in assessing the value of self-help activities.

Self-help organizations such as the BDA assume a responsibility for organizing activities which are thought to be beneficial to their members. Many of these activities are proposed by and ably assisted by members, but this category of organized 'corporate' activity should be distinguished from those generated by members for members – the self-help concept.

Table 37.1 Common characteristics of self-help groups.

1. Common experience	– 'all in the same boat'
2. Mutual support	– 'I'm not the only one in the world'
3. Shared experience	– 'help others to help yourself'
4. Reinforcement of normality	– 'it's not the end of the world' – 'there are others far worse off than me'
5. Collective action	– 'we're in this together'
6. Information resource	– sharing information – informal and formal education
7. Constructive activities	– building networks – group activities – new opportunities – making a contribution – expanding horizons – fund-raising

Table 37.2 Mechanisms for the success of self-help groups.

1. Identification of problems through informal contacts
2. Admission of problems by sharing
3. Relief on sharing problems
4. Loss of isolation
5. Fellowship: new friends
6. Bonding through common experience
7. Reduction of stigma
8. Exploring new ground: the independence factor
9. Feeling useful again
10. Fun

In the first category, associations have numerous and varied activities many of which have a long and distinguished history. For example, the BDA has published a lay magazine since 1935, in more recent decades appropriately entitled *Balance*. Similar news sheets, bulletins and newsletters are produced by many associations worldwide. In addition to lay magazines, the diabetic associations have been responsible for initiating the publication of prestigious professional journals such as *Diabetes* (ADA) and *Diabetic Medicine* (BDA), containing information not only of a high scientific nature but also studies related to self-help initiatives (Marteau *et al.*, 1987; North, 1990).

Arguably the most valuable work in the global context of diabetic associations has been to lobby governments, to identify supplies and to distribute (free or at discount prices) insulin, syringes and other life-saving essentials not only as a routine service but also in times of poverty, war and strife. The latter activity is still unfortunately a desperate requirement in certain areas of the world.

Diabetic associations have also been responsible for providing funds for the establishment of special hospitals, homes and hostels for patients and children with diabetes. In the UK, the need for community-based accommodation has evolved towards a more modern concept of purpose-designed District Diabetes Centres, often part-funded by local BDA branches. They function not only as medical facilities but also educational and social resource centres (Day & Spathis, 1988; Knight & Redmond, 1989).

A further fundamental objective of all diabetic associations is the promotion of all aspects of education. This involves many modalities of sharing information from teaching programs, production of educational materials and establishment of databases to the more personal development of contact networks. Educational meetings cover a wide spectrum ranging from huge international gatherings such as the triennial International Diabetes Federation (IDF) Congress to humble gatherings of patient groups in village halls around the world. IDF meetings include sessions for lay groups and diabetic associations as well as scientific meetings of the most specialized variety. Small local group activities include simple social evenings, formal lectures, group discussions, practical demonstrations, visits to research establishments and a wide variety of other activities the basis of which is to exchange information on an informal basis to improve understanding of diabetes.

Diabetic associations have helped to organize life and travel insurance for members when this has proved difficult (Songer *et al.*, 1991). Indeed the BDA has recently appointed an insurance broker with a formal contract to arrange insurance for members. Associations also inform members of government or state benefits available to parents of children with diabetes and try to ensure that employment and social necessities (e.g., driving vehicles) are not compromised by diabetes. In many countries there remains considerable stigma and prejudice against diabetes, although this varies in intensity (Baker *et al.*, 1992; Lloyd *et al.*, 1992). Increasing public awareness and projecting a favorable image of diabetes are vital roles of associations at local, national and international levels.

The social context of diabetes has recently been embodied in the St Vincent Declaration (Krans *et al.*, 1992) (see Appendix A). In 1989, representatives of government health departments and patients' organizations from all European countries met with diabetes experts under the aegis of the WHO and IDF in St Vincent, Italy. Many recommendations and targets for improving diabetes care were agreed including those directly relevant to young people:

- the promotion of self-sufficiency, independence and equity with full integration of the diabetic citizen into society.
- children and adolescents to have the same social rights in school, education and physical activity as their nondiabetic peers.
- parents to receive the necessary economic support to give their child adequate treatment.

To implement the St Vincent Declaration, Departments of Health in various contries have requested that diabetic associations set up task forces to determine the means by which the recommendations can be followed through and evaluated. Thus, in the UK, the BDA is being used by the government to help ensure improvement of care.

The BDA is able to take on this responsibility because it has developed into a highly complex organization which has recently drawn up its first formal Five-Year-Plan with well-defined policy statements (Balance, 1993). The structure of the BDA includes a management board to direct the strategic and executive functions. Other sections of the organization which influence children's diabetic services are:

- Executive Council – the central body of policy making and financial control. It has representatives from all BDA committees advising on the concerns of children and their families or their medical teams.
- Youth Department – responsible for organizing young people's educational holidays, parent-child weekends and school packs.
- Children and Young Persons Advisory Committee – usually chaired by a consultant pediatrician and concerned with the effective organization and standards of BDA children's holidays and has promoted the development of leaflets such as 'What professional supervision should children with diabetes and their parents expect?' (BDA publication, 1989), enabling parents to become more effective partners in the health care team.
- Parent's Advisory Committee – currently involved in establishing national parents' networks and has already developed lists of possible contacts for people with diabetes who have associated disorders or conditions e.g., pregnancy, celiac disease, Down Syndrome.

- Research Committee – considers research applications and allocates more than 2 million pounds per year for research, some of which inevitably impinges on the welfare of children.

At national and local levels diabetic associations, parent groups and branches around the world, working in close collaboration with professionals, organize a wide variety of initiatives.

One of the best-known activities for children with diabetes are camps or educational holidays described enthusiastically by a number of authors (Craig, 1977; Travis *et al.*, 1981) and they have become widely accepted as a source of support and education for thousands of children worldwide by many diabetic associations (see also Chapter 36). At camp the child sees others giving their own injections, they deal with problems similar to their own, they talk and play with confidence in a supervised environment or they may help a friend to reverse hypoglycemia. These and many other experiences away from home aim to boost self-confidence and independence. Camps have also been used for field research (Malone *et al.*, 1976a & 1976b; Frost *et al.*, 1986) but despite all these apparent benefits, some pediatricians remain sceptical of their value.

Critical evaluations have been reported, however, for a number of children's and parents group activities. The effects of camps have been studied in the US (McCraw & Travis, 1973; Moffatt & Pless, 1983) and Britain (Vyas *et al.*, 1987); as have parents' weekends (Marteau *et al.*, 1987) and Youth Diabetes projects (see Chapter 36). All these reports tend to portray positive effects on diabetes self-care and management.

Exciting holiday initiatives are organized in many countries adapted to all age groups, at all times in the year and in an infinite variety of environments. Some may be weekend breaks, some are 2- or 3-week organized programs in purpose-built holiday camps, some with specific activities such as skiing or sailboarding, some active and some quiet. The clinic-organized programs from big centres in the US stimulated the development of a district-based, BDA parent-organized annual 5-day holiday in Leicestershire (Swift & Waldron, 1990). This has some advantages over larger nationally organized camps because local clinic staff are able to incorporate information from the holiday into the clinic setting. The BDA Five-Year-Plan now describes an intention to devolve educational holidays to regions with the hope of increasing uptake and local involvement.

On a wider scale the Australian, Japanese and Pacific Island Diabetic Associations have, since 1989, organized biennial international summer camps in Japan, Australia and Hawaii to share experiences between children and staff from many countries. Similarly the International Society for the Study of Pediatric and Adolescent Diabetes (ISPAD) (see Appendix B) has promoted a number of youth camps for young people from Scandinavia and Europe.

On the quieter side, parents' groups and associations in many districts have initiated more sedentary but highly educational activities such as indoor hobbies and skills, video productions, cooking and dietary demonstrations, and quiz programs in addition to a multitude of fund-raising activities. Fundraising is a core activity which is often the motivating force behind many parents' involvement. Parents perceive that providing funds for research is of fundamental importance because only through research will come prevention or cure of diabetes (Posner, 1991).

37.5 SELF-HELP GROUPS

In 1991, a survey of parents of 500 newly-diagnosed children revealed that 82% had joined the BDA (Lessing *et al.*, 1992). It would appear therefore that most specialist nurses and pediatricians in the UK advise parents on the benefits of joining a nationally recognized self-help organization. The current membership of the BDA is 130 000, only a fraction of the estimated total UK diabetic population. Members who are under 18 years number about 8000 (6%), which is a slightly larger proportion than expected. This may be because young people with IDDM and their parents derive more benefit from membership than elderly patients with NIDDM. This large national membership is divided into district branches and it is at this level that local support networks and real self-help groups develop.

Initially, contacts may be established between parents at clinics or by informal conversations at local branch meetings. Unfortunately, clinics are seldom effective meeting places unless special efforts are made (Bloomfield *et al.*, 1990). More formalized contact systems have been described with variable results (Farquhar, 1989; Hirst, 1989) and over the last 5 years the BDA has encouraged the development of self-help groups by arranging regional training sessions. Residential and one-day training courses in group and listening skills have been organized for members wanting to start self-help groups or for those already involved in voluntary groups who wish to establish support networks (Kelleher, 1991; North, 1990). The rationale of a self-help group is that it should be distinctly different from the larger more structured meetings; it should enable parents to talk with each other on a more personal one-to-one basis preferably with one of the pairing having developed some skills in listening and communicating.

At a practical level, a proportion of parents request an early contact with another parent of a diabetic child soon after diagnosis. A greater number seem to make contacts at a later stage in their understanding of diabetes and this may be through the channels of a diabetic association. These differences in requirement need to be respected by the medical team and to facilitate 'diabetic contacts' a BDA Working Party has produced guidelines for members and branches (North, 1990).

The continuing success of voluntary organized activities depends upon the energy and enthusiasm of motivated individuals. Not surprisingly, self-help groups, networks, contacts and branches wax and wane – there are inevitable peaks and troughs. Activities are more likely to remain strong if there is a continuing stimulus from committed professionals such as specialist nurses, dietitians and doctors who are able to provide unwavering support for the group. A constructive trusting partnership between parents and professionals helps to unify the potentially divisive goals of self-management, self-help and medically-orientated diabetes care. Without partnership in care the child's diabetic management is likely to founder.

37.6 CONCLUSIONS

> Medical help provides a framework within which diabetes can be 'managed'. As far as living with the condition is concerned, parents and children need additional non-technical resources to give both practical and psychosocial support. (Posner, 1991, p. 22)

Diabetes may impose an unrelenting pressure on parents. When the diagnosis is made and insulin has been started, the subsequent management is most profoundly influenced not by the health care team but by parents, using their confidence and their skills. The team is important in providing the framework but parents must nurture the child and carry the burden of diabetes for 365 days a year. Many parents in this situation derive added support from external sources often coordinated by self-help organizations. Networks of support operate at family, neighborhood, district, regional, national and global levels, all of which help to enhance the status of the diabetic child in the family and in society.

REFERENCES

Baker, J., Scragg, R., Metcalf, P. *et al.* (1992) Diabetes Mellitus and employment: is there discrimination in the workplace. *Diabetic Medicine*, **10**, 362–65.

BDA (British Diabetic Association). (1989) What professional supervision should children with diabetes and their parents expect? BDA Publications, London WIM 0BD.

BDA (British Diabetic Association). (1992) About the BDA. BDA Publications, London WIM 0BD.

Beckman, H.B. and Frankel, R.M. (1984) The effect of physician behaviour on the collection of data. *Ann. Int. Med.*, **101**, 692–96.

Blau, J.N. (1989) Time to let the patient speak. *Brit. Med. J.*, **298**, 39.

Bloomfield, S., Calder, J.E., Chisholm, V. *et al.* (1990) A project in diabetes education for children. *Diabetic Med.*, **7**, 137–42.

Coles, C. (1990) Diabetes education: letting the patient into the picture. *Practical Diabetes*, **7**, 110–12.

Craig, J.O. (1977) 'Communication and education', in J. Apley (ed.). *Childhood diabetes and its management*, p. 74. Butterworths and Co (Publishers) Ltd, London.

Day, J.I. (1991) 'Diabetes education', in J.O. Pickup and G. Williams (eds). *Textbook of diabetes*. Blackwell Scientific Publications, London.

Day, J.I. and Spathis, M. (1988) District diabetes centres in the United Kingdom. *Diabetic Med.*, **5**, 372–80.

Farquhar, J.W. (1989) The use of a teleport system in parent and adolescent support. *Diabetic Med.*, **6**, 635–37.

Frost, G.J., Hodges, S. and Swift, P.G.F. (1986) Dietary carbohydrate deficits and hypoglycaemia in the young diabetic on holiday. *Diabetic Med.*, **3**, 250–52.

Hirst, J. (1989) Dialabetic. *Diabetic Med.*, **6**, 637–38.

Illich, I. (1975) *Medical Nemesis: the expropriation of health*, p. 11. Calder and Boyars Ltd, London.

Kaplan, S.H., Greenfield, S. and Ware, J.E. (1989) 'Impact of the doctor-patient relationship on the outcomes of chronic disease', in M. Stewart and D. Roter (eds). *Communicating with medical patients*, Sage, London.

Kelleher, D.J.A. (1991) Patients learning from each other: self-help groups for people with diabetes. *J. Roy. Soc. Med.*, **84**, 595–97.

Knight, A.H. and Redmond, S. (1989) District diabetes centres in the United Kingdom and Eire. *Diabetic Med.*, **6**, 639–42.

Krans, H.M.J., Porta, M. and Keen, H. (1992) Diabetes care and research in Europe: the St. Vincent Declaration action programme. *Giornale Italiano di Diabetologia*, **12** (suppl. 2).

Lawrence, R.D. (1925) 'The essentials of a diabetic education', Chapter XVIII in *The Diabetic Life*. J and A Churchill Ltd, London.

Lawrence, R.D. (1952) The beginning of the diabetic association in England. *Diabetes*, **1**, 420–21.

Lessing, D.N., Swift, P.G.F., Metcalfe, M.A. *et al.* (1992) Newly diagnosed diabetes: a study of parental satisfaction. *Arch. Dis. Child.*, **67**, 1011–13.

Lloyd, C.E., Robinson, N. and Fuller, J.H. (1992) Education and employment experiences in young adults with Type 1 diabetes mellitus. *Diabetic Med.*, **9**, 661–66.

Malone, J.I., Hellrung, J.M., Malphus, E.W. *et al.* (1976a) Good diabetic control – a study in mass delusion. *J. Pediatr.*, **88**, 943–47.

Malone, J.I., Rosenbloom, A.I., Grgic, A. *et al.* (1976b) The role of urine sugar in diabetic management. *Am. J. Dis. Child.*, **130**, 1324–27.

Marteau, T.M., Gillespie, C. and Swift, P.G.F. (1987) Evaluation of a weekend group for parents of children with diabetes. *Diabetic Med.*, **4**, 488–90.

McGraw, R.K. and Travis, L.B. (1973) Psychological effects of a special summer camp on juvenile diabetics. *Diabetes*, **22**, 275–78.

Moffat, M.E.K. and Pless, I.B. (1983) Locus of control in juvenile diabetic campers: changes during camp and relationship to camp assessments. *J. Pediatr.*, **103**, 146–50.

North, J. (1990) Diabetic contacts: an underutilised resource. *Diabetic Med.*, **7**, 933–36.

Posner, T. (1991) BDA membership survey: who are we? *Balance*, BDA magazine. Oct/Nov. London WIM OBD.

Robinson, D. (1985) Self-help groups. *Brit. J. Hosp. Med.*, **41**, 109–111.

Savage, D.C.L. (1991) Writing letters to patients: educational or pastoral?, *Diabetic Med.*, **8**, 590.

Songer, T.J., LaPorte, R.E., Dorman, J.S. *et al.* (1991) Health, life and automobile insurance characteristics in adults with IDDM. *Diabetes Care*, **14**, 318–24.

Sulway, M., Tupling, H., Webb, K. *et al.* (1980) New techniques for changing compliance in diabetes. *Diabetes Care*, **3**, 108–111.

Swift, P.G.F. and Waldron, S. (1990) Have diabetes – will travel. *Practical Diabetes*, **7**, 101–104.

Swift, P.G.F., Hearnshaw, J.R., Botha, J.T. *et al.* (1993) A decade of diabetes: keeping children out of hospital. *Brit. Med. J.*, **307**, 96–98.

Tattersall, R.B. (1990) Writing for and to patients. *Diabetic Med.*, **7**, 917–19.

Travis, L.B., Johnson, T., McMahon, P. *et al.* (1981) Camps for children with diabetes. *Texas Med.*, **77**, 36–40.

Vyas, S., Mullee, M.A. and Kinmonth, A.-L. (1987) British Diabetic Association holidays – what are they worth? *Diabetic Med.*, **5**, 88–92.

Walker, J.B. (1953) Field work of a diabetic clinic. *Lancet*, **ii**, 445–47.

PART FIVE

38

Prevention of IDDM

P.J. BINGLEY and E.A.M. GALE

38.1 INTRODUCTION

The prevention of IDDM demands a therapy and a strategy to apply it. This means that we need to understand the disease process both in order to identify points at which it might be possible to intervene, and in order to design screening programs to allow potential treatments to be used effectively.

38.2 THE DISEASE PROCESS

Insulin-dependent diabetes is the result of β cell destruction, the histological appearance at diagnosis suggesting that the clinical onset of disease does not occur until some 90% of the β cells have been destroyed (Gepts, 1965). There is abundant evidence that this is the result of autoimmune attack. First, IDDM is associated with other organ-specific autoimmune disease; second, insulitis with inflammatory cell infiltrate is found at the time of diagnosis and is present prior to diagnosis in animal models of IDDM, and third, antibodies and T cells directed against islet cell antigens can be detected prior to diagnosis.

The attack on the β cells appears to be a slow process; the associated humoral immune changes have been detected up to 15 years before the clinical onset of disease. Immune markers are detected in a much greater proportion of the general population than would ever be expected to develop diabetes (Bingley *et al.*, 1993) suggesting that initiation of the autoimmune process is relatively common but that the disease process only runs the full course in a minority. The time of onset of β cell damage in children is uncertain since few studies have followed subjects from confirmed islet cell antibodies (ICA) negativity to positivity. A small prospective study in children of women with diabetes demonstrated the appearance of anti-islet autoimmunity ICA and insulin autoantibodies (IAA) between 9 and 24 months of age (Ziegler *et al.*, 1993). Another study has reported that ICA always appeared for the first time in family members before age 6 though the levels often continued to rise thereafter (Pilcher *et al.*, 1991).

38.3 FEATURES OF DISEASE PROCESS

38.3.1 CHANGES IN HUMORAL IMMUNITY

Islet cell antibodies were first detected in the serum of patients with polyendocrine autoimmunity (Bottazzo *et al.*, 1974) and were subsequently found in a high proportion of patients with newly diagnosed IDDM (Lendrum *et al.*, 1974). They are detected

Childhood and Adolescent Diabetes
Published in 1994 by Chapman & Hall, London
ISBN 0 412 48610 5

by indirect immunofluorescence on human pancreas but the exact nature of the autoantigen to which they are directed remains unknown. Autoantibodies to a number of islet antigens have been identified – to a 64 kD antigen, subsequently identified as the GABA synthesizing enzyme glutamate decarboxylase (GAD); to insulin; and, more recently, antibodies to an islet ganglioside, heat-shock protein 65, the enzyme carboxypeptidase, and tryptic fragments of the 64kD protein have all been reported (Harrison, 1992). The role of these antibodies in the pathogenesis of IDDM seems limited. Although ICA, for example, have been shown to be cytotoxic to cultured islet cells *in vitro*, it is generally agreed that, *in vivo*, these autoantibodies probably represent an epiphenomenon and that β cell destruction is the result of cell-mediated immune processes. The presence of these autoantibodies many years prior to diagnosis has, however, provided the primary evidence for the long prodrome of IDDM and, in prospective studies, they have proved useful markers.

38.3.2 CHANGES IN CELL-MEDIATED IMMUNITY

Changes in cell-mediated immunity appear to play a more critical role in the pathogenetic process. *In vitro* peripheral blood leucocytes from newly-diagnosed patients can be shown to be sensitized to pancreatic antigens (Nerup *et al.*, 1974). The predominant cells in the inflammatory islet infiltrate seen at the time of diagnosis are T lymphocytes, the majority CD8-positive cytotoxic/suppressor T cells positive for markers of activation such as interleukin-2 receptors (Bottazzo *et al.*, 1985a). The number of circulating activated T cells is increased in newly-diagnosed diabetes (Bottazzo *et al.*, 1985b) and T lymphocyte clones expanded from the peripheral blood of newly-diagnosed patients have shown cytotoxic effects when exposed to HLA-matched islet cells in vitro (de Bernadinis *et al.*, 1988).

38.4 SUMMARY OF PATHOGENESIS

The precise sequence of events initiating autoimmune attack on the β cells remains unclear. Aberrant expression of HLA class II molecules by β cells, but not other islet cells, has been suggested to be the earliest abnormality. This is perhaps triggered by some environmental agent and, in turn, allows the target cell to behave as an antigen-presenting cell, 'suicidally' presenting its own surface antigens (Bottazzo, 1986). This would result in activation of T helper cells which then stimulate effector B and cytotoxic T lymphocytes. Cytokines may perpetuate a cycle of HLA gene activation or may play a more direct role in β cell destruction (Nerup *et al.*, 1989).

Cytotoxic T cells appear to play the pivotal role in the final selective destruction of β cells. When patients with long-standing IDDM received pancreatic transplants from their nondiabetic monozygotic cotwins, diabetes unexpectedly recurred rapidly in the recipients and histological examination of the pancreas revealed selective β cell destruction with insulitis in which cytotoxic T cells were the predominant cell type (Sibley & Sutherland, 1987).

One of the most important features of the process is its very slowness. Assuming that circulating autoantibodies reflect autoimmune activation, the process seems to be initiated early in life and may take many years to complete. This offers a large 'therapeutic window' for possible intervention.

38.5 TYPES OF PREVENTION

Strategies for the prevention of IDDM can be classified according the stage of the disease process at which intervention occurs. *Primary prevention* would avoid initiation of the autoimmune process and *secondary prevention* would slow or stop the established destructive process. The former has to be the final goal but, as discussed below, seems likely to be the last to be achieved.

38.6 TOWARDS PRIMARY PREVENTION

38.6.1 ETIOLOGY

The etiology of IDDM involves an interaction of genetic susceptibility with an environmental agent. Siblings of children with IDDM have a risk of developing IDDM about 15 times that of children from the general population (Bingley *et al.*, 1993), yet the concordance rate for IDDM in monozygotic twins is only 30–50% (Barnett *et al.*, 1981). The incidence of IDDM is rising sharply in many populations, equivalent to a doubling in 20–30 years in several European countries (Bingley & Gale, 1989); more rapidly than could be explained by alterations in the population gene pool.

38.6.2 GENETICS

Relatives of a child with IDDM have been shown to be at increased risk of developing diabetes. The lifetime risk for siblings is around 4–8%, while that in parents and offspring is slightly lower (Tillil & Kobberling, 1987).

Some 60% of the genetic susceptibility to insulin-dependent diabetes is estimated to be associated with genes in the Major Histocompatibility Complex (MHC) on the short arm of chromosome 6 (Rotter & Landaw, 1984). The strongest associations with IDDM are found in the genes encoding MHC class 2 antigens. DR3/DR4 heterozygosity is associated with a relative risk of 20 for the development of IDDM (Bertrams & Baur, 1984) and more specific associations are found with certain DQ alleles (Todd *et al.*, 1987). Susceptible DQB alleles all encode for an amino acid other than aspartate at position 57 (Todd *et al.*, 1987) which led to some enthusiasm in the late 1980s that this might be the diabetes gene. More recently it has become apparent that the effect of this gene is modulated by many other genes both within and beyond the MHC genes. The amino acid at position 52 of the DQα chain exerts an independent effect (Khalil *et al.*, 1990); the whole HLA haplotype affects the absolute risk associated with particular DQB1 and DQA1 types (Tienari *et al.*, 1992), and the discrepancy between the concordance between monozygotic twins and HLA-identical siblings implicates non-MHC genes in determining overall genetic susceptibility. Studies in the non-obese diabetic (NOD) mouse have identified non-MHC genes on several chromosomes that modulate the major effect of MHC genes; for example, a gene on chromosome 3 (analogous to human chromosome 1 or 4) determines frequency and severity of insulitis and another, on chromosome 11 (analogous to chromosome 17 in humans) may influence the progression from insulitis to overt diabetes in this animal model (Todd *et al.*, 1991). It seems probable that the situation in humans will prove at least as complex and the possibility of using genetic manipulation in such a polygenic disorder is limited.

38.6.3 ENVIRONMENTAL FACTORS

There is a considerable body of indirect evidence that environmental factors do play a role in the etiology of IDDM but their precise identity remains elusive. Studies correlating population exposure to an agent with the incidence of disease, have suggested many candidates ranging from coffee to rural isolation (Tuomilehto *et al.*, 1990; Patterson *et al.*, 1988). The environment is easy to manipulate in animal models and diabetes incidence is affected by, for example, diet, temperature and exposure to infection (Scott *et al.*, 1988;

Williams *et al.*, 1990; Himsworth, 1936). Certain environmental agents have been shown to produce disease in humans. Ingestion of the rat poison 'Vacor' results in an insulin-dependent form of diabetes (Prosser & Karam, 1978); maternal consumption of nitrosamine-rich foods such as smoked mutton around the time of conception is associated with an increased incidence of IDDM in the offspring (Helgasson & Jonasson, 1981), and intra-uterine infection with the rubella virus increases the risk of subsequent IDDM (Ginsberg-Fellner *et al.*, 1985). Our current understanding of the disease process suggests that environmental exposure is probably relevant many years before clinical presentation and that it may well be a 'hit and run' phenomenon with subsequent autoimmune destruction being an independent self-perpetuating process that proceeds long after the environmental agent has gone. It is also likely that, as the autoimmune process is triggered in only a minority of those with genetic susceptibility, so only a minority of those in whom the process is started will develop disease. These factors all act to 'dampen' differences between patients and controls and mitigate against easy identification of the relevant factors.

Currently, the main contenders for a role as environmental determinants of IDDM are infection or dietary factors.

38.6.4 INFECTIVE AGENTS

The rising incidence of IDDM (Bingley & Gale, 1989), a correlation between mean yearly temperature and the incidence of disease (DERIG, 1988) and the inverse relation between population density and disease found in some studies (Patterson *et al.*, 1988) would all be consistent with a infective etiology. The major problem at present is lack of a plausible candidate agent. A number of viruses can damage β cells *in vitro* or in experimental animals, or have been implicated in some cases of IDDM in humans. These include mumps, coxsackie B (Yoon *et al.*, 1979; Barrett-Conner, 1985), rubella (Ginsberg-Fellner *et al.*, 1985), and cytomegalovirus (CMV) (Ward *et al.*, 1979; Jenson *et al.*, 1980; Pak *et al.*, 1988). The long incubation of the disease however makes it necessary to look back over many years to early childhood, or perhaps even *in utero*. Viral infections also have a separate role in precipitating clinical onset of diabetes and evidence of such infections can complicate the picture. The idea that viral infection might be the initial trigger for the autoimmune process remains theoretically attractive, particularly since vaccination is one of the simplest imaginable means of primary prevention, but no progress can be made in this direction until the responsible agent is known.

38.6.5 DIETARY FACTORS

Diet is another factor that varies radically between countries and also changes over time. Alterations in diet have a profound effect on the incidence in animal models (Scott *et al.*, 1988; Daneman *et al.*, 1987). These observations have motivated a search for possible dietary causes of IDDM. One of these, cow's milk protein, has been the subject of considerable attention in recent years and its relevance is soon to be tested in the first primary prevention trial.

38.6.5.1 The cows' milk protein hypothesis

Alteration of the protein components of laboratory chow can alter the incidence of diabetes in the NOD mouse and BB rat models. Animals reared on a diet free of cow's milk for the first 3 months of life do not develop diabetes (Elliott & Martin, 1984). There is epidemiological evidence to support a role for these proteins in the etiology of IDDM. National *per capita* cow's milk consumption correlates with the incidence of diabetes (Dahl-Jorgansen *et al.*, 1991), and the risk of IDDM has been shown to be significantly lower in children who were exclusively breast-fed for three months (Virtanen *et al.*, 1991). Antibodies to bovine serum albumin were higher in children with newly-diagnosed IDDM than in normal children (Karjalainen *et al.*, 1992) and it has been suggested that an albumin peptide containing 17 amino acids (ABBOS) may be the reactive epitope. Antibodies to this peptide cross-react with a β cell specific surface antigen (p69) and an elegant hypothesis has been put foward whereby early exposure to bovine serum albumin, at a stage when it is able to cross the immature gut wall, triggers an immune reponse against the ABBOS peptide in genetically susceptible individuals. The p69 antigen is only expressed on the cell surface when it is induced by gamma-interferon during unrelated infectious events, but when these occur, the immune system is primed to attack the epitope that this antigen shares with the ABBOS protein. Delaying exposure to cow's milk until the gut is mature and therefore impermeable to large peptides such as this means that anti-ABBOS immunity (and therefore anti-p69 immunity) should be prevented. This hypothesis is soon to be tested in a study in which genetically susceptible neonates will be randomized to receive supplementary feeds with either normal formula or with formula modified to remove cows' milk protein for the first nine months of life (Skyler & Marks, 1993).

Table 38.1 Categories of intervention in type 1 diabetes (Harrison *et al.*, 1990).

I Nonspecific immunosuppression
e.g., Glucocorticoids, cytotoxic agents, anti-lymphocyte globulin or monoclonal antibody and total lymphoid or pancreatic irradiation.

II Nonspecific immunomodulation
e.g., plasma exchange, white cell transfusion, gamma-globulin, interferon-α or levamisole.

III Semispecific immunotherapy (targeted against particular components of the immune response)
e.g., anti-IL2 receptor monoclonal antibodies against activated T cell; Cyclosporin A against CD4+ helper-inducer cells; silica and methimazole against macrophages; Monoclonal antibodies against IL1, TNF or interferon gamma.

IV Specific immunotherapy
e.g., vaccination with disease/autoantigen-specific inactivated T cell clones or T cell receptors; anti-idiotypic monoclonal antibodies to T cell receptors; oral tolerization.

V Anti-inflammatory agents
e.g., Gold; anti-malarials such as hydrocychloroquine; cycloxygenase inhibitors; and anti-free radical agents such as superoxide dismutase, nicotinamide and vitamin E.

VI β cell modification
e.g., insulin and maintenance of euglycemia.

38.7 SECONDARY PREVENTION

Intervention to slow or stop an established process of β cell destruction is beginning to appear realistic, and trials of a number of agents designed to prevent or delay the clinical onset of IDDM in high-risk subjects are already starting (Skyler & Marks, 1993).

Using our current understanding of the disease process, Harrison and colleagues have produced a useful theoretical classification of potential points of intervention. The majority of these do not have immediate therapeutic potential in humans but the list does draw attention to the diversity of approaches that could be used (Table 38.1) (Harrison *et al.*, 1990).

38.7.1 NONSPECIFIC IMMUNOSUPPRESSION

Glucocorticoids were used in open pilot studies in newly-diagnosed diabetes with apparent benefit (Elliott *et al.*, 1981). Their use has been limited by their adverse metabolic effects but these studies did stimulate controlled trials of other nonspecific immunosuppressive agents.

In the first randomized controlled trial of azathioprine alone, remission occurred in 7 out of 13 adults with newly-diagnosed IDDM compared with 1 out of 11 controls (Harrison *et al.*, 1985). In the trial in children, however, no patients had complete remission though fasting C-peptide was significantly higher in the treated group at 3 and 6 months.

One trial combined azathioprine with initial short-term prednisolone. After 12 months 10 out of 20 treated patients and 3 out of 20 control patients were in partial remission (Silverstein *et al.*, 1988). Results were better in older patients and in those in whom the total lymphocyte count fell below the normal range.

38.7.1.1 Cyclosporin A

Cyclosporin A represents an example of semi-specific immunotherapy blocking the early stages of the immune response, in particular activation of CD4 positive helper/inducer T cells. It is the drug that first showed it was possible to alter the course of diabetes in humans, albeit transiently. In the first French controlled trial in adults with newly diagnosed IDDM, 24% of the cyclosporin treated group vs. 6% of the control group were in complete remission at 9 months. The result was significantly better in those with trough levels of at least 300 ng/ml (Feutren *et al.*, 1986). The Canadian-European trial confirmed these findings, and also showed that the results were better in those with a shorter duration of symptoms, less weight loss, higher C-peptide secretion and absence of ketoacidosis at diagnosis. The rate of non-insulin requiring remission was also higher at both 6 and 12 months in adults than in children. These observations suggest that, as would be predicted from its mode of action, the drug is more effective if given earlier in the disease process and less effective in the more rapid destructive process that occurs in children (Canadian-European Randomized Control Trial Group, 1988).

The use of cyclosporin prior to clinical onset is limited by its toxicity, particularly nephrotoxicity. This is dose-related and usually reversible but most clinicians would feel that, certainly with the relative lack of precision of current prediction, the risk–benefit ratio is too unfavorable to embark on long-term treatment in healthy subjects, most of whom will be children and some of whom might never develop IDDM even without intervention.

An alternative, more futuristic, approach is to use 'magic bullets' whereby highly toxic agents are carried to the attacking immune cells by attaching them to antibodies against markers of T cell activation. In pilot studies, ricin A-chain immunoconjugated with anti-CD5 monoclonal antibodies and IL-2 conjugated with diphtheria toxin, given at the time of diagnosis, have both been reported to improve glycemic control (Skyler *et al.*, 1991; Boitard *et al.*, 1992).

38.7.2 SPECIFIC IMMUNOTHERAPY

The overall aim of many investigators is the development of interventions that target disease- or antigen-specific immune changes. It may, for example, be possible to vaccinate with disease-specific T cells or perhaps with receptors that recognize disease-specific antigens. If T cell receptors can be characterized, it may be possible to target 'magic bullets' against them using anticlonotypic immunoglobulins.

Oral tolerization is a form of specific immunotherapy that has been found to be helpful in some autoimmune conditions. This is based on the observation that oral ingestion of soluble antigen can induce a state of immunological hyporesponsiveness or tolerance while parenteral administration causes sensitization. Most work has been done in animal models of autoimmune disease such as collagen-induced arthritis and experimental allergic encephalomyelitis (EAE) in which oral administration of the antigen (collagen and myelin basic protein (MBP) respectively) before conventional challenge reduces the incidence and severity of disease. There is also some reduction in severity of relapse if MBP is given after clinical onset of chronic relapsing EAE, an animal model of multiple sclerosis (Thompson & Staines, 1990).

Insulin, when given to young NOD mice, reduces insulitis and delays onset of disease (Zhong *et al.*, 1991). There is some evidence that administration of fragments of autoantigens that are not themselves autoimmunogenic may achieve the same degree of tolerance without risking sensitization and exacerbation of pre-existing disease. Thus, in pre-IDDM, it may be preferable to give an antigen such as insulin that is not likely to be the primary sensitizing antigen, and digestion of this peptide may even be beneficial. This theory is prompting a multicenter trial of oral insulin therapy in family members of children with IDDM.

38.7.3 NICOTINAMIDE

Nicotinamide (nicotinic acid amide or niacinamide) is a water-soluble group B vitamin, derived from nicotinic acid. Its effect in prevention of toxin-induced models of diabetes has been known for more than 40 years (Lazarow, 1947; Dulin *et al.*, 1969). It is also effective in preventing spontaneous diabetes in the NOD mouse, inhibits transplant allograft insulitis, another animal model of immune β-cell damage, preserves residual β cells in partially pancreatectomized rats, and promotes the growth of cultured human islet cells. It appears to act in the final stage of β-cell damage, preventing the cytotoxic effects of cytokines. There are two proposed mechanisms for its action: (1) that it acts as a free radical scavenger to reduce DNA damage, and (2) that it restores the islet cell content of nicotinamide adenine dinucleotide (NAD) towards normal by elevating intracellular NAD and by inhibiting poly ADP-Ribose polymerase, a major route of NAD metabolism (Pociot *et al.*, 1993). Further effects of nicotinamide that have been demonstrated recently include suppression of MHC Class II antigen expression on murine islet cells (Yamada *et al.*, 1982), implying that nicotinamide might reduce presentation of autoantigens to helper T cells by islet β cells in human Type I diabetes. It has also been shown to inhibit macrophage-mediated cytoxicity directed against rat islet cells (Kroncke *et al.*, 1991). There is therefore evidence to suggest that nicotinamide could offer a protective effect to human β cells, particularly if the drug were given at an early stage of the disease process.

Nicotinamide has been tried in humans with recently-diagnosed IDDM. The results have been variable but increased serum C-peptide concentrations and a longer remission period have been reported in treated individuals (Vague *et al.*, 1987; Mendola *et al.*, 1989), and similar effects were found in a longitudinal study of patients with established diabetes (Vague *et al.*, 1989). Pilot studies of its ability to prevent IDDM in first degree relatives have also been performed. Eight untreated historical controls under age 16 with high ICA levels were compared with another group of 14 children receiving nicotinamide (Elliott & Chase, 1991). Four out of eight historical controls developed diabetes within one year, as against none of nine in the treatment group. By two years, seven of eight in the untreated group and none of six on nicotinamide. Subsequently, one child on nicotinamide has developed diabetes, as had the last historical control.

In contrast, nicotinamide was ineffective in three first degree relatives with very low first phase insulin response (FPIR) (Dumont-Herskowitz *et al.*, 1989). These data suggest that nicotinamide may not work if the treatment begins at a time when FPIR is effectively lost. This observation needs to be confirmed, but suggests that nicotinamide should be most effective if started during the early phase of β-cell destruction.

The toxicity of nicotinamide is low (Hoffer, 1969) even if given at the pharmacological doses (100–150 times the recommended daily intake) used in pilot studies. The treatment has proved acceptable in large, open studies in New Zealand. Many investigators feel that a double-blind, randomized controlled trial of its efficacy in delaying or preventing the onset of Type 1 diabetes is indicated (Chase *et al.*, 1992). A large multinational European study is in progress.

38.7.4 INSULIN

Insulin therapy has been shown to delay the onset of insulitis in both the BB rat and NOD mouse and to prevent the adoptive transfer of diabetes in the NOD mouse (Gotfredson *et al.*, 1985; Vlahos *et al.*, 1991; Atkinson *et al.*, 1990). Proposed mechanisms are immune modulation (Peakman *et al.*, 1990), tolerance induction, or β cell rest, whereby reduced insulin secretion causes less antigen expression rendering the cells less susceptible to immune attack. Intensive insulin treatment (including two weeks of intravenous treatment given via biostator) at the time of diagnosis was associated with lower glycated hemoglobin levels and higher stimulated C-peptide after 12 months than in controls (Shah *et al.*, 1989).

A pilot trial of pre-emptive insulin treatment given to seven subjects predicted to have more than 90% risk of developing diabetes within three years has produced promising results (Keller *et al.*, 1993). This is prompting a multicenter study in first degree relatives in the United States (Skyler & Marks, 1993).

38.8 APPLICATION OF PREVENTIVE THERAPIES

Prevention of IDDM will involve the long-term treatment of ostensibly healthy individuals, many of whom will be children, a situation in which risk–benefit analysis becomes particularly critical. The balance for the individual is readily apparent – the likelihood that he or she will develop diabetes and the risk reduction that can be achieved have to be weighed against the likely adverse effects of the treatment (psychological as well as physical) and the probability that he or she may be treated unnecessarily. The accuracy of prediction and the acceptable degree of risk associated with treatment are related. A clinician would probably not be prepared to consider, for example, toxic immunosuppressive treatment unless very certain that the patient would develop IDDM, while a simple treatment such as avoidance of cow's milk protein for the first 3–4 months of life may be applicable in those whose risk of IDDM might be much lower. The overall aim is, however, to reduce the incidence of diabetes in the community and this raises other, less obvious considerations such as the proportion of cases that can be detected by screening. An intensive screening program which can identify only a few percent of the overall number of cases may be impossible to justify on economic grounds, even if they are certain to develop diabetes and the treatment can be 100% effective.

An individual's probability of developing diabetes can be set out in a series of steps known as a 'decision tree'. This illustrates that we are dealing with a complex and evolving body of information and that the risk cannot merely be assigned on the basis of a single test. The probability is refined at each successive step, with the outcome of each 'branching' determined by all of the previous steps so that the overall risk is built up layer by layer (Figure 38.1) (Bingley *et al.*, 1993a).

38.8.1 BASELINE RISK

The absolute risk of developing IDDM changes with age, rising to a peak around

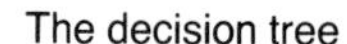

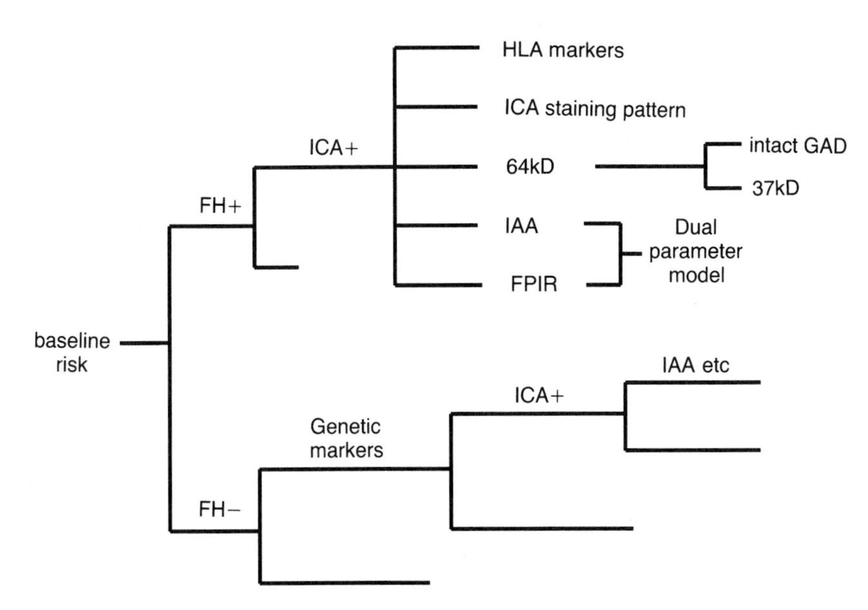

Figure 38.1 The decision tree.

puberty and receding gradually through adult life (Laakso & Pyorala, 1985). There are dramatic geographic differences, such that a child born in Finland has a ten times greater risk of developing diabetes than a child in northern Greece (Green *et al.*, 1992). There are changes within a given population over time; childhood diabetes is now some 2–3 times more common in much of Europe than it was in the 1950s and 1960s (Bingley & Gale, 1989). These considerations greatly modify the subsequent analysis; a test such as islet cell antibodies (ICA) would, for example, be expected to have a higher predictive value in children than in adults.

38.8.2 FAMILY HISTORY

Family history is the first major determinant of an individual's risk of IDDM. The lifetime risk in siblings of a child with IDDM in Europid populations is quoted at 5–8% (Tillil & Kobberling, 1987; Gamble, 1980), as against a background cumulative incidence of around 0.1–0.5%.

38.8.3 RISK ASSESSMENT IN FAMILY MEMBERS

Most information on risk markers of IDDM has been derived from family studies and we will consider this branch of the decision tree first (Figure 38.1), giving the risks over a 5-year period of follow-up. Siblings under the age of 20 have an average risk of developing IDDM within 5 years of 1.5%.

38.8.3.1 Islet cell antibodies

Islet cell antibodies (ICA) are detectable in 70–80% of new cases of childhood IDDM (Lardin-Olsson *et al.*, 1989). Their measurement has been the subject of a number of international workshops and they are now expressed in standardized Juvenile Diabetes Foundation (JDF) units. They are detected in

5–8% of first degree relatives, provided a sensitive assay is used, and in several prospective studies around 80% of future cases have detectable ICA. The risk of IDDM is directly proportional to the titer of ICA. Five percent of first degree relatives with ICA 4–19 JDF units, and 35% of those with ICA ⩾20 JDF units will develop IDDM within 5 years; 60–70% are likely to be on insulin within 10 years (Bonifacio *et al.*, 1990; Riley *et al.*, 1990).

38.8.4 ADDITIONAL MARKERS IN ICA POSITIVE RELATIVES

38.8.4.1 Genetic markers

Combining genetic markers with ICA can enhance the prognostic significance of ICA. In a French study, progression to IDDM over 8 years was 70% in ICA positive DR3,4 heterozygotes and 37% in those either HLA DR3 or DR4 alone (Deschamps *et al.*, 1992). A study by the Pittsburgh group found progression to IDDM in 33% of ICA positive relatives homozygous for Asp negativity in position 57 of the DQB chain, as against less than 5% in those with ICA alone, or with Asp-57 negativity alone (Lipton *et al.*, 1989). These studies have not, however, taken account of the level of ICA, and it is likely that the additional value of genetic markers will be very different in high and low levels of ICA. Until this is resolved, HLA typing still has a limited role in diabetes prediction in family members (American Diabetes Association, 1990).

38.8.4.2 ICA staining patterns

It has recently been demonstrated that some ICA stain predominantly β cells within islets (β-cell selective or restricted pattern) and are associated with a markedly lower risk of progression to diabetes than ICA that stain all types of islet cells (whole islet or nonrestricted pattern) (Genovese *et al.*, 1992; Gianini *et al.*, 1992; Timsit *et al.*, 1992).

38.8.4.3 Autoantibodies to insulin (IAA)

IAA appear to have little prognostic significance in the absence of ICA provided a sensitive ICA assay is used, but the combination is highly predictive (Ziegler *et al.*, 1989; Atkinson *et al.*, 1986). In the Boston-Sacramento family study, family members with IAA plus ICA ⩾40 JDF units have a 77% risk of diabetes within 5 years, as compared with 42% for those with ICA ⩾40 JDF units alone.

38.8.4.4 Antibodies to the 64 000 M_r islet antigen

Antibodies to the 64 000 M_r islet antigen, recently identified as GAD are found in around 80% of relatives studied before diagnosis (Harrison, 1992; Atkinson *et al.*, 1990; Thivolet *et al.*, 1992). High levels of GAD antibodies are, however, also found in the absence of diabetes. They were first described in 'stiff man syndrome', a rare neurological disorder (Solimena *et al.*, 1990), and GAD may be the autoantigen of β cell selective ICA, which as we have seen, carries a lower risk of progression to IDDM. Antibodies to a 50 000-M_r tryptic fragment of the islet antigen are found in most patients with IDDM but are also present in 15% of monozygotic twins who remain discordant for IDDM after prolonged follow-up and in all ICA positive polyendocrine patients who did not develop IDDM. In contrast, antibodies to 37 000/40 000-M_r tryptic fragments, distinct from GAD, are found in the majority of patients with IDDM, correlate well with whole islet ICA and seem to be highly specific risk markers (Christie *et al.*, 1991; Genovese *et al.*, 1991). The prognostic significance of these various antibodies remains to be evaluated.

38.8.4.5 Metabolic tests

The insulin response to an intravenous glucose load as measured in the intravenous glucose tolerance test (IVGTT) is the most widely used measure of β cell function used in the prediction of IDDM. A progressive decline in first phase insulin response prior to diabetes has been shown in prospective twin and family studies (Srikanta *et al.*, 1983; Chase *et al.*, 1987; Vialettes *et al.*, 1988). Unfortunately the test has proved highly variable, both within and between subjects, and there are major changes in the insulin response during puberty (Smith *et al.*, 1988a & 1988b) which make interpretation of changes within the normal range extremely difficult. This has limited the application of this finding in individual subjects.

Loss of first phase insulin secretion (defined as below the first centile of a control population) is highly predictive; in one study ICA positive relatives in this category developed diabetes at the rate of 0.48 per subject-year of follow-up, compared with only 0.05 per subject-year in those with first phase insulin release above this level (Vardi *et al.*, 1991). Comparison of results has been hindered by differences of method, but a new international standard for performance of the IVGTT has recently been agreed (Bingley *et al.*, 1992).

38.8.4.6 Predictive models

Combining the various available markers into a single model may well improve our ability to predict IDDM. The dual parameter model makes use of IAA and first phase insulin response to provide a broad estimate of time to predict diabetes in individuals who also have high levels of ICA (>40 JDF units). The model looks promising and gives highly specific prediction in end-stage prediabetes, with progression within 3–4 years in some 90% of those identified, but prediction beyond 3 years is less certain (Colman & Eisembarth, 1988). As yet it draws on data from very few subjects, and will need to be tested and modified by inclusion of many more cases.

38.8.4.7 What proportion of the future cases might be identified?

If screening is limited to family members of patients with IDDM, the scope of prediction is immediately reduced to around 10% of the at-risk population. Use of highly specific prediction as in the dual parameter model limits the scope considerably further. The model has been developed for use in those with ICA >40 JDF units, a level that will be detected in no more than 40–50% of future cases (Bonifacio *et al.*, 1990; Riley *et al.*, 1990). The model predicts early progression only in those with high IAA levels and/or impaired insulin secretion, representing perhaps 15% of the family population at risk. Thus, only 2% of all future cases are identified by this approach. Even highly effective intervention directed to this subgroup would obviously have little impact upon IDDM as a public health problem.

38.8.5 PREDICTION IN INDIVIDUALS WITH NO FAMILY HISTORY OF IDDM

Ninety per cent of patients with IDDM have no family history of diabetes and come from a population with a very low base rate of disease. Bayes' theorem dictates that markers applied in such a situation will have low predictive value and will generate a large proportion of false positives.

38.8.5.1 Risk of ICA in the general population

We compared the prevalence of ICA and the risk of diabetes in schoolchildren aged 9–13 years and age-matched nondiabetic siblings recruited for our family study and living in the same region. Siblings were twice as likely to have a given titer of ICA than schoolchildren, but were 14 times as likely to go on to diabetes. The predictive value of ICA in the general population would therefore fall to about one-seventh of that in siblings (Bingley *et al.*, 1993b). This indirect estimate has subsequently found support from prospective data collected from siblings and schoolchildren in Finland (Knip *et al.*, 1992), and indeed accords well with the theoretical estimate derived from Bayes' theorem. This correction factor implies that progression to diabetes within 5 years would occur in 2–3% of schoolchildren with detectable ICA and only 5–10% of those with ICA ≥20 JDF units. ICA alone therefore have limited prognostic value in the general population (Bingley *et al.*, 1993b).

38.8.5.2 Genetic markers in the general population

Genetic markers are subject to the same limitations. High sensitivity is relatively easy to achieve but current markers are so prevalent in the general population as to have low specificity. For example, in a recent Finnish study there was no aspartate residue at position 57 on either DQB chain in 74.5% of patients with IDDM and 18% of controls, giving an lifetime absolute risk of only 2%. A panel of four sequence-specific oligonucleotide probes was used to identify susceptible and protective DQ alleles. This achieved the best segregation of patients and controls yet described in IDDM, a high-risk combination was found in 82% of patients as against 3% of controls, but even this strategy could only assign a lifetime absolute risk of 13.7% (Reijonen *et al.*, 1991).

38.8.5.3 Combining predictive markers in the general population

This level of absolute risk still provides an inadequate basis for intervention, but a strategy combining genetic and immune markers in series would allow much higher levels of risk to be defined within the general population.

If ICA testing in the Finnish population were confined to those already identified as genetically susceptible by DQ typing, the expected positive predictive value would rise from 2% in 5 years in the whole population to 35% in 5 years, or more than 60% in 10 years – a level of risk at which intervention with a relatively non-toxic agent seems very reasonable (Bingley *et al.*, 1993a). This approach is, at present, purely theoretical and obviously needs testing.

38.8.5.4 The potential yield from screening in the general population

The oligonucleotide screen used in Finland identified 82% of cases, and low titer ICA has a sensitivity of around 80% in non-familial cases; 10% of cases have an affected first degree relative. A strategy involving screening of all family members of children with IDDM combined with sequential testing for genetic markers and ICA could thus potentially identify 65–70% of future cases.

38.9 CONCLUSION

Research has at last reached a stage where the findings of the last 20 years can be applied. The 1970s and 1980s were times of describing– investigators worked to understand the disease process, the long prodrome and markers of susceptibility, the genetics and the epidemiology of the disease. In the 1990s all these disciplines are coming together. We can identify family members more likely than not to develop diabetes within 10 years; we can envisage population screening programs; we can design intervention trials and have at least four distinct preventive strategies that are ready for large-scale testing. Prevention of childhood diabetes may not be imminent, but it is no longer inconceivable.

REFERENCES

American Diabetes Association. (1990) Position Statement. Prevention of Type 1 diabetes mellitus. *Diabetes*, **39**, 1151–52.

Atkinson, M.A., Maclaren, N.K., Riley, W.J. *et al.* (1986) Are insulin autoantibodies markers for insulin-dependent diabetes mellitus? *Diabetes*, **35**, 894–98.

Atkinson, M.A., Maclaren, N.K., Scharp, D.W. *et al.* (1990) 64 000 Mr autoantibodies as predictors of insulin-dependent diabetes. *Lancet*, **335**, 1357–60.

Atkinson, M.A., Maclaren, N.K. and Luchetta, R. (1990) Insulitis and insulin dependent diabetes in NOD mice reduced by prophylactic insulin therapy. *Diabetes*, **39**, 933–37.

Barnett, A.H., Eff, C., Leslie, R.D.G. *et al.* (1981) Diabetes in identical twins: a study of 200 pairs. *Diabetologia*, **20**, 87–93.

Barrett-Connor, E. (1985) Is insulin-dependent diabetes mellitus caused by coxsackie B infection? A review of the epidemiologic evidence. *Rev. Infect. Dis.*, **7**, 207–215.

Bertrams, J. and Baur, M.P. (1984) 'Insulin dependent diabetes mellitus', in E.D. Albert and W.R. Mayr (eds). *Histocompatibility testing 1984*, pp. 348–58. Springer-Verlag, Berlin.

Bingley, P.J., Bonifacio, E. and Gale, E.A.M. (1993a) Can we really predict IDDM? *Diabetes*, **42**, 213–20.

Bingley, P.J., Colman, P.G., Eisenbarth, G.S. *et al.* (1992) Standardization of IVGTT to predict IDDM. *Diabetes Care*, **15**, 93–102.

Bingley, P.J., Bonifacio, E., Shattock, M. *et al.* (1993b) Can islet cell antibodies predict IDDM in the general population? *Diabetes Care*, **16**, 45–50.

Bingley, P.J. and Gale, E.A.M. (1989) Rising incidence of IDDM in Europe. *Diabetes Care*, **12**, 289–95.

Boitard, C., Timsit, J., Assan, R. *et al.* (1992) Treatment of type 1 diabetes mellitus with DAB486-IL-2, a toxin conjugate which targets activated T-lymphocytes. *Diabetologia*, **35** (suppl. 1), A218.

Bonifacio, E., Bingley, P.J., Dean, B.M. *et al* (1990) Quantification of islet-cell antibodies and prediction of insulin-dependent diabetes. *Lancet*, **335**, 147–49.

Bottazzo, G.F. (1986) Death of a beta cell: Homicide or suicide? *Diabetic Med.*, **3**, 119–30.

Bottazzo, G.F., Dean, B.M., McNally, J.M. *et al.* (1985a) *In situ* characterisation of autoimmune phenomena and expression of HLA molecules in the pancreas in diabetic insulitis. *N. Engl. J. Med.*, **313**, 353–60.

Bottazzo, G.F., Florin-Christensen, A. and Doniach D. (1974) Islet-cell antibodies in diabetes mellitus with polyendocrine disease. *Lancet*, **ii**, 1279–83.

Bottazzo, G.F., Pujol-Borrell, R. and Gale, E.A.M. (1985b) 'Etiology of diabetes: the role of autoimmune mechanisms', in K.G.G.M. Alberti and L.P. Krall (eds). *The Diabetes Annual*, Vol. 1, pp. 16–52. Elsevier Science Publications, Amsterdam.

Canadian-European Randomized Control Trial Group. (1988) Cyclosporin-induced remission of IDDM after early intervention: association with enhanced insulin secretion. *Diabetes*, **37**, 1574–82.

Chase, H.P., Voss, M.A., Butler-Simon, N. *et al.* (1987) Diagnosis of pre-type 1 diabetes. *J. Pediatr.*, **111**, 807–12.

Chase, H.P., Dupre, J., Mahon, J. *et al.* (1992) Nicotinamide and the prevention of diabetes. *Lancet*, **339**, 1051–52.

Christie, M.R., Tun, R.Y.M., Lo, S.S.S. *et al.* (1991) Antibodies to GAD and tryptic fragments of the islet 64K antigen as distinct markers for development of IDDM: studies with identical twins. *Diabetes*, **41**, 782–87.

Colman, P.G. and Eisenbarth, G.S. (1988) 'Immunology of Type 1 diabetes – 1987', in K.G.G.M. Alberti and L.P. Krall (eds). *Diabetes Annual/4*, pp. 17–45. Elsevier, Amsterdam.

Dahl-Jorgansen, K., Joner, G. and Hanssen, K.F. (1991) Relationship between cow's milk consumption and the incidence of IDDM in childhood. *Diabetes Care*, **14**, 1081–83.

Daneman, D., Fishman, L., Calrson, C. *et al.* (1987) Dietary triggers of insulin-dependent diabetes in the BB rat. *Diabetes Res.*, **5**, 93–97.

de Bernadinis, P., Londei, M., James, R.F.L. *et al.* (1988) Do CD4-positive cytotoxic T cells damage islet β cells in Type 1 diabetes? *Lancet*, **ii**, 823–24.

Deschamps, I., Boitard, C., Hors, J. *et al.* (1992) Life table analysis of the risk of Type 1 (insulin-dependent) diabetes in siblngs according to islet cell antibodies and HLA markers. *Diabetologia*, **35**, 951–57.

Diabetes Epidemiology Research International Group. (DERIG) (1988) Geographic patterns of childhood insulin-dependent diabetes mellitus. *Diabetes*, **37**, 1113–19.

Dulin, W.E., Wyse, B.M. and Kalamazoo, M.S. (1969) Studies on the ability of compounds to block the diabetogenic activity of streptozotocin. *Diabetes*, **18**, 459–66.

Dumont Herskowitz, R., Jackson, R.A., Soeldner, J.S. *et al.* (1989) Pilot trial to prevent Type 1 diabetes: progression to overt IDDM despite oral nicotinamide. *J. Autoimmunity*, **2**, 733–37.

Elliott, R.B. and Chase, H.P. (1991) Prevention or delay of Type 1 (insulin-dependent) diabetes mellitus in children using nicotinamide. *Diabetologia*, **34**, 362–65.

Elliott, R.B., Crossly, J.R., Berryman, C.C. *et al.* (1981) Partial preservation of β cell function in children with diabetes. *Lancet*, **ii**, 1–4.

Elliott, R.B. and Martin, J.M. (1984) Dietary protein: a trigger of insulin-dependent diabetes in the BB rat? *Diabetologia*, **26**, 297–99.

Feutren, G., Papoz, L., Assan, R. *et al.* (1986) Cyclosporin increases the rate and length of remission in insulin-dependent diabetes of recent onset. *Lancet*, **ii**, 119–23.

Gamble, D.R. (1980) An epidemiological study of childhood diabetes affecting two or more siblings. *Diabetologia*, **19**, 341–44.

Genovese, S., Cassidy, D., Bonifacio, E. *et al.* (1991) Antibodies to 37/40kD tryptic fragments of 64kD antigen are markers of rapid progression to Type 1 insulin-dependent diabetes (abstract). *Diabetes Res. Clin. Prac.*, **14** (suppl. 1), S11.

Genovese, S., Bonifacio, E., Dean, B.M. *et al.* (1992) Distinct cytoplasmic islet cell antibodies with different risks for Type 1 (insulin-dependent) diabetes mellitus. *Diabetologia*, **35**, 385–88.

Gepts, W. (1965) Pathological anatomy of the pancreas in juvenile diabetes mellitus. *Diabetes*, **14**, 619–33.

Gianini, R., Pugliese, A., Bonner-Weir, S. *et al.* (1992) Prognostically significant heterogeneity of cytoplasmic islet cell antibodies in relatives of patients with Type 1 diabetes. *Diabetes*, **41**, 347–53.

Ginsberg-Fellner, F., Witt, M.E., Fedun, B. *et al.* (1985) Diabetes and autoimmunity in patients with the congenital rubella syndrome. *Rev. Infect. Dis.*, **7**, 5170–76.

Gotfredsen, G.F., Buschard, K. and Frandsen, E.K. (1985) Reduction of diabetes incidence of BB Wistar rats by early prophylactic insulin treatment of diabetes-prone animals. *Diabetologia*, **28**, 933–35.

Green, A., Gale, E.A.M., Patterson, C.C. *et al.* (1992) Incidence of childhood-onset diabetes mellitus: The EURODIAB ACE Study. *Lancet*, **339**, 905–909.

Harrison, L.C. (1992) Islet cell antigens in insulin-dependent diabetes: Pandora's box revisited. *Immunology Today*, **13**, 348–52.

Harrison, L.C., Colman, P.G., Dean, B. *et al.* (1985) Increased remission rate in newly diagnosed type 1 diabetic subjects treated with azathioprine. *Diabetes*, **37**, 1306–1308.

Harrison, L.C., Campbell, I.L., Colman, P.G. *et al.* (1990) Type 1 diabetes: immunopathology and immunotherapy. *Adv. Endocrin. Metab.*, **1**, 36–94.

Helgasson, T. and Jonasson, M.R. (1981) Evidence for a food additive as a cause of ketosis-prone diabetes. *Lancet*, **ii**, 716–20.

Himsworth, H.P., (1936) Diabetes mellitus, its differentiation into insulin-sensitive and insulin-insensitive types. *Lancet*, **i**, 127–30.

Hoffer, A. (1969) Safety, side effects and relative lack of toxicity of nicotinic acid and nicotinamide. *Schizophrenia*, **1**, 78–87.

Jenson, A.B., Rosenburg, H.S. and Notkins, A.L. (1980) Pancreatic islet cell damage in children with fatal viral infections. *Lancet*, **ii**, 354–58.

Karjalainen, J., Martin, J.M., Knip, M. *et al.* (1992) A bovine serum albumen peptide as a possible trigger of insulin-dependent diabetes mellitus. *N. Eng. J. Med.*, **327**, 302–307.

Keller, R.J., Eisenbarth, G.S. and Jackson, R.A. (1993) Insulin prophylaxis in individuals at high risk of type 1 diabetes. *Lancet*, **341**, 927–28.

Khalil, I., d'Auriol, L., Gober, M. *et al.* (1990) A combination of HLA-DQβ Asp 57-negative and HLA-DQα Arg 52 confers susceptibility to insulin-dependent diabetes mellitus. *J. Clin. Invest.*, **85**, 1315–19.

Knip, M., Vahasalo, P., Karjalainen, J. *et al.* (1992) Natural course of pre-type 1 diabetes in high risk individuals. *Diabetologia*, **35**, A32.

Kroncke, K.-D., Funda, J., Berschick, B. *et al.* (1991) Macrophage cytotoxicity towards isolated rat islet cells: neither lysis nor its protection by nicotinamide are β-cell specific. *Diabetologia*, **34**, 232–38.

Laakso, M. and Pyorala, K. (1985) Age of onset and type of diabetes. *Diabetes Care*, **8**, 114–17.

Landin-Olsson, M., Karlsson, A., Dahlquist, G. *et al*. (1989) Islet cell and other organ specific autoantibodies in all children developing Type 1 (insulin-dependent) diabetes in Sweden during one year and in matched control children. *Diabetologia*, **32**, 387–95.

Lazarow, A. (1947) Protection against alloxan diabetes. *Anatom. Res.*, **97**, 353.

Lendrum, R., Walker, G. and Gamble, D.R. (1975) Islet-cell antibodies in juvenile diabetes mellitus of recent onset. *Lancet.*, **i**, 880–83.

Lipton, R.B., Atchison, J.J. and Becker, D.J. (1989) Prediction of IDDM among first-degree relatives of children with IDDM. *Diabetes*, **38** (suppl. 2), 91A.

Mendola, G., Casamitjana, R., Gomis, R. (1989) Effect of nicotinamide therapy upon B-cell function in newly-diagnosed Type 1 (insulin-dependent) diabetic patients. *Diabetologia*, **32**, 160–62.

Nerup, J., Andersen, O., Bendixin, G. *et al*. (1974) Cell mediated immunity in diabetes mellitus. *Proc. Roy. Soc. Med.*, **67**, 506–513.

Nerup, J., Mandrup-Poulsen, T., Molvig, J. *et al*. (1989) 'On the pathogenesis of insulin-dependent diabetes – a discussion of three recently proposed models', in W. Creutzfeld and P.J. Lefebvre (eds). *Diabetes Mellitus: Pathophysiology and therapy*, pp. 39–50. Springer-Verlag, Berlin.

Pak, C.Y., Eun, H.M., McArthur, R.G. *et al*. (1988) Association of cytomegalovirus infection with autoimmune Type 1 diabetes. *Lancet*, **ii**, 1–5.

Patterson, C.C., Smith, P.G., Webb, J. *et al*. (1988) Geographical variation in the incidence of diabetes mellitus in Scottish children during the period 1977–1983. *Diabetic Med.*, **5**, 160–65.

Peakman, M., Hussain, M.J., Millward, B.A. *et al*. (1990) Effect of initiation of insulin therapy on T-lymphocyte activation in type 1 diabetes. *Diabetic Med.*, **7**, 327–30.

Pilcher, C., Dickens, K. and Elliott, R.B. (1991) ICA only develop in early childhood. *Diabetes Res. Clin. Prac.*, **14**, (suppl. 1), S82.

Pociot, F., Reimers, J.I. and Andersen, H.U. (1993) Nicotinamide – biological actions and therapeutic potential in diabetes prevention. IDIG Workshop, Copenhagen, Denmark, 4–5 December 1992. *Diabetologia*, **36**, 574–76.

Prosser, P.R. and Karam, J.H. (1978) Diabetes mellitus following rodenticide ingestion in man. *J. Am. Med. Assoc.*, **239**, 1148–50.

Reijonen, H., Ilonen, J., Knip, M. *et al*. (1991) HLA-DQB1 alleles and absence of Asp 57 as susceptibility factors of IDDM in Finland. *Diabetes*, **40**, 1640–44.

Riley, W.J., Maclaren, N.K., Krischer, J. *et al*. (1990) A prospective study of the development of diabetes in relatives of patients with insulin-dependent diabetes. *N. Eng. J. Med.*, **323**, 1167–72.

Rotter, J.I. and Landaw, E.M. (1984) Measuring the genetic contribution of a single locus to a multilocus disease. *Clin. Genet.*, **26**, 529–42.

Scott, F.W., Daneman, D. and Martin, J.M. (1988) Evidence for a critical role of diet in the development of insulin-dependent diabetes mellitus. *Diabetes Res.*, **7**, 153–57.

Shah, S.C., Malone, J.I. and Simpson, N.E. (1989) A randomized trial of intensive insulin therapy in newly diagnosed insulin-dependent diabetes mellitus. *N. Engl. J. Med.*, **320**, 550–54.

Sibley, R.K. and Sutherland, D.E.R. (1987) Pancreas Transplantation: an immunohistologic examination of 100 grafts. *Am. J. Path.*, **128**, 151–70.

Silverstein, J., Maclaren, N., Riley, W. *et al*. (1988) Immunosuppression with azathioprine and prednisolone in recent-onset insulin-dependent diabetes mellitus. *N. Engl. J. Med.*, **319**, 599–604.

Skyler, J.S., Byers, V., Einhorn, D. *et al*. (1991) Effects of an anti-CD5 immunoconjugate (H65-RTA) on pancreatic islet beta cell function in type 1 diabetes mellitus (abstract). *Diabetes Res. Clin. Prac.*, **14** (suppl. 1), S54.

Skyler, J.S. and Marks, J.B. (1993) Immune intervention in type 1 diabetes mellitus. *Diabetes Rev.*, **1**, 15–42.

Smith, C.P., Tarn, A.C., Thomas, J.M. *et al*. (1988b) Between and within subject variation of the first phase insulin response to intravenous glucose. *Diabetologia*, **31**, 123–25.

Smith, C.P., Archibald, H.R., Thomas, J.M. *et al*. (1988a) Basal and stimulated insulin levels rise with advancing puberty. *Clin. Endocrinol.*, **28**, 7–14.

Solimena, M., Folli, F., Aparisi, R. *et al*. (1990) Autoantibodies to GABA-ergic neurons and pancreatic β-cells in stiff-man syndrome. *N. Eng. J. Med.*, **322**, 1555–60.

Srikanta, S., Ganda, O.P., Eisenbarth, G.S. *et al.* (1983) Islet-cell antibodies and beta cell function in monozygotic triplets and twins initially discordant for Type 1 diabetes mellitus. *N. Eng. J. Med.*, **308**, 322–25.

Thivolet, C.H., Tappaz, M., Durand, A. *et al.* (1992) Glutamic acid decarboxylase (GAD) autoantibodies are additional predictive markers of Type 1 (insulin-dependent) diabetes in high risk individuals. *Diabetologia*, **35**, 570–76.

Thompson, H.S.G. and Staines, N.A. (1990) Could specific oral tolerance be a therapy for autoimmune disease? *Immunology Today*, **11**, 396–99.

Tienari, P.J., Tuomilehto-Wolf, E., Tuomilehto, J. *et al.* (1992) HLA haplotypes in Type 1 (insulin-dependent) diabetes mellitus: molecular analysis of the HLA-DQ locus. *Diabetologia*, **35**, 254–60.

Tillil, H. and Kobberling, J. (1987) Age-corrected empirical genetic risk estimates for first degree relatives of IDDM patients. *Diabetes*, **36**, 93–99.

Timsit, J., Caillat-Zucman, S., Blondel, H. *et al.* (1992) Islet cell antibody hetergoeneity among Type 1 (insulin-dependent) diabetic patients. *Diabetologia*, **35**, 792–95.

Todd, J.A., Bell, J.I. and McDevitt, H.O. (1987) HLA DQb gene contributes to susceptibility and resistance to insulin-dependent diabetes mellitus. *Nature*, **329**, 599–604.

Todd, J.A., Aitman, T.J., Cornall R.J. *et al.* (1991) Genetic analysis of autoimmune type 1 diabetes mellitus in mice. *Nature*, **351**, 542–47.

Tuomilehto, J., Tuomilehto-Wolf, E., Virtala, E. *et al.* (1990) Coffee consumption as trigger for isulin-dependent diabetes mellitus in childhood. *Diabetes Care*, **13**, 642–43.

Vague, P., Vialettes, B., Lassman-Vague, V. *et al.* (1987) Nicotinamide may extend remission phase in insulin-dependent diabetes. *Lancet*, **i**, 619–20.

Vague, P., Picq, R., Bernal, M. *et al.* (1989) Effect of nicotinamide on the residual insulin secretion of Type 1 (insulin-dependent) diabetic patients. *Diabetologia*, **32**, 316–21.

Vardi, P., Crisal, L. and Jackson, R.A. (1991) Predictive value of intravenous glucose tolerance test insulin secretion less than or greater than the first percentile in islet cell antibody positive relatives of Type 1 (insulin-dependent) diabetic patients. *Diabetologia*, **34**, 93–102.

Vialettes, B., Mattei-Zevaco, C., Badier, C. *et al.* (1988) Low acute insulin response to intravenous glucose. A sensitive but non-specific marker of early stages of Type 1 (insulin-dependent) diabetes. *Diabetologia*, **31**, 592–96.

Virtanen, S.M., Rasanen, L., Aro A. *et al.* (1991) Infant feeding in Finnish children <7 yr of age with newly diagnosed IDDM. *Diabetes Care*, **14**, 415–17.

Vlahos, W.D., Seemayer, T.A. and Yale, J.F. (1991) Diabetes prevention in BB rats by inhibition of endogenous insulin secretion. *Metabolism*, **40**, 825–29.

Ward, K.P., Galloway, W.H. and Auchterlonie, I.A. (1979) Congenital cytomegalovirus infection and diabetes. *Lancet*, **ii**, 497.

Williams, A.J.K., Krug, J.P., Lampeter, E.F. *et al.* (1990) Raised temperature reduces the incidence of diabetes in the NOD mouse. *Diabetologia*, **33**, 635–37.

World Health Organization. (1985) *Diabetes Mellitus*. Geneva: World Health Organization.

Yamada, K., Nonaka, K., Hanafusa, T. *et al.* (1982) Preventive and therapeutic effects of large-dose nicotinamide injections on diabetes associated with insulitis. *Diabetes*, **31**, 749–53.

Yoon, J-W., Austin, M., Onodera, T. *et al.* (1979) Virus-induced diabetes mellitus. Isolation of virus from the pancreas of a child with diabetic ketoacidosis. *N. Eng. J. Med.*, **300**, 1173–79.

Zhong, Z.J., Davidson, L., Eisenbarth, G.S. *et al.* (1991) Suppression of diabetes in nonobese diabetic mice by oral administration of porcine insulin. *Proc. Nat. Acad. Sci. USA*, **88**, 10252–56.

Ziegler, A.G., Ziegler, R., Vardi, P. *et al.* (1989) Life-table analysis of progression to diabetes of anti-insulin autoantibody-positive relatives of individuals with Type 1 diabetes. *Diabetes*, **38**, 1320–25.

Ziegler, A.G., Hillebrand, B., Rabl, W. *et al.* (1993) On the appearance of islet associated autoimmunity in offspring of diabetic mothers: a prospective study from birth. *Diabetologia*, **36**, 402–408.

39

Control and outcome: clinical and epidemiologic aspects

D.J. BECKER, T.J. ORCHARD and C.E. LLOYD

39.1 INTRODUCTION

Insulin-dependent diabetes mellitus (IDDM) diagnosed during childhood and adolescence results in major disruption of daily living with a constant threat of acute complications. The high risk of morbidity and mortality due to chronic complications which may occur as early as young adulthood (DERI Mortality Group, 1991) adds to the toll. In our own pediatric population evaluated in 1982 and diagnosed prior to the age of 17 years between 1950 and 1981, we documented a 11.5-fold increased risk of dying in females and 5.4-fold increased risk in males compared to an age-matched nondiabetic population (Dorman *et al.*, 1984). These increased mortality rates in relatively young populations persist despite the major advances in the treatment of the complications of diabetes in the past decades and increase with advancing age (Panzram, 1984). It has become obvious that the chronic complications of IDDM, once clinically overt, cannot be reversed, and at best treatment can slow their progression. This has led to increasing interest in the diagnosis and possible intervention of subclinical complications, both micro- and macrovascular, in the hope that subsequent mortality from chronic complications can be prevented and morbidity ameliorated. Increasingly sensitive techniques available for the detection of microvascular complications have demonstrated that these complications are already highly prevalent during childhood and adolescence. The major questions facing pediatricians and pediatric diabetologists are: 1) what is the prognostic significance of the subclinical complications? 2) Can intervention therapy controlling the metabolic abnormalities induced by insulin deficiency, prevent the progression from subclinical to clinical complications? 3) Are other intervention therapies safe and effective?

39.2 PREVALENCE OF CHRONIC COMPLICATIONS

Anecdotal observations suggest that the incidence of overt nephropathy, proliferative retinopathy and neuropathy have clearly decreased in adolescent IDDM patients over the past 25 years, so that these chronic complications are now relatively rare in pediatric diabetes practices. However, there have been no epidemiological studies to confirm the impression that improved therapies aimed mostly at glycemic control, have decreased

Childhood and Adolescent Diabetes
Published in 1994 by Chapman & Hall, London
ISBN 0 412 48610 5

the prevalence of overt microvascular complications during youth. By contrast, the advent of fluorescein angiography and fundus photography and the development of assays able to detect micro amounts of albumin in the urine, have revealed a high prevalence of subclinical complications of the eyes and kidneys compared to what was detectable 20 years ago. Smaller studies of motor nerve conduction and sensory changes also reveal very early alterations in nerve function. Tests for macrovascular disease are relatively crude, so that the prevalence of chronic changes that might lead to heart attacks and strokes is less readily apparent, but disturbed cardiovascular risk factors are already present (Cruickshanks *et al.*, 1985).

39.2.1 RETINOPATHY

The reported prevalence of retinopathy varies somewhat according to methodology used and the characteristics of the populations studied. We have shown, using fluorescein angiography, a 13% prevalence in children and adolescents diagnosed consecutively after 5 years' IDDM duration (D'Antonio *et al.*, 1989). Two very large population-based studies have examined cross-sectional prevalence rates of subjects with youth-onset IDDM. The Wisconsin Epidemiological Study of Diabetic Retinopathy (WESDR) found similar rates in presumed IDDM subjects with <4 years' duration (Klein *et al.*, 1985). In this study, which is based on subjects diagnosed before age 30 years, and the Pittsburgh Epidemiology of Diabetes Complications Study (EDC) (Orchard, 1990a), based on children diagnosed before age 17 years, the prevalence of any retinopathy at <18 years of age was 27% and 25% respectively (Lloyd & Orchard, 1993). The prevalence is, in general, slightly higher in populations which include young adults from a low of 27% (Frank *et al.*, 1982) to 47% (Burger *et al.*, 1986). In the WESDR and EDC studies, very similar prevalence rates of about 80% in patients age 18–29 years are reported (Orchard *et al.*, 1990b; Klein *et al.*, 1985). There is fairly remarkable consistency in prevalence rates in other more recent studies of retinopathy in young subjects with IDDM. If followed long enough, it appears that all IDDM patients diagnosed in childhood will eventually develop some degree of retinopathy (Orchard *et al.*, 1990a; Klein *et al.*, 1989).

Because of the absence of prolonged longitudinal studies, it is at yet unknown whether there is any degree of retinopathy which is predictive of proliferative retinopathy and vision impairment in the future. Proliferative retinopathy is found in 60–70% of IDDM subjects after 30 years' duration (Klein *et al.*, 1989; Orchard *et al.*, 1990; Krolewski *et al.*, 1986). The incidence of retinopathy has been examined in the Wisconsin (WESDR) and Pittsburgh (EDC) populations in the US. In the former, 10% developed proliferative retinopathy over a 4-year period (Klein *et al.*, 1988). In the latter, 11% developed proliferative disease in 2 years (Lloyd *et al.*, 1993).

39.2.2 NEPHROPATHY

Whereas retinopathy is defined as structural changes of the vasculature, subclinical nephropathy in the absence of renal biopsies is defined as functional changes in the excretion of large molecules by the kidneys. Interest in microalbuminuria has escalated since reports suggested that it may predict the later development of overt nephropathy (Mogensen & Christensen, 1984; Viberti *et al.*, 1982; Mathiesen *et al.*, 1984). This concept is still to be proven in large longitudinal studies in childhood cohorts with microalbuminuria. However, it is vitally important, as obviously all patients with renal failure will go through a phase of microalbuminuria and renal failure is 17 times more common in diabetic patients compared to a nondiabetic population (Lewitt & Yue, 1988). In addition, the presence of albumin in the urine is highly predictive of the other major cause of death in IDDM patients, cardiovascular disease (Borch-Johnsen *et al.*, 1985). Studies are urgently needed to determine which patients with established microalbuminuria in childhood will develop overt nephropathy and to establish the risk factors which influence this outcome e.g., the degree of metabolic control.

Like retinopathy, microalbuminuria increases with increasing duration of diabetes. Although it has been suggested by a number of investigators that microalbuminuria is extremely rare prior to 5 years' IDDM duration (Dahlquist & Rudberg, 1987; Mathiesen *et al.*, 1986), a study specifically examining a cohort of children at 5 years' duration revealed a prevalence of 21% (D'Antonio *et al.*, 1989). Prevalence rates in children and adolescents have varied from 4.3–37% partially because of differences in the definition of microalbuminuria, and the age and duration of the patients studied (Dahlquist & Rudberg, 1987; Mathiesen *et al.*, 1986; Mortensen *et al.*, 1990; Cook & Daneman, 1990; Davies *et al.*, 1985), with marked increases after puberty (Dahlquist & Rudberg, 1987; Mathiesen *et al.*, 1986). The prevalence of albumin excretion rates 20–200 μg/min in our 65 EDC children aged <18 years after 5 years' IDDM is 14% (Coonrod *et al.*, 1991a). In patients followed for longer periods, 20–40 years, 35% were found to have microalbuminuria (Krolewski *et al.*, 1985b). This prevalence is very similar to that of our own EDC population examined after 30 years' IDDM (32% for males and 25% for females). Combining both microalbuminuria and overt nephropathy (>200 μg/min), shows that 80% of males and over 50% of females have abnormal albumin excretion after 30 years' duration. Thus, with prolonged duration of IDDM, most patients have evidence of microvascular renal damage, but not all develop renal failure (Orchard *et al.*, 1990a). Both the Joslin Clinic and the Steno Hospital have reported major decreases in the prevalence of overt proteinuria from the 1950s to the 1980s with the prediction of large reductions in the development of renal failure (Krolewski *et al.*, 1985a; Kofoed-Enevoldsen *et al.*, 1987).

39.2.3 NEUROPATHY

The most common test to detect subclinical neuropathy in children with IDDM is motor nerve conduction velocity. Using this technique, abnormalities have been detected already very early after the onset of IDDM in children, suggesting a functional metabolic abnormality (Hoffman *et al.*, 1983). Prevalence rates of 50–72% are recorded (Hoffman *et al.*, 1983; Sosenko *et al.*, 1985; Barkai *et al.*, 1990; Young *et al.*, 1983; Dorchy *et al.*, 1985). By contrast, clinical distal asymmetric polyneuropathy, which may reflect metabolic or microvascular changes, was found by careful examination in 3% of 65 children in our EDC population under the age of 18 years and in 18% in those between 18 and 29 years (Maser *et al.*, 1989). This is similar to the 20% reported by Allen *et al.* (1992) for subjects age 16–29 years. The prevalence in all studies was associated with duration of diabetes and age (Allen *et al.*, 1992; Maser *et al.*, 1989). In fact, a study of vibration perception threshold showed abnormalities were more likely to occur in postpubertal children (Sosenko *et al.*, 1985).

Both impaired visual and auditory brain stem evoked potentials have been described in studies of small numbers of subjects. Abnormalities of visual evoked potentials were found in 30% of 37 children and this was unrelated to age (Cirillo *et al.*, 1984) and was similar to the prevalence in adult diabetic patients (Algan *et al.*, 1989). Abnormal auditory evoked potentials were found in 22% of adult IDDM patients (Martini *et al.*, 1987). Detailed studies of autonomic neuropathy are rare in pediatric populations. One such study revealed a prevalence of 15% of children with abnormal cardiovascular reflex tests, increasing to 31% when only teenage subjects were included (Ewing & Clarke, 1986). In our own population of childhood-onset IDDM patients, 38% of those age 25–34 years had signs of autonomic neuropathy (Maser *et al.*, 1992). These prevalence rates are important as autonomic neuropathy has been described to be associated with increased mortality (Sampson *et al.*, 1990; Navarro *et al.*, 1991), with a 5-year cumulative mortality rate more than five times greater compared to those without autonomic neuropathy in an adult population of diabetic subjects (O'Brien *et al.*, 1991).

39.3 CONTROL AND COMPLICATIONS

The pathogenesis of diabetes complications is discussed in other chapters. It is very logical that the metabolic abnormalities induced by insulin deficiency (with or without excessive circulating peripheral insulin concentrations) must in some way play a role in the development of the chronic complications associated with IDDM. Controversies regarding the role played by glycemic control over the years are largely due to our inability to fully measure and correct the metabolic milieu. In addition, because some patients with apparently very poor metabolic control never develop overt clinical complications, while others with apparently good control are devastated by severe complications, factors other than glycemic control have been implicated. These include a genetic susceptibility to the development of complications as these tend to cluster in families (Seaquist *et al.*, 1989; Dorman *et al.*, 1991). Other environmental factors such as smoking and lack of exercise have been shown in epidemiologic studies to increase the risk for complications (Moy *et al.*, 1993; Chase *et al.*, 1991). In addition, sex hormones appear to be important in the expression of complications as demonstrated by the gender differences in mortality risks and risks for nephropathy (Dorman *et al.*, 1984; Orchard *et al.*, 1990a; Mortensen *et al.*, 1990; Andersen *et al.*, 1983). However, it is also possible that these gender differences may reflect lifestyles, including diet, rather than hormones. The observation that the postpubertal years of diabetes are more predictive of both subclinical and clinical complications than the prepubertal years, also raises the possibility of a major role for sex hormones (Kostraba *et al.*, 1989). However, there are also increases in growth hormone and IGFI during this period. Both these hormones are thought to have pathogenic influences on the development of microvascular complications (Merimee, 1990).

It has become increasingly clear that the major nonmetabolic risk factor for the development of complications is blood pressure. Hypertension has been described as a very important risk factor for the development of diabetes complications and mortality in IDDM (Christlieb *et al.*, 1981). Even slightly increased blood pressure levels, not defined as hypertension, have been associated with the incidence of retinopathy and the progression of retinopathy and nephropathy (Cruickshanks *et al.*, 1985; Orchard *et al.*, 1990b; Lloyd *et al.*, 1993; Teuscher *et al.*, 1988; Chase *et al.*, 1990; Parving *et al.*, 1983; Coonrod *et al.*, 1993). Although control of hypertension is not conventionally included in discussion of the role of 'control' of IDDM and its complications, it may be as great a predictor of overt clinical complications as glycemic control (Orchard *et al.*, 1990b). Therefore, very close and accurate monitoring of blood pressure measurements must be an essential part of diabetes care. Therapeutic interventions are necessary as soon as sustained hypertension is detected. The dilemma for the pediatrician comes when blood pressure levels are raised slightly above normal, but are not in the defined hypertensive ranges. These 'non-normal' blood pressure levels are shown in epidemiologic studies to be associated with both retinopathy and microalbuminuria. Intervention studies with antihypertensive therapies in children with microalbuminuria are to date, small and short (Rudberg *et al.*, 1990; Cook *et al.*, 1990). As increased blood pressure may be a result of renal disease rather than its cause (Mathiesen *et al.*, 1990), it is possible that improved metabolic control may be associated with the prevention, or even decrease of mildly elevated blood pressure levels. This has not been evaluated.

39.4 METABOLIC CONTROL

The most obvious metabolic abnormality induced by insulin deficiency is hyperglycemia. Therefore, by convention, metabolic control is usually defined as glycemic control. However, insulin deficiency also results in major abnormalities of lipid and amino acid metabolism, together with elevations of ketones and other intermediary metabolites as well as many hormones. Glucose is the most easily measured metabolite. But it was not until the availability of glycosylated hemoglobin measurements that glycemic control could be accurately monitored over long periods of time (Koenig *et al.*, 1976). Therefore, measurements of glycosylated hemoglobin have become the surrogate for determining metabolic control. However, abnormalities of cholesterol, triglycerides, and lipoprotein composition are not infrequently seen in IDDM. Raised LDL cholesterol and reduced HDL cholesterol are well-established as important risk factors for the development of cardiovascular disease in the general population (Jarrett, 1985), although prospective studies in populations with IDDM are limited (Krowleski *et al.*, 1987; Maser *et al.*, 1991). In addition, cross-sectional studies have shown an association between increased lipid levels and microalbuminuria (Jones *et al.*, 1989; Jay *et al.*, 1991). In our EDC study of 256 IDDM patients 10% of whom developed microalbuminuria during a 2-year follow-up, LDL cholesterol levels were significantly higher in males and triglycerides in females (Coonrod *et al.*, 1991b). In addition, in this population, abnormal lipid profiles were associated cross-sectionally with diabetic neuropathy, with these patients showing significantly higher LDL cholesterol and lower HDL cholesterol and increased serum triglycerides (Maser *et al.*, 1989). Similar associations were seen in autonomic neuropathy (Maser *et al.*, 1990).

High-risk lipid profiles may be a result of poor glycemic control or may be induced by factors other than those related to diabetes (D'Antonio *et al.*, 1989; Sosenko *et al.*, 1980). Although there have been no intervention studies to show that improvement of the lipid profile will decrease diabetes complications, regular monitoring of cholesterol levels is advocated (American Diabetes Association, 1993b). In addition, most groups suggest diets contain 30% of the calories as fat with limitations of cholesterol and saturated fatty acid intake to 300 mg/day and less than 10% of the total fat, respectively (American Diabetes Association, 1993a; Nutrition Subcommittee of the British Diabetic Association's Professional Advisory Committee, 1992). There are currently no clear guidelines based on scientific data to assist the pediatrician in deciding when to undertake more stringent dietary restrictions or pharmacological intervention. Pharmacological strategies are introduced when dietary maneuvers fail to decrease hypercholesterolemia to attempt that LDL cholesterol levels are decreased below 3.4–4.1 mmol. The level of LDL cholesterol, which would stimulate the introduction of pharmacological agents, has not been clearly established in childhood diabetes.

39.5 GLYCEMIC CONTROL

The animal studies of the 1970s showed that in these IDDM models, microvascular complications could be prevented by keeping plasma glucose levels close to normal with insulin injections (Engerman *et al.*, 1977; Rasch, 1979). Because the microvascular complications in rats and dogs showed different pathology and clinical progression to lesions seen in humans, these data were not directly extrapolated to a cause and result mechanism of complications in humans. Studies in humans were limited by the lack of an objective measure of glycemic control and our inability to monitor plasma glucose in the home environment so that tight glycemic control could be attempted safely. The advent of glycosylated hemoglobin assays allowed meaningful epidemiologic studies to be initiated, and with home blood glucose monitoring, intervention studies affecting long-term glycemic control. The absence of these two important requirements prior to the 1980s is the major reason that clinical studies until now have not conclusively demonstrated that metabolic control affects the micro- and macrovascular complications of IDDM. In addition, epidemiologic studies such as those of Pirart and others in which decreased microvascular complications and neuropathy were reported in patients with 'good glycemic control' and vice versa, assessment of control could not be documented, many patients dropped out and other factors were not taken into account (Pirart, 1978; Miki *et al.*, 1969; Job *et al.*, 1976). The deficiencies in many of the studies of the time were reviewed by Raskin (1978). Subsequent to this, a number of epidemiologic studies have demonstrated an association between glycemic control, as measured by glycosylated hemoglobin, and retinopathy, nephropathy and neuropathy (Strowig & Raskin, 1992). After 25 years of diabetes in our EDC population, the 19% of subjects who had avoided major clinical complications, had a significantly lower glycosylated hemoglobin at the time of study. However, data for the prior years were not available (Orchard *et al.*, 1990b).

39.5.1 RETINOPATHY

In both adults and children, glycosylated hemoglobin has been shown to be an important risk factor for the initiation and progression of diabetic retinopathy (Klein *et al.*, 1988). We showed that glycosylated hemoglobin measured over a prior 3-year period in 58 adolescents, aged 14–18 years, with IDDM with duration of more than 8 years, was a significant independent predictor of early retinopathy (Doft *et al.*, 1984). Similar data have been reported in other large pediatric populations (Burger *et al.*, 1986; Chase *et al.*, 1989). The development of microaneurysms was delayed by 4.5 years in a population of young IDDM subjects in 'good' compared with 'poor' control (Weber *et al.*, 1986). In addition, long-term glycemic control correlates with the progression of retinopathy in this and other studies of adults (Burger *et al.*, 1986; McCance *et al.*, 1989; Friberg *et al.*, 1985). In a 40-year follow-up study at the Joslin Clinic, the risk for proliferative retinopathy was strongly related to the level of glycemic control over the previous 4 years (Krolewski *et al.*, 1986). In the large Wisconsin study, glycosylated hemoglobin at baseline was a significant predictor of the incidence of any retinopathy, progression of retinopathy and progression to proliferative retinopathy during a 4-year follow-up period (Klein *et al.*, 1988). The EDC study has confirmed this observation over a 2-year follow-up period. However, the incidence of any new retinopathy did not appear to be significantly associated with glycosylated hemoglobin, but was more strongly related to blood pressure (Lloyd *et al.*, 1993).

39.5.2 NEPHROPATHY

The Wisconsin study has also shown that glycemic control is a risk factor for the development of microalbuminuria, with the risk of developing microalbuminuria being twice as high in patients in the highest quartile of glycosylated hemoglobin distribution compared to those in the lowest quartile (Klein *et al.*, 1992). Studies of children attending a diabetes clinic also demonstrated a significant relationship between glycemic control and microalbuminuria (Chase *et al.*, 1989; Norgaard *et al.*, 1989), and this was confirmed by a population-based study in Norway (Joner *et al.*, 1992). One report suggested that the maintenance of glycosylated hemoglobin level at less than 1.5 times the normal range or 4 standard deviation (SD) above the normal mean, resulted in a significantly lower risk for developing nephropathy (Rose *et al.*, 1991). This association between level of glycemic control and microalbuminuria has not been found by a number of other investigators in the pediatric population (Dahlquist & Rudberg, 1987; Mathiesen *et al.*, 1986; Cook & Daneman, 1990).

A gender difference for the relationship between prior glycemic control and microalbuminuria was demonstrated in our study of adolescents at five years' IDDM duration. Girls with microalbuminuria had a significantly higher glycosylated hemoglobin than those with normal albumin excretion rates. This relationship was not found in boys. In girls, there was a correlation between current glycosylated hemoglobin and albumin excretion rate (D'Antonio *et al.*, 1989). This gender difference was also found in the very large population-based study in Denmark (Mortensen *et al.*, 1990). In our EDC study of 65 patients under the age of 18 years, with greater than five years' duration, there was a low order, but significant correlation between glycosylated hemoglobin and microalbuminuria ($R = 0.28$, $p < 0.05$), but this significance was lost when boys and girls were analyzed separately. When the total cohort of EDC subjects which included adults and children was evaluated by multiple logistic regression, there was a significant relationship between glycosylated hemoglobin and microalbuminuria in both males and females ($p < 0.01$) (Becker *et al.*, 1992). In a recent follow-up of 256 of the EDC IDDM subjects who had normal albumin excretion at baseline, glycosylated hemoglobin was a significant independent predictor of the development of microalbuminuria over two years (Coonrod *et al.*, 1991b). It should be noted that lipid profiles were also predictive of microalbuminuria in this study.

39.5.3 NEUROPATHY

Although clinical neuropathy has been more closely related to duration of diabetes than glycemic control, a significant correlation with glycosylated hemoglobin was reported in 75 adolescents age 16–19 years (Young *et al.*, 1983 & 1986). The relatively rare adolescents with overt polyneuropathy improve with appropriate insulin therapy (White *et al.*, 1981). Studies of nerve conduction and glycemic control in children and adolescents have also demonstrated a significant relationship (Dorchy *et al.*, 1985; Maser *et al.*, 1989; Kaar *et al.*, 1983; Duck *et al.*, 1991). A prospective study of 32 patients aged 12–36 years for five years after diagnosis, showed that nerve conduction was slower and temperature (but not vibration) thresholds were higher in the group with poorer glycemic control (Ziegler *et al.*, 1991). Surprisingly, the initial baseline cross-sectional evaluation of the DCCT showed few, if any, relationships between measures of nerve conduction and clinical neuropathy and glycosylated hemoglobin (DCCT Research Group, 1988a).

39.5.4 OTHER COMPLICATIONS

Other chronic complications of IDDM detectable in childhood and adolescence are not found to correlate with glycosylated hemoglobin, e.g., abnormalities of visual and auditory evoked potentials (Cirillo *et al.*, 1984; Martini *et al.*, 1987), cardiopathy (Lababidi &

Goldstein, 1983; Friedman *et al.*, 1980) and some, but not all, cardiovascular risk factors (Cruickshanks *et al.*, 1985).

39.6 GLYCEMIC CONTROL INTERVENTION STUDIES

Although there are numerous epidemiologic studies showing a correlation between glycemic control and progression of microvascular complications, these associations do not prove cause and effect. Many of these studies have shown associations of microvascular complications with a number of other factors including age, duration of IDDM, blood pressure and lipid profiles which are also significant risk factors. Using multiple logistic regression, some of these other factors appear to be more significant risk predictors than glycemic control (Orchard *et al.*, 1990a; Becker *et al.*, 1992). In addition, correlations with glycemic control are of relatively low order and do not explain all of the risks for chronic complications. It is, therefore, mandatory to prove the role of glycemic control in the pathogenesis of microvascular complications in humans by an intervention strategy that nearly normalizes long-term blood glucose levels, in a study that is of sufficient duration to assess incidence and progression of microvascular changes.

Successful pancreatic transplantation may result in long-term normoglycemia in humans, although concomitant immunosuppressive therapy, with its attendant complications, is always required. Pancreatic transplantation has been shown to be associated with absence of progression of structural abnormalities of the glomeruli in renal biopsies of transplanted kidneys, with less mesangial expansion compared to an age-matched group of subjects who did not receive a pancreas transplant (Bilous *et al.*, 1989). In another report, studies of neurologic function, including clinical examination, nerve conduction and autonomic function, improved after pancreas transplantation, whereas a control group of subjects without pancreas transplants, showed some (but not significant) deterioration during a 42-month period (Kennedy *et al.*, 1990). However, the neuropathy was only slightly improved, suggesting that changes may be irreversible once they have developed. Changes in autonomic indices did not improve appreciably. Pancreas transplantation has also been reported to reverse or arrest the progression of retinopathy in some but not all patients with IDDM (Landgraf *et al.*, 1986; Abendroth *et al.*, 1989; Ramsay *et al.*, 1988). Unfortunately, none of these studies were adequately controlled with simultaneous similarly treated subjects without pancreas transplants. However, it does suggest that normoglycemia can prevent the progression of very early microvascular complications, but more severe lesions are unaffected. Because of the risks of surgery and immunosuppression, pancreas transplantation is not undertaken in young patients, particularly those who are in relatively good health. In addition, the shortage of donor organs at present precludes the possibility of transplanting all young IDDM patients. Therefore, the progress of research involving transplantation with encapsulated or otherwise protected islets is anticipated with much hope (see Chapter 45).

The ability to monitor blood glucose levels frequently at home, was the most important factor in allowing the performance of controlled intervention studies to examine the effect of optimization of glycemic control on the chronic complications of diabetes. Intensive insulin therapy, consisting of multiple daily injections or continuous subcutaneous insulin infusion, greatly assisted patients in achieving these goals. The earliest studies included very small numbers of patients for only short periods of time (Hanssen *et al.*, 1992). As described below, the longest of these studies are six and seven years' duration with numbers of subjects decreasing because of dropouts and cross-over of treatment groups. In all these studies, intensive insulin therapy improved, but did not normalize glycemic control for any length of time. Even when mean blood glucose levels are normalized, glycemic excursions persist to varying degrees in different patients. Most of these studies included few, if any, children and adolescents, probably because of the known difficulties with compliance, particularly in adolescents, as well as the risks including hypoglycemia and ketoacidosis in young children.

39.6.1 RETINOPATHY

No published controlled intervention study has shown that improved glucose control has resulted in clear improvement of retinopathy. In fact, two of the first publications from the Kroc and the Steno groups reported an increased incidence of microaneurysms and soft exudates in the intensive insulin therapy group during the first year of improved glycemic control (Kroc Collaborative Study Group, 1984; Lauritzen *et al.*, 1983). This was confirmed by the Oslo Study (Dahl-Jorgensen *et al.*, 1985). This initial deterioration of retinopathy was shown to regress over the follow-up period so that overall there was no difference in the degree of retinopathy between conventionally and intensively treated patients (Brinchmann-Hansen *et al.*, 1988; Feldt-Rasmussen *et al.*, 1991). Only when two studies were combined were any statistical differences found between conventionally and intensively treated groups (Hanssen *et al.*, 1986). In the Stockholm Study, after five years, there was a small but significantly greater degree of retinopathy in the conventional, than the multiple injection group due to slowing of the progression of the lesions in the multiple injection group (Reichard *et al.*, 1991). These statistical differences are of questionable clinical importance. The recent publication of the seven-year follow-up of the Oslo studies gives the longest follow-up data available (Brinchmann-Hansen *et al.*, 1992). Because of treatment crossovers, the data could not be analyzed according to the intent to treat, so that the control group was lost. However, those patients who maintained improved glycosylated hemoglobin levels showed slower progression of retinopathy, with a cutoff of glycosylated hemoglobin (HbA_1) of 8.7% for this effect to be demonstrable. Those with HbA_1 >10% had an increased risk of progression. The authors suggest that long periods of improved glycemic control are necessary to demonstrate any beneficial effect.

39.6.2 NEPHROPATHY

The results from the glycemic control intervention studies of kidney disease are more encouraging. Two years of tight metabolic control were reported to prevent the progression of established microalbuminuria (Kroc Collaborative Study Group, 1984; Feldt-Rasmussen *et al.*, 1986). At this time, there was no reduction of urinary albumin excretion in the normal range in the Oslo Study, but there was a decrease after four years of continuous subcutaneous insulin infusion (CSII), but not multiple injections (Dahl-Jorgensen *et al.*, 1988). Beneficial effects of improved metabolic control have also been reported using other markers of renal function such as glomerular filtration rate and kidney size (Wiseman *et al.*, 1985). Intensive insulin therapy did not improve established proteinuria (Viberti *et al.*, 1983) although one group reported delayed deterioration of creatinine clearance in patients with proteinuria selected because of background retinopathy (Holman *et al.*, 1983).

A recent update of the Steno studies includes 69 of 70 patients with IDDM diagnosed prior to 30 years of age and followed for 5–8 years. Of these, 51 patients had microalbuminuria (albumin excretion rates 30–300 mg/

24 hrs) and the others were normoalbuminuric. There was initial significant improvement in glycosylated hemoglobin in subjects treated with CSII but there were minimal differences between these subjects and those with conventional therapy at the end of the study. This was attributed to the fact that 18 patients crossed over to intensive insulin therapy after three years of follow-up. There was a slight increase in the number of patients who progressed to clinical nephropathy, proliferative retinopathy or developed hypertension in the conventionally treated groups. However, the difference compared to the intensively treated group was not statistically significant. There was a significantly increased systolic blood pressure in the conventionally treated group ($p < 0.05$) but no change in those on CSII. The differences in urine albumin excretion between the CSII and conventionally treated groups were also not significant, and some patients in both groups reverted to normal after having microalbuminuria. When only those subjects with albumin excretion rates of greater than 100 mg/24 hrs were analyzed, two of nine had developed overt nephropathy in the CSII group compared with ten of ten in the control group ($p < 0.01$). In these patients, glycosylated hemoglobin was significantly higher in the conventional than in the CSII group ($p < 0.001$). In this subgroup treated with conventional therapy arterial hypertension was more frequent than in the CSII group ($p < 0.01$). The rate of decline of glomerular filtration rate was also significantly slower in the CSII group compared with conventionally treated patients with initially higher rates of albumin excretion. This study demonstrates the difficulties in analyzing a long-term study where patients have crossed over and no clear differences are seen in metabolic control between conventional and intensively treated patients. However, the small numbers of subjects with higher albumin excretion rates did appear to have beneficial effects on an intent to treat basis with CSII over the 5–8-year period (Feldt-Rasmussen *et al.*, 1991).

Improved glycemic control may also have an effect on the hemodynamic response of the kidney to an intravenous amino acid load. The exaggerated increase in GFR compared to nondiabetic subjects, was returned to the normal range after several weeks of tightened glycemic control (Tuttle *et al.*, 1991). These data can be extrapolated to the potential improvement of handling of a high protein meal in subjects with near normoglycemia.

39.6.3 NEUROPATHY

There have been fewer glycemic intervention studies with neuropathy as a primary endpoint. However, most reports have included some measures of neuropathy status. In the Stockholm Study, nerve conduction velocities were lower in three nerves in a conventional insulin-treated group compared to an intensified insulin-treatment group. No differences were found in vibration and temperature threshold (Reichard *et al.*, 1991). In the Oslo Study, the group treated with CSII showed improvement of motor nerve conduction velocities (Dahl-Jorgensen, 1987). Because of cross-overs, these groups could not be analyzed in their 8-year follow-up studies. However, those subjects with a mean HbA_1 of more than 10% over this time, had marked deterioration in nerve conduction velocity which was significantly greater than those with a glycosylated hemoglobin of less than 10% (Hanssen *et al.*, 1992). There is no evidence that these results translate into the prevention of clinical neuropathy.

Autonomic nervous system function was assessed by heart rate variation during deep respiration by two groups. A deterioration and heart rate variation was reported in the conventionally treated patients of the Steno Study compared to no change in those on CSII (Lauritzen *et al.*, 1985). Similar observations after two years of CSII have also been reported in another study (Jakobsen *et al.*, 1988).

39.7 LESSONS FROM GLYCEMIC INTERVENTION STUDIES

Inspection of the glycosylated hemoglobin levels of most of the intervention studies, shows that even in the conventionally treated groups, mean levels are usually lower than those described in the epidemiologic studies. Thus, highly motivated subjects who would be willing to be randomized into an intervention study, will be relatively well-controlled at the outset of the study and also show a 'study effect' with improvement in glycemic control in the absence of this intention. By contrast, the intensively treated groups did not achieve normoglycemia, although there was improvement in glycosylated hemoglobin. The maintenance of euglycemia over long periods of time with current forms of therapy seems almost impossible, even in adults. The effects of these two factors together with patients crossing over treatment groups, made the differences in glycosylated hemoglobin between intensively and conventionally treated subjects very small in the longer studies. In all studies it was clear that some patients showed progression of measures of complications while others with similar glycemic levels showed improvement or no change. Thus, individual factors other than improvement in glycemia, apparently affect the progression of the complications of diabetes. However, it does appear that hyperglycemia may be important in the development of the complications in tissues that are made susceptible by other factors such as genetic changes, hemodynamic influences and environmental factors.

Most studies failed to show clear benefits of improved glycemic control on the progression of retinopathy. Despite initial deterioration of the lesions during the first year of improved glycemic control, intensively treated patients were not different from their conventionally treated counterparts after 4–7 years. The reasons for the lack of effect of improved glycemic control may be the small differences between the groups or that structural damage to the blood vessels was irreversible.

By contrast, almost all reports showed a benefit of tight glycemic control for the kidney in those subjects with established microalbuminuria, prior to the presence of overt nephropathy. There were minimal differences in microalbuminuria between the intensively treated and conventionally treated groups in the presence of normoalbuminuria or minor degrees of abnormalities of albumin excretion. There were some reports of beneficial effects of glycemic control on glomerular filtration rates but long-term effects are uncertain.

Motor nerve conduction did improve, but studies of peripheral neuropathy and clinical autonomic neuropathy are not yet available. Lipid abnormalities are also reported to improve with glycemic control interventions with the hope that this may be related to the decreased risk of cardiovascular disease in the future. However, this link has not been proven. Cardiovascular risk factors, particularly the abnormal lipid profile, have been reported to improve with near normoglycemia within weeks (Dunn *et al.*, 1981) and persisting for up to three years (Rosenstock *et al.*, 1987).

Most investigators agree that established complications of IDDM are not affected by alterations in glycemic control. While measures of subclinical complications appear to improve or show decreased rates of progression, none of these studies have proven that complications can ultimately be prevented. Because of the relatively small size and short duration of the studies described above, the results of the large Diabetes Control and Complications Trial, which includes over 1400 subjects, have been eagerly awaited (DCCT Research Group, 1986). This multi-center

United States study (DCCT Research Group, 1993) (discussed below) was designed to assess whether near normal glycemic control can prevent retinopathy in patients without retinopathy at baseline (primary prevention group) and prevent the progression of retinopathy in patients with some background lesions.

Although retinopathy is a primary endpoint, nephropathy, neuropathy and macrovascular disease have also been assessed. The results of this study, which should be large enough and long enough to arrive at clear conclusions, will help determine glycemic therapeutic goals in the future. Hopefully, additional analyses will answer other crucial questions such as the probability of a threshold effect of blood glucose for the chronic complications or a dose response relationship between glycemic control over time and microvascular disease. There will be some specific analyses of the adolescents who were recruited into the study. However, this study will not be able to assess the role of puberty and the need for tight glycemic control prior to puberty as the youngest age of participants was 13 years.

39.8 THE PROS AND CONS OF TIGHT GLYCEMIC CONTROL IN CHILDHOOD: CURRENT STATUS

Despite the advances in insulin delivery and glucose monitoring over the past 15 years, the majority of patients with IDDM are not able safely to achieve normoglycemia. Only 17% of the intensively treated patients taking part in the DCCT were able to achieve normal glycosylated hemoglobin levels during the first year of the study (DCCT Research Group, 1987). Attempts at normoglycemia carry a variety of risks, the most important being hypoglycemia. The initial analyses of the DCCT confirmed the increased risk of severe hypoglycemia experienced by patients treated with intensive therapy in previous studies (Kroc Collaborative Study Group, 1984; Reichard *et al.*, 1991; Feldt-Rasmussen *et al.*, 1986). In the DCCT, intensively treated subjects had a three-fold increase in severe hypoglycemia compared to the conventionally treated groups (DCCT Research Group, 1991). There was also an increase in the frequency of mild hypoglycemia. Intensive insulin therapy appears to increase the risk for hypoglycemia by lowering the mean blood glucose levels as well as changing the threshold for neurogenic warning symptoms as well as counterregulatory hormonal responses (Amiel *et al.*, 1987; Simonson *et al.*, 1985). Failure of glucose counter-regulation in response to hypoglycemia may be life-threatening and it has been suggested that tight glycemic control not be attempted in patients with this disorder (Santiago *et al.*, 1984). Our own data in children show that even mild hypoglycemia, with arterialized plasma glucose levels of 3.3 mmol, can induce significant decreases in cognitive function in children and adolescents with IDDM (Ryan *et al.*, 1990). These frequently asymptomatic episodes are likely to compromise school performance if they occur often enough. Treatment of frequent hypoglycemic episodes may be part of the cause of significant weight gain which has been seen in subjects undergoing intensive insulin therapy (Reichard *et al.*, 1991; DCCT Research Group, 1988b). This elicits not only a cosmetic problem, particularly in adolescents, but also may increase the risk of future blood presure elevations and abnormal lipids. Treatment of diabetes with insulin infusion pumps carries with it the additional risk of increased frequency of diabetic ketoacidosis (Kroc Collaborative Study Group, 1984; Feldt-Rasmussen *et al.*, 1991). This is due to the lack of a depot of long-acting insulin which could act as a reservoir if the delivery of regular insulin by the pump is interrupted for any reason. Under these conditions, glucose and ketones rise extremely rapidly.

The financial burden of intensive insulin

therapy may be prohibitive in some areas around the world. Not only are insulin delivery systems expensive, but frequent daily blood sugar monitoring, laboratory tests and frequent contact with the health care professionals are very costly. It is important to realize that merely injecting insulin more frequently does not necessarily improve glycemic control. Probably the most important aspect of intensified therapy is patient education and support requiring many hours of health care professional time and effort. Successful near normalization of glycemic control requires an inordinate amount of effort on the part of the patient and the family.

This brings us to the last, but maybe most important aspect of intensified diabetes therapy. The psychological toll exacted by the tyranny of an extremely demanding regimen is unacceptable and intolerable in many individuals or families. While the parents of young children frequently find that working hard at diabetes control relieves their concerns somewhat, others are unable to cope with these necessities together with the other demands of a young family. The most challenging time for the pediatrician is during adolescence when diabetes is particularly difficult to control, partially due to rebellion and loss of compliance and partially related to hormonal changes. Theoretically, the increased insulin requirements seen during this period should be easily met, if other lifestyle aspects could be overcome (see also Chapters 5 and 26).

Many hoped that the results of the DCCT would allow us to say honestly to our patients that 'good' glycemic control will prevent complications of diabetes. Our handling of the pediatric population will probably be very different if we can remove the specter of blindness, amputations and renal failure. In addition, many older adolescents are reported to feel a sense of control when they are able to manipulate their lifestyles and eating habits with varying doses of insulin given multiple times a day. This liberalization has been shown, however, to result in no improvement of glycemic control and sometimes in deterioration. In addition, the best of efforts often results in failure with associated incredible frustration.

How do pediatricians and pediatric diabetologists achieve a balance? Even before the results of the DCCT, most of us believed that very poor metabolic control is associated with a high risk of diabetic chronic complications. Thus, our aim should always be improvement in patients with glycosylated hemoglobins that are high. But how high? What we need is an accurately determined glycemic threshold below which patients are safe and which hopefully is not normoglycemia. We need some markers to determine which patients are at greater risk for the detrimental effects of hypoglycemia. We also need even longer studies than the DCCT in order to determine which subclinical abnormalities of the micro- and macrovasculature and nerves will develop into manifest complications with confirmation of the attendant risk factors that determine their cause.

In the meanwhile, dogmatic approaches to the treatment of IDDM in childhood and adolescence do not yet have a basis. Treatment has to be individualized, and in all patients we should try to achieve the best balance of risks and benefits, while trying to maintain blood glucose levels as close to normal as that individual is able to achieve without too many adverse effects.

39.9 ADDENDUM: RESULTS OF THE DIABETES CONTROL AND COMPLICATIONS TRIAL

The DCCT results were announced in June, 1993 and published three months later (DCCT Research Group, 1993). This study was terminated one year earlier than anticipated because the benefits of intensive diabetes therapy had become clear to the noninvestigator monitoring group. Final analyses showed that intensive therapy effectively delays the onset and slows the progression of diabetic retinopathy, nephropathy and neuropathy in all patients with IDDM irrespective of age, age of onset, gender and baseline glycosylated hemoglobin values. Despite the confirmation of transient deterioration of retinopathy with the initiation of intensive therapy, the risk of developing retinopathy in the primary cohort (those without retinopathy at baseline) was reduced by 76% compared with conventional therapy and the progression of retinopathy in the secondary cohort (those with mild baseline retinopathy) was slowed by 54%. The development of proliferative or severe nonproliferative retinopathy was reduced by 47%.

Thus, this study was large enough and long enough to show that despite the fact that normoglycemia and normal glycosylated hemoglobin could not be achieved in the majority of subjects, there was a clear beneficial effect of intensive diabetes therapy. Less than 5% of the patients in the intensive therapy group managed to maintain a glycosylated hemoglobin in the normal range throughout the study, although 44% of the patients achieved this goal at least once during the study. Unfortunately, an analysis of the relationship between mean glycosylated hemoglobin and the rate of development of retinopathy did not show a specific breakpoint below which retinopathy did not progress. Instead, there was a relatively linear relationship between glycosylated hemoglobin and progression of retinopathy. This relationship does have some degree of optimism in that even in the ranges of poor glycemic control, there is a benefit of sustained decrease in glycosylated hemoglobin. Thus, we should not give up even in those patients with the poorest glycemic control.

The benefits of intensive diabetes therapy were also evident when examining markers of nephropathy and neuropathy. Intensive therapy reduced microalbuminuria by 39% and overt nephropathy by 54%. Clinical neuropathy was decreased by 60% in the intensive therapy group. All these conclusions are very similar to those reported from the smaller Stockholm Diabetes Intervention Study, which was initiated in 1982 and reported about the same time (Reichard, 1993).

The DCCT included 195 adolescent patients between the ages of 13 and 18 years. Results were essentially the same as those of the total cohort, although the mean glycosylated hemoglobin values achieved throughout the study were higher than those for the adults and less than 2% were able to maintain the HbA_{1C} within the normal range. Although too few patients developed advanced retinopathy, nephropathy or clinical neuropathy to achieve statistically different results between intensive and conventional therapy, the differences in subclinical markers of retinopathy, nephropathy and neuropathy were very similar to those of the total cohort.

These DCCT results confirm the previous report of a significantly increased risk of severe hypoglycemia and any hypoglycemia in intensively treated patients. The three-fold increase of severe hypoglycemia, which was previously reported (DCCT Research Group, 1991) was similar in adults and adolescents. However, this adverse effect was not related to any important changes in neuropsychological function. There was an almost linear inverse relationship between the number of severe hypoglycemic episodes and glycosylated hemoglobin levels. In addition, there was a 33% increase in the risk of becoming overweight in the intensive therapy group compared to 9% in the conventional therapy group. This translated to a mean weight gain of 4.6 kg more in the intensive than conventional treatment group.

When assessing the risk:benefit ratio of intensive therapy, there was no clear glycemic level at which the benefits of intensive therapy were maximized with the least amount of hypoglycemia. Thus, glycemic targets will have to be individualized by all physicians for their individual patients. The overall conclusion has to be that intensive therapy is warranted and that improved glycemic control, as measured by glycosylated hemoglobin, can delay or prevent both subclinical and clinical microvascular complications of IDDM. This study did not include enough macrovascular events in order to make a similar conclusion. Results in the adolescent age group show that the benefits of intensive therapy appear to outweigh the long-term results of increased risk of hypoglycemia. Younger children may be more vulnerable to the effects of hypoglycemia, but it appears that efforts at improvement of glycemic control are warranted in children irrespective of their age, but with careful attention to the prevention of hypoglycemia. Probably, glycemic target levels will have to be raised compared to those of adolescents and adults.

REFERENCES

Abendroth, D., Landgraf, R., Illner, W.D. *et al.* (1989) Evidence for reversibility of diabetic microangiopathy following pancreas transplantation. *Transplant Proc.*, **21**, 2850–51.

Algan, M., Ziegler, O., Getin, P. *et al.* (1989) Visual evoked potentials in diabetic patients. *Diabetes Care*, **12**, 227–29.

Allen, C., Duck, S.C., Sufit, R.L. *et al.* (1992) Glycemic control and peripheral nerve conduction in children and young adults after 5–6 months of IDDM. *Diabetes Care*, **15**, 502–507.

American Diabetes Association. (1993a) Nutritional recommendations and principals for individuals with diabetes mellitus. Position Statement. *Diabetes Care*, **16** (suppl. 2), 22–29.

American Diabetes Association. (1993b) Standards of medical care for patients with diabetes mellitus. Position Statement. *Diabetes Care*, **16** (suppl. 2), 10–13.

Amiel, S.A., Tamborlane, W.V., DeFronzo, R.A. *et al.* (1987) Defective glucose counterregulation after strict glycaemic control of insulin dependent diabetes mellitus. *N. Eng. J. Med.*, **316**, 1376–83.

Andersen, A.R., Christiansen, J.S., Andersen, J.K. *et al.* (1983) Diabetic nephropathy in Type I (insulin dependent) diabetes: An epidemiologic study. *Diabetol.*, **25**, 496–501.

Barkai, L., Madacsy, L. and Kassay, L. (1990) Investigation of subclinical signs of autonomic neuropathy in the early stages of childhood diabetes. *Horm. Res.*, **34**, 54–59.

Becker, D.J., Coonrod, B.A., Ellis, D. *et al.* (1992) 'Influence of age, sex, blood pressure and glycemic control on microalbuminuria in children and adolescents with IDDM', in B. Weber, W. Burger and T. Danne (eds). *Structural and Functional Abnormalities in Subclinical Diabetic Angiopathy*, Vol. 22, pp. 95–107. Pediatr. Adolesc. Endocrinol. Basel, Karger.

Bilous, R.W., Mauer, S.M., Sutherland, D.E.R. *et al.* (1989) The effects of pancreas transplantation on the glomerular structure of renal allografts in patients with insulin-dependent diabetes. *N. Eng. J. Med.*, **321**, 8–85.

Borch-Johnsen, K., Andersen, P.K. and Deckert, T. (1985) The effect of proteinuria on relative mortality in Type I (insulin dependent) diabetes mellitus. *Diabetol.*, **28**, 590–96.

Brinchmann-Hansen, O., Dahl-Jorgensen, K., Sandvik, L. *et al.* (1992) Blood glucose concentrations and progression of diabetic retinopathy: The seven year results of the Oslo study. *Brit. Med. J.*, **304**, 19–22.

Brinchmann-Hansen, O., Dahl-Jorgensen, K., Hanssen, K.F. *et al.* (1988) The response of diabetic retinopathy to 41 months of multiple insulin injections, insulin pumps and conventional insulin therapy. *Arch. Ophthalmol.*, **106**, 1242–46.

Burger, W., Hovener, G., Dustertrus, R. *et al.* (1986) Prevalence and development of retinopathy in children and adolescents with Type I (insulin dependent) diabetes mellitus. A longitudinal study. *Diabetol.*, **29**, 17–22.

Chase, H.P., Jackson, W.E., Hoops, L. *et al.*, (1989) Glucose control and the renal and retinal complications of insulin-dependent diabetes. *J. Am. Med. Assoc.*, **261**, 1155–60.

Chase, H.P., Garg, S.K., Jackson, W.E. *et al.* (1990) Blood pressure and retinopathy in Type I diabetes. *Ophthalmol.*, **97**, 155–59.

Chase, H.P., Garg, S.K., Marshall, G. *et al.* (1991) Cigarette smoking increases the risk of albuminuria among subjects with Type I diabetes. *J. Am. Med. Assoc.*, **265**, 614–17.

Christlieb, A.R., Warram, J.H., Krolewski, A.S. *et al.* (1981) Hypertension: The major risk factor in juvenile-onset insulin-dependent diabetics. *Diabetes*, **30**, 90–96.

Cirillo, D., Gonfiantini, E., Grandis, D.D. *et al.* (1984) Visual evoked potentials in diabetic children and adolescents. *Diabetes Care*, **7**, 273–75.

Cook, J. and Daneman, D. (1990) Microalbuminuria in adolescents with insulin dependent diabetes mellitus. *Am. J. Dis. Child.*, **144**, 234–37.

Cook, J., Daneman, D., Spiro, M. *et al.* (1990) Angiotensin converting enzyme inhibitor therapy to decrease microalbuminuria in normotensive children with insulin-dependent diabetes mellitus. *J. Pediatr.*, **117**, 39–45.

Coonrod, B.A., Becker, D.J., Ellis, D. *et al.* (1991a) Unpublished data.

Coonrod, B., Orchard, T.J., Ellis, D. *et al.* (1991b) Lipids and glycemic control may be stronger risk factors than blood pressure for progression to microalbuminuria. Epidemiology of diabetes and its complications. *Proceedings of Satellite Symposium*, 14th IDF Williamsburg, **29**.

Coonrod, B., Ellis, D., Becker, D.J. *et al.* (1993) Predictors of microalbuminuria in individuals with insulin dependent diabetes mellitus. The Pittsburgh Epidemiology of Diabetes Complications Study. *Diabetes Care*, **16**, 1376–83.

Cruickshanks, K.J., Orchard, T.J. and Becker, D.J. (1985) The cardiovascular risk profile of adolescents with insulin dependent diabetes mellitus. *Diabetes Care*, **8**, 118–24.

D'Antonio, J.A., Ellis, D., Doft, B.H. *et al.* (1989) Diabetes complications and glycemic control. The Pittsburgh prospective insulin dependent diabetes cohort study. Status report after five years of IDDM. *Diabetes Care*, **12**, 694–700.

Dahl-Jorgensen, K. (1987) Near-normoglycemia and late diabetic complications: The Oslo study. *Acta. Endocrinol.*, **284** (Suppl.), 1–38.

Dahl-Jorgensen, K., Brinchmann-Hansen, O., Hanssen, K.F. *et al.* (1985) Rapid tightening of blood glucose control leads to transient deterioration of retinopathy in insulin-dependent diabetes mellitus. The Oslo Study. *Brit. Med. J.*, **290**, 811–14.

Dahl-Jorgensen, K., Hanssen, K.F., Kierul, F.P. *et al.* (1988) Reduction of urinary albumin excretion after four years of continuous subcutaneous insulin infusion in insulin dependent diabetes. *Acta. Endocrinol. (Copenh.)*, **117**, 19–25.

Dahlquist, G. and Rudberg, S. (1987) The prevalence of microalbuminuria in diabetic children and adolescents and its relation to puberty. *Acta Paed. Scand.*, **76**, 795–800.

Davies, A.G., Postlethwaite, R.J., Addison, G.M. *et al.* (1985) Renal function in diabetes mellitus. *Arch. Dis. Child.*, **60**, 299–304.

The DCCT Research Group. (1986) The Diabetes Control and Complications Trial (DCCT). Design and methodologic considerations for the feasibility phase. *Diabetes*, **35**, 530–45.

The DCCT Research Group. (1987) The Diabetes Control and Complications Trial (DCCT): Results of feasibility study. *Diabetes Care*, **10**, 1–19.

The DCCT Research Group. (1988a) Factors in the development of diabetic neuropathy. Baseline analysis of neuropathy in feasibility phase of Diabetes Control and Complications Trial (DCCT). *Diabetes*, **37**, 476–81.

The DCCT Research Group. (1988b) Weight gain associated with intensive therapy in the Diabetes Control and Complications Trial. *Diabetes Care*, **11**, 567–73.

The DCCT Research Group. (1991) Epidemiology of severe hypoglycemia in the Diabetes Control and Complications Trial. *Am. J. Med.*, **90**, 450–59.

The DCCT Research Group. (1993) The effect of intensive treatment of diabetes on the development and progression of long-term complications in insulin dependent diabetes mellitus. *N. Eng. J. Med.*, **329**, 977–86.

Diabetes Epidemiology Research International Mortality Study Group. (1991) Major cross-country differences in risk of dying for people with IDDM. *Diabetes Care*, **14**, 49–54.

Doft, B.H., Kingsley, L.A., Orchard, T.J. *et al.* (1984) The association between long-term diabetic control and early retinopathy. *Ophthalmology*, **91**, 1–7.

Dorchy, H., Noel, P., Kruger, M. *et al.* (1985) Peroneal motor nerve conduction velocity in diabetic children and adolescents. *Eur. J. Pediatr.*, **144**, 310–15.

Dorman, J.S., LaPorte, R.E. and Kuller, L.H. (1984) The Pittsburgh Insulin-dependent diabetes mellitus (IDDM) mortality study: Mortality results. *Diabetes*, **33**, 271–76.

Dorman, J.S., O'Leary, L., Kramer, M. *et al.* (1991) Concordance of microvascular complications among IDDM sib pairs. Epidemiology of Diabetes and its complications *Proceedings of Satellite Symposium*, 14th IDF Williamsbury, **25**.

Duck, S.C., Wei, F., Parke, J. *et al.* (1991) Role of height and glycosylated hemoglobin in abnormal nerve conduction in pediatric patients with Type I diabetes mellitus after 4–9 years of disease. *Diabetes Care*, **14**, 386–92.

Dunn, F.L., Pietri, A. and Raskin, P. (1981) Plasma lipid and lipoprotein levels with continuous subcutaneous insulin infusion in Type I diabetes mellitus. *Ann. Int. Med.*, **95**, 426–31.

Engerman, R., Bloodworth Jr., J.M. and Nelson, S. (1977) Relationship of microvascular disease in diabetes to metabolic control. *Diabetes*, **26**, 760.

Ewing, D.J. and Clarke, B.F. (1986) Diabetic autonomic neuropathy: present insights and future prospects. *Diabetes Care*, **9**, 648–65.

Feldt-Rasmussen, B., Mathiesen, E.R. and Deckert, T. (1986) Effect of two years of strict metabolic control on progression of incipient nephropathy in insulin-dependent diabetes. *Lancet*, **i**, 1300–1304.

Feldt-Rasmussen, B., Mathiesen, E.R., Jensen, T. *et al.* (1991) Effect of improved metabolic control on loss of kidney function in insulin-dependent diabetic patients. *Diabetol.*, **34**, 164–70.

Frank, R.N., Hoffman, W.H., Podgor, M.J. *et al.* (1982) Retinopathy in juvenile onset Type I diabetes of short duration. *Diabetes*, **31**, 874–82.

Friberg, T.R., Rosenstock, J., Sanborn, G. *et al.* (1985) The effect of long-term near normal glycemic control on mild diabetic retinopathy. *Ophthalmology*, **92**, 1051–58.

Friedman, N.E., Levitsky, L.L., Edidin, D.V. *et al.* (1980) Echocardiographic evidence for impaired myocardial performance in children with Type I diabetes mellitus. *Am. J. Med.*, **64**, 221.

Hanssen, K.F., Bangstad, H.J., Brinchman-Hansen, O. *et al.* (1992) Blood glucose control and diabetic microvascular complications: Long-term effects of near-normoglycemia. *Diabetic Med.*, **9**, 697–705.

Hanssen, K.F., Dahl-Jorgensen, K., Lauritzen, T. *et al.* (1986) Diabetic control and microvascular complications: The near-normoglycemic experience. *Diabetol.*, **29**, 677–84.

Hoffman, W.H., Hart, Z.H. and Frank, R.N. (1983) Correlates of delayed motor nerve conduction and retinopathy in juvenile-onset diabetes mellitus. *J. Pediatr.*, **102**, 351–56.

Holman, R.R., Dorman, T.L., Mayon-White, V. *et al.* (1983) Prevention of deterioration of renal and sensory-nerve function by more intensive management of insulin-dependent diabetic patients: A two year randomized prospective study. *Lancet*, **2**, 204–208.

Jakobsen, J., Christiansen, J.S., Kristoffersen, I. *et al.* (1988) Autonomic an somatosensory nerve function after two years of continuous subcutaneous insulin infusion in Type I diabetes. *Diabetes*, **37**, 452–55.

Jarrett, R.J. (1985) Risk factors of macrovascular disease in diabetes mellitus. *Hormone and Metabolic Research*, **15**, 1–3.

Jay, R.H., Jones, S.L., Hill, C.E. *et al.* (1991) Blood rheology and cardiovascular risk factors in Type I diabetes: Relationship with microalbuminuria. *Diabetic Med.*, **8**, 662–67.

Job, D., Eschwege, E., Guyot-Argentan, C. *et al.* (1976) Effect of multiple daily insulin injections on the course of diabetic retinopathy. *Diabetes*, **251**, 463–69.

Joner, G., Brinchmann-Hansen, O., Torres, C.G. *et al.* (1992) A nationwide cross-sectional study of retinopathy and microalbuminuria in young Norwegian Type I (insulin-dependent) diabetic patients. *Diabetol.*, **35**, 1049–54.

Jones, S.L., Close, C.F., Mattock, M.B. *et al.* (1989) Plasma lipid and coagulation factor concentrations in insulin dependent diabetics with microalbuminuria. *Brit. Med. J.*, **298**, 487–90.

Kaar, M.L., Saukkonen, A.L., Pitkaren, M. *et al.* (1983) Peripheral neuropathy in diabetic children and adolescents. A cross-sectional study. *Acta Paed. Scand.*, **72**, 373–78.

Kennedy, W.R., Navarro, X., Goetz, F.C. *et al.* (1990) Effects of pancreatic transplantation on diabetic neuropathy. *N. Eng. J. Med.*, **322**, 1031–37.

Klein, R., Klein, B.E.K. and Lintonk, L.P. (1992) Microalbuminuria in a population-based study of diabetes. *Arch. Intern. Med.*, **152**, 53–58.

Klein, R., Klein, B.E.K., Moss, S.E. *et al.* (1988) Glycosylated hemoglobin predicts the incidence and progression of diabetic retinopathy. *J. Am.*

Med. Assoc., **260**, 2864–71.

Klein, R., Klein, B.E.K. and Moss, S.E. (1989) The Wisconsin epidemiological study of diabetic retinopathy: A review. *Diab. Metab. Rev.*, **5**, 559–70.

Klein, R., Klein, B.E.K. and Moss, S.E. (1985) A population based study of diabetic retinopathy in insulin using patients diagnosed before 30 years of age. *Diabetes Care*, **8**, 71–76.

Koenig, R.J., Peterson, C.M., Jones, R.L. *et al.* (1976) Correlation of glucose regulation and hemoglobin $A1_c$ in diabetes mellitus. *N. Eng. J. Med.*, **295**, 417.

Kofoed-Enevoldson, A., Borch-Johnsen, K., Kreiner, S. *et al.* (1987) Declining incidence of persistent proteinuria in Type I (insulin dependent) diabetic patietns in Denmark. *Diabetes*, **36**, 205–209.

Kostraba, J.N., Dorman, J.S., Orchard, T.J. *et al.* (1989) Contribution of diabetes duration before puberty to development of microvascular complications in IDDM subjects. *Diabetes Care*, **12**, 686–93.

Kroc Collaborative Study Group. (1984) Blood glucose control and the evolution of diabetic retinopathy and albuminuria. *N. Eng. J. Med.*, **311**, 365–72.

Krolewski, A.S., Warram, J.H., Christlieb, A.R. *et al.* (1985) The changing natural history of nephropathy in Type I diabetes. *Am. J. Med.*, **78**, 785–94.

Krolewski, A.S., Warram, J.H., Cupples, A. *et al.* (1985) Hypertension, orthostatic hypotension and the microvascular complications of diabetes. *J. Chron. Dis.*, **38**, 319–26.

Krolewski, A.S., Wantam, J.H., Randl, I. *et al.* (1986) Risk of proliferative diabetic retinopathy in juvenile Type I diabetes: A 40 year follow up study. *Diabetes Care*, **9**, 443–52.

Krolewski, A.S., Kosurski, E.J., Warram, J.H. *et al.* (1987) Magnitude and determinants of coronary artery disease in juvenile onset insulin-dependent diabetes mellitus. *Am. J. Cardiol.*, **59**, 750–55.

Lababidi, Z.A. and Goldstein, D.E. (1983) High prevalence of echocardiographic abnormalities in diabetic youths. *Diabetes Care*, **6**, 18–22.

Landgraf, R., Landgraf-Leurs, M.M.C., Burg, D. *et al.* (1986) Long-term follow-up of segmental pancreas transplantation in Type I diabetics. *Transplant Proc.*, **18**, 1118–24.

Lauritzen, T., Frost-Larsen, K., Larsen, H.W. *et al.* (1985) The Steno Study Group. Two-year experience with continuous subcutaneous insulin infusion in relation to retinopathy and neuropathy. *Diabetes*, **34** (suppl. 3), 74–79.

Lauritzen, T., Frost-Larsen, K., Larsen, H.W. *et al.* (1983) Effect of one year of near normal blood glucose levels on retinopathy in insulin-dependent diabetics. *Lancet*, **i**, 200–203.

Lewitt, M. and Yue, D. (1988) Macrovascular and microvascular disease in diabetes: an overview. *World Book of Diabetes in Practice*, **3**, 278–82.

Lloyd, C.E., Klein, R., Maser, R.E. *et al.* (1993) The progression of retinopathy over two years: The Pittsburgh epidemiology of diabetes complications (EDC) study. *J. Diab. Comp.*, Submitted.

Lloyd, C. and Orchard, T.J. (1993) 'Insulin dependent diabetes mellitus in young people: Physical and psychosocial complications', in P. Home, S. Marshall, K.G.M.M. Alberti *et al.* (eds). *Diabetes Annual 7*, pp. 211–44. Elsevier, Netherlands.

Martini, A., Comacchio, F., Fedele, D. *et al.* (1987) Auditory brainstem evoked responses in the clinical evaluation and follow-up of insulin dependent diabetic subjects. *Acta Otolaryngol.* (Stockh), **103**, 620–27.

Maser, R.E., Steekiste, A.R., Dorman, J.S. *et al.* (1989) Epidemiological correlates of diabetic neuropathy. A report from Pittsburgh epidemiology of diabetes complications study. *Diabetes*, **38**, 1456–61.

Maser, R.E., Pfeifer, M.A., Dorman, J.S. *et al.* (1990) Diabetic autonomic neuropathy and cardiovascular risk. *Arch. Int. Med.*, **150**, 1218–1222.

Maser, R.E., Wolfson, S.K., Ellis, D. *et al.* (1991) Cardiovascular disease and arterial calcification in insulin dependent diabetes mellitus: interrelations and risk profiles. *Arteriosclerosis and Thrombosis*, **11**, 958–65.

Maser, R.E., Becker, D.J., Drash, A.L. *et al.* (1992) Pittsburgh Epidemiology of Diabetes Complications Study: Measuring diabetic neuropathy. Follow-up study results. *Diabetes Care*, **15**, 525–27.

Mathiesen, E.R., Oxenboll, B., Johansen, K. *et al.* (1984) Incipient nephropathy in Type I (insulin dependent) diabetes. *Diabetol.*, **26**, 406–10.

Mathiesen, E.R., Saurbrey, N., Hommel, E. *et al.*

(1986) Prevalence of microalbuminuria in children with Type I (insulin dependent) diabetes mellitus. *Diabetol.*, **29**, 640–63.

Mathiesen, E.R., Ronn, B., Jensen, T. *et al.* (1990) Relationship between blood pressure and urinary albumin excretion in development of microalbuminuria. *Diabetes*, **39**, 245–49.

McCance, D.R., Hadden, D.R., Atkinson, A.B. *et al.* (1989) Long-term glycaemic control and diabetic retinopathy. *Lancet*, **II**, 824–28.

Merimee, T.J. (1990) Diabetic retinopathy. A synthesis of perspectives. *N. Eng. J. Med.*, **322**, 978–83.

Miki, E., Fukuda, M., Kuzuya, T. *et al.* (1969) Relation of the course of retinopathy to control of diabetes, age and therapeutic agents in diabetic Japanese patients. *Diabetes*, **18**, 773.

Mogensen, C.E. and Christensen, C.K. (1984) Predicting diabetic nephropathy in insulin-dependent patients. *N. Eng. J. Med.*, **311**, 89–93.

Mortensen, H.B., Marinelli, K., Norgaard, K. *et al.* (1990) The Danish study group of diabetes in childhood. A nationwide cross-sectional study of urinary albumin excretion rate, arterial blood pressure and blood glucose control in Danish children with Type I diabetes mellitus. *Diabetic Med.*, **7**, 887–97.

Moy, C.S., Songer, T.J., LaPorte, R.E. *et al.* (1993) Insulin dependent diabetes mellitus physical activity and death. *Am. J. Epidemiol.*, **137**, 74–81.

Navarro, X., Kennedy, W.R. and Sutherland, D.E.R. (1991) Autonomic neuropathy and survival in diabetes mellitus: Effect of pancreas transplantation. *Diabetol.*, **34** (suppl. 1), 108–112.

Norgaard, K., Storm, B., Graae, M. *et al.* (1989) Elevated albumin excretion and retinal changes in children with Type I diabetes are related to long-term poor glucose control. *Diabetic Med.*, **6**, 325–28.

Nutrition Subcommittee of the British Diabetic Association's Professional Advisory Committee. (1992) Dietary recommendations for people with diabetes: An update for the 1990s. *Diabetic Med.*, **9**, 189–202.

O'Brien, I.A., McFadden, J.P. and Corral, R.J.M. (1991) The influence of autonomic neuropathy on mortality in insulin dependent diabetes. *Quart. J. Med.*, **79**, 495–502.

Orchard, T.J., Dorman, J.S., Maser, R.E. *et al.* (1990a) Factors associated with the avoidance of severe complications after 25 years of IDDM. Pittsburgh epidemiology of diabetes complications study I. *Diabetes Care*, **13**, 741–47.

Orchard, T.J., Dorman, J.S., Maser, R.E. *et al.* (1990b) Prevalence of complications in IDDM by sex and duration. Pittsburgh Epidemiology of Diabetes Complications Study II. *Diabetes*, **39**, 1116–24.

Panzram, G. (1984) Epidemiologic data on excess mortality and life expectancy in insulin dependent diabetes mellitus – critical review. *Exp. Clin. Endocrinol.*, **83**, 93–100.

Parving, H.H., Andersen, A.R., Smidt, U.M. *et al.* (1983) Diabetic nephropathy and arterial hypertension. *Diabetol.*, **24**, 10–12.

Pirart, J. (1978) Diabetes mellitus and its degenerative complications: A prospective study of 4400 patients observed between 1947 and 1973. *Diabetes Care*, **1**, 168–88.

Ramsay, R.C., Goetz, F.C., Sutherland, D.E.R. *et al.* (1988) Progression of diabetic retinopathy after pancreas transplantation for insulin-dependent diabetes mellitus. *N. Eng. J. Med.*, **318**, 208–14.

Rasch, R. (1979) Prevention of diabetic glomerulopathy in streptococcus diabetic rats by insulin treatment: The mesangial regions. *Diabetol.*, **17**, 243.

Raskin, P. (1978) Diabetic regulation and its relationship to microangiopathy. *Metab.*, **27**, 235.

Reichard, P., Berglund, B., Britz, A. *et al.* (1991) Intensified conventional insulin treatment retards the microvascular complications of insulin dependent diabetes mellitus (IDDM). The Stockholm Diabetes Intervention Study after five years. *J. Int. Med.*, **230**, 101–108.

Reichard, P., Nilsson, B.Y. and Rosenquist, U. (1993) The effect of long-term intensified insulin treatment on the development of microvascular complications of diabetes mellitus. *N. Eng. J. Med.*, **329**, 304–309.

Roe, T.F., Costin, G., Kaufman, F.R. *et al.* (1991) Blood glucose control and albuminuria in Type I diabetes mellitus. *J. Pediatr.*, **119**, 178–82.

Rosenstock, J., Strowig, S., Cercone, S. *et al.* (1987) Reduction in cardiovascular risk factors with intensive diabetes treatment in insulin-dependent diabetes mellitus. *Diabetes Care*, **10**, 729–34.

Rudberg, S., Apena, A., Freyschuss, U. *et al.* (1990)

Enalapril reduces microalbuminuria in young normotensive type I (insulin dependent) diabetic patients irrespective of its hypotensive effect. *Diabetol.*, **33**, 470–76.

Ryan, C.M., Atchison, J., Puczynski, S. *et al.* (1990) Mild hypoglycemia associated with deterioration of mental efficiency in children with insulin dependent diabetes mellitus. *J. Pediatr.*, **117**, 32–38.

Sampson, M.J., Wilson, S., Karagiannis, P. *et al.* (1990) Progression of diabetic autonomic neuropathy over a decade in insulin-dependent diabetics. *Quart. J. Med.*, **75**, 635–46.

Santiago, J.V., White, N.H., Skor, D.A. *et al.* (1984) Defective counterregulation limits intensive therapy of diabetes mellitus. *Am. J. Physiol.*, **247**, E215–20.

Seaquist, E.R., Goetz, F.C., Rich, S. *et al.* (1989) Familial clustering of diabetic kidney disease. Evidence for genetic susceptibility to diabetic nephropathy. *N. Eng. J. Med.*, **320**, 1161–65.

Simonson, D.C., Tamborlane, W.V., DeFronzo, R.A. *et al.* (1985) Intensive insulin therapy reduces counterregulatory response to hypoglycemia in patients with Type I diabetes. *Am. Int. Med.*, **103**, 184–90.

Sosenko, J.M., Boulton, A.J.M., Kubrusly, D.B. *et al.* (1985) The vibratory perception threshold in young diabetic patients: Associations with glycemia and puberty. *Diabetes Care*, **8**, 605–607.

Sosenko, J.M., Breslow, J.L., Miehinen, O.S. *et al.* (1980) Hyperglycemia and plasma lipid levels: A prospective study of young insulin-dependent diabetic patients. *N. Eng. J. Med.*, **302**, 650–54.

Strowig, S. and Raskin, P. (1992) Glycemic control and diabetic complications. *Diabetes Care*, **15**, 1126–40.

Teuscher, A., Schnell, H. and Wilson, P.W.F. (1988) Incidence of diabetic retinopathy and relationship to baseline plasma glucose and blood pressure. *Diabetes Care*, **11**, 246–51.

Tuttle, K.R., Bruton, J.L., Perusek, M.C. *et al.* (1991) Effect of strict glycemic control on renal hemodynamic response to amino acids and renal enlargement in insulin-dependent diabetes mellitus. *N. Eng. J. Med.*, **324**, 1626–32.

Viberti, G.C., Bilous, R.W., Mackintosh, D. *et al.* (1983) Long-term correction of hyperglycemia and progression of renal failure in insulin-dependent diabetes. *Brit. Med. J.*, **286**, 598–602.

Viberti, G.C., Jarrett, R.J., Matimud, U. *et al.* (1982) Microalbuminuria as a predictor of clinical nephropathy in insulin-dependent diabetes mellitus. *Lancet*, **i**, 1430–32.

Weber, B., Burger, W., Hartman, R. *et al.* (1986) Risk factors for the development of retinopathy in children and adolescents with Type I (insulin dependent) diabetes mellitus. *Diabetol.*, **29**, 23–29.

White, N.H., Saltman, S.R., Krupin, T. *et al.* (1981) Reversal of neuropathic and gastrointestinal complications related to diabetes mellitus in adolescents with improved metabolic control. *J. Pediatr.*, **99**, 41.

Wiseman, M., Saunders, A.J., Keen, H. *et al.* (1985) Effect of blood glucose control on increased glomerular filtration rate and kidney size in insulin dependent diabetes. *N. Eng. J. Med.*, **312**, 617–21.

Young, R.J., Ewing, D.J. and Clarke, B.F. (1983) Nerve function and metabolic control in teenage diabetics. *Diabetes*, **32**, 142–47.

Young, R.J., MacIntyre, C.C.A., Martyn, C.N. *et al.* (1986) Progression of subclinical polyneuropathy in young patients with Type I (insulin dependent) diabetes: associations with glycemic control and microangiopathy. *Diabetol.*, **29**, 56–61.

Ziegler, D., Moyer, P., Mühlen, H. *et al.* (1991) The natural history of somatosensory and autonomic nerve dysfunction in relation to glycaemic control during the first 5 years after diagnosis of Type I (insulin-dependent) diabetes mellitus. *Diabetol.*, **34**, 822–29.

40

Screening for complications in adolescence and beyond

B.F. CLARKE

40.1 INTRODUCTION

Diabetes mellitus is associated with a considerable morbidity from a variety of complications, which tend to worsen over time, and carries a significant premature mortality risk. Many of the complications have a prolonged subclinical asymptomatic phase and their natural history has become increasingly understood in recent years. Epidemiological studies have shown the value of screening for pre-symptomatic complications such as retinopathy (Klein *et al.*, 1984) and microalbuminuria (Mogensen, 1982). Diabetic complications therefore represent an ideal model for the application of screening procedures.

Screening in human disease should ideally include most of the following principles:

- the detection of a potentially serious condition with a recognizable pre-symptomatic phase in a population at risk.
- the means of detection should be relatively quick, easy to perform and acceptable to the patient, as well as being reasonably sensitive and specific.
- any treatment stemming from the earlier diagnosis should effectively modify the known natural history of the condition.
- the costs of detection and earlier treatment should be economically balanced against both the fiscal and human costs of the consequences of leaving the condition untreated.

It is generally not considered appropriate to introduce screening in childhood diabetes. With regard to adolescent diabetics and beyond, the ongoing care of the majority will usually continue within the context of the hospital diabetic clinic. The setting-up of clinic screening for complications requires a clearly identified program with definite aims and objectives, as well as a logistical strategy involving available resources. There should also be a clear policy for subsequent intervention and treatment objectives. General guidelines and targets for the standards of care of childhood and adolescent diabetics became recently established as part of the St Vincent Declaration action program (St Vincent Declaration, 1992) (see Appendix A). The recently published results of the Diabetes Control and Complications Trial (1993) have shown the benefits of intensive treatment of hyperglycemia with substantially less risk of the development and progression of diabetic retinopathy, microalbuminuria and abnormal nerve function.

Childhood and Adolescent Diabetes
Published in 1994 by Chapman & Hall, London
ISBN 0 412 48610 5

Screening for complications should be carried out at diagnosis, and then, having established a baseline, should be conveniently incorporated in the clinic annual review scheme. Any defaulter appearing at the clinic should be screened immediately. The collection and storage of data is best carried out by computerization to allow (a) processing and inclusion of other data such as glycemic control, (b) updated printouts on individual patients and (c) flagging of patients for annual screening.

What to screen for? The remainder of this chapter will provide an outline of the basis for screening and the practical techniques that are available for the following: hypertension, retinopathy, microalbuminuria, hyperlipidemia, neuropathy, and foot problems.

40.2 HYPERTENSION

Hypertension in diabetes is an important risk factor for cardiovascular disease (Christlieb *et al.*, 1981) and is associated with an increased incidence of retinopathy (Knowler *et al.*, 1980). In controlled studies, elevation of the blood pressure, although not of hypertensive proportions, occurs in childhood and adolescent diabetics (Moss, 1962; Young *et al.*, 1986). The prevalence of hypertension rises with the duration of Type 1 diabetes. In a multinational study of vascular disease in diabetes, 34% of patients aged 35–54 years qualified for the WHO designation of hypertension (Diabetes Drafting Group, 1985). Hypertension is closely associated with microalbuminuria (Wiseman *et al.*, 1984) and in Type 1 diabetes may be related to the development of clinical nephropathy (Christensen & Mogensen, 1985). In some individuals treatment of hypertension will be required by the late teens. There is evidence that such treatment has a beneficial effect on diabetic retinopathy (Teuscher *et al.*, 1988) and allows for the protection of renal function (Mogensen, 1982; Parving *et al.*, 1983). The importance of early detection of hypertension by regular and careful screening of all patients, irrespective of age, cannot therefore be over-emphasized.

The diagnosis of hypertension in adults is based on WHO criteria (World Health Organization Multinational Study, 1985). These define normal blood pressure, 'borderline' hypertension and hypertension (Table 40.1). The criteria may be inappropriately high for young Type 1 patients when blood pressure should be interpreted with respect to the normal for their age and sex (Drury & Tarn, 1985). In those with microalbuminuria, it has been recommended that blood pressure values should be kept below 135/85 which means that patients defined by the World Health Organization criteria as having borderline hypertension should be treated (Mogensen, 1988).

40.2.1 SCREENING

In most diabetic clinics blood pressure is measured with a conventional mercury sphyg-

Table 40.1 World Health Organization criteria for hypertension.

	Systolic pressure (mmHg)	Diastolic pressure (mmHg)
Normal blood pressure	<140	<90
'Borderline' hypertension	140–160	90–95
Hypertension	>160	>95

momanometer using, in those who are not overweight, a standard 12 cm cuff. The measurement is made after resting for at least 2 minutes in either the sitting or supine position. Postural hypotension occurs only in the presence of advanced diabetic autonomic neuropathy and in younger diabetics measurement in the erect posture is not required. The mean of two or three measurements of systolic and diastolic pressure to the nearest 2 mmHg should be obtained. The diastolic pressure should be recorded at the 5th Korotkov phase. Following the initial visit the blood pressure, if normal, should be checked at least annually but more frequently at each visit should retinopathy or microalbuminuria develop.

There is current interest in 24-hour ambulatory blood pressure monitoring using automated portable devices. In Type 1 diabetic patients with microalbuminuria, the mean blood pressure is higher than in controls with normal albumin excretion, both during the day and night but without significant alteration of the diurnal pattern. It has been suggested that ambulatory blood pressure reflects the association between urine albumin excretion and blood pressure more precisely than clinical measurements and may be preferable for identifying candidates for antihypertensive treatment (Hansen *et al.*, 1992).

40.3 RETINOPATHY

The natural history of diabetic retinopathy is well-known and its sight-threatening stages can be readily identified. The prevalence of retinopathy is highest in young-onset insulin treated patients, and steadily increases with duration of diabetes (Klein *et al.*, 1984). Murphy *et al.* (1990) reported the onset of retinopathy at puberty which correlated with the children's pubertal development. A fluorescein angiography study in children found no evidence of retinopathy under the age of 12 years and at least three years of diabetes had to elapse before the first features appeared. Retinopathic lesions could appear from puberty onwards with a mean age of occurrence at 16 years (Verougstraete *et al.*, 1991). A high rate of appearance of clinical retinopathy in the late teens was reported by Palmberg *et al.* (1981). In general, background retinopathy is unusual before five years duration of diabetes and proliferative retinopathy before ten years, even in teenage diabetics (Krolewski *et al.*, 1987).

The first aim of screening for diabetic retinopathy should be its detection at the very earliest stages when attention to glycemic control together with other possible risk factors (smoking, hypertension) may modify further progress. Thereafter the aim should be to detect the appearance of high risk retinopathy, which often occurs in patients who are still asymptomatic, and at a stage when it can be effectively treated by laser therapy.

Eye examination before the age of 12 years is thought to be unnecessary. In adolescent patients and thereafter the eyes are examined preferably at yearly intervals as part of the clinic annual review scheme. If retinopathy develops, the patient should be 'flagged' and examined more frequently as appropriate. In women planning pregnancy, the eyes should be examined at pre-conception, at confirmation of pregnancy and thereafter every three months.

40.3.1 SCREENING

40.3.1.1 Visual acuity

This is a simple test of central retinal function and measures distance visual acuity with the Snellen Chart and near vision with a standard reading test type card. Where appropriate, the patient's spectacles should be worn to obtain the best visual acuity. Poor distance visual acuity should be checked with a

Table 40.2 Screening for diabetic retinopathy. Recommended classification of data for each eye.

- Visual acuity
- No retinopathy
- Non-proliferative retinopathy not requiring referral
- Non-proliferative retinopathy requiring referral
- Macular involvement
- Pre-proliferative retinopathy
- Proliferative retinopathy
- Photocoagulated maculopathy
- Photocoagulated proliferative retinopathy
- Advanced diabetic eye disease
- Legal blindness
- Other eye disease (specify)

Reproduced from Retinopathy Working Party (1991) with permission from *Diabetic Medicine*.

pinhole device to detect whether the reduction is due to a refractive problem.

40.3.1.2 Ophthalmoscopy

Fundal examination should be carried out in a darkened room with the pupils dilated. The most commonly used short-acting mydriatic is tropicamide 0.5% or 1.0%, the weaker concentration being more suitable for children.

In the diabetic clinic the fundus is usually examined by direct ophthalmoscopy and this remains the recommended test to screen for diabetic retinopathy (Retinopathy Working Party, 1991). It is essential that this is undertaken by well-trained and experienced medical staff since it is not feasible for diabetic retinopathy screening to be carried out by ophthalmologists.

The Retinopathy Working Party (1991) in Europe have recommended a classification of the data collected on each eye in the course of screening (Table 40.2).

40.3.1.3 Retinal photography

Retinal photography, where available, is a useful adjunct to ophthalmoscopy. It provides a permanent objective record and is helpful for subsequent comparisons. As a screening tool, however, retinal photography may sometimes fail to detect serious retinopathy, because of technical and other problems (Bron & Cheng, 1986; Barrie & MacCuish, 1986).

Fundus photography may be undertaken by means of standard or non-mydriatic cameras. If using a 45° or 50° angle camera, photography of at least two fields is recommended: (1) the first field is centered on the macula to show the macular area, optic disc and temporal vascular arcades, (2) the second field is nasal to disc to show the optic disc and the nasal vascular arcades. Retinal cameras are operated by technical personnel and the photographs are assessed later by a specialist. Protocols for standardization in retinal photography have been recommended by the Retinopathy Working Party (1991).

40.4 MICROALBUMINURIA

The detection of microalbuminuria is well-established as the earliest clinical means of identifying diabetic renal disease (Viberti *et al.*, 1982). This stage, so-called 'incipient nephropathy', occurs when renal function is still normal (Mogensen *et al.*, 1983) and precedes the onset of positive proteinuria using Albustix(TM) (Ames, Stokes Poges), or other commercially available dipstix. Like retinopathy, microalbuminuria is rare in prepubertal children (Norgaard *et al.*, 1989) but may appear in adolescence (Cooke & Daneman, 1990). It usually does not occur until after five years' duration of diabetes (Nathan *et al.*, 1987).

Prospective studies have confirmed that microalbuminuria is highly predictive of subsequent proteinuria and overt nephropathy in Type 1 diabetes (Viberti *et al.*, 1982; Parving *et al.*, 1982; Mogensen & Christensen, 1984). Microalbuminuria also closely predicts the majority of early deaths in Type 1 diabetes not only from end-stage renal disease but also from cardiovascular causes (Jensen *et al.*, 1987; Gatling *et al.*, 1988a). It is clearly correlated with poor glycemic control (Norgaard *et al.*, 1989), with higher levels of blood pressure (Wiseman *et al.*, 1984) and the presence of retinopathy (Barnett *et al.*, 1985; Norgaard *et al.*, 1989) and in general can be regarded as a marker for microvascular disease.

40.4.1 DEFINITION AND MEASUREMENT

Microalbuminuria has been defined by consensus as a urinary albumin excretion rate (AER) of 30–300 mg/24 hours (or 20–200 μg/minute) in two out of three timed collections obtained over a six-month period (Mogensen, 1987). The latter proviso was made because of the considerable day-to-day variation in an individual patient having AER coefficients of variation of around 40% (Feldt-Rasmussen & Mathiesen, 1984). This variation depends particularly on physical activity, but also on posture and state of hydration. The AER derived from the 24-hour collection is regarded as the 'gold standard' against which other methods should be compared although a timed overnight collection may be equally reliable.

More simplified and practical screening tests have been developed which avoid the inconvenience of timed (24 hours, overnight or 2–3 hours) urine collections. The concentration of albumin (mg/l) in the early morning specimen, which is less subject to variation than occurs in later random samples, correlates reasonably well with the AER derived from 24-hour (Cowell *et al.*, 1986) and timed overnight (Hutchison *et al.*, 1988) urinary collections. An albumin concentration >20 mg/l in the early morning specimen has a sensitivity of 86–91% and a specificity of 74–97% of predicting an overnight AER of >30 μg/min (Gatling *et al.*, 1985; Marshall & Alberti, 1986).

The predictive value of early morning, and also to some extent random, specimens of urine, can be improved further by the simultaneous measurement of urinary creatinine, thereby correcting for the flow rate, with calculation of the albumin (mg/l) : creatinine (mmol/l) ratio (ACR). The ACR in early morning samples was shown to have a correlation coefficient of 0.91 with timed overnight AER (Gatling *et al.*, 1985). An early morning ACR of >3.5 mg/mmol has a sensitivity of 88–100% and a specificity of 95–99% of predicting a timed overnight AER of >30 μg/min (Gatling *et al.*, 1985 & 1988b). An early morning ACR of >10 mg/mmol will identify the majority of patients with an AER >100 mg/24 hours and at most risk of progressing to end-stage renal disease (Mathiesen *et al.*, 1984).

If no laboratory immunoassay is available then one of the commercially produced semi-quantitative side-room tests can be used for albumin concentration in an early morning specimen of urine. The recently introduced immunochemical Micral-Test™ strip (Boehringer Mannheim, UK) is specific for albumin and detects concentrations ⩾20 mg/l (Marshall & Shearing, 1991).

40.4.2 SCREENING

All patients over the age of 12 years who have had diabetes for five years or more should be screened for microalbuminuria. The measurement of ACR in an early morning urine sample brought to the clinic by the patient is probably the most reliable and simple screening test for microalbuminuria. If the patient fails to comply with the above a random urine sample for ACR can be obtained during the clinic visit.

Marshall (1991) has suggested a screening plan for microalbuminuria based on the known correlation of early morning ACR with 24-hour AER. Those patients having an initial ACR ≤3.5 mg/mmol should continue to be checked annually. Those with an ACR ≥10 mg/mmol should have a timed AER measurement to confirm the presence of microalbuminuria before appropriate treatment is begun. Of those with an ACR in the intermediate range 3.6–9.9 mg/mmol, probably almost half will have an AER >30 μg/min, and ACR should be re-checked every 3–6 months.

40.5 HYPERLIPIDEMIA

Macrovascular (atherosclerotic) complications, especially premature coronary artery disease, increase with the duration of Type 1 diabetes and carry a high morbidity and mortality. Along with hypertension and smoking, dyslipidemia is one of the three major risk factors for the development of atherosclerosis and it is generally accepted that early and frequent lipid screening in Type 1 diabetic patients is mandatory (American Diabetes Association, 1989).

Lipid risk factors for cardiovascular disease in the general population and probably also the diabetic population are (1) elevated total cholesterol, (2) elevated low density lipoprotein (LDL), (3) lowered high density lipoprotein (HDL)-cholesterol and (4) raised triglycerides. With regard to the latter, this is considered a high risk for coronary artery disease unless the total cholesterol to HDL-cholesterol ratio is less than 4.5 (Castelli, 1986). It should be emphasized that there are different mechanisms with different patterns of dyslipidemia in Type 1 and Type 2 diabetes. Hypertriglyceridemia in Type 2 diabetes results from a different defect in the triglyceride pathway with increased hepatic production of very low density lipoprotein (VLDL) and apoprotein B associated with a corresponding decreased HDL-cholesterol. This follows excessive calorie intake and hyperinsulinemia (Ginsberg, 1991) and may be independent of glycemic control.

A hyperlipidemic pattern is common at diagnosis in Type 1 diabetic patients, at all ages, with the finding of a raised triglycerides but usually normal HDL-cholesterol. The lipid profile should usually return to normal following improvement of glycemic control as confirmed by the glycated hemoglobin (HbA_1) and recent self-monitored blood glucose (SMBG) values. Raised triglyceride concentrations will invariably be found in Type 1 patients who have persistent poor glycemic control. This is consequent on reduced activity of the insulin-dependent enzyme lipoprotein lipase with decreased hydrolysis of triglyceride-rich lipoproteins and reduced clearance of VLDL. This in turn results in elevated circulating levels of highly atherogenic LDL precursors (Ginsberg, 1991).

Occasionally, and despite good glycemic control (HbA_1 and SMBG values) an elevated cholesterol without or with an elevated triglyceride may be found on screening in Type 1 diabetics. This may be due to the chance detection of an inherited disorder such as familial hypercholesterolemia (approximately 1 in 500 subjects) and familial combined hyperlipidemia (approximately 1 in 100–300 subjects).

Guidelines for intervention with diet and drugs have been recommended by the European Atherosclerosis Society Study Group (1988). There are, however, no reports, so far, of the effect of long-term intervention on morbidity and mortality from macrovascular complications in Type 1 diabetes.

40.5.1 SCREENING

The most widely recommended lipid profile for initial screening in Type 1 (and Type 2) diabetic patients comprises measurement of (1) total cholesterol, (2) HDL-cholesterol, (3) triglycerides in a random non-fasting specimen and (4) calculation of LDL cholesterol.

Table 40.3 Values for blood lipids.

	Concentration (mmol/liter)		
	Good	Acceptable	Poor
Total cholesterol	$\leqslant 5.2$	5.2–6.5	$\geqslant 6.5$
HDL-cholesterol	$\geqslant 1.1$	0.9–1.1	$\leqslant 0.9$
Fasting triglycerides	$\leqslant 1.7$	1.7–2.2	$\geqslant 2.2$

Reproduced from St Vincent Declaration (1992). Adopted from the European NIDDM Policy Group, International Diabetes Federation Brussels, 1989.

The latter which is one of the principal targets for therapy can be obtained from the Friedewald calculation (Friedewald *et al.*, 1972):

$$\text{LDL cholesterol (mmol/l)} = \text{total cholesterol} - \text{HDL cholesterol} - (\text{triglycerides}/2.2)$$

Recommended values for blood lipids are shown in Table 40.3.

Both total cholesterol and HDL-cholesterol remain relatively stable throughout the day and fasting has little effect on the values. Triglyceride concentrations, however, rise after meals and if elevated should be repeated after an overnight fast. Where an abnormal lipid profile is associated with poor glycemic control the measurements should be repeated following the establishment of improved control. Repeat lipid screening should be undertaken as part of the clinic annual review scheme.

40.6 NEUROPATHY

A diffuse polyneuropathy involving somatic (sensory and motor) and autonomic nerve fibers is a frequent complication of diabetes (Pirart, 1978; Clarke *et al.*, 1979). Diabetic polyneuropathy is fiber-length related and at first predominantly sensory, affecting small fibers. It is associated with different clinical syndromes especially painful neuropathy, which may be acute following metabolic upsets and often reversible, or chronic, when it is usually irreversible (Young *et al.*, 1986). A syndrome of painless neuropathy associated with recurrent foot ulcers may gradually develop.

Neuropathy in children became increasingly recognized following the report of Lawrence and Locke (1963) which described 13 children aged under 16 years with peripheral neuropathy, five of whom had painful features. Subclinical abnormalities of motor, sensory and autonomic nerve function are common in teenage Type 1 diabetic patients, even of short duration. Young *et al.* (1983) in a study of 79 teenage patients aged 16–19 years found abnormal electrophysiologic tests in 72% and abnormal tests of cardiovascular reflex function in 31%, these abnormalities correlating with poor glycemic control. Prospective studies for periods of up to five years in young diabetics have shown progression of subclinical polyneuropathy with deterioration of somatic and autonomic nerve function (Young *et al.*, 1986; Ziegler *et al.*, 1991).

The pathogenesis remains unclear but there is probably a variable combination of two major abnormalities. The first of these is diffuse metabolic changes in axons consequent on hyperglycemia with increased polyol pathway activity as proposed by Greene *et al.* (1987). This involves alterations of phosphoinositide metabolism and sodium-potassium ATPase activity with disturbance of normal nerve conduction and axonal transport mechanisms. The second hypothesis has proposed a widespread 'multifocal' loss of nerve fibers resulting from microvascular changes (Dyck *et al.*, 1986) with, especially, involvement of endoneurial capillaries (Britland *et al.*, 1990a).

Neurophysiologic studies, including electrophysiology which reflects large myelinated fiber function and autonomic nerve tests which reflects small unmyelinated fiber function, together with morphometric studies of sural nerves from selected groups of patients, have provided a clearer understanding of the clinical syndromes. In young diabetics there may be a predominantly small fiber neuropathy associated with painful neuropathy (Brown *et al.*, 1976) and abnormal cardiovascular reflex tests (Young *et al.*, 1986). The pain may be related to the ability of the damaged fibers to regenerate (Britland *et al.*, 1990b). In some patients there may be a gradual onset of a predominant large fiber neuropathy with the syndrome of painless polyneuropathy and recurrent foot ulceration (Young *et al.*, 1986; Tsigos *et al.*, 1992). These patients have severe large fiber, as well as small fiber losses probably with less effective nerve fiber regeneration (Britland *et al.*, 1990b). To determine whether these two neuropathic syndromes (small fiber loss, small plus large fiber loss) are distinct entities requires further prospective study (Tsigos *et al.*, 1992).

40.6.1 SCREENING

Clinical screening for diabetic neuropathy should be undertaken at diagnosis and then repeated annually. The most simple screening procedure of the peripheral nervous system should include:

1. The tendon reflexes in the lower limbs (knee and ankle jerks) using reinforcement when indicated. The results can be graded as present, diminished or absent.
2. Testing of sensory modalities: The modalities should include light touch perception by cotton wool, vibration perception using a low frequency 128 Hz tuning fork and proprioception by testing position sense of the first toe. These modalities reflect large nerve fiber function. Pain sensation by pinprick and temperature perception by metal tubes (ice, water at about 45°C) reflect small nerve fiber function. Sensory screening is confined to the lower limbs and testing should commence distally at the toes. The anatomical level in the feet or legs below which the sensory modality is impaired is recorded and can be scored.

This simple clinical assessment, although less objective and reproducible than obtained from more sophisticated methods, nevertheless provides useful information (Neuropathy Consensus Statement, 1988) and can help identify patients at risk of later developing symptomatic neuropathy and foot problems.

40.6.1.1 Measurement of cutaneous sensory thresholds

Some clinics are equipped with instruments for the specialized testing of cutaneous sensory thresholds. Although more reproducible than clinical assessment and allowing for quantification these methods are time-consuming and not suitable for screening purposes.

1. Vibration perception threshold: This is assessed by electromechanical instruments such as the Vibrameter™ (Somedic, Stockholm, Sweden) and the Biothesiometer™ (Bio-medical Instrument Company, Newbury, OH, USA). Their use has been fully described (Goldberg & Lindblom, 1979; Lowenthal & Hockaday, 1987; Masson & Boulton, 1990). As an alternative the Rydel-Seiffer graduated tuning fork (Firma Martin, Tuttingler, FRG) which allows scoring of vibration on an arbitrary 0–8 scale may be a suitable tool for neurological screening (Liniger *et al.*, 1990).
2. Thermal discrimination threshold: Devices such as the Marstock stimulator (Fruhstorfer *et al.*, 1976) and the Middlesex computer-assisted thermostimulator (Fowler *et al.*, 1987) provide standardized methods of detecting raised thermal

perception thresholds and reflect disturbance of small fiber function.

40.6.1.2 Autonomic nerve function tests

Tests based on cardiovascular autonomic reflexes are widely accepted for both the diagnosis and research assessment of diabetic autonomic neuropathy. A battery of five simple non-invasive tests has been recommended (Ewing *et al.*, 1985; Neuropathy Consensus Statement, 1988).

These tests comprise (a) the heart rate responses to the Valsava maneuver (Valsava ratio), standing up (30:15 ratio) and deep breathing (maximum-minimum heart rate) which reflect mainly parasympathetic function and (b) the blood pressure responses to standing up (systolic BP fall) and sustained handgrip (diastolic BP rise) which reflect mainly sympathetic function. A flow-plan for performing these tests is shown in Table 40.4. The minimum equipment needed are a sphygmomanometer, EKG machine, aneroid pressure gauge attached to a mouthpiece by a rigid or flexible tube and a handgrip dynamometer (Telephonics, Edinburgh, UK). Data can be handled either by a ruler and electrocardiogram strip or a computer program which measures R-R intervals and calculates the results. A package specifically designed for the tests is *Autocraft*™ (UnivEd Technologies Limited, Edinburgh, UK).

Each of the five tests has a range of normal, borderline and abnormal values (Table 40.5) and can be scored (Ewing & Clarke, 1982; Ewing *et al.*, 1985). The heart rate tests, reflecting parasympathetic function, indicate earlier nerve damage and are more useful in young diabetics (Young *et al.*, 1983; Ziegler *et al.*, 1992). Although simple and easily carried out in the clinic, these tests are still not widely used for screening purposes.

40.6.1.3 Electrophysiologic measurements

These require an electromyograph with measurement of motor and sensory nerve conduction velocities (MNCV, SNCV) and sensory nerve potential amplitude (SPA) as well as other measures. Nerve electrophysiology reflects the function of large myelinated axons which make up only about 25% of fibers in peripheral nerves.

Electrophysiologic testing is not practical in the clinic setting and unsuitable for screening.

Table 40.4 Flow-plan for performing cardiovascular autonomic function tests.

Test (in following order)	Position	Approximate time of test (min)	Apparatus required
Heart rate response to valsalva maneuver	Sitting	5	Aneroid manometer Electrocardiograph
Heart rate response to deep breathing	Sitting	2	Electrocardiograph
Blood pressure response to sustained handgrip	Sitting	5	Handgrip dynamometer Sphygmomanometer
Heart rate response to standing	Lying, then standing	3	Electrocardiograph
Blood pressure response to standing			Sphygmomanometer

Reproduced from Ewing and Clarke (1982) with permission from *British Medical Journal*.

Table 40.5 Values for cardiovascular autonomic function tests.

Test	Expressed as	Normal	Borderline	Abnormal
Heart rate (HR) tests:				
HR response to valsalva manoeuvre	Valsalva ratio	>1.21	1.11–1.20	⩽1.0
HR response to deep breathing	Maximum minus minimum HR (beats/minute)	⩾15	11–14	⩽10
HR response to standing up	30:15 ratio	⩾1.04	1.01–1.03	⩽1.0
Blood pressure tests:				
BP response to sustained handgrip	Rise in diastolic BP (mmHg)	⩾16	11–15	⩽10
BP response to standing up	Fall in systolic BP (mmHg)	⩽10	11–29	⩾30

Reproduced from Ewing *et al.* (1985) with permission from *Diabetes Care.*

Its use is for assessment of diagnostic problems such as isolated limb mononeuropathies and for research purposes.

40.7 FOOT PROBLEMS

Although a common cause of morbidity in adults, diabetic foot problems are not usually seen in young diabetic patients. However, minor foot deformities often have their beginnings in childhood and adolescence and may provide a source of future problems. Sensory neuropathy, an important risk factor, is undoubtedly developing imperceptibly and progressing during these earlier years (Young *et al.*, 1986; Ziegler *et al.*, 1992).

Regular screening of the feet especially with the aim of identifying risk factors is therefore highly important in young diabetic patients and management should concentrate on prevention. Advice should be given on smoking and education given on foot care and appropriate footwear. This should commence early despite the difficulty often encountered in motivating younger diabetic patients because of their perceived invulnerability at this age.

The success of screening and appropriate management depends very much on the inclusion of a podiatrist as a member of the diabetes care team (Chiropodial Care Report, 1990).

40.7.1 SCREENING

The screening of the feet in younger patients is preferably carried out by the clinic podiatrist in close collaboration with the clinician. Routine screening should be undertaken at diagnosis, and thereafter on an annual basis, with inclusion of the following:

1. footwear inspection
2. examination for early foot deformities
3. examination for nail problems (ingrowing nails, paronychia, etc.) and for fungal infection
4. palpation of pedal pulses (posterior tibial and dorsalis pedis)
5. screening for peripheral neuropathy (tendon jerks and sensory modalities).

40.8 CONCLUSION

Evidence has accrued that regular screening in young Type 1 diabetic patients may help identify those who are more liable to severe complications in future years. Several recent studies have suggested that improved quality of care initiated at an early stage, especially with regard to blood glucose control, treatment of hypertension, correction of dyslipidemia, skilled foot care and avoidance of smoking may modify the course of microvascular and macrovascular complications.

It is therefore essential that every diabetic clinic should develop a comprehensive screening program to detect complications while still at a subclinical phase together with a policy of appropriate intervention.

REFERENCES

American Diabetes Association. (1989) Consensus statement: role of cardiovascular risk factors in prevention and treatment of macrovascular disease in diabetes. *Diabetes Care*, **12**, 573–79.

Barnett, A.H., Dallinger, K., Jennings, P. *et al.* (1985) Microalbuminuria and diabetic retinopathy. *Lancet*, **i**, 53–54.

Barrie, T. and MacCuish, A.C. (1986) Assessment of non-mydriatic fundus photography in detection of diabetic retinopathy. *Brit. Med. J.*, **293**, 1304–1305.

Britland, S.T., Young, R.J., Sharma, A.K. *et al.* (1990a) Relationship of endoneurial capillary abnormalities to type and severity of diabetic polyneuropathy. *Diabetes*, **39**, 909–13.

Britland, S.T., Young, R.J., Sharma, A.K. *et al.* (1990b) Association of painful and painless diabetic polyneuropathy with different patterns of nerve fiber degeneration and regeneration. *Diabetes*, **39**, 898–908.

Bron, A.J. and Cheng, H. (1986) Cataract and retinopathy: screening for treatable retinopathy. *Clin. Endocrinol. Metab.*, **4**, 971–99.

Brown, M.J., Martin, J.R. and Asbury, A.K. (1976) Painful diabetic neuropathy, a morphometric study. *Arch. Neurol.*, **33**, 164–71.

Castelli, W.P. (1986) The triglyceride issue: a view from Framingham. *Amer. Heart J.*, **112**, 432–37.

Chiropodial Care Report. (1991) *Diabetes and Chiropodial Care*. Report on the findings by a joint working party of the British Diabetic Association and the Society of Chiropodists – 1990. *Brit. Diabetic Assoc.*, London.

Christensen, C.K. and Mogensen, C.E. (1985) Correlation between blood pressure and kidney function in insulin-dependent diabetics. *Diabetic Nephropathy*, **4**, 34–40.

Christlieb, A.R., Warram, J.H., Krolewski, A.S. *et al.* (1981) Hypertension: the major risk factor in juvenile-onset insulin-dependent diabetics. *Diabetes*, **30** (suppl. 2), 90–96.

Clarke, B.F., Ewing, D.J. and Campbell, I.W. (1979) Diabetic autonomic neuropathy. *Diabetologia*, **144**, 234–37.

Cook, J. and Daneman, D. (1990) Overnight versus 24 hour urine collections in detection of microalbuminuria. *Diabetes Care*, **13**, 813.

Cowell, C.T., Rogers, S. and Silink, M. (1986) First morning urinary albumin excretion in children with Type 1 (insulin-dependent) diabetes. *Diabetologia*, **29**, 97–99.

Diabetes Control and Complications Trial Research Group. (1993) The effect of intensive treatment of diabetes on the development and progression of long term complications in insulin-dependent diabetes mellitus. *N. Eng. J. Med.*, **3**, 977–86.

Diabetes Drafting Group. (1985) Prevalence of small and large vessel disease in diabetic patients from 14 centres. The World Health Organization Multinational Study of Vascular Disease in Diabetes. *Diabetologia*, **28**, 615–40.

Drury, P.L. and Tarn, A.C. (1985) Are the WHO criteria for hypertension appropriate in young insulin-dependent diabetics? *Diabetic Med.*, **2**, 79–82.

Dyck, P.J., Lais, A., Karnes, J.L. *et al.* (1986) Fiber loss is primary and multifocal in sural nerves in diabetic neuropathy. *Ann. Neurol.*, **19**, 425–39.

European Atherosclerosis Society Study Group (1988) The recognition and management of hyperlipidaemia in adults: a policy statement of the European Atherosclerosis Society. *Eur. Heart J.*, **9**, 571–600.

Ewing, D.J. and Clarke, B.F. (1982) Diagnosis and management of diabetic autonomic neuropathy. *Brit. Med. J.*, **285**, 916–18.

Ewing, D.J., Martyn, C.N., Young, R.J. *et al.* (1985)

The value of cardiovascular autonomic function tests, 10 years experience in diabetes. *Diabetes Care*, **8**, 491–98.

Feldt-Rasmussen, B.F. and Mathiesen, E.R. (1984) Variability of urinary albumin excretion in incipient diabetic retinopathy. *Diabetic Nephropathy*, **3**, 101–103.

Fowler, C.J., Carroll, M.B., Burns, D. *et al.* (1987) A portable system for measuring cutaneous thresholds for warming and cooling. *J. Neur., Neurosurg. Psychiat.*, **50**, 1211–15.

Friedewald, W.T., Levy, R.I. and Frederickson, D.S. (1972) Estimation of the concentration of low density lipoprotein cholesterol in plasma without use of the preparative ultracentrifuge. *Clin. Chem.*, **18**, 499–502.

Fruhstorfer, H., Lindblom, U. and Schmidt, W.G. (1976) Method for quantitative estimation of thermal thresholds in patients. *J. Neurol., Neurosurg. Psychiat.*, **39**, 1071–75.

Gatling, W., Knight, C. and Hill, R.D. (1985) Screening for early diabetic nephropathy: which sample to detect microalbuminuria? *Diabetic Med.*, **2**, 451–55.

Gatling, W., Mullee, M.A., Knight, C. *et al.* (1988a) Microalbuminuria in diabetes. Relationship between urinary albumin excretion and diabetes related variables. *Diabetic Med.*, **5**, 348–51.

Gatling, W., Knight, C., Mullee, M.A. *et al.* (1988b) Microalbuminuria in diabetes: a population study of the prevalence and assessment of three screening tests. *Diabetic Med.*, **5**, 343–47.

Ginsberg, H.N. (1991) Lipoprotein physiology in nondiabetic and diabetic states: relationship to atherosclerosis. *Diabetes Care*, **14**, 839–55.

Goldberg, J.M. and Lindblom, U. (1979) Standardised method of determining vibratory perception threshold for diagnosis and screening in neurological investigation. *J. Neurol., Neurosurg. Psychiat.*, **42**, 793–803.

Greene, D.A., Lattimer, S.A. and Sima, A.F.F. (1987) Sorbitol, phosphoinositides and sodium-potassium-ATPase in the pathogenesis of diabetic complications. *N. Eng. J. Med.*, **316**, 599–606.

Hansen, K.W., Christensen, C.K., Andersen, P.H. *et al.* (1992) Ambulatory blood pressure in microalbuminuric type 1 diabetic patients. *Kidney International*, **41**, 847–54.

Hutchison, A.S., O'Reilly, D.S. and MacCuish, A.C. (1988) Albumin excretion rate, albumin concentrations and albumin/creatinine ratio compared for screening diabetics for slight albuminuria. *Clin. Chem.*, **34**, 2019–21.

Jensen, J., Borch-Johnsen, K., Kofoed-Enevoldsen, A. *et al.* (1987) Coronary heart disease in young Type 1 (insulin-dependent) diabetic patients with and without diabetic nephropathy: incidence and risk factors. *Diabetologia*, **30**, 144–48.

Klein, R., Klein, B.E.K., Moss, S.E. *et al.* (1984) The Wisconsin epidemiological study of diabetic retinopathy. II. Prevalence and risk of diabetic retinopathy when age at diagnosis is less than 30 years. *Arch. Ophthalmol.*, **102**, 520–26.

Knowler, W.C., Bennett, P.H. and Ballantine, G.J. (1980) Increased incidence of retinopathy in diabetics with elevated blood pressure. *N. Eng. J. Med.*, **302**, 645–50.

Krolewski, A.S., Warram, J.H., Rand, L.I. *et al.* (1987) Epidemiologic approach to the etiology of Type 1 diabetes mellitus and its complications. *N. Eng. J. Med.*, **137**, 1390–98.

Lawrence, D.G. and Locke, S. (1963) Neuropathy in children with diabetes mellitus. *Brit. Med. J.*, **i**, 784–86.

Liniger, C., Albeanu, A., Bloise, D. *et al.* (1990) The tuning fork revisited. *Diabetic Med.*, **7**, 859–64.

Lowenthal, L.M. and Hockaday, T.D.R. (1987) Vibration sensory thresholds depend on pressure applied stimulus. *Diabetes Care*, **10**, 100–104.

Marshall, S.M. (1991) Screening for microalbuminuria: which measurement. *Diabetic Med.*, **8**, 706–711.

Marshall, S.M. and Alberti, K.G.M.M. (1986) Screening for early diabetic nephropathy. *Ann. Clin. Biochem.*, **23**, 195–97.

Marshall, S.M. and Shearing, P.A. (1991) Assessment of Micral-Test strips as a screening tool for microalbuminuria. *Diabetic Med.*, **8** (suppl. 1), 111.

Masson, E.A. and Boulton, A.J.M. (1990) Calibration problems with the biosthesiometer. *Diabetic Med.*, **7**, 261–62.

Mathiesen, E.R., Oxenboll, B., Johansen, K. *et al.* (1984) Incipient nephropathy in Type 1 (insulin-dependent) diabetes. *Diabetologia*, **26**, 406–410.

Mogensen, C.E. (1982) Long-term antihypertensive therapy inhibiting progression of diabetic nephropathy. *Brit. Med. J.*, **285**, 685–88.

Mogensen, C.E. (1987) Microalbuminuria as a predictor of clinical diabetic nephropathy. *Kidney International*, **31**, 673–89.

Mogensen, C.E. (1988) Management of diabetic renal involvement and disease. *Lancet*, **i**, 867–70.

Mogensen, C.E., Christensen, C.K. and Vittinghus, E. (1983) The stages in diabetic renal disease. With emphasis on the stage of incipient diabetic nephropathy. *Diabetes*, **32** (suppl. 2), 64–78.

Mogensen, C.E. and Christensen, C.K. (1984) Predicting diabetic nephropathy in insulin-dependent patients. *N. Eng. J. Med.*, **311**, 89–93.

Moss, A.J. (1962) Blood pressure in children with diabetes mellitus. *Paediatrics*, **30**, 932–36.

Murphy, R.P., Nanda, M., Plotnick, L. *et al.* (1990) the relationship of puberty to diabetic retinopathy. *Arch. Ophthalmol.*, **108**, 215–18.

Nathan, D.M., Rosenbaum, C. and Prostasowicki, V.D. (1987) Single void urine samples can be used to estimate quantitative microalbuminuria. *Diabetes Care*, **10**, 414–18.

Neuropathy Consensus Statement. (1988) Report and recommendations of the San Antonio conference on diabetic neuropathy. *Diabetes*, **37**, 1000–1004.

Norgaard, K., Storm, B., Graae, M. *et al.* (1989) Elevated albumin excretion and retinal changes in children with Type 1 diabetes are related to long term poor blood glucose control. *Diabetic Med.*, **6**, 325–28.

Palmberg, P., Smith, M., Waltman, S. *et al.* (1981) The natural history of retinopathy in insulin dependent juvenile-onset diabetes. *Ophthalmology*, **88**, 613–18.

Parving, H-H., Oxenball, B., Svendsen, P.A. *et al.* (1982) Early detection of patients at risk of developing diabetic nephropathy. A longitudinal study of urinary albumin excretion. *Acta Endocrinologica (Copenh.)*, **100**, 550–55.

Parving, H-H., Anderson, A.R., Smidt, U. *et al.* (1983) Early aggressive antihypertensive treatment reduces rate of decline in kidney function in diabetic nephropathy. *Lancet*, **i**, 1175–79.

Pirart, J. (1978) Diabetic mellitus and its degenerative complications: a prospective study of 4000 patients observed between 1947 and 1973. *Diabetes Care*, **1**, 168–88.

Retinopathy Working Party (1991) A protocol for screening for diabetic retinopathy in Europe. *Diabetic Med.*, **8**, 263–67.

St Vincent Declaration (1992) *Diabetes Care and Research in Europe: the St Vincent Declaration action programme*, in H.M.J. Krans, M. Porta and H. Keen (eds). WHO Regional Office for Europe, Copenhagen.

Teuscher, A., Schnell, H. and Wilson, P.W.F. (1988) Incidence of diabetic retinopathy and relationship to baseline plasma glucose and blood pressure. *Diabetes Care*, **11**, 246–51.

Tsigos, C., White, A. and Young, R.J. (1992) Discrimination between painful and painless diabetic neuropathy based on testing large somatic nerve and sympathetic nerve function. *Diabetic Med.*, **9**, 359–65.

Verougstraete, C., Toussaint, D., De Schepper, J. *et al.* (1991) First microangiopathic abnormalities in childhood diabetes-types of lesion. *Graefe's Arch. Clin. Experi. Ophthalmol.*, **229**, 24–32.

Viberti, G.C., Jarrett, R.J., Mahmud, U. *et al.* (1982) Microalbuminuria as a predictor of clinical nephropathy in insulin-dependent diabetes mellitus. *Lancet*, **i**, 1430–32.

Wiseman, M., Viberti, G.C., Mackintosh, D. *et al.* (1984) Glycaemia, arterial pressure and microalbuminuria in Type 1 (insulin dependent) diabetes. *Diabetologia*, **26**, 401–405.

World Health Organization Multinational Study (1985) Prevalence of small vessel and large vessel disease in diabetic patients from 14 centres. *Diabetologia*, **28** (Suppl.), 615–40.

Young, R.J., Ewing, D.J. and Clarke, B.F. (1983) Nerve function and metabolic control in teenage diabetics. *Diabetes*, **32**, 142–47.

Young, R.J., Macintyre, C.C.A., Martyn, C.N. *et al.* (1986) Progression of subclinical polyneuropathy in young patients with Type 1 (insulin-dependent) diabetes: associations with glycaemic control and microangiopathy (microvascular complications). *Diabetologia*, **29**, 156–61.

Ziegler, D., Mayer, P., Mühlen, H. *et al.* (1991) The natural history of somatosensory and autonomic nerve dysfunction in relation to glycaemic control during the first 5 years after diagnosis of Type 1 (insulin-dependent) diabetes mellitus. *Diabetologia*, **34**, 822–29.

41

Prevention of complications

R.J. YOUNG

41.1 INTRODUCTION

If one allows that the 'complications of diabetes' embrace all of the acute metabolic disturbances and psychosocial responses which may accompany diabetes, as well its physical or 'structural' consequences, then prevention of complications may subsume the whole of diabetes management. In this chapter, however, we will address only those 'complications' which may lead to long-term morbidity and, in some cases, by extension of the same pathological process, early mortality.

For health professionals, just as much as children, young people and their parents, such diabetes 'endpoints' or 'outcomes' often seem somewhat remote, and hence irrelevant, to more immediate matters. This is understandable. It is difficult to address logically and with appropriate weight the unseen and the unknown; fortunately photocoagulation, blindness, pain, foot ulceration, amputation, chronic ambulatory peritoneal dialysis (CAPD), renal transplantation, cardiac failure, myocardial infarction, stroke, and death virtually never intrude on pediatric or adolescent clinics. As a result, attitudes and fears have tended to veer from the inappropriately dismissive (denial?) to the over-reactive histrionic. Furthermore, until quite recently there has been little clear evidence to suggest that the approach to treatment in early life has any major long-term sequelae. It has to be said that in many respects direct evidence, from studies in childhood through to adult life, is still lacking. But there is now a small amount of sound natural historical evidence, an improving understanding of those aspects of care organization which influence long-term outcomes, and a recent explosion of knowledge in adults which can, if interpreted with caution, be extrapolated to children and adolescents.

This discussion, therefore, will try to present a reasoned case for certain practical, achievable and justifiable measures which, in the light of current knowledge seem certain to be associated with complications prevention, focusing particularly on those consequences which may become manifest before the age of 40. Where appropriate, probable future directions will also be mentioned.

41.2 PRIMARY VS. SECONDARY PREVENTION

A distinction must be made between primary and secondary prevention. Primary prevention relates to those aspects of treatment which may, in the context of living with

Childhood and Adolescent Diabetes
Published in 1994 by Chapman & Hall, London
ISBN 0 412 48610 5

rather than curing diabetes, stop or delay the onset of a complication. Secondary prevention, on the other hand, refers to interventions which impede or halt the development of already established complications.

Though primary prevention is the ideal, current evidence and the practical realities of present-day treatment strategies would suggest that secondary prevention, which can prevent or attenuate much of the most serious morbidity, will retain an important role in diabetes treatment programs for some time to come.

41.3 RETINOPATHY

41.3.1 NATURAL HISTORICAL CONSIDERATIONS

Long-term follow-up studies have shown fundoscopically detectable diabetic retinopathy to be a virtually invariable accompaniment of conventionally managed childhood-onset IDDM. However, although retinopathy is the hallmark of the diabetes specific microvascular complications (indeed so much so that it was chosen as the threshold abnormality for the 1978 WHO definition of diabetes, and as the primary endpoint for the landmark Diabetes Control and Complications Trial (DCCT, 1993)), retinopathy *per se* is not a cause of serious morbidity. This is because although, pathologically, diabetic retinopathy is a continuum, there is a fundamental difference between minimal ('background' or 'non-visually threatening') and more advanced (maculopathy and proliferative) retinopathy in respect of their clinical implications. The former does not threaten vision and may remain stable and harmless indefinitely. The latter, which is always preceded by the former, can cause blindness. Proliferative retinopathy causes blindness through non-clearing vitreous hemorrhage or by inducing pre-retinal fibrosis and retinal detachment and is by far the commonest form of visually-threatening retinopathy in young people.

The earliest detection of retinopathy depends on the sensitivity of the technique being used. DCCT and other studies have shown that a few microaneurysms or dot hemorrhages may manifest within a year or two of the clinical onset of IDDM in a small minority of subjects (<10% of conventionally treated) but visually threatening retinopathy is almost exclusively associated with diabetes duration >10 years. Whether the prepubertal period 'counts' or whether the risk attaches only to the duration of diabetes after puberty is still uncertain but, unquestionably, visually threatening retinopathy is a post-pubertal phenomenon even in those very rare individuals with early onset retinopathy.

In historical series, proliferative retinopathy has been documented in 60–70% of childhood-onset IDDM after 20 years duration, with a lifetime risk of blindness/visual impairment of up to 50%. Many of these studies have shown, with increasing degrees of sophistication, an association between poor glycemic control and the risks both of the onset and the progression of retinopathy. Now that DCCT (1993), the Oslo study (Brinchmann-Hanson *et al.*, 1988) and others have reported there can be no doubt that, in post-pubertal young patients, interventions which improve glycemic control reduce both of these risks. Although in adults with both IDDM and NIDDM, hypertension is associated with progression of retinopathy, this is uncommon in young people and intervention data at all ages are lacking.

41.3.2 PRIMARY PREVENTION

Preventing the onset of retinopathy must be the ultimate goal but it is probably outwith our grasp at present. DCCT (1993) has shown that, in patients with duration of diabetes less than five years, improving glycemic control as reflected in HBA_{1C}, from 2.5% ('conventionally' treated) to 1.0% ('intensively' treated) above the upper limit of the reference range, markedly reduces the incidence of the very earliest manifestations of retinopathy, but it does not abolish them: after nine years of study the prevalence of retinopathy in the 'conventional' group was >50% compared with 10% in the 'intensive' group; no one in either group developed visually threatening retinopathy during the study. The suspicion remains, therefore, that glycemia may need to be restored to normal if retinopathy is to be prevented completely.

DCCT (1993) also shows us, however, that such a goal is unrealistic and, with current modes of treatment, undesirable, because of the inverse relationship between average blood glucose and the frequency of severe hypoglycemia. Nevertheless, if non-visually threatening retinopathy was the only consequence of 'good' glycemic control there would be no serious detriment to the health of young people with IDDM. Reducing the incidence of visual loss to zero is, arguably, the more important and certainly the more immediate prize.

It is at present unknown how the recent knowledge about the role of glycemia in complications development should be applied to prepubertal children. As indicated above it is not clear whether there is true prepubertal 'protection', or whether sex steroids simply play a permissive role in allowing underlying damage to become manifest. It would seem sensible to 'optimize' glycemic control at all ages but bearing in mind that the long-term neurological cost of severe hypoglycemia is probably much greater in the developing than in the mature brain (Chapter 25).

41.3.3 SECONDARY PREVENTION

41.3.3.1 Glycemic control

Once again DCCT (1993) provides the critical evidence. For about a decade the rather gloomy view had prevailed that once early retinopathy was established, further progression was inexorable irrespective of the metabolic milieu. This was founded on studies (Engerman & Kern, 1987) in diabetic dogs which had suggested a role for improved glycemia in primary but not secondary prevention, and on natural history observations (Krowlewski *et al.*, 1986) which implied a constant rate of progression from 'background' to proliferative retinopathy irrespective of the duration of diabetes albeit with some influence from prevailing glycemia. Now it is clear that better glycemia is associated with a reduced rate of progression of established non-proliferative retinopathy.

As in previous studies, patients in the DCCT 'intensive' group showed a slight initial deterioration in the grade of their retinopathy, but after two years the 'conventional' group had caught up and after nine years, at the end of the study, 50% had deteriorated among the latter as against 20% among the former. Furthermore, laser treatment was needed for visually threatening retinopathy in 2.3/100 patient-years of the 'conventional' group as compared with 0.9/100 patient-years of the 'intensive' group. This accords with clinical experience since glycosylated hemoglobin measurements made assessment of glycemia reliable.

The message is clear. It is never too late to anticipate benefits from improved glycemic control.

41.3.3.2 Screening and retinal photocoagulation

A strategy for diabetic retinopathy screening must be predicated on the knowledge that timely photocoagulation can prevent virtually all visual loss in those patients who have progressed to the stage of visually threatening retinopathy. The evidence is particularly clear in respect of proliferative disease, the most common form of severe retinopathy in young patients. Thus secondary prevention of diabetic retinopathy must encompass a system which detects reliably all eyes which have reached any of the Early Treatment Diabetic Retinopathy Study (ETDRS) thresholds and ensures that appropriate laser treatment is given.

Current knowledge would suggest, therefore, that a combination of good glycemic control, secure screening and laser photocoagulation could prevent virtually all blindness and/or visual impairment in young patients with IDDM. When to start screening is perhaps the only contentious issue. In my opinion, a reasonable approach in childhood is to examine the fundi shortly after diagnosis, to pick up the very rare occurrence of early-onset retinopathy, and then to examine the eyes annually from puberty onwards.

41.3.3.3 Other interventions?

At this time there is no evidence that non-glycemic treatments or alternatives to photocoagulation have anything to contribute to the primary or secondary prevention of diabetic retinopathy. Trials of aldose reductase inhibitors and aspirin have not demonstrated any benefit (Frank, 1994). These studies presupposed an understanding of the pathogenesis and a pharmacological mechanism for inhibiting a critical pathogenetic step. Whether lack of pathological knowledge or pharmacological ineffectiveness were responsible for the lack of success is uncertain.

41.4 CATARACT

Cataract is uncommon in young patients. A very small number develop the diabetes-specific acute 'snowflake' cataract usually within a year or two of diagnosis. These can be troublesome to treat and there is no known method of prevention though there is an anecdotal impression that prolonged prediagnosis hyperglycemia may be a factor.

Cataracts later in life probably represent acceleration of an underlying genetic or acquired susceptibility. The role of glycemia has not been elucidated.

41.5 NEUROPATHY

41.5.1 TYPES OF NEUROPATHY AND NATURAL HISTORY

The clinical and subclinical manifestations of diabetic neuropathy are protean. Important differences must be recognized between mononeuropathies and polyneuropathy, and between acute and chronic polyneuropathies. Non-pressure mononeuropathies probably have an occlusive vascular etiology; they are very uncommon below the age of 40 and there are no clear-cut risk factors. Pressure-related mononeuropathies, e.g., carpal tunnel syndrome, are most likely due to a combination of soft tissue damage and increased susceptibility from underlying asymptomatic polyneuropathy. Acute polyneuropathy is generally related to a well-defined acute metabolic disturbance (e.g., diabetic ketoacidosis (DKA), severe anorexia or bulimia); although the severe (sometimes extremely severe) neuropathic pain and/or motor weakness usually remits, permanent nerve damage may ensue. Chronic polyneuropathy is, ultimately, by far the most common clinical problem: asymptomatic neuropathy with severe sensory deficits may lead to neuropathic ulceration or osteopathy, secondary infection, gangrene and amputation; painful neuropathic symptoms may cause severe discomfort. Clinical chronic polyneuropathy has affected up to 25% of young postpubertal IDDM cohorts and historic series have reported amputation rates of >10%. Duration of diabetes and poor glycemic control have been identified as important risk factors; in those who develop severe neuropathic deficits pre-existing functional foot abnormalities and poor foot care/hygiene often contribute to the severity of the clinical problem (Young, 1987).

As with retinopathy, clinical neuropathy before puberty is very rare. Although clinical expressions become more prevalent in the third decade (and towards the end of the second) they are less frequent at this age than visually threatening retinopathy. Nonetheless, subclinical nerve dysfunction can be found in most (50–70%), its severity probably predicts subsequent clinical problems and it too is clearly related to average glycemic control.

41.5.2 PRIMARY PREVENTION

It has been known for many years that nerve dysfunction is common at the clinical presentation of IDDM and that some improvement follows during the first few months of treatment. Subsequent evidence has shown that further decline in nerve function and the early manifestations of clinical neuropathy are also associated with poor glycemic control. Now, in its primary prevention arm, DCCT (1993) has demonstrated a 69% reduction in the appearance of neuropathy in the 'intensive' as compared to the 'conventional' group. Significantly, however, in the 'intensive' group where HBA_{1C} was only on average 1% above the reference range, 3% of those with no neuropathy at baseline had developed evidence of neuropathy after five years. (It was 10% in the 'conventional' group where HBA_{1C} was 2.5% above the reference range.)

As for retinopathy, complete primary prevention of chronic polyneuropathy may require metabolic normalization. Similarly, also, if the only manifestations of neuropathy were a few asymptomatic mild nerve deficits this would be clinically trivial but we know much less about the stability of this degree of neuropathy than for background retinopathy. Primary prevention of the acute polyneuropathies of course depends on all those practical, educational and organizational measures which can be effected to minimize the occurrence of DKA, etc.

41.5.3 SECONDARY PREVENTION

41.5.3.1 Glycemic control

DCCT (1993) also found a similar benefit in preventing the appearance of clinical neuropathy in their 'secondary intervention' cohort. It must be remembered, however, that patients were assigned to these groups on the basis of their retinopathy status not their neuropathy status. What is not known at present is whether improving glycemic control modifies the progression of established neuropathy. Anecdotal clinical experience suggests that it does, at least in the case of chronic polyneuropathy but acute polyneuropathies have been observed to continue to improve after a secondary deterioration in glycemia. This sort of behavior, the apparently different susceptibilities of individuals at equivalent levels of glycemia and, perhaps, the much less satisfactory secondary prevention measures available for chronic polyneuropathy (as compared to laser photocoagulation for retinopathy) have driven a very wide-ranging search for non-glycemic interventions.

41.5.3.2 Non-glycemic interventions

Controversy has raged for more than 20 years between those favoring a 'vascular' versus those favoring a 'metabolic' etiology for diabetic polyneuropathy. Recently, both animal and clinical experimental work has inclined to reconciliation of the erstwhile opposing camps (Cameron & Cotter, 1993). Thus the notion is developing that the consequences of metabolic (glycemic) insults may be mediated by a number of diverse biochemical pathways (excess polyol pathway activity, altered *myo*-inositol and phosphoinositide metabolism, the formation of advanced glycosylation products, and oxidative stress) all of which lead to a final common pathway of neuronal damage through disruption of the nerve vascular supply. Furthermore, it is becoming apparent that nerve growth and regeneration may be compromised in diabetes so that the ultimate nature and degree of the pathology is influenced by the balance between degenerative and regenerative forces.

Potentially, therefore, the opportunities for pharmacological interventions based on these accumulating pathophysiologic insights are almost limitless. Indeed in diabetic rodents this has been borne out with *myo*-inositol, aldose reductase inhibitors (which reduce polyol pathway activity by inhibiting the rate limiting enzyme), aminoguanidine (which inhibits the formation of advanced glycoslation products), anti-oxidants, direct vasodilators (e.g., calcium channel blockers, ace inhibitors, and vasomodulator prostanoids or their precursors) and nerve growth agents (e.g., ORG 2766, gangliosides) all proving to be effective in preventing or reversing early nerve dysfunction (Cameron & Cotter, 1993). It is not known whether similar benefits would accrue in human diabetes. So far, individual trials of these drugs have been disappointing, possibly because they have concentrated on patients with quite advanced nerve damage and numbers have been small. Meta-analysis suggests that even in such patients aldose reductase inhibitors may have a small but significant effect, sufficient to prevent or at least postpone major adverse outcomes such as neurotrophic ulceration. But, conceivably, non-glycemic treatments of this sort may prove to be more valuable as primary rather than as secondary interventions.

41.6 NEPHROPATHY

41.6.1 NATURAL HISTORICAL CONSIDERATIONS

Unlike retinopathy and neuropathy, diabetic nephropathy seems not to be an inevitable accompaniment of sustained hyperglycemia. Rather, it would appear that there are subpopulations of diabetic patients with intrinsic susceptibility and resistance. Nevertheless the degree of hyperglycemia does influence expression of the inherited or acquired tendency; some hypotheses suggest that hyperfiltration induced very early in the course of clinical diabetes is important. Microalbuminuria (24 hr urinary albumin excretion >30 mg but <300 mg) is now generally recognized as the earliest manifestation of nephropathy detectable in routine clinical practice; most microalbuminuric subjects will progress to albuminuria (24 hr urinary albumin excretion >300 mg) whence declining renal function is inexorable, albeit at individually specific rates (Marshall, 1991). Hypertension is a virtually invariable accompaniment of diabetic nephropathy and is often apparent at the microalbuminuric stage; in young people, of course, blood pressures within the normal range for middle-aged adults are often significantly above the normal age-related range. As in all renal diseases, hypertension accelerates the decline in renal function, the effect being proportional to its degree.

Diabetic nephropathy patients have a much higher mortality than other patients with IDDM. Historically, most have not survived to require treatment for end-stage renal failure but have died of macrovascular disease, mainly coronary artery disease. Hyperlipidemia is another common accompaniment of diabetic nephropathy and may be an important contributory factor.

41.6.2 PRIMARY PREVENTION

Once again the best evidence comes from DCCT (1993). In the primary intervention, limb intensive therapy reduced the risk of microalbuminuria by 34% (from 27% to 15%) but the number progressing to albuminuria was similar in each group (2%). This is both encouraging, in the sense that optimizing glycemic control is worthwhile, but discouraging in that so many patients with the best glycemic control currently achievable develop early nephropathy. Perhaps this emphasizes the dominant role of other susceptibility factors. As for neuropathy, aldose reductase inhibitors and vasoactive agents, particularly ace inhibitors, have shown promise in animal studies but no human primary prevention data has yet been reported.

41.6.3 SECONDARY PREVENTION

41.6.3.1 Glycemic control

At the end of the nine-year DCCT (1993) study, 'intensive therapy' reduced the adjusted mean risk of microalbuminuria by 43% (22% vs. 41%) and albuminuria by 56% (4% vs. 10%) among patients in the secondary intervention cohort (selected for the presence of 'background' retinopathy; 5% had microalbuminuria at entry but were excluded from analysis). These and other less comprehensive data would suggest that there is benefit to be gained from improving glycemia at any stage in the development of nephropathy.

41.6.3.2 Non-glycemic intervention

Nephropathy is the complication for which the value of non-glycemic intervention has been established beyond all doubt. Right up to and including the stage of declining renal function, it has been clear for some time that blood pressure control and protein restriction reduce the rate of progression even if they do not actually halt the process.

It seems to be beneficial to lower raised blood pressure with any conventional hypotensive drugs. The first studies were carried out before the advent of angiotensin 1-converting enzyme (ACE) inhibitors. It does appear, however, that ACE inhibitors may have specific advantages: they tend to correct the abnormal glomerular hemodynamics; they reduce proteinuria by more than any other agent; and it is assumed that this reflects benefit to the glomerular pathology. Clinical trial evidence has now shown that, for captopril at least, the protection against deterioration in renal function afforded by ACE inhibitor treatment is significantly greater than that conferred by blood pressure control alone; and there is early evidence to suggest that treating even normotensive microalbuminuric patients may slow progression (Lewis *et al.*, 1993). Wherever blood pressure is raised, the optimum impact of hypotensive therapy is dependent on complete normalization of blood pressure.

In common with other renal diseases when renal function has already started to decline, protein restriction (to approximately 1 g/kg body weight) reduces hyperfiltration in intact glomeruli and hence further deterioration. It is not known how early in the course of diabetic nephropathy such restriction may be valuable; pragmatically there seems good reason to advise at least against excessive protein intake in patients with microalbuminuria, perhaps setting a target of 1 g/kg body weight after puberty.

The possible role of other interventions such as aldose reductase inhibitors is unknown at this time. It is conventional to treat even mild degrees of hyperlipidemia vigorously in view of the hugely increased risk of macrovascular disease (up to 100-fold greater than their non-proteinuric peers in some studies).

41.7 MACROVASCULAR DISEASE

41.7.1 NATURAL HISTORICAL CONSIDERATIONS

The hugely increased risk of coronary artery disease, peripheral disease and stroke in patients with IDDM is a consequence of enhanced atherosclerosis. Although the earliest clinical manifestations do not appear until late in the third decade the mortality rate due to coronary artery disease by age 55 years may be as high as 35%. The evolution of atherogenesis, however, starts in the first and second decades, the period we are considering, and it is here that preventative measures may be most effective.

41.7.2 PRIMARY PREVENTION

41.7.2.1 Glycemia

Until DCCT (1993) the role of improved glycemic control within the currently practicable target range has seemed unlikely to have much impact on the excess risk of atherosclerosis attributable to diabetes. After all, even impaired glucose tolerance has been shown to be associated with an increased likelihood of atheromatous disease. Furthermore, hyperinsulinemia (an inevitable accompaniment of near normoglycemia in IDDM) is held by many to be an important mediator of atherosclerosis. In DCCT, however, intensive therapy reduced the development of hypercholesterolemia (here defined as increased low-density lipoprotein (LDL) cholesterol) and, although the numbers were very small, there were appreciably fewer major vascular events in the intensive therapy group. At this time, therefore, the case may be said to be not proven.

41.7.2.2 Lipids

It is now well-established that the risk of coronary artery disease is considerably increased if total cholesterol, LDL cholesterol or triglyceride levels are high or if high-density lipoprotein (HDL) cholesterol levels are low. In patients with IDDM, HDL cholesterol levels tend to be raised but so are LDL cholesterol and triglyceride. Regrettably, there are no clinical trial data to guide the practising clinician regarding the value of trying to modify such abnormalities. At the present time, a pragmatic approach would be to concentrate intensive lipid-lowering therapy on the microalbuminuric sub-population, who have such a hugely increased risk, and on the very small number of individuals with gross lipid disturbances. In these patients, if diet and best achievable glycemic control are insufficient, the use of fibrates, statins and nicotinic acid can be considered.

41.7.2.3 Hypertension

In contrast to the undoubted benefit with respect to cerebrovascular disease, primary prevention of coronary artery disease by treating hypertension in nondiabetic populations has not been shown to be conspicuously effective. Nonetheless, in young patients with IDDM, almost all of those with blood pressure appreciably above the age-related reference range will, as for hyperlipidemia, have microalbuminuria and so hypotensive therapy will be central to their management plan anyway. Clinical trial data are much needed here as well.

41.7.2.4 Lifestyle measures

The risk of coronary artery disease in diabetes mellitus displays extraordinary geographical variation being much less in, for example, Japanese and Mediterranean populations. Probably this reflects dietary variations more than anything else. By deduction, rather than on the basis of clinical trial evidence, it is presumed that diets high in complex high fiber carbohydrate, poly/monounsaturated fats, marine oils, and anti-oxidants (beta-carotene, vitamins C and K) would be protective. Avoidance of obesity would also be expected to yield benefit.

Smoking, of course, compounds all other macrovascular risk factors. Finally, there is exercise which is possibly underestimated as a modifiable risk factor and which carries the added value of improving insulin sensitivity so reducing the peripheral insulin levels needed to obtain any given level of glycemic control.

41.8 ORGANIZATION OF CARE

It is clear from the above that though knowledge is far from complete and the available interventions are far from ideal, there is nevertheless a huge amount that can already be done to prevent the complications of diabetes in young patients. Whether it is done, however, and whether the potential benefits of future developments are realized, depends fundamentally on the organization of care. It has been known for some time that simply attending a service which offers organized diabetes care is associated with improved survival. Nowadays one would expect such services to work in partnership with young people who have diabetes to achieve the best possible individual and overall outcomes.

Increasingly it is being recognized that 'ensuring the quality of care' in this way requires not only a service tuned to the values, attitudes and aspirations of young people but a system which documents key processes (e.g., eye screening) and intermediate outcomes (e.g., absent ankle jerks, microalbuminuria) in a manner which informs, appropriately, both patients and health care professionals so that no practicable opportunity for the application of effective preventive measures is delayed or overlooked. The sensible use of information technology, application of the simple principles of continuous quality improvement, and sharing information with young patients are all possible. A marked reduction in the long-term morbidity and mortality of IDDM is now achievable and the outlook for future improvements is very promising.

REFERENCES

Brinchmann-Hanson, O., Dahl-Jorgensen, K., Hanssen, K.F. *et al.* (1988) The response of diabetic retinopathy to 41 months of multiple insulin injections, insulin pumps and conventional insulin therapy. *Arch. Opthalmol.*, **106**, 1242–46.

Cameron, N.E. and Cotter, M.A. (1993) Potential therapeutic approaches to the treatment or prevention of diabetic neuropathy: evidence from experimental studies. *Diabetic Med.*, **10**, 593–605.

The DCCT Research Group. (1993) The effect of intensive treatment of diabetes on the development and progression of long-term complications in insulin-dependent diabetes mellitus. *N. Eng. J. Med.*, **329**, 977–86.

Engerman, R.L. and Kern, T.S. (1987) Progression of incipient diabetic retinopathy during good glycaemic control. *Diabetes*, **36**, 808–812.

Frank, R.N. (1994) The aldose reductase controversy. *Diabetes*, **43**, 169–72.

Krowlewski, A.S., Warram, J.M., Rand, L.I. *et al.* (1986) Risk of proliferative diabetic retinopathy in juvenile onset type 1 diabetes: A 40-year follow-up study. *Diabetes Care*, **9**, 443–52.

Lewis, E.J., Hunsicker, L.G., Bain, R. *et al.* (1993) The effect of angiotensin-converting-enzyme inhibition on diabetic nephropathy. *N. Eng. J. Med.*, **329**, 1456–62.

Marshall, S.M. (1991) Screening for microalbuminuria: which measurement? *Diabetic Med.*, **8**, 706–711.

Young, R.J. (1987) 'Identification of the foot "at risk" of ulceration', in H. Connor, A.J.M. Boulton and J.D. Ward (eds). *The Diabetic Foot.* John Wiley & Sons, Chichester.

PART SIX

42
New insulins

A.B. KURTZ

42.1 INTRODUCTION

Ever since the 1920s when insulin was first used, there have been continuing efforts to produce insulin preparations with new and special properties; the search has not stopped in the 1990s even though human insulin is now widely used and could be viewed as the ultimate insulin. In 1987, concluding his monograph, Brange (1987) wrote, 'Introducing pure human insulin for the treatment of diabetes has finally made it possible to substitute diabetics' lack of endogenous insulin with an identical molecule.'

There are several problems with insulin. First, as a protein it faces destruction if exposed to digestive enzymes, so that administration is by injection – fortunately, with nearly 100% bioavailability. Second, the time-course of the appearance of insulin in the circulation after injection is rather variable and distinctly unphysiologic. Third, the currently available formulations of insulin are not ideal for sub-cutaneous administration; short-acting insulin is absorbed too slowly to provide an insulin 'bolus' to match carbohydrate absorption following a meal and long-acting insulins are absorbed both too rapidly and too variably to provide a stable 'basal' insulin supply. Although considerable effort has been invested in developing alternative routes for insulin administration (see Chapter 43), insulin will continue to be administered subcutaneously for nearly all insulin-requiring diabetics in the foreseeable future. The current pharmaceutical preparations of short, intermediate and long-acting human insulins are similar to their bovine and porcine counterparts (Brange, 1987; Owens *et al.*, 1991).

What are the clinical limitations of current insulins? There is considerable variability in absorption rate; a coefficient of variation of 25% is probably the best that can be achieved by an individual patient injecting insulin subcutaneously under 'laboratory' conditions (Binder, 1969). Variability of insulin absorption increases with the long-acting insulin formulations. The between patient variation in insulin absorption is so great that the way in which individuals respond to particular formulations of insulin is rather unpredictable. Short-acting insulins are rather slowly absorbed with a pronounced lag-phase, lasting approximately 30 minutes, before the maximal rate of absorption is reached; the peak concentration of circulating insulin is achieved at approximately 90 minutes. This pattern of absorption explains the need for a diabetic to inject insulin half-an-hour before eating rather than at the start of a meal. The duration of action of short-acting insulins is

Childhood and Adolescent Diabetes
Published in 1994 by Chapman & Hall, London
ISBN 0 412 48610 5

sufficiently prolonged to make hypoglycemia a problem between three and five hours after food intake. Long-acting insulins still produce insulin peaks, often at night with resultant hypoglycemia, rather than level circulating insulin concentrations. The difficulty is that humans have periods of feeding – the absorptive state, interspersed with periods of fasting – the post-absorptive state; current insulins are not ideal for either state.

What improvements could one wish for? Theoretically it would be desirable to have an insulin that could be taken orally (Damgé, 1991; Roques *et al.*, 1992) – possibly nasally (Lassmann-Vague, 1991) – with a meal to provide a short-lived peak of circulating insulin that would both maintain postprandial euglycemia and avoid subsequent hypoglycemia. A slowly absorbed insulin is also needed to provide the low level of circulating insulin appropriate to the post-absorptive state. As far as injected insulin goes, we need an insulin without an absorptive lag-phase and with more rapid absorption and clearance than current short-acting insulins. This would allow injection immediately before food with reduced risk of later hypoglycemia, i.e., a 'bolus' of insulin could be closely tuned to food absorption. A very slowly absorbed insulin, with full bioavailability and little variability of absorption, would provide ideal 'basal' insulin. The clinical aim is to make it easier to normalize metabolism with less risk of hypoglycemia. In addition to good pharmacokinetics, a modified insulin might exert a differential effect between the liver and the periphery (Tompkins *et al.*, 1981); probably an unrealizable goal.

Recognizing these clinical aims, the First World Conference on Diabetes Research in 1985 recommended that monomeric insulins and derivatives should be tested.

Many modified insulins have been developed in the past; the idea is not new but certainly the scope is much increased by current techniques of protein engineering. Past modifications include phenylcarbamoyl insulin, sulfated beef insulin, heat-treated lente insulin, desalanine (B30) porcine insulin, desphenylalanine (B1) insulin, tetranitrotyrosine insulin, despentapeptide (B26–B30) insulin and despentapeptide (B26–B30) insulin amide (Figure 42.1) (Brange, 1987; Owens *et al.*, 1991)

For research purposes a series of insulins,

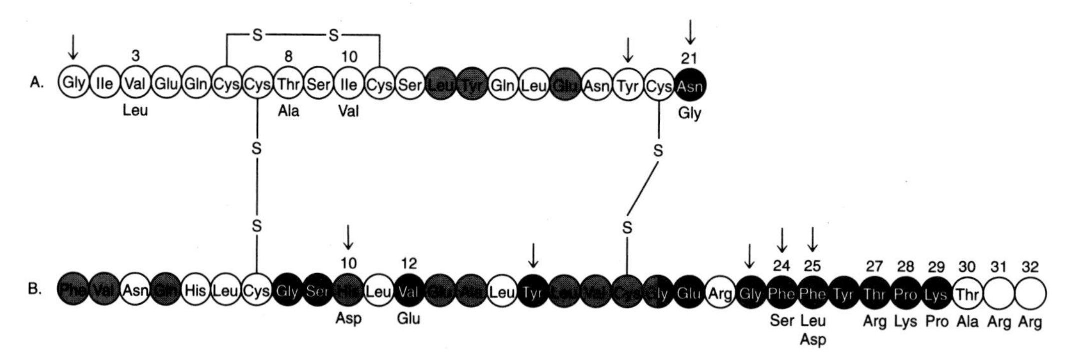

Figure 42.1 Primary structure of human insulin with indications of amino acid residues involved in association of 2 insulin molecules into dimer (black residues) and assembly of 3 dimers and 2 Zn^{2+} into Zn^{2+}-insulin hexamer (gray residues). Putative sites interacting with receptor are indicated by arrows. Sites and types of mutation in different analogues are also shown. (Reprinted with permission from Brange *et al.*, 1990, *Diabetes Care.*, **13**, Sept. 1990. Copyright © 1990 by American Diabetes Association, Inc.)

modified by conventional chemical techniques, were tested for *in vitro* and *in vivo* activity and it was concluded that over a range of receptor affinity the *in vivo* potency remained 100%, implying that clearance is receptor-mediated, i.e., an insulin with low affinity for the receptor is cleared more slowly and therefore circulates at a higher concentration which compensates for its lower affinity and vice versa (Jones *et al.*, 1976).

The list of adjuvants used to extend the action of insulin is also long. Epinephrine, cholesterol and lecithin, tried in the 1920s, did not work; protamine, globin, surfen, protamine with excess zinc and excess zinc alone have all been used in insulin formulations. Only protamine and zinc have survived: the current isophane and lente insulins. These insulins are crystalline with insulin hexamers contained within the crystals. Although, over many years, many attempts have been made to prepare insulin formulations suitable for administration by routes avoiding injection none have had significant success. Nasal insulin administration has possibly been closer to success than others. Using human insulin at 200 or 500 U/ml with detergents such as deoxycholic acid a good, and rapid, time course of absorption can be achieved; however, the bioavailability is low at around 20–25% at best (Lassmann-Vague, 1991).

It is worth bearing in mind the normal products of the β-cell: not just insulin and C-peptide but also proinsulin and the intermediates in the conversion of proinsulin to insulin – split (65–66) proinsulin, des (64,65) proinsulin, split (32–33) proinsulin and des (31,32) proinsulin. Insulin is stored and secreted by β-cells as a hexamer which rapidly dissociates to dimer and then monomer at the low insulin concentration found in the circulation (<1 nmol/l). Several genetic variants of insulin have been detected. Mutant human insulin genes produce Insulin Chicago (Leu^{B25}), Insulin Los Angeles (Ser^{B24}) and Insulin Wakagama (Leu^{A3}). The presence of an abnormal insulin is often associated with diabetes which is unexpected given the presence of a normal insulin allele with co-production of normal insulin. Several mutants block the conversion of proinsulin to insulin, yielding mutant proinsulin as the abnormal secretory product. Proinsulin is the most studied 'analog' of insulin and the experience from clinical studies using proinsulin should temper our expectations of analog insulins (Galloway *et al.*, 1992).

When soluble human insulin is injected the high concentration (100 U/ml or 0.59 mmol/l) ensures that the insulin is mostly in the hexameric state (Figure 42.2) (Brange, 1990). Dissociation of the hexamer to dimer and monomer is a rate-limiting step. Small monomers are able to enter capillaries much more readily than the large hexamers. The hexamers diffuse from the injection site with dissociation occurring when the local insulin concentration falls, i.e., the insulin becomes diluted as it diffuses and dissociates as it becomes diluted. This explains the lag-phase of insulin absorption and also the effect of insulin concentration – 40 U/ml insulin is absorbed faster than 100 U/ml insulin – and massage at the injection site. The lente and isophane insulin preparations are retarded as the crystals have to break up and release the hexameric insulin before the process of diffusion can begin. Crystal size therefore has an obvious effect on retardation as can be seen in the lente series with amorphous crystals (semi-lente) being absorbed more rapidly than large crystals (ultralente).

42.2 INSULINS DESIGNED FOR RAPID ABSORPTION

The insulin molecule has been extensively studied and the areas of the molecule interacting with the insulin receptor, with another insulin molecule in dimer formation and with other dimers in hexamer formation have been mapped (Figure 42.2); several amino acids are

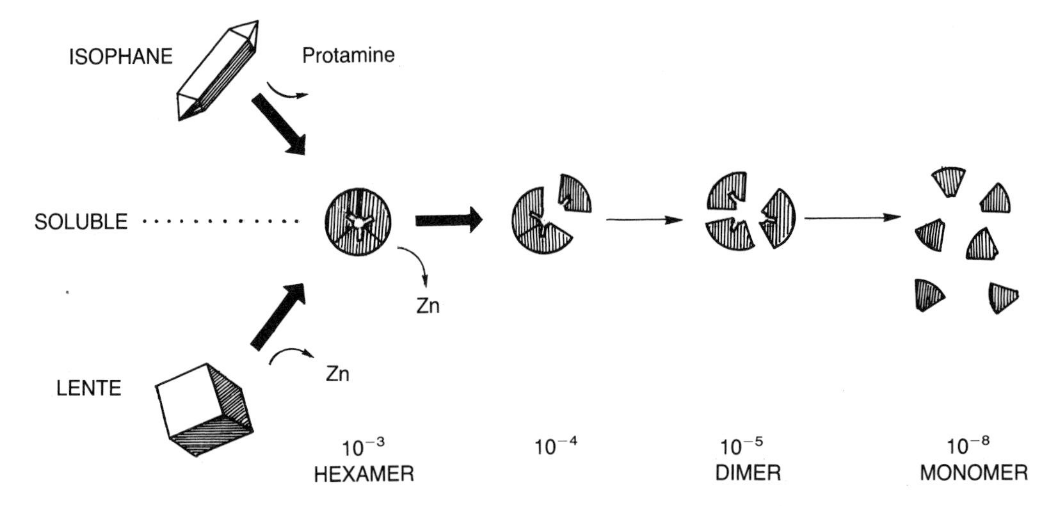

Figure 42.2 Dissociation of the zinc-insulin hexamer into dimeric and monomeric insulin. (Reprinted with permission from Brange *et al.*, 1990, *Diabetes Care.*, **13**, Sept. 1990. Copyright © 1990 by American Diabetes Association, Inc.)

metal ion binding sites. These functions can be selectively altered by protein engineering and insulins produced which cannot form hexamers. This can be achieved by, for example, producing charge repulsion in the dimerizing area (switching B28 proline, B29 lysine to B28 lysine, B29 proline), producing steric hindrance (substitution of B12 valine with isoleucine) or removing a metal binding site (substitution of B10 histidine with aspartate). Substitutions that would make the molecule similar to IGF1 have been avoided both to avoid IGF1 activity and to avoid binding to IGF1 binding proteins.

It should be pointed out that the despentapeptide (B26–B30) insulin is monomeric having lost much of the dimerizing area.

The amino acid 'substitutions' by which bovine (Ala^{A8}, Val^{A10}, Ala^{B30}) and porcine (Ala^{B30}) insulins differ from human insulin alter the strength of the association of the monomers in hexameric insulin. Human insulin has the weakest association and is absorbed the most rapidly, bovine insulin the strongest association and is absorbed the most slowly. An additional factor which may be of some relevance is that human insulin is more hydrophilic than porcine insulin. Guinea pig insulin is also monomeric but with very low affinity for other mammalian insulin receptors.

There have been many novel insulins manufactured. Very few have survived to clinical trial; most have been useful only as research tools. Some have very low affinity for the insulin receptor, e.g., Asp^{B25} at 0.05%, and some very high affinity – Glu^{B12} + Des^{B30} at 600%. *In vivo* potency for modified insulins with reasonable receptor affinity (>25% as compared with human insulin) is usually near 100% as expected.

Asp^{B10} insulin is largely monomeric and has high receptor affinity (560%). Clinical trial has confirmed that its pharmacokinetic attributes are satisfactory. Lys^{B28}, Pro^{B29} insulin has been reported to have a similar satisfactory pharmacokinetic profile and is undergoing clinical trial. Absorption after subcutaneous injection is rapid with no lag phase. The rate of absorption is monoexponential. The peak insulin concentration in the circulation is achieved about three times more quickly than with neutral soluble human insulin, with suitably rapid clearance. The high affinity Asp^{B10} insulin was withdrawn from clinical trial as animal studies showed that it could cause cancer; possibly a consequence of the high receptor-binding affinity promoting mitogenic rather than metabolic effects. No mammalian insulins have affinity over 100% for the human insulin receptor; however, chicken and turkey insulin do have affinity of >100%. It would seem important that negative cooperativity is retained in a modified insulin in order to retain 'normal' function. It is the metabolic effect of insulin that is required and relative enhancement of its mitogenic actions are likely to be undesirable.

Over the last 60 years much effort has been invested in producing insulin formulations which possess a high degree of stability. Hexameric insulin is less prone to polymerization into fibrils than monomeric insulin. New insulins may well have problems of stability.

42.3 INSULINS DESIGNED FOR EXTENDED ACTION

The isoelectric point (pK) of insulin is at pH 5.4. This means that at pH 5.4 the insulin is at its most insoluble. Protein engineering can, by the addition of positive charges, alter the pK to around 7 which renders the insulin much less soluble in the extra-cellular fluid at subcutaneous injection sites. This has been achieved with the substitution of arginine for threonine at B27, the conversion of threonine at B30 to the amide or by adding an extension to the B chain of Arg^{B31}, Arg^{B32}. The substitution of glycine for aspartate at A21 makes the molecule more hydrophobic and the crystal, with less water, more dense and less soluble.

These insulins are soluble when in solution at pH 3.0 to 4.0. After injection, the acid is neutralized and the insulin precipitated; subsequent absorption is slow. Acid-soluble insulins were used in the past, before neutral insulins were developed, and were relatively immunogenic – a pitfall to be avoided for the future.

The use of a retardant such as zinc or protamine would be expected to further retard some varieties of 'slow' insulin-analog. Many clinicians would settle for a revamped protamine zinc insulin – possibly using human insulin rather than an analog. A porcine protamine zinc insulin was tested some years ago with apparently satisfactory results – and low immunogenicity. I would anticipate that new formulations of human insulin will provide clinically valuable preparations in the foreseeable future. Clinicians and patients are conservative by nature and I do not foresee analog insulins having similar impact.

One interesting insulin, used only in the research area for laboratory animals, is heat-treated lente insulin. At pH 5.5 prolonged gentle heating causes the formation of a small number of covalent links between hexamers. The increased stability of the crystals greatly retards absorption.

42.4 CONCLUSION

The clinical performance of an insulin preparation is dependent on a very large number of factors in addition to the amino acid structure which genetic engineering can provide. Insulin is a protein and it interacts with, and is affected by, most of the constituents of the preparation – salts, glycerol, preservatives and retardants. Protein engineering can merely provide new building blocks on which new formulations of modified insulins may ultimately be based.

Over the years insulin preparations have evolved in an almost Darwinian fashion. Many preparations and formulations are no longer with us; in the future I expect that we shall see many more come – and go.

REFERENCES

Binder, C. (1969) *Absorption of injected insulin, a clinical-pharmacological study*. Munksgaard, Copenhagen, pp. 37–49.

Brange, J. (1987) *Galenics of insulin*, Springer-Verlag, Berlin Heidelberg.

Brange, J., Owens, D.R., Kang, S. *et al.* (1990) Monomeric insulins and their experimental and clinical implications. *Diabetes Care*, **13**, 923–54.

Damgé, C. (1991) 'Oral insulin', in J.C. Pickup (ed.). *Biotechnology of Insulin Therapy*, pp. 97–112. Blackwell Scientific Publications, Oxford.

Galloway, J.A., Hooper, S.A., Spradlin, C.T. *et al.* (1992) Biosynthetic human proinsulin. Review of chemistry, *in vitro* and *in vivo* receptor binding, animal and human pharmacology studies, and clinical trial experience. *Diabetes Care*, **15**, 666–92.

Jones, R.H., Dron, D.I., Ellis, M.J. *et al.* (1976) Biological properties of chemically modified insulins. *Diabetologia*, **12**, 601–608.

Lassmann-Vague, V. (1991) 'The intranasal route for insulin administration', in J.C. Pickup (ed.). *Biotechnology of Insulin Therapy*, pp. 113–25. Blackwell Scientific Publications, Oxford.

Owens, D.R., Vora, J.P. and Dolben, J. (1991) 'Human insulin and beyond: semi-synthesis and recombinant DNA technology reviewed', in J.C. Pickup (ed.). *Biotechnology of Insulin Therapy*, pp. 24–41. Blackwell Scientific Publications, Oxford.

Roques, M., Damgé, C., Michel, C. *et al.* (1992) Encapsulation of insulin for oral administration preserves interaction of the hormone with its receptor *in vitro*. *Diabetes*, **41**, 451–56.

Tompkins, C.V., Brandenburg, D., Jones, R.H. *et al.* (1981) Mechanism of action of insulin and insulin analogues. *Diabetologia*, **20**, 94–101.

43

New routes and means of insulin delivery

G.M. DANIELSEN, K. DREJER, L. LANGKJÆR and A. PLUM

43.1 INTRODUCTION

The administration of insulin by alternative routes is not, in fact, a new concept, and has been considered for almost as long as injectable insulin has been available. First attempts addressed intranasal, oral, vaginal and rectal administration (Woodyatt, 1922). Although many well-conceived and ingenious approaches have been investigated in the ensuing years, no alternative administration forms are yet in routine clinical use. The scope of this review is therefore to provide an evaluation of the present status and future perspectives for new routes of insulin administration.

Administration forms covered in this chapter include non-invasive routes via the epithelial surfaces – nasal, gastrointestinal, pulmonary, ocular and buccal, together with transdermal delivery (iontophoresis) and insulin implants, but exclude biofeedback systems, which are covered in Chapter 44. Many of these subjects have been reviewed recently (Pickup, 1991a). Not all approaches are equally realistic, and an attempt has been made here to evaluate the various routes in terms of clinical feasibility and desirability. During the last decade, developments in production of recombinant peptides and proteins have promoted a surge of interest in non-parenteral delivery systems (Lee, 1991). Often, insulin is used as a model peptide, and it is not always taken into consideration that insulin administration has stringent demands in terms of pharmacokinetics, reproducible bioavailability and the effects of chronic administration, including the effects of penetration enhancers.

The main impetus for development of new insulin therapies must be that they confer a real advantage compared to existing regimens. The current subcutaneous insulin therapy is far from ideal (Pickup, 1991b), and is not able to normalize glycemia despite improvements in insulin preparations and introduction of multiple injection regimens. When injected subcutaneously, unmodified insulin is absorbed too slowly to mimic the effects of endogenously secreted insulin in response to a meal. The relatively slow and sustained subcutaneous absorption gives rise to prandial hyperglycemia and carries a risk of postprandial hypoglycemia, necessitating snacks between meals. For the protracted insulin suspensions, the main problem is the great inter- and intra-patient variability in absorption, which can be responsible foı

Childhood and Adolescent Diabetes
Published in 1994 by Chapman & Hall, London
ISBN 0 412 48610 5

poor metabolic control, especially during the night. Furthermore, local discomfort and perceived disruption of a normal lifestyle deter many IDDM patients from accepting intensive insulin treatment regimens. In addition, many NIDDM patients refuse insulin therapy entirely because of their unwillingness to accept the physical and social trauma involved with insulin injections. For children, a conventional regimen with multiple injection therapy creates special problems – apart from being stressful, it is also difficult to administer small doses accurately.

A more convenient insulin therapy would be expected to result in improved patient compliance, and, together with more physiologic insulin levels, lead to better metabolic control, and thereby reduced risk of late diabetic complications. Ideally, an insulin delivery system should also aim for a hepatic portal, rather than systemic delivery, to reduce peripheral hyperinsulinemia.

43.2 MEAL-RELATED INSULIN – NASAL INSULIN

43.2.1 THE NASAL ROUTE FOR INSULIN ADMINISTRATION

The nasal mucosa is an attractive potential site for peptide administration, with the epithelial surface covering a rich network of submucosal blood capillaries facilitating systemic delivery. For nasal drug delivery, there are three physical barriers to systemic absorption: 1) penetration of the mucus layer covering the epithelial surface, 2) mucociliary clearance, with constant, co-ordinated beating of cilia resulting in a flow of mucus towards the pharynx, and 3) absorption over the epithelial layer itself. In addition, enzymatic clearance may play a role. Nasal delivery of peptides has been reviewed recently (Edman & Björk, 1992).

Research aimed at developing a clinically acceptable form of insulin, either as spray, drops, gel or powder, has concentrated on two approaches: first, to increase the time of contact between insulin and the mucosa, e.g., by incorporation in starch microspheres exhibiting reduced mucociliary clearance (Illum *et al.*, 1987; Farraj *et al.*, 1989) and second, the use of additives to enhance penetration of the mucosa, with focus on achieving maximal bioavailability and minimal mucosal damage and irritation. For this more intensively studied approach, many surfactant enhancers have been investigated, including bile salts (sodium glycocholate and sodium deoxycholate), non-ionic polyoxyethylene ether (Laureth-9), a derivative of fusidic acid, sodium tauro-24,25-dihydrofusidate, and combination preparations, e.g., Tween 80/polyoxyethylene ethers (Hirai *et al.*, 1978 & 1981; Pontiroli *et al.*, 1982; Moses *et al.*, 1983; Bruce *et al.*, 1991; Kimmerle *et al.*, 1991). These compounds are effective, with a variety of proposals as to the mechanism of enhancement (Gizurarson & Bechgaard, 1991; Lassmann-Vague, 1991; Muranishi, 1990). However, for most of the enhancers, mucosal irritation has been a major problem.

An effective, almost non-irritating enhancer is didecanoyl-L-alpha phosphatidylcholine (DDPC), a medium-chain phospholipid closely related to naturally occurring cell membrane phosholipids. For insulin given nasally in combination with this phospholipid, immunohistochemistry shows insulin localized in the epithelial layer, predominantly in ciliated cells (Guldhammer *et al.*, 1988), but the prevailing mechanism for increase in flux across the epithelial barrier has been suggested to involve a reversible opening of tight junctions, allowing paracellular transport (Carstens *et al.*, 1991).

43.2.2 PHARMACOKINETICS OF INTRANASALLY ADMINISTERED INSULIN

Following intranasal administration of insulin preparations (incorporating various absorption enhancers) to normal volunteers, plasma insulin levels increase rapidly and in a dose-dependent manner, with a corresponding swift, dose-dependent decline in blood glucose (Pontiroli *et al.*, 1982; Moses *et al.*, 1983; Salzman *et al.*, 1985; Nolte *et al.*, 1990).

In a pharmacokinetic study using Novolin Nasal® U200 spray with DDPC as enhancer, these previous findings were confirmed (Drejer *et al.*, 1992). Eleven fasting subjects received 0.05 IU/kg insulin intravenously, 0.08 IU/kg subcutaneously or three doses intranasally (approx. 0.3 IU/kg, 0.6 IU/kg, 0.8 IU/kg) in random order on five separate days. The plasma glucose concentration following insulin administration (Figure 43.1) shows a decline after 20 min with nadir reached at 44 min and return to baseline within 120–180 min. Intranasal administration caused a dose-dependent reduction in plasma glucose, the nadir occurring at the same time for all doses (Table 43.1), and with a significantly smaller variation in time compared with subcutaneous administration. The peak insulin concentration was reached 23 min after intranasal spraying and had returned to baseline after 60–90 min (Figure 43.2). Following subcutaneous administration a much less pronounced peak, calculated to 86 min, was observed (Table 43.1).

Bioavailability for the nasal formulation was 8.3% relative to an intravenous bolus injection when plasma insulin was corrected for endogenous insulin production as estimated by plasma C-peptide (Drejer *et al.*, 1992). In contrast to previous reports with alternative enhancers, the short-term local irritation of this preparation was absent or slight (Table 43.2).

Preliminary results indicate that intra-

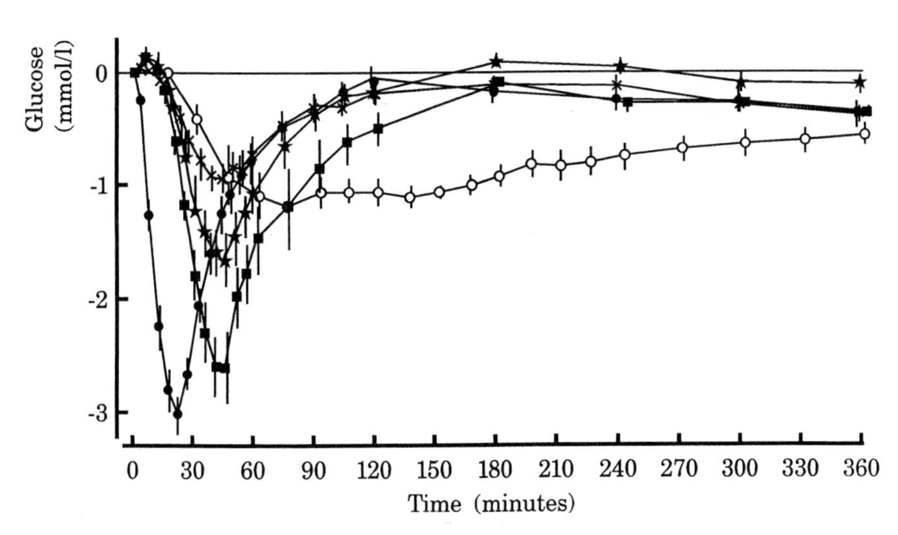

Figure 43.1 Plasma glucose levels in 11 fasting normal subjects after graded doses of intranasal insulin with phospholipid enhancer and intravenous and subcutaneous insulin.

●: intravenous, 0.05 IU kg^{-1}; x: nasal, 0.28 IU kg^{-1}; ★: nasal, 0.59 IU kg^{-1}; ■: nasal, 0.77 IU kg^{-1} ($n = 7$ due to intravenous glucose administration to 4 hypoglycemic subjects); ○: subcutaneous, 0.081 IU kg^{-1}.

Table 43.1 Time from insulin administration until maximum plasma insulin concentration, and from insulin administration until maximum effect on plasma glucose.

	Glucose nadir (min)	Peak insulin (min)
Intravenous	25 ± 3	5 ± 0
Intranasal low dose	45 ± 6	26 ± 7
Intranasal medium dose	44 ± 7	23 ± 7
Intranasal high dose	45 ± 6	22 ± 8
Intranasal average	44 ± 6	23 ± 7
Subcutaneous	131 ± 72	86 ± 38

Mean ± SE (n = 11).

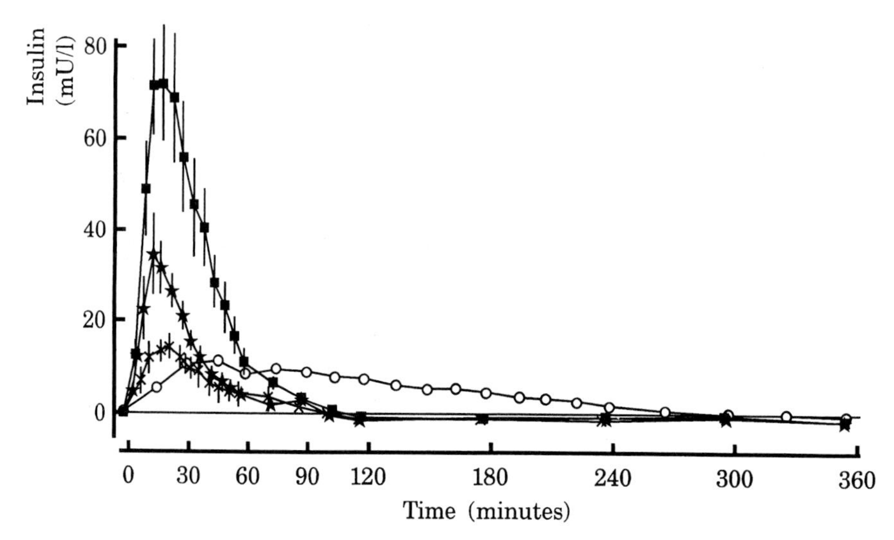

Figure 43.2 Plasma insulin levels in 11 fasting normal subjects after graded doses of intranasal insulin with phospholipid enhancer or subcutaneous insulin.
x: nasal, 0.28 IU kg^{-1}; ★: nasal, 0.59 IU kg^{-1}; ■: nasal, 0.77 IU kg^{-1}; ○: subcutaneous 0.081 IU kg^{-1}.

patient variability in absorption is similar to that for soluble, fast-acting subcutaneous insulin preparations (Sinay *et al.*, 1990; Holman & Steemson, 1991). However, due to the pharmacokinetic profile of nasal insulin, fewer clinical disturbances may be expected, as the variability appears in the first hour after nasal insulin administration, i.e., within the post-prandial period.

Pharmacokinetic studies in diabetic patients have revealed changes in plasma insulin levels similar to studies in normal volunteers (Pontiroli *et al.*, 1982; Moses *et al.*, 1983; Salzman *et al.*, 1985; Frauman *et al.*, 1987; Kimmerle *et al.*, 1991; Thow & Home, 1992). A double blind, placebo-controlled dose-response study of Novolin Nasal® U500 in relation to a standard meal in NIDDMs con-

Table 43.2 Local nasal irritation resulting from insulin spray.

	Nasal irritation score			
	None 0	Slight 1	Moderate 2	Severe 3
Low dose	9	3	0	0
Medium dose	6	6	0	0
High dose	4	6	2	0

0: no irritation; 1: slight irritation of no significance for use of the spray; 2: intermediate irritation; 3: unacceptable for practical use.

cluded that nasal insulin was well-tolerated, did not cause hypoglycemia and that nasal insulin improved meal-related blood glucose control in a dose-dependent manner in well-controlled, insulin sensitive type II subjects (Thow & Home, 1992).

Euglycemic clamp studies show pharmacodynamic profiles supporting the quick onset of action of nasal insulin and a short duration of action (Nolte *et al.*, 1990; Jacobs *et al.*, 1991).

43.2.3 CLINICAL EXPERIENCES WITH NASAL INSULIN

Long-term use of intranasal insulin administration in IDDM patients has been reported. In a 3-month study by Salzman *et al.* (1985), eight IDDM patients received preprandial intranasal insulin (containing Laureth-9 as absorption enhancer) as a supplement to Ultralente insulin. Glycemic control was comparable to that observed during a subsequent 3-month period of conventional subcutaneous insulin treatment. The authors concluded that intranasal insulin has potential as an adjunct to subcutaneous insulin in diabetes therapy, but the extent of its usefulness will depend on the development of new surfactants. Frauman *et al.* (1987) studied the long-term use of an intranasal insulin preparation containing another enhancer, sodium glycocholate. Injections of fast-acting insulin preparations were replaced by intranasal insulin for a 4-month period and glycemic control was compared to that obtained during a period of conventional insulin treatment as well as a period with an intensified insulin regimen. A significant rise in glycated hemoglobin was seen during the intranasal phase, but not in plasma or urinary glucose levels. The authors state that intranasal insulin satisfactorily controlled blood glucose levels in approximately half the subjects studied. This group also concluded that intranasal insulin has the potential to replace short-acting insulin in some IDDM patients, but that clinical use will require new adjuvants.

Novolin Nasal® U500 was tested in an open, randomized, crossover study in 19 patients with type I diabetes on basal and prandial insulin therapy (Holman & Steemson, 1992). U500 Novolin Nasal® insulin given with meals was compared with U100 soluble subcutaneous insulin given 30 min before meals with 4-week outpatient treatment periods. It was concluded that U500 Novolin Nasal® insulin, given as a single administration immediately before meals, was effective in treating type I diabetic outpatients but a less satisfactory glycemic control was achieved with the limited dose range available.

43.2.4 NASAL INSULIN – CONCLUSIONS

In addition to the advantage of convenience, the pharmacokinetic profile of intranasal insulin, showing a rapid increase in plasma insulin levels, mimics the normal response to a meal more precisely than conventional subcutaneous soluble fast-acting insulin preparations. Consequently, nasal insulin can be administered immediately prior to meals, in contrast to subcutaneous insulin, which is usually given 30 min before meals. Supplementary sprays administered postprandially may offer the possibility of greater freedom with respect to meal size. Furthermore, the short duration of the insulin peak would be expected to reduce the risk of late and unpredictable hypoglycemic episodes seen in IDDM patients.

Although the initial studies with intranasal administration of insulin with phospholipid as absorption enhancer have been encouraging, displaying desirable absorption kinetics, precise timing of absorption and only slight irritation, it should also be emphasized that the bioavailability of the preparation is not sufficient to cover the meal-related insulin requirements in many diabetic patients. Further long-term studies addressing potential adverse effects on the nasal mucosa, and the influence of viral and allergic rhinitis on insulin absorption remain to be performed.

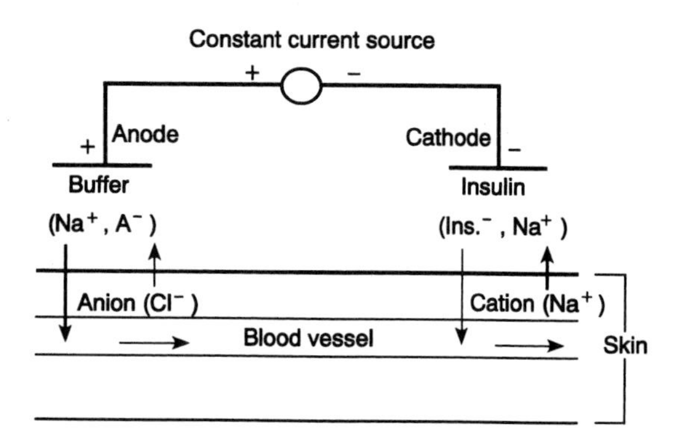

Figure 43.3 A diagrammatic outline of an iontophoretic system for transdermal delivery of insulin. Forced by an electric field, the negatively charged ions in the cathode reservoir will migrate in the direction of the anode into the skin, where they will reach the capillary system. Concurrently, there is an outward migration of ions from the tissue, mainly Cl^- and Na^+, towards the anode and cathode respectively (modified from Burnette, 1989).

43.3 BASAL ADMINISTRATION – TRANSDERMAL INSULIN

43.3.1 IONTOPHORESIS

Of the various alternative administration forms for peptide drugs currently being investigated, one main focus of interest is the transdermal route. The skin is an efficient barrier to the penetration of ionic and hydrophilic substances and large molecules. However, by applying an electric current it is possible to transport ionic substances across the skin. This technique, iontophoresis, which has been known for about a century, is presently receiving considerable attention from both academia and industry because of the need for a non-invasive and nonparenteral administration form for new peptide drugs. For several years, short-term iontophoresis has been used in the diagnosis of cystic fibrosis, for treatment of hyperhidrosis, and for local treatment of joints with steroids and non-steroidal anti-inflammatory drugs. The clinical experience regarding impact on the skin has recently been reviewed by Ledger (1992).

An iontophoretic device consists of two electrode chambers and a power supply, e.g., a battery (Figure 43.3). The donor electrode, which can be either the anode or the cathode depending on the charge of the drug, contains the drug to be transdermally delivered. The two electrodes are placed on the skin a few centimeters apart. The current carries the drug into the skin, the pathways most likely being the sweat-glands and the hair-follicles (Cullander, 1992).

The delivery rate is dependent on current density, electrode area and drug concentration and can preferably be controlled by adjusting the current (Sage & Riviere, 1992). When current is turned off, delivery stops. Factors of importance for iontophoretic delivery of a drug include molecular size, charge, and hydrophobicity, with small, charged and hydrophilic substances having the highest delivery rate (Yoshida & Roberts, 1992; DelTerzo *et al.*, 1989). Generally, anodal delivery is considered more efficient than cathodal delivery, due to the additional electro-osmotic volume flow from the anode to the cathode (Pikal, 1992).

43.3.2 *IN VITRO* AND *IN VIVO* STUDIES

Several *in vivo* experiments with iontophoresis of insulin have been reported (Stephen *et al.*, 1984; Kari, 1986; Siddiqui *et al.*, 1987; Liu *et al.*, 1988; Meyer *et al.*, 1989; Chien, 1991). Transdermal delivery in diabetic pigs, rabbits and hairless rats was investigated using variable current densities, formulation and donor polarity. Insulin has an isoelectric point of pH 5.4 and is soluble below pH 4 and above pH 6.5. It can therefore be iontophoresed from the anodal as well as from the cathodal side at pH levels compatible with the skin. Siddiqui *et al.* (1987) found greater glucose-lowering effect with anodal as compared to cathodal delivery, which was explained by the difference in association state – dimeric at acid pH and hexameric at neutral pH. Using pulsed current, Chien (1991) observed significant lower blood glucose in diabetic hairless rats than with constant current. This phenomenon has been explained by depolarization of the skin during the 'off' state. Stephen *et al.* (1984) could not detect any effect after cathodal iontophoresis of porcine (hexameric) insulin, whereas with a monomeric highly-ionized insulin (presumably sulfated insulin), therapeutic insulin plasma levels were obtained in one diabetic pig. In common for the experiments are the use of relatively large electrode areas and high current densities, thus the obtained insulin transport rates are not clinically relevant.

Recently it has been shown *in vitro*, that by cathodal iontophoresis monomeric human insulin analogs, produced by site-directed mutagenesis (Brange *et al.*, 1990) can be delivered 50–100 times more efficiently across hairless mouse skin than hexameric, zinc-free human insulin (Langkjær *et al.*, 1983, 1984). The preliminary data indicate that for a 10 cm^2 electrode area a delivery rate of around 1 IU per hour – enough to cover basal insulin need – is theoretically possible, when specially designed monomeric insulin analogs are used.

43.3.3 POTENTIAL AND CONCLUSIONS

Iontophoretic transdermal delivery of insulin has several potential advantages. In addition to being non-invasive and replacing injections, thereby increasing compliance, controlled delivery will be possible by changing the current (either preprogrammed or on demand), thus allowing adjustment of delivery rates to individual needs. The delivery rate can be pulsatile, which is more physiologic and efficient (Waldhäusl, 1986). Another important factor is that the insulin depot is outside the body. Thus, increased bloodflow due to, e.g., high muscle activity, will not induce hypoglycemia, and termination of insulin delivery is possible. Finally, for NIDDM patients, nocturnal basal insulin can reduce overnight plasma-free fatty acids as well as blood glucose (Taskinen *et al.*, 1989). For these patients, who may not get accustomed to, or accept, traditional hypodermic insulin therapy, a transdermal iontophoretic patch would be more acceptable and convenient.

The concurrent development of technology relating to patch-materials, microprocessors and miniaturized batteries makes iontophoretic delivery of peptides, including insulin, within the realm of possibilities, although great efforts must still be put into research and development programs. An insulin analog exhibiting optimal transport characteristics and acceptable stability and biological features needs to be identified. Ideally, a transdermal insulin patch could deliver basal as well as bolus insulin in a reproducible and reliable manner. The product should be esthetic, easy to apply and remove, and not induce skin irritation or allergy. It should also be preprogrammable and easy to adjust on demand. The ultimate goal would be a closed-loop system comprising a non-invasive blood glucose monitor and automatic adjustment of insulin delivery rate.

43.4 GASTROINTESTINAL ADMINISTRATION – AN UNREALISTIC GOAL?

43.4.1 ORAL INSULIN – RATIONALE

Oral administration of insulin, or an 'insulin pill' is superficially an attractive proposition, with two main advantages over parenteral administration: first, convenience, and thereby patient compliance; and second, the possibility of delivery via hepatic portal drainage, allowing for first-pass liver extraction, mimicking the physiologic situation and reducing peripheral hyperinsulinemia. These attributes are, however, overshadowed by two main barriers to insulin delivery – enzymatic degradation in the intestinal lumen, and limited penetration of this relatively large, hydrophilic peptide over the epithelial surface (Davis, 1990). This results in a very limited bioavailability (0.5%) of native insulin when orally administered in humans (Crane *et al.*, 1968). Design concepts for oral insulin delivery formulations are thus rather complex, and are largely based on various combinations of three factors: physical protection from the gastrointestinal milieu, chemical protection by co-formulation with enzyme inhibitors, and enhancement of penetration of the mucosa. Presented below are three very different approaches to oral insulin. For a more detailed review, see Damgé (1991), or for general oral peptide administration, Smith *et al.* (1992).

43.4.2 ORAL INSULIN – THREE APPROACHES

In 1986, Saffran *et al.* proposed an oral insulin formulation theoretically designed to release insulin in the colon, a part of the intestine 'devoid of secreted digestive enzymes'. An insulin formulation was coated with polymers cross-linked with azoaromatic groups to form an impervious film to protect orally administered drugs from digestion in the stomach and small intestine. On reaching the large intestine, indigenous microflora reduce the azo bonds, degrading the polymer film, and thus releasing the drug into the lumen of the colon. Subsequent trials in pancreatectomized dogs (Saffran *et al.*, 1991) with the additional additive of 5-methoxysalicylic acid, an absorption enhancer, did show a dose-dependent fall in plasma glucose and decrease in hepatic glucose production, but also demonstrated three general deficits in oral insulin preparations – a very low bioavailability (<1%), irreproducible effects and lack of controlled timing, being dependent in this case on mouth-to-cecum transit time, assuming release in the colon.

A second approach, aimed at an extremely protracted, basal insulin release, has been pursued by Damgé and co-workers, and comprises a biodegradable polymeric colloidal drug carrier composed of polyalkylcyanoacrylates. In this case, the insulin-containing microcapsules are apparently absorbed through the mucosa, and are distributed throughout the body, followed by a progressive degradation of polymer by hydrolysis of ester side-chains and concomitant release of insulin to target organs (Damgé, 1991). In studies in normal dogs, using decrease in peak hyperglycemia induced by oral glucose load, maximal effect was observed at day 9, with control values reached again by day 21 (Damgé *et al.*, 1990). Many questions remain to be answered regarding the mechanism of action of these preparations, and safety issues would probably exclude such preparations as clinical candidates.

The most visibly commercial approach regarding an oral insulin preparation to date is based on a delivery system comprising insulin formulated in a water-in-oil emulsion together with lecithin, non-esterified fatty acids and cholesterol, together with aprotinin, a serine protease inhibitor, and an inert carrier (Cho & Flynn, 1989). From the very limited data presented (with no control data), no conclusions of the efficacy of this preparation can be drawn. It is unknown if the route of insulin absorption is via hepatic portal drainage or via the lymphatics.

43.4.3 RECTAL INSULIN

Rectal administration, designed for either basal or bolus profiles, would reduce the number of necessary injections, but hardly attain the same degree of convenience as afforded by nasal or oral administration. Three routes of drainage occur from the rectum: from the middle and lower rectum via the iliac veins to the inferior vena cava (systemic delivery), to the upper rectum via the hepatic portal system (with the same advantage as for the small intestine with reduction of peripheral hyperinsulinemia), and finally, the possibility for lymphatic drainage (de Boer *et al.*, 1992). The rectum is largely a non-turbulent area for administration; however the dose will be affected by defecation, especially periprandial defecation in the case of children. As for oral administration, design concepts are based on physical and chemical protection, and absorption enhancement, and the formulation could conceivably be applied as suppositories or gel.

In the rabbit, the most frequently used *in vivo* model, the rectum is practially impervious to insulin (Yamamoto *et al.*, 1992) and the use of penetration enhancers is obligate, either as single entities or in synergistic combinations, e.g., Na glycocholate/EDTA (Yamamoto *et al.*, 1992). A range of other enhancers have been studied (Aungst & Rogers, 1988; van Hoogdalem *et al.*, 1990; Nishihata *et al.*, 1987). A goal of reproducible and realistic bioavailability with no loss of mucosal integrity has not yet been proven, and, to the authors' knowledge, no pharmaceutical developments are in progress.

43.4.4 GASTROINTESTINAL INSULIN – CONCLUSIONS

Even if a pharmacologically active basal or bolus gastrointestinal insulin preparation is demonstrated in animal models or clinical trials, it is far from certain that a clinically and commercially realistic preparation can be achieved. The need to design a delivery system which both protects insulin and enhances absorption over the gastrointestinal mucosa, together with the strict requirements for reproducibility, bioavailability, timing and safety in chronic administration means that this route of administration is more easily achievable for delivery of therapeutic peptides with less restriction on delivery patterns, and a wider therapeutic index.

43.5 OTHER ADMINISTRATION FORMS

43.5.1 PULMONARY DELIVERY

In comparison to the nasal mucosa, skin and the gastrointestinal tract, the lungs represent an alternative administration route (defined as the upper airways and alveoli, accessed by oral inhalation) exhibiting significant rates of peptide absorption in the absence of enhancers following aerosol inhalation. Conjectures on the mechanism of uptake of peptides across the alveolar epithelial type 1 cells, representing a surface area up to 140 m^2, have been discussed recently (Patton & Platz, 1992), and determinants of polypeptide bioavailability reviewed (Byron, 1990).

In a short-term clinical study (Elliott *et al.*, 1987), with normal individuals and diabetic children (n = 6), an efficiency of insulin absorption of 20–25% was estimated in normal subjects, based on *in vivo* C-peptide response. Absorption efficiency in diabetic children was difficult to calculate, due to poor matching of results on days with subcutaneous administration as compared to days with nebulized insulin delivery. Several patients appeared to have significant functional alterations in flow parameters of lung function over the study period. In another clinical study (Köhler *et al.*, 1987) with healthy volunteers (smokers and non-smokers), a bioavailability of 25% was claimed for non-smokers and 75% for smokers, with a plasma insulin peak reached after 15–20 min. However, appropriate controls and C-peptide values were not shown. As for nasal insulin, pulmonary insulin absorption profiles exhibit a rapid onset, sharp plasma insulin peak, compatible with meal-related insulin delivery (Patton & Platz, 1992).

If the pulmonary route were to be accepted as a potential delivery site for clinical use, considerable effort must be put into two lines of research: first, device technology, to develop a portable and convenient device exhibiting reproducible administration, and second, safety aspects, including local immune response, induction of allergic response, and chronic effect on pulmonary function, especially as pulmonary dysfunction is an early measurable complication in IDDM (Sandler, 1990; Sandler *et al.*, 1986).

43.5.2 OCULAR DELIVERY

Delivery of insulin via the eyes is the least desirable administration route for such a systemic chronic drug delivery, and unlikely to be a clinical possibility. Undoubtedly, it is possible to obtain systemic absorption of polypeptides via this route, with absorption occurring via both conjunctival mucosa and, after drainage, the nasal mucosa (Yamamoto *et al.*, 1989). Nomura *et al.* (1990) showed a peak plasma insulin at approx. 30 min postadministration, and a calculated 'bioavailability' of between 1–7% (dose-dependent) in diabetic dogs, and <0.5% in normal dogs in the absence of enhancers, and with no histological changes after 2 months' administration. Yamamoto *et al.* (1989) showed poor absorption of insulin alone to the systemic circulation in a rabbit model, and studied the effect of various absorption promoters. The authors concluded that the ocular route was unlikely to be widely accepted 'because of the innate aversion to instilling drugs to the eye, and because of perceived sensitivity of the eye, notably the corneal epithelium, to external insult (p. 255).

43.5.3 BUCCAL ADMINISTRATION

Mucous membranes (buccal, sublingual) of the oral cavity are used as sites for systemic drug delivery. The sublingual area is apparently more permeable to low molecular weight drugs, but not so convenient a site for attachment of retentive/occluding delivery systems, necessary to reduce salivary clearance of the drug (Harris & Robinson, 1992). For insulin, buccal administration has been most studied. Human buccal mucosa is a highly vascularized, stratified squamous epithelium, about 100–400 μm in thickness, with penetrant drugs entering the systemic circulation. Buccal delivery has recently been reviewed as a route for delivery of proteinaceous substances (Ho *et al.*, 1992). For insulin, bioavailability in the absence of enhancers is very low, despite the relatively low peptidase activity. In a rabbit study, no hypoglycemic response could be demonstrated in the absence of absorption enhancers (Oh & Ritschel, 1990), with insulin administered via a buccal cell. Another study quoted an efficiency of 'less than 4% (3.6%)', compared to intramuscular administration (Aungst & Rogers, 1989). However, this value is based on fall of blood glucose alone, and shows a large statistical variation. Absorption of insulin can be increased in the presence of enhancers (Aungst & Rogers, 1989; Oh & Ritschel, 1990). A wide variety of devices for drug delivery in the oral cavity have been suggested, although no published clinical data are available for insulin.

43.5.4 IMPLANTS

Several systems for small, sustained release implants designed for basal insulin therapy have been tested over the years, and have been reviewed in depth by Wang (1991a). These include both non-biodegradable and biodegradable/erodable systems, and a wide range of variable dose implants. Ethylene-vinyl acetate co-polymer matrices, implanted subcutaneously into diabetic rats, achieved normoglycemia for 100 days with one implant (Brown *et al.*, 1986a & 1986b), and palmitic acid implants achieved glycemic control over a period of 33 days (Wang, 1991b). Development of these invasive approaches for clinical consideration must include reproducible and accurate prediction of sustained insulin release, absence of hypoglycemic events related to the presence of a large insulin depot in the body and absence of local reaction, e.g., fibrous overgrowth.

43.6 CONCLUSIONS

At the present time, it is difficult to evaluate which 'new routes' will show the greatest progress clinically over the next decade. Undoubtedly, for children, a regimen combining nasal (bolus) and transdermal (basal) delivery, would represent a more convenient, non-invasive therapy, with possible improvement in metabolic control and intrapatient variability, although still achieving systemical delivery. To achieve the full benefit, this regimen would have to be used in combination with a noninvasive glucose determination. However, it is still questionable whether these administration forms can be satisfactorily clinically and commercially developed.

REFERENCES

Aungst, B.J. and Rogers, N.J. (1988) Site dependence of absorption-promoting actions of Laureth-9, Na salicylate, Na_2EDTA, and aprotinin on rectal, nasal, and buccal insulin delivery. *Pharmacol. Res.*, **5**, 305–308.

Aungst, B.J. and Rogers, N.J. (1989) Comparison of the effects of various transmucosal absorption promoters on buccal insulin delivery. *Int. J. Pharmaceutics*, **53**, 227–35.

Brange, J., Owens, D.R., Kang, S. *et al.* (1990) Monomeric insulins and their experimental and clinical implications. *Diabetes Care*, **13**: 9, 923–54.

Brown, L., Munoz, C., Siemer, L. *et al.* (1986a) Controlled release of insulin from polymer martrices. Control of diabetes in rats. *Diabetes*, **35**, 692–97.

Brown, L., Siemer, L., Munoz, C. *et al.* (1986b) Controlled release of insulin from polymer matrices. *In vitro* kinetics. *Diabetes*, **35**, 684–91.

Bruce, D.G., Chisholm, D.J., Storlien, L.H. *et al.* (1991) Meal-time intranasal insulin delivery in Type 2 diabetes. *Diabetic Med.*, **8**, 336–70.

Burnette, R.R. (1989) 'Iontophoresis', in J. Hadgraft and R.H. Guy (eds). *Transdermal Drug Delivery: Developmental Issues and Research Initiatives*, pp. 247–91. Marcel Dekker, New York.

Byron, P. (1990) Determinants of drug and poly peptide bioavailability from aerosols delivered to the lung. *Adv. Drug Deliv. Rev.*, **5**, 107–132.

Carstens, S., Danielsen, G., Guldhammer, B. *et al.* (1991) 'Transport mechanisms for phospholipid-induced insulin absorption across the *in vitro* rabbit nasal mucosa (abstract)', in D. Duchêne (ed.). *Buccal and Nasal Administration as an Alternative to Parenteral Administration*, p. 264. Editions De Santé, Paris.

Chien, Y.W. (1991) 'Transdermal route of peptide and protein drug delivery', in V.H.L. Lee (ed.). *Peptide and Protein Drug Delivery*, pp. 667–89. Marcel Dekker; New York, Basel, Hong Kong.

Cho, Y.W. and Flynn, M. (1989) Oral delivery of insulin. *Lancet*, **ii**, 1518–19.

Crane, C.W., Path, M.C. and Luntz, G.R.W.N. (1968) Absorption of insulin from the human small intestine. *Diabetes*, **17**, 625–27.

Cullander, C. (1992) What are the pathways of iontophoretic current flow through mammalian skin? *Adv. Drug Deliv. Rev.*, **9**, 119–35.

Damgé, C. (1991) 'Oral insulin', in J.C. Pickup (ed.). *Biotechnology of Insulin Therapy*, pp. 97–112. Blackwell Scientific Publications, London.

Damgé, C., Michel, C., Aprahamiam, M. *et al.* (1990) Nanocapsules as carriers for oral peptide delivery. *J. Controlled Release*, **13**, 233–39.

Davis, S.S. (1990) Overcoming barriers to the oral administration of peptide drugs. *Trends in Pharmacological Sciences*, **11**, 353–55.

de Boer, A.G., van Hoogdalem, E.J. and Breimer, D.D. (1992) Rate-controlled rectal peptide drug absorption enhancement. *Adv. Drug Deliv. Rev.*, **8**, 237–51.

DelTerzo, S., Behl, C.R. and Nash, R.A. (1989) Iontophoretic transport of a homologous series of ionized and nonionized model compounds: Influence of hydrophobicity and mechanistic interpretation. *Pharm. Res.*, **6**, 85–90.

Drejer, K., Vaag, A., Bech, K. *et al.* (1992) Intranasal administration of insulin with phospholipid as absorption enhancer: Pharmacokinetics in normal subjects. *Diabetic Med.*, **9**, 335–40.

Edman, P. and Björk, E. (1992) Nasal delivery of peptide drugs. *Adv. Drug Deliv. Rev.*, **8**, 165–77.

Elliott, R.B., Edgar, B.W., Pilcher, C.C. *et al.* (1987) Parenteral absorption of insulin from the lung in diabetic children. *Austral. Paediatr. J.*, **23**, 293–97.

Farraj, N.F., Jørgensen, H., Johansen, B.R. *et al.* (1989) Insulin delivery via the nasal route using bioadhesive microspheres. *Diabetes*, **38** (suppl. 2), A604.

Frauman, A.G., Cooper, M.E., Parsons, B.J. *et al.* (1987) Long-term use of intranasal insulin in insulin-dependent diabetic patients. *Diabetes Care*, **10**, 573–78.

Gizurarson, S. and Bechgaard, E. (1991) Intranasal administration of insulin to humans. *Diabetes Res. Clin. Prac.*, **12**, 71–84.

Guldhammer, B., Drejer, K., Engesgaard, A. *et al.* (1988) The absorption of intranasally administered insulin demonstrated by immunohistochemistry (abstract). *Diabetes Res. Clin. Prac.*, **5** (suppl. 1), 164.

Harris D. and Robinson, J.R. (1992) Drug delivery via the mucous membranes of the oral cavity. *J. Pharmaceutical Sciences*, **81**:1, 1–10.

Hirai, S., Ikenaga, T. and Matsuzawa, T. (1978) Nasal absorption of insulin in dogs. *Diabetes*, **27**, 296–99.

Hirai, S., Yashiki, T. and Mima, H. (1981) Mechanisms for the enhancement of the nasal absorption of insulin by surfactants. *Int. J. Pharmaceutics*, **9**, 173–84.

Ho, N.F.H., Barsuhn, C.L., Burton, P.S. *et al.* (1992) Mechanistic insights to buccal delivery of proteinaceous substances. *Adv. Drug Delivery Rev.*, **8**, 197–235.

Holman, R.R. and Steemson, J. (1991) Nasal insulin in type I diabetes. *Diabetic Med.*, **8** (suppl. 1), A5.

Holman, R.R. and Steemson, J. (1992) Nasal insulin outpatient study in type I diabetes. *Diabetologia*, **35** (suppl. 1), A14.

Illum, L., Jørgensen, H., Bisgaard, H. *et al.* (1987) Bioadhesive microspheres as a potential nasal drug delivery system. *Int. J. Pharmaceutics*, **39**, 189–99.

Jacobs, M.A.J.M., Schreuder, R.H., Jap-a-Joe, H.K. *et al.* (1991) Euglycaemic clamp study on the pharmacodynamics of intranasal insulin. *Diabetologia*, **34** (suppl. 2), A182.

Kari, B. (1986) Control of blood glucose levels in alloxan-diabetic rabbits by iontophoresis of insulin. *Diabetes*, **35**, 217–21.

Kimmerle, R., Griffing, G., McCall, A. *et al.* (1991) Could intranasal insulin be useful in the treatment of non-insulin-dependent diabetes mellitus? *Diabetes Res. Clin. Prac.*, **13**, 69–76.

Köhler, D., Schlüter, K.J., Kerp, L. *et al.* (1987) Nicht radioactives Verfahren zur Messung der Lungepermeabilität: Inhalation von Insulin. *Atemw.-Lungenkrkh.*, **13**:6, 230–32.

Langkjær, L., Brange, J., Grodsky, G.M. *et al.* (1993) Basal-rate transdermal delivery of monomeric insulins by iontophoresis. *Diabetalogia*, **36** (suppl. 1), A161.

Langkjær, L., Brange, J., Grodsky, G.M. *et al.* (1994) Transdermal delivery of monomeric insulin analogues by iontophoresis. *Proc. Int. Symp. Control. Rel. Bioact. Mater.*, **21**, 172–73.

Lassmann-Vague, V. (1991) 'The intranasal route for insulin administration', in J.C. Pickup (ed.). *Biotechnology of Insulin Therapy*, pp. 113–25. Blackwell Scientific Publications, London.

Ledger, P.W. (1992) Skin biological issues in electrically enhanced transdermal delivery. *Adv. Drug Delivery Rev.*, **9**, 289–307.

Lee, V.H.L. (ed.). (1991) *Peptide and Protein Drug Deliv.*, Marcel Dekker; New York, Basel, Hong Kong.

Liu, J.-C., Sun, Y., Siddiqui, O. *et al.* (1988) Blood glucose control in diabetic rats by transdermal iontophoretic delivery of insulin. *Int. J. Pharmaceutics*, **44**, 197–204.

Meyer, B.R., Katzeff, H.L., Eschbach, J.C. *et al.* (1989) Transdermal delivery of human insulin to albino rabbits using electrical current. *Am. J. Med. Sciences*, **297**, 321–25.

Moses, A.C., Gordon, G.S., Carey, M.C. *et al.* (1983) Insulin administered intranasally as an insulin-bile salt aerosol: Effectiveness and reproducibility in normal and diabetic subjects. *Diabetes*, **32**, 1040–47.

Muranishi, S. (1990) Absorption enhancers. *Critical Reviews™ in Therapeutic Drug Carrier Systems*, **7**:1, 1–33.

Nishihata, T., Sudoh, M., Inagaki, H. *et al.* (1987) An effective formulation for an insulin suppository; examination in normal dogs. *Int. J. Pharmaceutics*, **38**, 83–90.

Nolte, M.S., Taboga, C., Salamon, E. *et al.* (1990) Biological activity of nasally administered insulin in normal subjects. *Horm. Metab. Res.*, **22**, 170–74.

Nomura, M., Kubota, M.A., Sekiya, M. *et al.* (1990) Insulin absorption from conjunctiva studied in normal and diabetic dogs. *J. Pharmacy and Pharmacology*, **42**, 292–94.

Oh, C.K. and Ritschel, W.A. (1990) Biopharmaceutic aspects of buccal absorption of insulin. *Meth. Find. Exp. Clin. Pharmacol.*, **12**:3, 205–212.

Patton. J.S. and Platz, R.M. (1992) Pulmonary delivery of peptides and proteins for systemic action. *Adv. Drug Deliv. Rev.*, **8**, 179–96.

Pickup, J.C. (ed.). (1991a) *Biotechnology of Insulin Therapy*. Blackwell Scientific Publications, London.

Pickup, J.C. (1991b) 'An introduction to the problems of insulin delivery', in J.C. Pickup (ed.). *Biotechnology of Insulin Therapy*, pp. 1–23. Blackwell Scientific Publications.

Pikal, M.J. (1992) The role of electro-osmotic flow in transdermal iontophoresis. *Adv. Drug Deliv. Rev.*, **9**, 201–237.

Pontiroli, A.E., Alberetto, M., Secchi, A. *et al.* (1982) Insulin given intranasally induces hypoglycaemia in normal and diabetic subjects. *Brit. Med. J.*, **284**, 303–306.

Saffran, M., Kumar, G.S., Savariar, C. *et al.* (1986) A new approach to the oral administration of insulin and other peptide drugs. *Science*, **233**, 1081–84.

Saffran, M., Field, J.B., Peña, J. *et al.* (1991) Oral insulin in diabetic dogs. *J. Endocrinol.*, **131**, 267–78.

Sage, B.H. and Riviere, J.E. (1992) Model systems in iontophoresis – transport efficacy. *Adv. Drug Deliv. Rev.*, **9**, 265–87.

Salzman, R., Manson, J.E., Griffling, G.T. *et al.* (1985) Intranasal aerosolized insulin: Mixed meal studies and long-term use in type I diabetes. *N. Eng. J. Med.*, **312**, 1078–84.

Sandler, M. (1990) Is the lung a 'target organ' in diabetes mellitus? *Arch. Int. Med.*, **150**, 1385–88.

Sandler, M., Bunn, A.E. and Stewart, R.I. (1986) Pulmonary function in young insulin-dependent diabetic subjects. *Chest*, **90**, 670–75.

Siddiqui, O., Sun, Y., Liu, J.-C. *et al.* (1987) Facilitated transdermal transport of insulin. *J. Pharm. Sciences*, **76**:4, 341–45.

Sinay, I.R., Schlimovich, S., Damilano, S. *et al.* (1990) Intranasal insulin administration in insulin dependent diabetes: Reproducibility of its absorption and effects. *Horm. Metab. Res.*, **22**, 307–308.

Smith, P.L., Wall, D.A., Gochoco, C.H. *et al.* (1992) Oral absorption of peptides and proteins. *Adv. Drug Deliv. Rev.*, **8**, 253–90.

Stephen, R.L., Petelenz, T.J. and Jacobsen, S.C. (1984) Potential novel methods for insulin administration: I. Iontophoresis. *Biomedica Biochim. Acta*, **43**, 553–58.

Taskinen, M.-R., Sane, T., Helve, E. *et al.* (1989) Bedtime insulin for suppression of overnight free-fatty acid, blood glucose, and glucose production in NIDDM. *Diabetes*, **38**, 580–88.

Thow, J.C. and Home, P.D. (1992) A double blind, placebo controlled dose response study of nasal insulin in relation to a standard meal in type 2 diabetic subjects. *Diabetologia*, **35** (suppl. 1), A14.

van Hoogdalem, E.J., Heijliers-Feijen, C.D., Verhoef, J.C. *et al.* (1990) Absorption enhancement of rectally infused insulin by sodium tauro-24,25-dihydrofusidate (STDHF) in rats. *Pharmacol. Res.*, **7**, 180–83.

Waldhäusl, W.K. (1986) The physiological basis of insulin treatment – clinical aspects. *Diabetologia*, **29**, 837–49.

Wang, P.Y. (1991a) 'Sustained-release implants for insulin delivery', in J.C. Pickup (ed.). *Biotechnology of Insulin Therapy*, pp. 42–74. Blackwell Scientific Publications, London.

Wang, P.Y. (1991b) Palmitic acid as an excipient in implants for sustained release of insulin. *Biomaterials*, **12**, 57–62.

Woodyatt, R.T. (1922) The clinical use of insulin. *J. Metab. Res.*, **2**, 793–801.

Yamamoto, A., Luo, A.M., Dodda-Kashi, S. *et al.* (1989) The ocular route for systemic insulin delivery in the albino rabbit. *J. Pharmacol. Exper. Therapeutics*, **249**:1, 249–55.

Yamamoto, A., Hayakawa, E., Kato, Y. *et al.* (1992) A mechanistic study on enhancement of rectal permeability to insulin in the albino rabbit. *J. Pharmacol. Exper. Therapeutics*, **263**:1, 25–31.

Yoshida, N.H. and Roberts, M.S. (1992) Structure-transport relationships in transdermal iontophoresis. *Adv. Drug Deliv. Rev.*, **9**, 239–64.

44

Biosensors and feedback-controlled systems

J.C. PICKUP

44.1 INTRODUCTION

Biosensors are miniature analytical probes in which a biological recognition molecule such as an enzyme, antibody, receptor, lectin, etc. is coupled to an electronic transducer (Figure 44.1). Binding of an analyte to the receptor is detected by the transducer and the electronic signal is processed and displayed to give a measure of analyte concentration (Pickup, 1985a; Turner *et al.*, 1987).

The special advantages of biosensors compared to conventional methods of analysis are: (a) no added reagent is needed, (b) no sample manipulation such as centrifugation is necessary, (c) the sample is not consumed, so that very small volumes can be measured, (d) the response is rapid (usually within seconds), (e) the small size of the probe enables the device to be portable or to monitor at sites within the body (organs, tissues, blood vessels) and (f) analyte measurement can be continuous.

Biosensors are generally employed in three ways (Figure 44.2). *In vitro* sensing is where the probe is placed in a sample of biological fluid such as blood, serum, plasma or urine outside of the body, for example, in a bench-top blood glucose analyzer or a portable meter for home monitoring of capillary blood glucose levels. *In vivo* sensors monitor changes within the body using an implanted or surface detector. *Ex vivo* sensors are incorporated into a flow-through cell outside of the body, through which blood (or perhaps breath or urine) is pumped or otherwise directed.

In the context of diabetes, the particular application for an *in vivo* sensor which comes most readily to mind is an implanted glucose sensor which forms part of a closed-loop insulin delivery system (artificial endocrine pancreas). Equally important though, is the requirement for a hypoglycemia alarm to alert the patient to dangerously low glucose levels and the need to take corrective action. This type of *in vivo* sensor could be used over a relatively short time, say 12–24 hours, and has no need for complicated automatic feedback mechanisms. Its introduction into clinical practice in the near future is therefore more feasible than for an artificial pancreas.

Ex vivo sensors will most probably be of use in diabetes for short-term metabolic monitoring during surgery, parturition and in the intensive care setting.

Diabetes is, in fact, considered by clinicians of all medical specialities to be the condition

Childhood and Adolescent Diabetes
Published in 1994 by Chapman & Hall, London
ISBN 0 412 48610 5

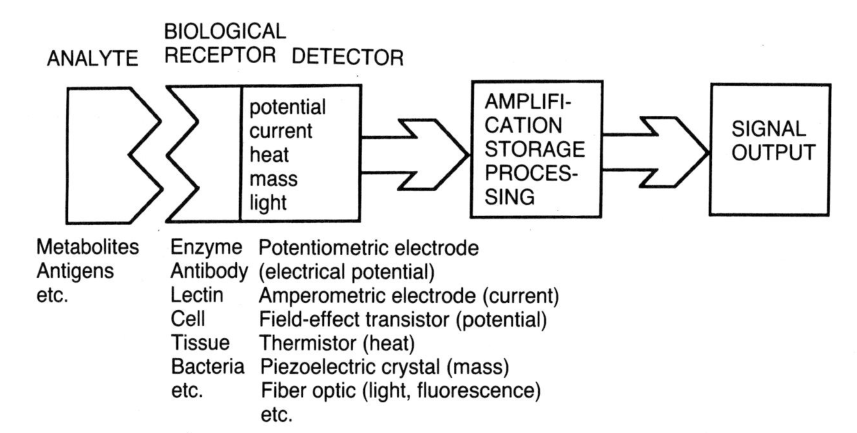

Figure 44.1 The principle of biosensor operation. An analyte binds to a biological receptor which is immobilized on a detector. The receptor may be an enzyme, antibody, lectin, etc. and the detector an electrode, thermistor, piezoelectric crystal or fiber optic. The resulting signal is amplified, stored and processed to produce an output which is a measure of the analyte concentration.

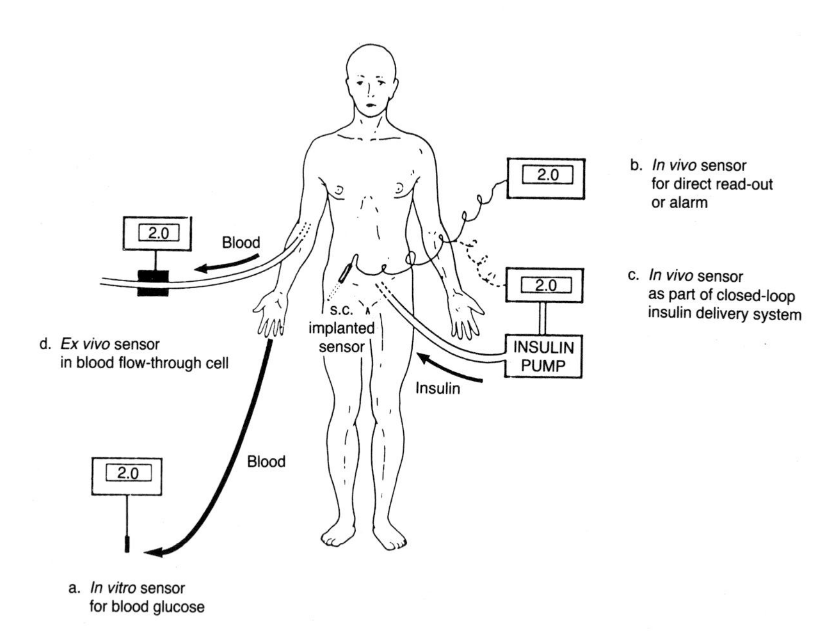

Figure 44.2 Uses for biosensors in medicine, for example, a glucose sensor – (a) an *in vitro* device such as a meter for home blood glucose monitoring; (b) an *in vivo* sensor comprising a subcutaneously-implanted electrode connected to a meter, for example, a hypoglycemia alarm; (c) an *in vivo* sensor used as part of a closed-loop insulin delivery system – insulin delivery is controlled by a computer according to pre-set algorithms; (d) an *ex vivo* system where blood is pumped from a peripheral vein through a cell containing the sensor.

where *in vivo* or *ex vivo* biosensors are most likely to be of clinical use in the future (Pickup & Alcock, 1991). Glucose is the analyte which is thought to be most appropriate for sensing in diabetes, of course, but a case might be made for continuous monitoring of other substances such as hydrogen ion, potassium, lactate, blood gases and perhaps ketone bodies. The number of potential applications for *in vitro* biosensors in diabetes is enormous and could include most of the assays for metabolites and hormones currently performed in clinical practice and research.

Finally, it should be said that the development of biosensors has particular relevance for pediatric practice for a number of reasons: either very small blood samples, or in the case of *in vivo* probes, no sample at all, need be taken; feedback-controlled insulin delivery systems and alarms for hypo- and hyperglycemia will be especially useful in the unpredictably brittle diabetic patient, who is often in the adolescent age group (Pickup, 1985b); and sensors implanted over an extended period of time may be preferable to those patients, often children, who dislike frequent intermittent finger pricks for home blood glucose monitoring.

44.2 BIOSENSOR TECHNOLOGY: A BRIEF GUIDE

44.2.1 ENZYME ELECTRODES

In these devices, an enzyme is immobilized over a detector or 'base' electrode (Figure 44.3) which monitors the accumulation of a reaction product or the diminution of substrate. The glucose oxidase-based glucose sensor is a good example, where the following reaction occurs:

$$\text{glucose} + \text{oxygen} \xrightarrow{\text{glucose oxidase}} \text{gluconic acid} + \text{hydrogen peroxide}$$

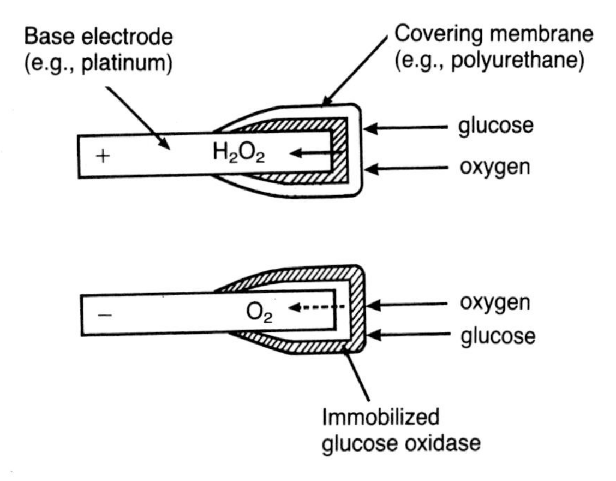

Figure 44.3 Two types of enzyme electrode for monitoring glucose. Upper: glucose oxidase is immobilized over a platinum electrode. Hydrogen peroxide produced by the oxidation of glucose is detected by the positively-charged base electrode. Lower: similar construction except that the base electrode is negatively charged. Oxygen consumption is monitored by the base electrode (from Pickup, 1993a).

Glucose may be monitored by detecting at a positively-charged platinum electrode the hydrogen peroxide which is produced:

$$H_2O_2 \xrightarrow{+700\ \text{mV}} O_2 + 2H^+ + 2e^-$$

This is an example of an amperometric or current-measuring sensor, where the potential is held constant. The Yellow Springs Instrument Glucose Analyser (YSI Ltd, Farnborough, UK) operates on this principle. Another amperometric glucose sensing strategy involves detecting the consumption of oxygen at a negatively-charged platinum electrode:

$$O_2 + 4e^- + 4H^+ \xrightarrow{-700\ \text{mV}} 2H_2O$$

The Beckman Glucose Analyser (Beckman Instruments, High Wycombe, UK) uses this strategy.

With amperometric sensors, the current is

directly proportional to the analyte concentration. However, some products such as the hydrogen ions in the above glucose oxidase-catalyzed reaction can be detected potentiometrically i.e., via a voltage change. Here, the relationship between analyte and signal is logarithmic, according to the Nernst equation:

$$E = E^{\circ} + \frac{RT}{nF} \ln \text{(analyte)}$$

Where E° is a constant, R the gas constant, T the absolute temperature, n the charge number and F the Faraday constant. The commonly-used glass pH electrode is a potentiometric device, but a device which is thought to have special application in biomedicine is the enzyme-coated field effect transistor (ENFET) (Van der Schoot & Bergveld, 1987 & 1988). Here, an enzyme such as glucose oxidase is coated onto the gate of an ion-selective transistor. H^+ production in the enzyme-catalyzed reaction alters the field in the transistor substrate and produces a potential change. These miniaturized sensors can be mass produced using established integrated circuit technology and might enable multiple sensors for different analytes to be built onto one chip. However, at the moment ENFETs have a number of practical difficulties which have prevented their development, such as the fact that the buffering capacity of biological samples decreases the glucose-induced pH changes, there is high output drift and there may be

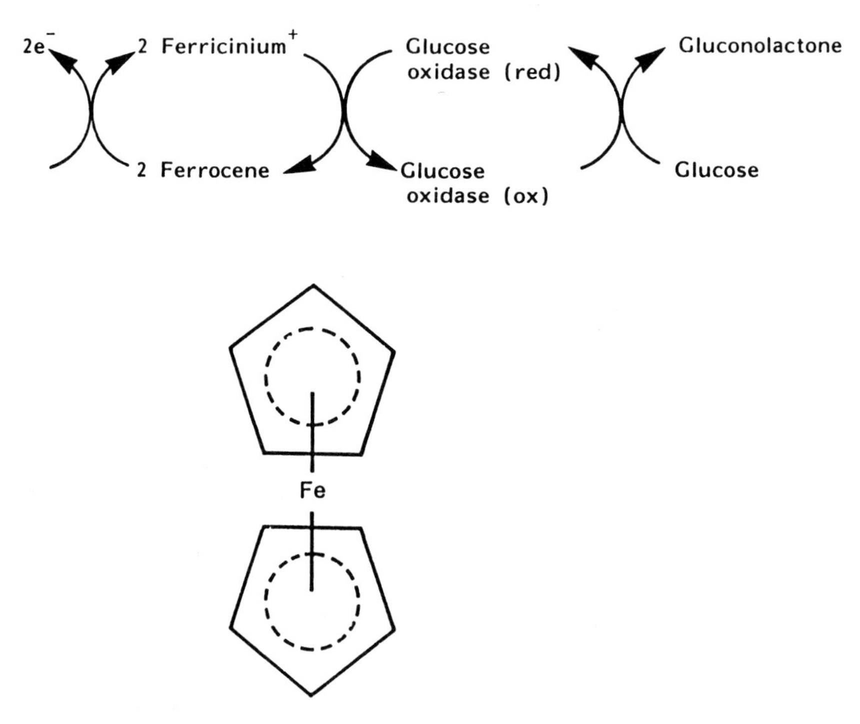

Figure 44.4 The principle of ferrocene-mediated glucose sensors. Ferrocene (lower) in its ferricinium ion form accepts electrons from reduced glucose oxidase and transfers them to a base electrode. Oxygen is not the final electron acceptor and sensors of this type are therefore relatively oxygen insensitive. This principle is used in the Exactech Pen™.

poor sealing of the electrical connections *in vivo*.

A variation of the amperometric enzyme electrode is the 'mediated sensor' (Cass *et al.*, 1984; Claremont *et al.*, 1986; Pickup *et al.*, 1989). Here, a small molecular weight redox couple such as ferrocene shuttles electrons between the enzyme and the base electrode (Figure 44.4). Since oxygen is not the final electron acceptor, the sensor is relatively insensitive to changes in oxygen tension, a major difficulty with unmodified glucose oxidase-based sensors which detect hydrogen peroxide production or oxygen consumption. The Exactech Pen(TM) (Medisense Ltd., Coleshill, UK) is an example of a mediated glucose sensor which has been commercialized as a device for home blood glucose monitoring (Matthews *et al.*, 1987). So-called 'organic metals' such as tetrathiafulvalene tetracyanoquinodimethane ($TTF^{+}TCNQ^{-}$) also form the basis of amperometric sensors. These are organic substances with a high conductivity which act in a similar way to mediators and have been used as enzyme electrodes for glucose assay (Albery *et al.*, 1985; Kulys, 1986).

Most enzyme electrodes are also covered by polymer membranes such as polyurethane and cellulose acetate which play a crucial role in encapsulating the enzyme, restricting the access of inhibitors or co-reactant, increasing the linear range of the sensor and decreasing oxygen dependence (Pickup, 1991).

44.2.2 OPTICAL SYSTEMS

Fiber-optic biosensors have some advantages over electrochemical devices in a clinical setting since they are small, relatively inexpensive, do not require a reference electrode and are electrically isolated from the patient (Seitz, 1984). Glucose oxidase may be immobilized at a fiber optic and gluconic acid detected by a color change in a dye (Goldfinch & Lowe, 1984), or oxygen consumption monitored by an oxygen-sensitive fluorescent dye (Schaffer & Wolfbeis, 1990) and hydrogen peroxide by, for example, a chemiluminescent system (Abdel-Latif & Guilbaut, 1988). A 'bioaffinity probe' is an alternative optical sensor in which the lectin concanavalin A is bound to the inner wall of a hollow dialysis fiber (Mansouri & Schultz, 1984). Competition between glucose and a fluorescently-labeled dextran for binding to the lectin displaces the fluorescent probe into the field of view of the fiber optic.

44.3 PROGRESS TOWARDS *IN VIVO* GLUCOSE SENSING

Although sensing in the vascular compartment would be ideal, the subcutaneous site has received the most attention because of its greater safety, the avoidance of thrombosis and septicemia, and because of the supposed close relationship between interstitial fluid and plasma glucose concentrations. Studies with implanted wicks and perfused microdialysis fibers show that subcutaneous glucose levels are very close to those in blood, except when the blood glucose is changing very rapidly (Fischer *et al.*, 1987; Jansson *et al.*, 1988; Bolinder *et al.*, 1992).

Many glucose sensor designs have been implanted in the subcutaneous tissue of animals and humans and have demonstrated a reasonably good correspondence between the sensor-recorded values and either spontaneous changes in blood glucose concentration or induced increases or decreases which occur with glucose or insulin administration (Claremont *et al.*, 1986; Pickup *et al.*, 1989; Moatti-Sirat *et al.*, 1992; Matthews *et al.*, 1988; Abel *et al.*, 1984; Koudelka *et al.*, 1991). A delay between the peak blood and subcutaneous reading is usual, varying between about 5–30 min (Figure 44.5). It is uncertain whether the magnitude of this delay is dependent on the species in which the sensor is implanted, the sensor design, some charac-

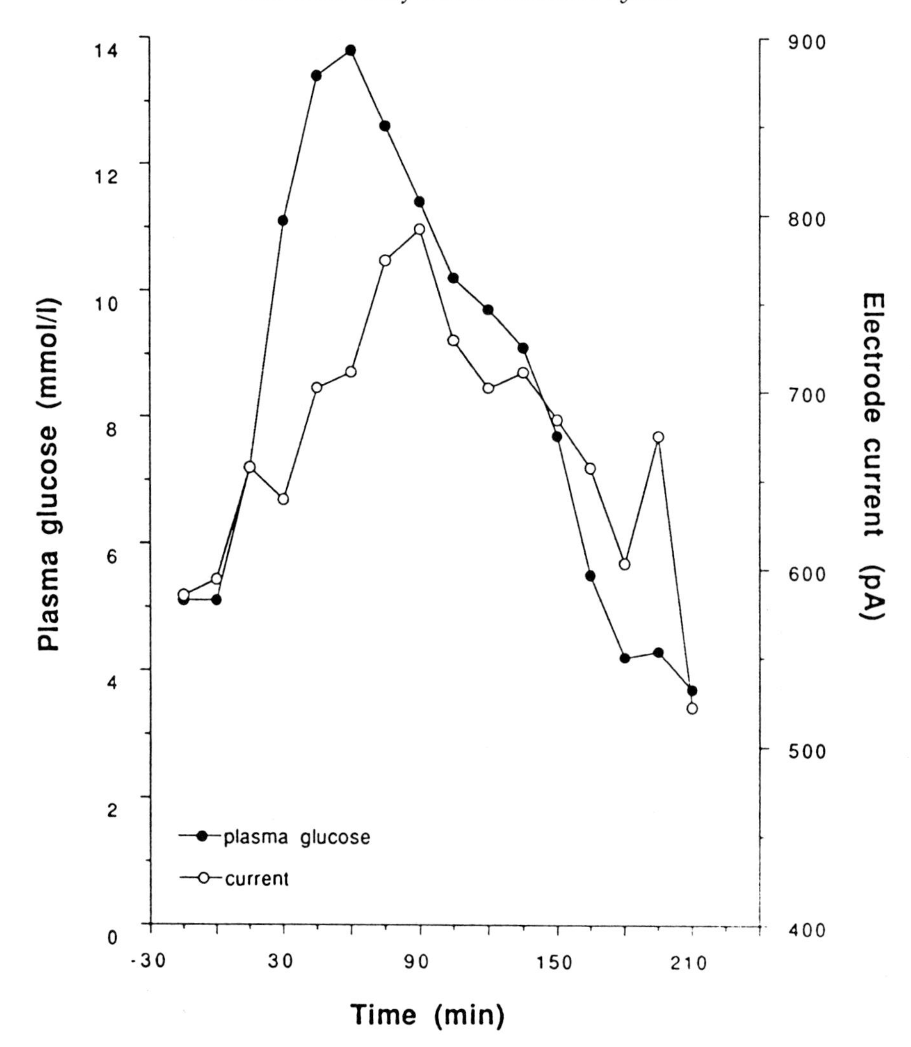

Figure 44.5 Plasma glucose concentration in a nondiabetic volunteer after a 75 g oral glucose load and current output from a subcutaneously-implanted glucose sensor. The sensor was based on glucose oxidase immobilized in a polymer (polyhydroxyethylmethacrylate) at a platinum electrode (Shaw *et al.*, 1991).

teristic of the animal or human such as degree of obesity, or is entirely random. Nevertheless, most investigators consider the delay still to be compatible with a clinically-useful device.

The most serious problem with implanted glucose sensors is a diminished *in vivo* response compared to the sensitively *in vitro*. *In vivo* sensitivities of 20–90% of those *in vitro* are routinely obtained (Bessman *et al.*, 1981; Abel *et al.*, 1984; Shichiri *et al.*, 1984; Claremont *et al.*, 1986) and occasionally almost no response at all is found on implantation (Pickup *et al.*, 1993). This necessitates an *in vivo* calibration procedure which estimates the *in vivo* sensitivity such as by comparing

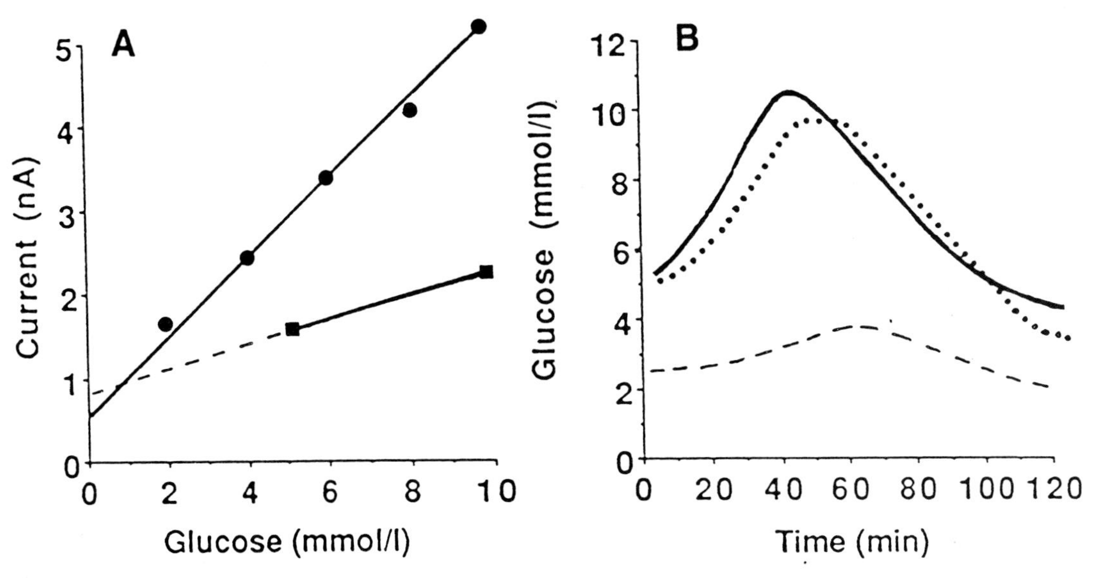

Figure 44.6 (A) *In vitro* calibration of a glucose sensor (●) and later *in vivo* calibration (■) showing reduced sensivity. (B) Plasma glucose after a 75 g oral glucose load in nondiabetics (——); subcutaneous glucose concentrations recorded by a sensor calibrated *in vitro* (------); subcutaneous glucose levels calculated using *in vivo* calibration curve in A (……). (From Pickup, 1993b, with permission of the American Diabetes Association.)

the sensor current and simultaneously-measured blood glucose value at a basal level and after an intravenous or oral glucose load or after insulin administration (Velho *et al.*, 1989; Pickup *et al.*, 1993) (Figure 44.6).

The reason for the impaired sensitivity *in vivo* is unknown. The possibilities include consumption of glucose by the sensor itself in the micro-environment of the device, coupled with slow mass transport of glucose through the interstitial gel. There may also be interfering substances *in vivo* which alter the electrochemistry of the sensor.

Although sensors can now be constructed which are stable in operation *in vitro* for several days, implanted glucose sensors may suffer unpredictable oscillations or drift in response (Rebrin *et al.*, 1992; Moatti-Sirat *et al.*, 1992). It has been suggested that inflammatory cells at the site of implantation may metabolize glucose and contribute to the impaired response (Rebrin *et al.*, 1992).

Difficulties with biocompatibility of sensors have stimulated recent research in the technique of microdialysis. Here, a fine hollow fiber of cellulose or similar dialysis membrane is implanted in the tissue and perfused with isotonic fluid (Mascini *et al.*, 1992; Meyerhoff *et al.*, 1992). Glucose diffusing into the perfusate from the interstitial space can be monitored by a sensor outside of the body, thus avoiding direct contact between the sensor and the tissues. Such devices function well over the course of a day or so (Meyerhoff *et al.*, 1992) but the long-term practicability for routine patient use is uncertain.

44.4 CLOSING THE LOOP

Feedback-controlled systems were first developed from adapted laboratory autoanalyzers some 30 years ago (Kadish, 1964). In the 1970s, bedside apparatuses were introduced

(Albisser *et al.*, 1974; Pfeiffer *et al.*, 1974) with computer control and at least one was commercialized as the Biostator™. In the latter, diluted blood from a peripheral vein was pumped through an *ex vivo* flow-through sensor based on hydrogen peroxide detection at a glucose oxidase sensor. Algorithms were used to set the insulin infusion rate according to the absolute glucose concentration and the rate of change, thus ensuring rapid delivery at meal-times, attenuation with falling blood glucose levels and a correction for the delay between blood withdrawal and sensing. A smaller artificial pancreas has been introduced more recently (Betalike™, Esaote Biomedical, Genoa, Italy) where blood is ultrafiltered and sensing achieved by the membrane system from the Yellow Springs Glucose Analyser.

Early work employed the artificial pancreas in a variety of research studies examining, for example, the effect of glycemic normalization on hormones and intermediary metabolites (Horwitz *et al.*, 1979; Nosadini *et al.*, 1982) and possible therapeutic uses such as management of diabetes during surgery, childbirth and ketoacidosis (Nattrass *et al.*, 1978; Schwartz *et al.*, 1979; Pfeiffer & Kerner, 1981). However, the device has never become a routine in clinical practice because of its size, complexity and cost, and the use of venous route for blood sampling and insulin delivery, which restricts studies to a day or so. Instead, efforts have turned to development of implantable glucose sensors and miniaturization of the artificial pancreas.

The introduction of continuous subcutaneous insulin infusion in the late 1970s (Pickup *et al.*, 1978) established open-loop insulin delivery with a portable pump as a safe and effective means of achieving long-term near normoglycemia in diabetic patients. Linking of subcutaneously-implanted glucose sensors to insulin pumps has been reported by at least two groups on an experimental basis (Shichiri *et al.*, 1983; Rebrin *et al.*, 1989), but the notion has not yet progressed to clinical application, primarily because of the limited and unpredictable lifetime of the sensing component, rather than because of faults with the insulin delivery system.

44.5 PROSPECTS FOR NON-INVASIVE SENSING

In the near-infrared region of about 700–1000 nm, radiation passes through several centimeters of biological tissue (Jöbsis, 1977). Glucose has a number of absorption peaks in this range which might be used for non-invasive sensing, though water also has a large peak and other metabolites also absorb in the near-infrared region (Zeller *et al.*, 1989; Arnold & Small, 1990). Variable light scattering in the tissues may also produce unpredictable alterations in the optical pathlength (Alcock *et al.*, 1992). In spite of these potential difficulties, three groups have recently reported encouraging first studies of non-invasive sensing of glucose with near-infrared spectroscopy (Rosenthal & Paynter, 1991; Noda *et al.*, 1992; Robinson *et al.*, 1992). A particularly promising approach uses multivariate calibration methods with the index finger as the sensing site (Robinson *et al.*, 1992).

44.6 CONCLUSIONS

In vitro biosensors have already entered routine clinical practice. Although several problems remain with the bioperformance of *in vivo* sensors such as those for glucose monitoring, a simple short-term alarm for altered blood glucose levels (e.g., hypoglycemia) is now feasible within the next few years. In order to extend operation of sensors to several days, more understanding of the host response to the implanted electrode must be gained and, probably, new techniques must be developed for improving biocompatibility.

Non-invasive sensing is in its infancy. It is not known whether a portable, continuously-operating monitor for metabolites such as glucose can be developed. But first studies are encouraging and indicate that work should continue in this potentially exciting area.

REFERENCES

Abdel-Latif, M.S. and Guilbaut, G.G. (1988) Fiber-optic sensor for the determination of glucose using micellar enhanced chemiluminescene of the peroxyoxalate reaction. *Anal. Chem.*, **60**, 2671–74.

Abel, P., Müller, A. and Fischer, U. (1984) Experience with an implantable glucose sensor as a prerequisite of an artificial β-cell. *Biomed. Biochim. Acta*, **43**, 577–84.

Albery, W.J., Bartlett, P.N. and Craston, D.H. (1985) Amperometric enzyme electrodes. II. Conducting salts as electrode materials for the oxidation of glucose oxidase. *J. Electroana. Chem.*, **194**, 223–35.

Albisser, A.M., Leibel, B.S., Ewart, J.G. *et al.* (1974) Clinical control of diabetes by the artificial pancreas. *Diabetes*, **23**, 396–404.

Alcock, S.J., Danielsson, B. and Turner, A.P.F. (1992) Advances in the use of *in vivo* sensors. *Biosensors and Bioelectronics*, **7**, 243–54.

Arnold, M.A. and Small, G.W. (1990) Determination of physiological levels of glucose in an aqueous matrix with digitally filtered Fourier transform near infrared spectra. *Anal. Chem.*, **62**, 1457–64.

Bessman, S.P., Thomas, L.J., Kojima, H. *et al.* (1981) The implantation of a closed loop artificial β-cell in dogs. *Trans. Am. Soc. Artif. Int. Org.*, **27**, 7–18.

Bolinder, J., Ungerstedt, U. and Arner, P. (1992) Microdialysis measurement of the absolute glucose concentration in subcutaneous adipose tissue allowing glucose monitoring in diabetic patients. *Diabetologia*, **35**, 1177–80.

Cass, A.E.G., Davis, G., Francis, G.D. *et al.* (1984) Ferrocene-mediated enzyme electrode for amperometric determination of glucose. *Anal. Chem.*, **56**, 667–71.

Claremont, D.J., Sambrook, I.E., Penton, C. *et al.* (1986) Subcutaneous implantation of a ferrocene-mediated glucose sensor in pigs. *Diabetologia*, **29**, 817–21.

Fischer, U., Ertle, R., Abel, P. *et al.* (1987) Assessment of subcutaneous glucose concentrations: validation of the wick technique as a reference for implanted electrochemical sensors in normal and diabetic dogs. *Diabetologia*, **30**, 940–45.

Goldfinch, M.J. and Lowe, C.R. (1984) Solid-phase optoelectronic sensors for biochemical analysis. *Anal. Biochem.*, **138**, 430–36.

Horwitz, D.L., Gonen, B., Jaspan, J.B. *et al.* (1979) An 'artificial beta cell' for control of diabetes mellitus: effect on plasma glucagon levels. *Clin. Endocrin.*, **11**, 639–44.

Jansson, P.A., Smith, J.F.U. and Lönnroth, P. (1988) Characterization by microdialysis of intercellular glucose level in subcutaneous tissue in humans. *Am. J. Physiol.*, **255**, E218–20.

Jöbsis, F.F. (1977) Non-invasive infrared monitoring of cerebral and myocardial oxygen insufficiency and circulatory parameters. *Science*, **198**, 1264–67.

Kadish, A.H. (1964) Automation control of blood sugar. *Am. J. Med. Electronics*, **3**, 82–86.

Koudelka, M., Rohner-Jeanrenaud, F., Terrattaz, J. *et al.* (1991) *In vivo* behaviour of hypodermically implanted microfabricated glucose sensors. *Biosensors and Bioelectronics*, **6**, 31–36.

Kulys, J.H. (1986) Enzyme electrodes based on organic metal. *Biosensors*, **2**, 3–13.

Mansouri, S. and Schulz, J.S. (1984) A miniature optical glucose sensor based on affinity binding. *Biotechnology*, **2**, 885–90.

Mascini, M., Moscone, D. and Bernard, L. (1992) *In vivo* continuous monitoring of glucose by microdialysis and a glucose sensor. *Sensors and Actuators B*, **6**, 143–45.

Matthews, D.R., Bown, E., Beck, T.W. *et al.* (1988) An amperometric needle-type glucose sensors tested in rats and man. *Diabetic Med.*, **5**, 248–52.

Matthews, D.R., Holman, R.R., Bown, E. *et al.* (1987) Pen-sized digital 30-second blood glucose meter. *Lancet*, **i**, 778–79.

Meyerhoff, C., Bischof, F., Sternberg, F. *et al.* (1992) On line continuous monitoring of subcutaneous tissue glucose in men by combining portable glucosensor with microdialysis. *Diabetologia*, **35**, 1087–92.

Moatti-Sirat, D., Capron, F., Poitout, V. *et al.* (1992) Towards continuous glucose monitoring: *in vivo* evaluation of a miniaturized glucose sensor implanted for several days in rat subcutaneous tissue. *Diabetologia*, **35**, 224–30.

Nattrass, M., Alberti, K.G.M.M., Dennis, K.J. *et al.* (1978) A glucose controlled insulin infusion system for diabetic women during labour. *Brit. Med. J.*, **2**, 599–601.

Noda, M., Taniguchi, N., Kimura, M. *et al.* (1992) Completely non-invasive measurements of human blood glucose *in vivo* using near infrared waves. *Diabetologia*, **35** (suppl. 1), 204A.

Nosadini, R., Noy, G., Nattrass, M. *et al.* (1982) The metabolic and hormonal response to acute normoglycaemia in type 1 (insulin-dependent) diabetes: Studies with a glucose controlled insulin infusion system (artificial endocrine pancreas). *Diabetologia*, **23**, 220–28.

Pfeiffer, E.F. and Kerner, W. (1981) The artificial endocrine pancreas: its impact on the pathophysiology and treatment of diabetes mellitus. *Diabetes Care*, **4**, 11–26.

Pfeiffer, E.F., Thum, C. and Clemens, A.H. (1974) The artificial beta cell. A continuous control of blood sugar by external regulation of insulin infusion (glucose controlled insulin infusion system). *Horm. Metab. Res.*, **6**, 339–42.

Pickup, J.C. (1985a) Biosensors: a clinical perspective. *Lancet*, **ii**, 817–20.

Pickup, J.C. (ed.). (1985b) *Brittle Diabetes*. Blackwell Scientific Publications, Oxford.

Pickup, J.C. (1991) 'Glucose sensors and closed-loop insulin delivery', in J.C. Pickup (ed.). *Biotechnology of Insulin Therapy*, pp. 126–53. Blackwell Scientific Publications, Oxford.

Pickup, J.C. (1993a) Developing glucose sensors for *in vivo* use. *Trends in Biotechnology*, **11**, 285–91.

Pickup, J.C. (1993b) *In vivo* glucose monitoring: sense and sensorbility. *Diabetes Care*, **16**, 535–39.

Pickup, J.C. and Alcock, S. (1991) Clinicians' requirements for chemical sensors for *in vivo* monitoring: a multinational survey. *Biosensors and Bioelectronics*, **6**, 639–46.

Pickup, J.C., Claremont, D.J. and Shaw, G.W. (1993) Responses and calibration of amperometric glucose sensors implanted in the subcutaneous tissue of man. *Acta Diabetologica*, **30**, 143–48.

Pickup, J.C., Keen, H., Parsons, J.A. *et al.* (1978) Continuous subcutaneous insulin infusion: an approach to achieving normoglycaemia. *Brit. Med. J.*, **1**, 204–207.

Pickup, J.C., Shaw, G.W. and Claremont, D.J. (1989) *In vivo* molecular sensing in diabetes mellitus: an implantable glucose sensor with direct electron transfer. *Diabetologia*, **32**, 213–17.

Rebrin, K., Fischer, U., von Woedtke, T. *et al.* (1989) Automatic feedback control of subcutaneous glucose concentration in diabetic dogs. *Diabetologia*, **32**, 573–76.

Rebrin, K., Fischer, U., Hahn von Dorsche, H. *et al.* (1992) Subcutaneous glucose monitoring by means of electrochemical sensors: fiction or reality? *J. Biomed. Engin.*, **14**, 33–40.

Robinson, M.R., Eaton, R.P., Haaland, D.M. *et al.* (1992) Non-invasive glucose monitoring in diabetic patients: a preliminary evaluation. *Clin. Chem.*, **38**, 1618–22.

Rosenthal, R.D. and Paynter, L.N. (1991) A portable non-invasive blood glucose meter. *Diabetes*, **40** (suppl. 1), 312A.

Schaffer, B.P.H. and Wolfbeis, P.S. (1990) A fast responding fibre optic glucose biosensor based on an oxygen optrode. *Biosensors and Bioelectronics*, **5**, 137–48.

Schwartz, S.S., Horwitz, D.L., Zehfus, B. *et al.* (1979) Use of glucose-controlled insulin infusion system (artificial beta cell) to control diabetes during surgery. *Diabetologia*, **16**, 157–64.

Seitz, W.R. (1984) Chemical sensors based on fiber optics. *Anal. Chem.*, **56**, 16A–34A.

Shaw, G.W., Claremont, D.J. and Pickup, J.C. (1991) *In vitro* testing of a simply constructed, highly stable glucose sensor suitable for implantation in diabetic patients. *Biosensors and Bioelectronics*, **6**, 401–406.

Shichiri, M., Goriya, Y., Yamasaki, Y. *et al.* (1983) Glycaemic control in pancreatectomized dogs with a wearable artificial pancreas. *Diabetologia*, **24**, 179–84.

Shichiri, M., Kawamori, R., Hakui, N. *et al.* (1984) Closed-loop glycemic control with a wearable artificial pancreas. *Diabetes*, **33**, 1200–1202.

Turner, A.P.F., Karube, I. and Wilson, G.S. (eds). (1987) *Biosensors: Fundamentals and Applications*. Oxford University Press, Oxford.

Van der Schoot, B.H. and Bergveld, P. (1987/88) ISFET based enzyme sensors. *Biosensors*, **3**, 161–86.

Velho, G., Froguel, P., Thévenot, D.R. *et al.* (1989) Strategies for calibrating a subcutaneous glucose sensor. *Biomed. Biochim. Acta*, **48**, 957–64.

Zeller, H., Novak, P. and Landgraf, R. (1989) Blood glucose measurement by infrared spectroscopy. *Inter. J. Artificial Organs*, **12**, 129–35.

45

Islet transplantation

N.J.M. LONDON, G.S.M. ROBERTSON, D. CHADWICK, R.F.L. JAMES and P.R.F. BELL

45.1 INTRODUCTION

In theory, there are three ways to treat diabetes by the transplantation of adult insulin-producing tissue: first, the transplantation of intact vascularized pancreas, second, the transplantation of purified islets of Langerhans, and third, the transplantation of purified β cells. The last technique has not been shown to work in animals other than small rodents and will not therefore be further discussed. The results of clinical vascularized pancreas transplantation have continued to improve since the first case in 1966 (Kelly *et al.*, 1967), with the most recent International Pancreas Transplant Registry analysis (Sutherland, 1992) showing overall one-year patient and graft survivals of 92% and 72% respectively. The majority of these vascularized pancreas transplants have been performed in patients who have previously received, or who are simultaneously receiving a kidney transplant. Although the results of vascularized pancreas transplantation have markedly improved, it remains a major surgical procedure with a significant morbidity and a small, but definite mortality (Nathan *et al.*, 1991). In addition, vascularized pancreas transplant recipients require profound long-term immunosuppression. For these reasons, it is unlikely that vascularized pancreas transplantation will ever be applicable to childhood diabetes – for any one child it will be impossible to predict whether the surgical and immunosuppressive risks will be less than the problems posed by their diabetes (London & Bell, 1992).

The advantages of islet transplantation are that the transplant itself is a minor procedure, and that, because it is a cellular transplant, it may be possible to pre-treat the islets prior to transplantation so that they are less likely to be rejected (immunomodulation). It is the potential for immunomodulation which has stimulated so much research in the field of islet transplantation, because it should be possible, using immunomodulated islets to restore normoglycemia in children or young adults with diabetes without the need for long-term immunosuppression. However, because islet transplantation is not life-saving in the same way that a liver or heart transplant may be, the safety and efficacy of the procedure has to be proven in patients who already require immunosuppression. Therefore the majority of human islet transplants performed so far, have been in patients who are already immunosuppressed for another

Childhood and Adolescent Diabetes
Published in 1994 by Chapman & Hall, London
ISBN 0 412 48610 5

organ transplant (usually the kidney). Immunomodulated human islets have not yet been transplanted and much work remains to be done in this area before the technique can be reasonably applied to children with diabetes.

45.2 ISLET ISOLATION

The fundamental techniques of islet isolation were developed in animal models (Ballinger & Lacy, 1972) and applied to the human pancreas in 1984 (Gray *et al.*, 1984). The isolation of human islets of Langerhans has proven particularly challenging and it is only in the last three years that it has been possible regularly to isolate large numbers of purified islets. The human pancreas contains between 4350 and 21 350 islets of 150 μm diameter equivalent per gram of tissue, corresponding to between 0.8% and 3.8% of the total pancreatic volume (Hellman, 1959; Saito *et al.*, 1978). The average human pancreas, weighing 70 g, therefore contains between 304 000 and 1.5 million islets of 150 μm equivalent diameter. The problems posed by human islet isolation are those of successfully separating intact islets, which form only 1% of the total tissue volume, from the remaining 99% of unwanted exocrine tissue and the fact that during the isolation process, the exocrine tissue releases proteolytic enzymes that may autodigest the islets. A further problem in the human is that, unlike standardized animal models, the human pancreas can be adversely affected by a number of pre organ donation events which subsequently impair islet purification.

Islet isolation consists of two basic steps, first the release of islets from the surrounding exocrine tissue by enzymatic collagenase digestion of the gland, and second the purification of the islets using density gradient centrifugation. The principle behind density gradient centrifugation is that the pancreatic digest is placed onto a density gradient medium such as bovine serum albumin or Ficoll, and after centrifugation, because islets are less dense than exocrine tissue, they migrate through the density gradient to their area of buoyant density and can thus be separated from the denser exocrine tissue.

Human islet isolation takes place as follows. The pancreas is excised at the time of multiple organ donation and must be processed as soon as possible, preferably within 6 hours. The pancreas is taken back to the islet isolation laboratory, cleaned of fat and vascular tissue and the pancreatic duct cannulated. Collagenase solution is injected through the cannula until the pancreas is fully distended. The pancreas is then placed into a stainless steel chamber (Ricordi *et al.*, 1988) through which medium recirculates and is slowly warmed from 4°C to 37°C. As the pancreas is warmed, the collagenase becomes active and the organ is converted from a solid organ into a suspension. As the digestion proceeds, biopsies are taken from the effluent of the chamber and stained with dithizone in order to identify the islets (dithizone binds to the zinc in beta granules and turns them red). As soon as intact islets are seen in the chamber effluent, the digestion is slowly stopped by cooling back to 4°C and the pancreatic digest collected (Plate 3). The crucial issue during this stage of the process is to allow the collagenase digestion to proceed to a point such that the islets are liberated from the surrounding exocrine tissue, but not allowing the digestion to go so far that the islets themselves are fragmented.

Once the collagenase digestion phase is completed, the digest is collected, pooled together and placed onto a density gradient. The total volume of digest from a human pancreas may be up to 80 ml and a recent advance has been the use of the COBE cell processor (Lake *et al.*, 1989) to form quickly large-scale density gradients that would otherwise have to be formed in large numbers of test tubes. The most commonly used density gradient media are Ficoll (polymeric sucrose), and bovine serum albumin. The purity of the final islet preparation varies from 30–95% (Plate 4) and the islet yield from a single pancreas ranges from 150 000–600 000 islets of 150 μm diameter equivalent.

45.3 ISLET TISSUE CULTURE AND CRYOPRESERVATION

After purification, islets can be aliquoted into petri dishes containing tissue culture medium and placed into humidified incubators at 37°C. Although, for experimental purposes, it is possible for human islets to remain viable in tissue culture for up to 2 years (Nielsen, 1981) there is the constant risk of bacterial and fungal contamination, and as each week passes there is a gradual loss of tissue. Tissue culture is only suitable therefore for the short-term storage of islets and it is for this reason that for long-term storage (in theory, millennia), islets have been cryopreserved. The basic technique of islet cryopreservation (Rajotte *et al.*, 1988) is slow equilibration with dimethylsulphoxide (a widely-used cyroprotectant), cooling at a rate of 0.25°C per minute to −40°C and then plunging into liquid nitrogen (−196°C). When required, the islets are rapidly thawed (200°C/min) and placed back into tissue culture for a short time prior to transplantation. The functional tissue recovery after cryopreservation is approximately 60%.

45.4 ISLET TRANSPLANTATION

Although it would seem logical to transplant islets back into the pancreas, the islets do not receive sufficient vascularization at this site. It is for this reason that the majority of human islet transplants have been performed by embolizing the islets into the liver via the portal vein (Scharp *et al.*, 1990) where they lodge in the portal triads and receive their vascular supply by ingrowth of recipient capillaries. Although in experimental animal models islets have also been successfully transplanted into the spleen or under the kidney capsule (Hayek *et al.*, 1990), in the case of the human, these sites have not been successful. An advantage of the hepatic site is that the insulin delivery is portal. After transplantation it takes up to 6 weeks for the islets fully to develop their new blood supply and they may take up to 6 months for transplanted human islets to reach their full functional potential (Warnock *et al.*, 1992).

In the case of islet transplants performed at the same time as a kidney transplant, the islets are embolized into the liver by cannulating a mesenteric vein and infusing the islets throughout the whole liver. In the case of islet transplants being performed after kidney transplants, a percutaneous transhepatic technique has been successfully used (London *et al.*, 1992). This is a local anesthetic technique and the transplant can be performed within half-an-hour. Recent evidence from human islet autotransplants performed in patients undergoing pancreatic resection for chronic pancreatitis shows that islets embolized into the liver via the portal vein have normal pulsatile insulin secretion (Pyzdrowski *et al.*, 1992).

45.5 ISLET IMMUNOMODULATION

There is a wealth of experimental evidence suggesting that the endocrine cells within islets provoke only a minimal rejection response in allograft recipients and that it is lymphoid cells within the islet, so-called 'dendritic cells' (Plate 5), that initiate the rejection response (Lafferty *et al.*, 1983). Each islet contains up to 20 of these dendritic cells which fortunately are exquisitely sensitive to modalities such as low-dose (2.5 Gray) gamma-irradiation (James *et al.*, 1989), ultraviolet irradiation (Kanai *et al.*, 1989) and low-temperature (24°C) tissue culture (Lacy *et al.*, 1979). The basic principle behind islet immunomodulation, therefore, is to treat purified islets prior to transplantation by one of the modalities above and then, provided a short course (roughly two weeks) of recipient immunosuppression is given at the time of transplantation, the islets are accepted long-term without the need for continued immunosuppression. This theoretical approach has been validated in rodent models and currently, much research is devoted to applying these principles to large animal and human islets.

45.6 THE RESULTS OF HUMAN ISLET TRANSPLANTATION

The majority of human islet transplants performed so far have been in patients with established kidney transplants or patients undergoing simultaneous kidney transplantation. As explained above, this is because the safety and efficacy of islet transplantation needs to be established in patients who require to be immunosuppressed anyway. During the three years 1990, 1991 and 1992, seventy-two cadaveric adult islet allografts were performed in thirteen centers (Scharp *et al.*, 1991; Socci *et al.*, 1991; London *et al.*, 1992; Ricordi *et al.*, 1992; Warnock *et al.*, 1992). The majority of these transplants used the intraportal site, most used multiple donors, and seventeen (24%) used a mixture of fresh and cryopreserved islets. All of the recipients were C-peptide negative prior to transplantation and all were performed in recipients concurrently immunosupressed for another organ transplant (usually the kidney). Sixteen (22%) of the recipients were rendered insulin-independent for variable periods, and forty-four (61%) had evidence of maintained graft function as measured by serum C-peptide levels. The longest period of insulin independence has been 30 months in a patient from Edmonton (Warnock *et al.*, 1992). This patient received a combination of fresh and cryopreserved islets from five donors.

45.7 AUTOIMMUNE DISEASE RECURRENCE

An important consideration in islet transplantation is the possibility of recurrent autoimmune β-cell destruction of transplanted islets. Valuable information concerning this issue comes from cases of vascularized pancreas transplantation between monozygotic twins, where the non-diabetic sibling has donated a hemi-pancreas to the diabetic partner (Sutherland *et al.*, 1989). Because the donor and reipient were major histocompatibility (MHC) identical, these transplants were initially performed without immunosuppression. It was found however, that although the pancreas transplants were technically successful and reversed diabetes, hyperglycemia returned within a few weeks. Biopsies from the recipients' pancreata revealed β cell destruction within the islets, presumably as a result of autoimmune disease recurrence. Subsequent identical twin pancreas transplant recipients were therefore immunosuppressed and this prevented recurrent β cell autoimmune destruction. There is no doubt therefore that autoimmune disease recurrence can occur but, fortunately, the majority of experimental evidence suggests that this process is MHC-restricted (Markmann *et al.*, 1991), i.e., the autoimmune process is directed only against cells with an identical MHC type to that of the recipient. In the case of allogeneic islet transplantation, the donor islets will never be truly identical with the recipients' and the transplanted islets should not therefore be susceptible to autoimmune β-cell destruction.

45.8 FUTURE PROSPECTS

45.8.1 ISLET ENCAPSULATION

There has been a great deal of interest in the technique of islet microencapsulation (Plate 6) because it offers the potential for islet transplantation without the need for recipient immunosuppression (O'Shea *et al.*, 1984). The basic principle is that islets are placed into a microcapsule (approximately 500 μm in diameter) formed from a wall that is permeable to insulin and glucose but impermeable to immunoglobulins and the cells that mediate rejection. The substances most commonly used to form the wall of the capsule are alginates (a complex polysaccharide derived from seaweed) combined with a poly-amino-acid such as poly-l-lysine.

Surprisingly, the insulin-release characteristics of these encapsulated islets are excellent (Clayton *et al.*, 1990). The commonest site for the transplantation of encapsulated islets is the peritoneal cavity and although there have been reports of successful reversal of diabetes, the major hurdle at the present time is biocompatibility. It is a common experience that although the capsules may initially function very well, within a period of weeks the capsules become enveloped in a fibrous reaction that has all the features of a foreign body response (Wijsman *et al.*, 1992). Further progress in this field will depend on determining the precise cause of this foreign body response and developing highly-purified alginates.

45.8.2 ISLET XENOTRANSPLANTATION

It is apparent that when the problems of human islet transplantation are solved and it is in a position to be applied clinically on a larger scale, there will never be sufficient cadaveric human pancreata to provide islets for the number of potential diabetic recipients. With this in mind, there has been much recent research into islet xenotransplantation. The most suitable donor for islet xenotransplantation is undoubtedly the pig (Thomas, 1991), and with recent advances it is now possible to isolate large numbers of purified porcine islets (Ricordi *et al.*, 1990). The major hurdle to xenotransplantation is the presence in humans of natural anti-endothelial cell antibodies that, after transplantation of vascularized xenogeneic organs, produce an immediate rejection response directed at the donor vasculature (Platt & Bach, 1991). Because islets are not immediately vascularized this problem may prove to be less profound than with solid organ transplants and there is experimental evidence to suggest that, providing the initial phase of antibody-mediated rejection can be abrogated, it is possible for xenografts to be accepted in the long term, a process called 'accommodation' (Platt *et al.*, 1990). The challenge of islet xenotransplantation is not therefore islet yield, but the immunology of xenograft rejection.

45.9 SUMMARY

The rationale behind islet transplantation is that it should be possible, using immunomodulated human islets, to safely transplant young diabetic patients soon after the onset of their diabetes without the need for long-term immunosuppression and hopefully, thereby prevent the long-term complications of the disease. In recent years, the safety and efficacy of human islet transplantation have been validated in diabetic patients who already have to receive immunosuppression for another organ transplant, and there is now a need to develop and adapt the techniques for islet immunomodulation which have worked so well in the rodent and apply them to larger animals and humans. Only when these techniques have been perfected, will it be possible safely to transplant highly purified, immunomodulated islets into diabetic children at an early stage of the disease process.

REFERENCES

Ballinger, W.F. and Lacy, P.E. (1972) Transplantation of intact pancreatic islets in rats. *Surgery*, **72**, 175–86.

Clayton, H.A., London, N.J.M., Colloby, P.S. *et al.* (1990) A study of the effect of capsule composition on the viability of cultured alginate/poly-l-lysine – encapsulated islets. *Diabetes Res.*, **14**, 127–32.

Gray, D.W.R., McShane, P., Grant, A. *et al.* (1984) A method for isolation of islets of Langerhans from the human pancreas. *Diabetes*, **33**, 1055–61.

Hayek, A., Lopez, A.D. and Beattie, G.M. (1990) Factors influencing islet transplantation: number, location, and metabolic control. *Transplantation*, **49**, 224–25.

Hellman, B. (1959) The frequency distribution of the number and volume of the islets of Langerhans in man. *Acta Societatus Medicorum Upsaliensis*, **64**, 432–60.

James, R.F.L., Lake, S.P., Chamberlain, J. *et al.* (1989) Gamma irradiation of isolated rat islets pretansplantation produces indefinite allograft survival in cyclosporine-treated recipients. *Transplantation*, **47**, 929–33.

Kanai, T., Porter, J., Gotoh, M. *et al.* (1989) Effect of γ-irradiation on mouse pancreatic islet allograft survival. *Diabetes*, **38**, 154–56.

Kelly, W.D., Lillehei, R.C., Merkel, F.K. *et al.* (1967) Allotransplantation of the pancreas and duodenum along with the kidney in diabetic nephropathy. *Surgery*, **61**, 827–37.

Lacy, P.E., Davie, J.M. and Finke, E.N. (1979) Prolongation of islet allograft survival following *in vitro* culture (24°C) and a single injection of ALS. *Science*, **204**, 312–13.

Lafferty, K.J., Prowse, S.J. and Simeonovic, C.J. (1983) Immunobiology of tissue transplantation: A return to the passenger leucocyte concept. *Ann. Rev. Immunol.*, **1**, 143–73.

Lake, S.P., Bassett, P.D., Larkins, A. *et al.* (1989) Large-scale purification of human islets utilising discontinuous albumin gradient on IBM 2991 cell separator. *Diabetes*, **38** (suppl. 1), 143–45.

London, N.J.M. and Bell, P.R.F (1992) Pancreas and islet transplantation. *Brit. J. Surg.*, **79**, 6–7.

London, N.J.M., James, R.F.L., Robertson, G.M. *et al.* (1992) 'Human Islet Transplantation: The Leicester Experience', in C. Ricordi (ed.) *Pancreatic Islet Transplantation*, pp. 454–62. RG Landes, Austin.

Markmann, J.F., Posselt, A.M., Bassiri, H. *et al.* (1991) Major-histocompatibility-complex restricted and nonrestricted autoimmune effector mechanisms in BB rats. *Transplantation*, **52**, 662–67.

Nathan, D.M., Fogel, H., Norman, D. *et al.* (1991) Long-term metabolic and quality of life results with pancreatic/renal transplantion in insulin-dependent diabetes mellitus. *Transplantation*, **52**, 85–91.

Nielsen, J.H. (1981) 'Human pancreatic islets in tissue culture', in K. Federlin and R.G. Bretzel (eds.). *Islet isolation, culture and cryopreservation: Giessen Workshop 1980*, pp. 69–83. Thieme Verlag, Stuttgart.

O'Shea, G.M., Goosen, M.F.A and Sun, A.M. (1984) Prolonged survival of transplanted islets of Langerhans encapsulated in a biocompatible membrane. *Biochimica Biophysica Acta*, **804**, 133–36.

Platt, J.L. and Bach, F.H. (1991) The barrier to xenotransplantation. *Transplantation*, **52**, 937–47.

Platt, J.L., Vercelloti, G.M., Dalmasso, A.P. *et al.* (1990) Transplantation of discordant xenografts: A review of progress. *Immunology Today*, **11**, 450–57.

Pyzdrowski, K.L., Kendall, D.M., Halter, J.B. *et al.* (1992) Preserved insulin secretion and insulin independence in recipients of islet autografts. *N. Eng. J. Med.*, **327**, 220–26.

Rajotte, R.V., Warnock, G.L. and Coulombe, M.G. (1988) 'Islet cryopreservation: methods and experimental results in rodents, large mammals and humans', in R. van Schilfgaarde and M.A. Hardy (eds). *Transplantation of the endocrine pancreas in diabetes*, pp. 125–35. Elsevier Science Publishers, Amsterdam.

Ricordi, C., Lacy, P.E., Finke, E.H., *et al.* (1988) Automated method for isolation of human pancreatic islets. *Diabetes*, **37**, 413–20.

Ricordi, C., Socci, C., Davalli, A.M. *et al.* (1990) Isolation of the elusive pig islet. *Surgery*, **107**, 688–94.

Ricordi, C., Tzakis, A.G., Carroll, P.B. *et al.* (1992) Human islet isolation and allotransplantation in 22 consecutive cases. *Transplantation*, **53**, 407–14.

Saito, K., Iwama, N. and Takahashi, T. (1978) Morphometric analysis on topographical difference in size distribution, number and volume of islets in the human pancreas. *Tohoku J. Exper. Med.*, **124**, 177–86.

Scharp, D.W., Lacy, P.E., Santiago, J.V. *et al.* (1990) Insulin independence after islet transplantation into Type 1 diabetic patients. *Diabetes*, **39**, 515–18.

Scharp, D.W., Lacy, P.E., Santiago, J.V. *et al.* (1991) Results of our first nine intraportal islet allografts in Type 1, insulin-dependent diabetic patients. *Transplantation*, **51**, 76–85.

Socci, C., Falqui, L., Davalli, A.M. *et al.* (1991) Fresh human islet transplantaion to replace pancreatic endocrine function in type 1 diabetic patients. *Acta Diabetologica*, **28**, 151–57.

Sutherland, D.E.R. (1992) Pancreatic transplantation: State of the art. *Transplantation Proceedings*, **24**:3, 762–66.

Sutherland, D.E.R., Goetz, F.G. and Sibley, R.K. (1989) Recurrence of disease in pancreas transplants. *Diabetes*, **38** (suppl. 1), 85–87.

Thomas, F.T. (1991) 'Isolated pancreas islet xenografting', in D.K.C. Cooper, E. Kemp, K. Reemtsma *et al.* (eds). *Xenotransplantation*, pp. 275–96. Springer-Verlag, Berlin.

Warnock, G.L., Kneteman, N.M., Ryan, E.A. *et al.* (1992) Long-term follow-up after transplantation of insulin-producing pancreatic islets into patients with Type 1 (insulin-dependent) diabetes mellitus. *Diabetologica*, **35**, 89–95.

Wijsman, J., Atkinson, P., Mazaheri, R. *et al.* (1992) Histological and immunopathological analysis of recovered encapsulated allogeneic islets from transplanted diabetic BB/W rats. *Transplantation*, **54**, 588–92.

46

Current controversies in the management of the diabetic child and adolescent

Z. LARON and O. KALTER-LEIBOVICI

46.1 INTRODUCTION

Although the treatment of diabetic children seems straightforward – insulin replacement, regular meals, no simple sugars, and exercise – it is astonishing how many related issues are matters of different approaches. Childhood diabetes is a very complex disease, both in its etiopathology, in its requirements for long-term control and in its prognosis (Laron & Karp, 1990). Often not medical but social, economic and political factors dictate differences in the medical care of young and even older diabetics.

The following is an attempt to highlight a series of definitions, approaches and issues on which there is no general agreement. Some of the comments present the personal viewpoint of the authors.

We wish to start with a few notions or definitions which are often used incorrectly.

46.1.1 CHILDHOOD DIABETES

In the colloquial sense, childhood diabetes is synonymous with autoimmune insulin-dependent diabetes (IDDM); however, there are also non-insulin dependent (NIDDM) forms of diabetes in childhood, some associated with genetic diseases – muscular dystrophies, gonadal dysgenesis, cystic fibrosis, leprechaunism, etc. (Rimoin, 1975) (see Chapter 29). In several populations such as in Japanese (Tajima & LaPorte, 1992) and American Indians (Dean *et al.*, 1992), NIDDM is relatively common. Also MODY (mature onset diabetes in youth) may start in puberty (Fajans *et al.*, 1992). Therefore even childhood diabetes should be classified.

46.1.2 PREDIABETES

Prediabetes (correctly the state before the pathogenetic process has started) is often confounded with 'early diabetes' – a state in which β cell insufficiency of any cause is already present. Thus, positive genetic markers may indicate susceptible individuals before they have a β cell insult or insulin receptor resistance, i.e., 'prediabetes' but a positive immunological or biochemical marker indicates 'early diabetes'.

Childhood and Adolescent Diabetes
Published in 1994 by Chapman & Hall, London
ISBN 0 412 48610 5

46.2 WHO SHOULD TREAT THE DIABETIC CHILD AND ADOLESCENT?

Children and adolescents, up to approximately 18 years, i.e., the age at which most of the population have reached the end of puberty, should be treated by pediatricians and those with diabetes by pediatric endocrinologists. Physicians trained in adult medicine are not versed in normal growth, puberty and child-parent relationships (Laron & Galatzer, 1982).

The care of diabetes requires much time: listening to the problems of the patient and the family, as well as offering counseling to provide solutions. Often, the overworked pediatrician and GP has no time available. Thus, much of the burden falls on the education nurse and the dietician. As diabetes evokes many psychological problems, a psychologist and a social worker are worthy partners in the treatment team to help solve problems at home and at school (Laron *et al.*, 1979; Galatzer *et al.*, 1982).

The conclusion that a multidisciplinary team is needed to treat effectively IDDM patients was reached by the large DCCT (Diabetes Control and Complication Trial) performed over a period of nine years in the US and concluded recently (DCCT Research Group, 1993). Regretfully not everybody agrees with the above conclusions; on the other hand, authorities do not readily provide the means for multidisciplinary personnel even in large diabetes clinics.

46.3 EDUCATION OF THE DIABETIC CHILD AND THE FAMILY: WHEN, WHERE AND BY WHOM?

At diagnosis the young patients (if old enough) and their families (usually only the parents, and often only one of them) receive oral explanations on diabetes and its management, and printed information in the form of books (Chase, 1992; Hurter & Travis, 1991) or leaflets. During follow-up, depending upon existing services and size of the treating team, often instructions rather than education are provided. For many of the diabetic youngsters, follow-up education occurs during a vacation camp. It should be noted that camps do not accept very young children, that they last only a few days and do not provide teaching for the parents, other family members, and for the personnel of the school which the patients attend.

During our 30 years' experience we have reached the following conclusions concerning the needs of education (Laron, 1981).

46.3.1 PREVENTIVE EDUCATION

Education of the public on the presenting signs and symptoms of diabetes mellitus so that an early approach to the physician is made, enables diagnosis at a stage when β-cell function is not severely reduced. There is evidence that IDDM is better controlled when a greater β cell reserve is present at diagnosis (Shah *et al.*, 1989).

Education will also help the public and especially relatives of diabetic patients combat fear of the condition (Halloran, 1992).

46.3.2 EDUCATION AT DIAGNOSIS

As a whole family is in shock when the diagnosis is pronounced, practical instructions and information related to acute and chronic complications given during the first week or two after diagnosis are not efficiently perceived and have to be repeated again and again, often over long periods of time (Laron, 1984; Galatzer *et al.*, 1982).

46.3.3 CONTINUOUS EDUCATION

As many practical problems, both medical and social, arise continuously throughout treatment, it is useful to have 3–4 education courses per year for patients and their parents. One whole-day course per year for health visiting and school nurses and a whole-day update course for pediatricians and school physicians has been well-received and highly frequented (Laron, 1981).

Reading offers general education but counselling for personal problems has to be done by the members of the treatment team.

46.3.4 EDUCATION DURING THE YEARLY VACATION CAMP

The camp is ideal in showing children that many others have the same disease and that a child with diabetes can cope also in situations of intensified physical exertion (Wentworth, 1987). However, the camp, a once, or at the most, twice-yearly short period cannot replace basic or continuing education programs. If the camp is attended by children treated by many physicians their therapeutic routines may differ. The correction of wrong habits does not guarantee that they will continue to be followed at home.

A camp should be a real vacation for both patients and parents and cannot be a school for education. Education should be provided throughout the year for the patients and their families, and during the camp the children should have their supervised recreation program. They should be taught how to cope and after two to three diabetic camps be able to participate in regular camps. Large diabetes centers should have their own camps, a situation which eliminates the need for basic diabetes education.

In certain instances, juvenile diabetic camps are organized by voluntary organizations or parent associations which hire personnel not belonging to clinics which treat children. They do not know the children and vice versa; they have different viewpoints on diabetes management; these conditions can lead to conflicts, misunderstandings, lack of confidence and often to over- or undertreatment.

46.4 NUTRITION

Nutrition is one of the basic components of diabetes control, but there are several controversial issues. The first relates to the percentage of carbohydrates as an energy source. In northern Italy (Pinelli, 1993) the usual quantity of 45–55% carbohydrates was increased to 55–60%, but this is not accepted by others. However, there is agreement that animal (saturated) fats should be decreased in favor of unsaturated vegetable fats (Laron & Karp, 1990). Despite this the polyunsaturated/saturated fatty acid (P/S) ratio in northern Europe remains 0.4:0.6 (Mozin *et al.*, 1978; Virtanen *et al.*, 1987) whereas in the Mediterranean area it reaches 1:1.2 (Faiman *et al.*, 1979). The proposition to reduce protein intake to decrease the load to the kidneys cannot be accepted in growing children. The number of meals, timing and food distribution between meals has been found to be important in diabetes management. There are discrepancies between habits of 3 meals, multiple meals or meals on demand, using multiple injections of short-acting insulin (Jenkins *et al.*, 1989). Our experience is that regular meals (3 main meals and 3–5 snacks) and adjustment to exercise, are best to maintain good control (Laron *et al.*, 1988). A user-friendly microcomputer system (DIACON) has been found useful in nutrition education (Laron *et al.*, 1990). The high association between celiac disease and diabetes (Koletzko *et al.*, 1988) complicates nutritional counseling.

46.5 AMBULATORY CARE VS. HOSPITALIZATION

In most countries the newly-diagnosed diabetic patient is hospitalized for 1–2 or more weeks to treat ketoacidosis and for education, together with the parents. This disrupts family life and has economical sequelae (Munoz *et al.*, 1989; Sutton *et al.*, 1990). It is our belief that as most patients do not need special care after 1–2 days, the treatment and education can be effectively performed on an ambulatory basis.

Depending upon the distance of the family's domicile from the treatment center, any facility is preferable to a hospital; home being best (McNally *et al.*, 1991; Paton *et al.*, 1991). In addition to the negative psychosocial aspect, hospitalization presents a very heavy economic burden on the health services. Also during the follow-up years, hospitalization should be avoided or be as short as possible.

46.6 MICROVASCULAR COMPLICATIONS

Long-term diabetic microvascular complications are associated with increased morbidity and mortality and put a heavy financial burden on public health and welfare funds.

There are a series of controversies regarding strategies for early detection, primary prevention and secondary intervention in diabetic microvascular complications.

46.6.1 SCREENING FOR MICROVASCULAR COMPLICATIONS

46.6.1.1 Diabetic retinopathy

Diabetic retinopathy is relatively infrequent in prepubertal insulin-dependent diabetes mellitus (IDDM) patients (Frank *et al.*, 1982; Klein *et al.*, 1985) and in the first years of IDDM (Frank *et al.*, 1982; Burger *et al.*, 1986). Hence, the American Diabetes Association (ADA) suggested annual screening for retinopathy in patients 18–30 years of age, starting with their fifth year of diabetes (ADA, 1991a). However, some investigators reported an earlier appearance of diabetic retinopathy (Palmberg *et al.*, 1981; Klein *et al.*, 1984; McCance *et al.*, 1989), including the proliferative form (O'Hara, 1990).

Early stages of non-proliferative diabetic retinopathy have been observed in 8–19% of prepubertal IDDM patients (Klein *et al.*, 1985; Lund-Andersen *et al.*, 1987; Murphy *et al.*, 1990). Although the appearance of sight-threatening retinopathy is exceptional during the first five years of insulin-dependent diabetes and in prepubertal diabetic children, the diagnosis of any degree of retinopathy indicates the need for careful ophthalmologic follow-up and efforts to improve glycemic control.

The cost-benefit issue of early screening for diabetic retinopathy was recently addressed (Javitt *et al.*, 1991). The authors suggest that the costs of annual screening since diagnosis of all IDDM patients might be lower than those caused by the increased rate of severe visual loss developing in patients who are lost to follow-up by the current screening guidelines.

The ADA guidelines do not refer to the issue of who should perform the screening for diabetic retinopathy and what methods should be used. According to Singer *et al.* (1992) who summarized current data on different screening strategies, the sensitivity of an ophthalmologic evaluation performed by personnel other than trained ophthalmologists (i.e., diabetologists, internists, nurses, etc.) was unsatisfactory in most instances. While photographs of seven standard fields of the retina serve as the gold standard for the detection and staging of diabetic retinopathy, the costs are considerable. The sensitivity of direct and indirect ophthalmoscopy performed by an ophthalmologist through dilated pupils is generally fair. Such an examination should be aided by fundus photographs when possible. Retinal photographs also provide accurate and objective data for the application of laser therapy (Singer *et al.*, 1992).

46.6.1.2 Diabetic nephropathy

The hallmark of overt diabetic nephropathy is macroalbuminuria with urinary albumin excretion (UAE) >300 mg/24 hr, which can be easily detected using dipsticks in spot urine tests (Mogensen *et al.*, 1983). After the appearance of macroalbuminuria, progression to renal failure is almost inevitable and half of the patients reach this stage within the following ten years (Krolewski *et al.*, 1985). The detection of diabetic nephropathy in its incipient stage when various therapeutic interventions may arrest or delay its progression is therefore of great importance. Persistent microalbuminuria, defined as increased UAE >30 mg/24 hr and <300 mg/24 hr, was found to precede and predict the development of macroalbuminuria (Viberti *et al.*, 1982; Mogensen & Christensen, 1984). Persistent microalbuminuria is also associated with an increased risk of cardiovascular mortality (Massent *et al.*, 1992). Recently, Försblom *et al.* (1992) challenged the predictive value of microalbuminuria. They found that in their patients with longstanding IDDM (>15 years), microalbuminuria was not a good predictor for the subsequent development of overt nephropathy during a 10-year follow-up. Lane *et al.* (1992) described a small subgroup of female IDDM patients with a reduced creatinine clearance rate and pathological findings compatible with diabetic nephropathy on kidney biopsy who had a normal UAE. It might be, therefore, that for some subgroup of IDDM patients, microalbuminuria alone may not be a good predictor for subsequent nephropathy and therefore other kidney functions such as glomerular filtration rate (GFR) should be followed as well.

Urinary albumin excretion was originally measured in a 24-hr urine collection and Mogensen (1987) proposes at least three urine collections for an accurate determination of microalbuminuria because of the day-to-day variation in UAE (C.V. > 45%). Such tests may be cumbersome, especially in small children; therefore overnight collections or even spot urine tests may be used, but these methods were reported to miss up to 30–60% of patients with microalbuminuria (Stehouwer *et al.*, 1990; Kouri *et al.*, 1991).

Overt diabetic nephropathy is rare in the first five years of IDDM and its incidence thereafter until the fifteenth or sixteenth year of diabetes and declines afterwards (Andersen *et al.*, 1983; Krolewski *et al.*, 1985). Borch-Johnsen *et al.* (1993) recently published the result of a cost-benefit analysis of a screening program for microalbuminuria using a computer simulation program. Their calculations showed that a yearly screening starting from the fifth year of IDDM for the following 30 years is expected to result in a significant delay of overt nephropathy due to early initiation of anti-hypertensive treatment. The calculated saving per patient lifespan increases using such screening ranges from 800–7700 US$/year (depending also on different expected treatment effect and depending on the treatment regimen). The authors did not refer to the possible effect and costs of intensified insulin treatment in patients with early detected microalbuminuria

46.6.1.3 Diabetic neuropathy

Current available data on the prevalence of diabetic neuropathy are inconsistent mainly due to the lack of uniform methods for the diagnosis of its various forms (Green *et al.*, 1990).

In the Pittsburgh Epidemiology of Diabetes Complications Studies II, clinical distal symmetric polyneuropathy was not observed in patients with a duration of IDDM of less than ten years (Orchard *et al.*, 1990). On the other hand, the DCCT reported a 39% prevalence of clinical distal symmetric polyneuropathy in patients with 1–15 years of IDDM, despite the exclusion of subjects with severe symptomatic diabetic polyneuropathy. The mean duration of disease in affected IDDM patients in the DCCT group was 8 ± 4 (SD) years (DCCT Research Group, 1988a). Ziegler *et al.* (1991) reported a high incidence rate (62.5%) of subclinical and clinical diabetic polyneuropathy in the first five years of poorly controlled insulin-dependent diabetes. Said *et al.* (1992) also reported the unusual appearance of severe diabetic polyneuropathy in five young adult IDDM patients within the first three years of diabetes. As in the patients of Ziegler *et al.* (1991) these patients also had poorly controlled IDDM. Subclinical diabetic neuropathy was reported in late pubertal adolescent IDDM patients (Sosenko *et al.*, 1985).

A careful clinical assessment of diabetic neuropathy is recommended for epidemiological and clinical studies (ADA, 1991b). The clinical significance of an early diagnosis of subclinical neuropathy, using expensive equipment for electrodiagnostic studies and quantitative sensory and autonomic function testing, is not indicated considering the low prevalence of diabetic neuropathy in the pediatric age group, and the lack of specific therapy at present. One may agree, however, that an early intervention at a subclinical stage by improving glycemic control may be more beneficial than in the clinical and less reversible phase. There are as yet no available data on cost-benefit calculations in this issue. For an accurate diagnosis of subclinical diabetic neuropathy each laboratory must use its own normal reference values from its age-matched nondiabetic population (ADA, 1991b).

46.6.2 TREATMENT

46.6.2.1 Intensive insulin therapy

Poor glycemic control in insulin-dependent diabetes is a major risk factor for diabetic retinopathy (Klein *et al.*, 1984; McCance *et al.*, 1989; Krolewski *et al.*, 1986; Joner *et al.*, 1992), nephropathy (Krolewski *et al.*, 1985; Klein *et al.*, 1991 & 1992), and neuropathy (DCCT Research Group, 1988a; Orchard *et al.*, 1990). These findings are the rationale for intensive insulin therapy aimed to achieve near normoglycemia and to modify the cause of diabetic microvascular complications. The main criticism of these trials was the small number of pediatric patients included and the short-term follow-up in some, and the lack of conclusive results (DCCT Research Group, 1988b). A meta-analysis of 16 randomized clinical trials of intensive insulin therapy showed that after two years of intensive insulin therapy the risk for progression of diabetic retinopathy was significantly lower (odds ratio (OR) 0.49 [95% confidence interval 0.28–0.85] $p = 0.011$). The risk for nephropathy progression also decreased significantly in the intensive treatment group (OR 0.34 [0.2–0.58] $p < 0.001$) (Wang *et al.*, 1993).

The DCCT was designed as a large-scale study testing the effect of long-term intensive insulin therapy on the appearance and progression of diabetic microvascular complications. A total number of 1441 patients were allocated to either intensive or conventional insulin treatment. The study included both patients with short duration of IDDM and no signs of diabetic nephropathy or retinopathy and patients with longer duration of diabetes and minimal ocular and renal complications (DCCT Research Group, 1988b & 1990). The recently reported preliminary results showed that improved glycemic control achieved in the intensive treatment group caused a significant risk reduction in the progression of diabetic retinopathy, nephropathy and neuropathy in the primary prevention and the secondary intervention subgroups, compared to patients on the conventional insulin regimen (DCCT Research Group, 1993). A major risk associated with intensive insulin treatment is the increased frequency of severe hypoglycemia (DCCT Research Group, 1991; Wang *et al.*, 1993). In the DCCT, the risk was about three times higher in the intensive insulin treatment group, even after the modification of the study protocol (DCCT Research Group, 1991) and the exclusion of patients with clinically significant diabetic neuropathy – who were *a priori* more prone to severe hypoglycemia (DCCT Research Group, 1988a). Intensive insulin treatment delivered through continuous insulin infusion pumps is associated with increased frequency of diabetic ketoacidosis. This complication was not reported, however, when multiple insulin injections were used for intensive insulin treatment (Wang *et al.*, 1993). Intensive insulin treatment is also associated with significant weight gain with an increase of 33% in the mean adjusted risk of becoming overweight (DCCT Research Group, 1993).

The clinical trials of intensive insulin treatment included patients with minimal or no involvement of microvascular complications. The benefit of such treatment in more advanced stages of microvascular complications is doubtful. In fact, the restoration of near normoglycemia does not retard the deterioration of renal function patients with overt diabetic nephropathy (Viberti *et al.*, 1983). Successful pancreas transplantation apparently does not improve advanced diabetic retinopathy (Ramsay *et al.*, 1988). Pancreas transplantation causes some improvement in neurophysiologic tests but no change in clinical evaluation scores in IDDM patients with advanced diabetic neuropathy (Kennedy *et al.*, 1990). Only about 14% of the patients included in the DCCT protocol were adolescents, 13–18 years of age (18% in the primary prevention phase and 9.5% in the secondary intervention phase); children below 13 years of age were not included (DCCT Research Group, 1993). There is as yet no answer to whether intensive insulin therapy is associated with a similar risk reduction for microvascular complications when given to younger children or to the degree of risk especially for severe hypoglycemic episodes associated with such treatment in young IDDM patients. One should keep in mind that these trials on intensive insulin treatment were performed in selected highly-motivated IDDM patients and do not necessarily reflect the clinic population as a whole.

Thus, the outcome of such treatment regimens in terms of risks and benefits when implemented in a general clinic and with less capable and motivated patients may be very different. The application of intensive insulin therapy is associated with substantial financial costs for trained personnel (diabetologists, dieticians, education nurses and psychosocial consultants), clinic organization for frequent visits, telephone counseling and an increased need for medical supplies such as blood glucose strips, needles and syringes. The cost benefit issue of implementing such treatment strategies on a large scale has to be addressed by health authorities. An alternative strategy may be to make particular efforts to decrease the magnitude of hyperglycemia in patients with poor glycemic control, in whom the risk for severe microvascular complications is very high (Kalter-Leibovici *et al.*, 1991; Krolowski *et al.*, 1985 & 1986).

46.6.2.2 Anti-hypertensive treatment

There is still a debate whether a genetic predisposition to essential hypertension, expressed by increased sodium-lithium countertransport in erythrocytes, is a risk factor for diabetic nephropathy (Elving *et al.*, 1991; Krolewski *et al.*, 1988; Magilli *et al.*, 1988; Norgaard *et al.*, 1990). There is no doubt, however, that hypertension is detrimental to renal function once diabetic nephropathy exists and that anti-hypertensive treatment can modify the cause of progression to end-stage renal disease (Parving *et al.*, 1983 & 1987). The guidelines for the implementation of anti-hypertensive treatment in patients with diabetic nephropathy are as yet not well-defined.

Patients with microalbuminuria have higher values of blood pressure compared to normoalbuminuric subjects (Klein *et al.*, 1992; Mathiesen *et al.*, 1984). Furthermore, 24-hour monitoring of blood pressure in IDDM patients may demonstrate loss of the normal diurnal variation with relative nocturnal hypertension that can be missed in morning blood pressure measurements taken in the clinic (Hansen *et al.*, 1992; Wiegmann *et al.*, 1990). Mogensen *et al.* (1991) suggested that values of blood pressure >130/85 mmHg should indicate the initiation of anti-hypertensive treatment in microalbuminuric patients since values above this threshold are associated with an increased risk for the progression of diabetic nephropathy. This threshold is considerably lower than >160/90 mmHg, the WHO definition of hypertension. Similar data on blood pressure cut-off points for the initiation of anti-hypertensive treatment in IDDM children are not available. The basic question is whether the indications for anti-hypertensive treatment in diabetic nephropathy are the blood pressure values or the detection of an increased UAE, regardless of the blood pressure.

Studies with angiotensin-converting enzyme (ACE) inhibitors given to normotensive IDDM patients with micro- (Marre *et al.*, 1988; Mathiesen *et al.*, 1991) and macroalbuminuria (Parving *et al.*, 1989) demonstrated a beneficial effect of these drugs on UAE and renal function independent of their antihypertensive properties. These effects may be explained by modifications of the intraglomerular hemodynamics and basal membrane properties (Morelli *et al.*, 1990; Wiegmann *et al.*, 1992). Although various anti-hypertensive agents were reported to be of therapeutic value, there is as yet no agreement on the preferred antihypertensive regime in diabetic nephropathy. The effect of ACE inhibitors on diabetic nephropathy was thoroughly investigated in the last decade (Marre *et al.*, 1988; Mathiesen *et al.*, 1991; Morelli *et al.*, 1990; Parving *et al.*, 1989; Wiegmann *et al.*, 1992). Some authors claim that ACE inhibitors exhibit special properties in diabetic nephropathy which make them advantageous over other anti-hypertensive agents such as calcium channel blockers (Holdaas *et al.*, 1991; Romanelli *et al.*, 1990). Other investigators, however, failed to demonstrate such an advantage (Melbourne Diabetic Nephropathy Study Group, 1991).

46.7 ALDOSE REDUCTASE INHIBITORS

One of the mechanisms suggested in the pathogenesis of diabetic microvascular complications is the activation of the polyol-pathway with sorbitol formation and alteration in the intracellular *myo*-inositol content and phosphoinositides metabolism (Green *et al.*, 1987). Various aldose-reductase inhibitors (ARIs) which interfere with sorbitol formation were tried in clinical diabetic neuropathy with conflicting results (Boulton *et al.*, 1990; Florkowski *et al.*, 1991; Sima *et al.*, 1988). No effect of ARIs was demonstrated in diabetic retinopathy (Sorbinil Retinopathy Trial Research Group, 1990). ARIs caused a reduction of hyperfiltration in IDDM patients (Pedersen *et al.*, 1991). The lack of a straightforward benefit and the significant side-effects associated with the use of ARIs make these agents unlikely to be in clinical practice in the near future, certainly not in a young population.

46.8 THE POLEMIC RELATED TO SCREENING FOR FIRST-DEGREE FAMILY MEMBERS AT RISK TO BECOME DIABETIC AND EARLY INTERVENTION TRIALS

Advances in the genotyping of individuals susceptible to IDDM (Cambon-Thomsen *et al.*, 1992), the recent availability of immunological markers considered specific for the autoimmune process destroying the β cells (Wilkin, 1992; Palmer, 1993) and the development of immunomodulatory or suppressive drugs (Skyler & Marks, 1993) have led to the initiation of trials both for screening the individual at risk (Bingley *et al.*, 1993; Kitagawa *et al.*, 1993; Knip *et al.*, 1993) as well as for performing active intervention trials to either stop the disease at diagnosis (Silverstein *et al.*, 1988; Bougneres *et al.*, 1990) or prevent its full expression (Bach *et al.*, 1990; Skyler, 1992; Bingley and Gale, 1993, Bingley *et al.*, 1993; Pociot *et al.*, 1993). These trials, in their initial stages, evoked a series of polemics on feasibility (Pozzilli *et al.*, 1992; Lernmark, 1993) and ethical issues (Gil *et al.*, 1993; Guthrie, 1993; Ludvigsson, 1993; Shapira, 1993).

Our point of view (Laron, 1993) is that the treatment team is confronted with a great dilemma as to whether to participate in one of the presently open or randomized trials, or to wait and see their results. What and how should the patient and family be told? How should they be persuaded to participate in a placebo-control study?

At present we know the limited availability of the very specific markers on the one hand and on the other hand the difficulties in the treatment of IDDM. The family will ask 'If there is evidence that the drug tested is effective, then why treat the subject at risk with a placebo?' This is especially true with oral nicotinamide which even if not effective may not be harmful (Pociot *et al.*, 1993). With injectable or oral insulin the questions may be 'If insulin, then why not wait for the full-blown disease? What are the known advantages of treating before the disease has presented, especially considering the potential danger of insulin?'

Children and many older subjects hate to be different from their peers. Early and repeated testing interferes with school attendance and work and also leads to difficult psychosocial situations within the family, for example, feelings of guilt, accusations of hereditary responsibility. Thus, psychosocial counselling may be indicated before screening for each IDDM marker is started.

To ease this heavy burden of responsibility we favour the route of 'polypragmatism' – let us do all we can using present-day knowledge:

1) genotype family members: those found to be Asp 57 negative, Arg 52 positive should be followed closely.
2) test for any immune markers, and at the earliest sign of autoimmune disease, begin with the administration of nicotinamide (Pociot *et al.*, 1993).
3) If during follow-up, the titer of the immune marker rises, maybe even before the first phase of insulin during an iv GTT decreases or disappears, start small doses of oral insulin adding subcutaneous or intravenous boosters. Although this may not seem a very scientific approach, it may be a practical one which could save the physician many sleepless nights and give family members the feeling that the utmost is being done.

A fall in the incidence of newly-onset IDDM within 3–5 years of such a polypragmatic approach could prove or disprove its usefulness. In the meantime, more specific markers and more specific therapeutic agents will become available. At a time when all young children and all older patients take vitamins daily, why should a certain population not take also nicotinamide today, or another harmless, but possibly effective, drug in the future, when the least risk of IDDM arises?

REFERENCES

ADA Position Statement. (1991a) Eye care guidelines for patients with diabetes mellitus. *Diabetes Care*, **14** (suppl. 2), 16–17.

ADA Consensus Statement. (1991b) Diabetic neuropathy. *Diabetes Care*, **14** (suppl. 2), 63–68.

Andersen, A.R., Sandahl-Christiansen, J., Andersen, J.K. *et al.* (1983) Diabetic nephropathy in type 1 (insulin-dependent) diabetes: An epidemiologic study. *Diabetologia*, **25**, 496–501.

Bach, J.F., Dupre, J., Eisenbarth, G.S. *et al.* (1990) Immunotherapy in pre-type 1 diabetes mellitus. *Diabetologia*, **33**, 741.

Bingley, P.J. and Gale, E.A.M. (1993) 'Prediction of IDDM', in Z. Laron and M. Karp (eds). *Prediabetes – Are We Ready to Intervene? Pediatric and Adolescent Endocrinology*, Vol. 23, pp. 65–70. Karger, Basel.

Bingley, P.J., Knip, M. and Gale, E.A.M. (1993) 'Designing an intervention study to delay or prevent the clinical onset of IDDM', in Z. Laron and M. Karp (eds). *Prediabetes – Are We Ready to Intervene? Pediatric and Adolescent Endocrinology*, Vol. 23, pp. 147–56. Karger, Basel.

Borch-Johnsen, K., Wenzel, H., Viberti, C.G. *et al.* (1993) Is screening and intervention for microalbuminuria worthwhile in patients with insulin dependent diabetes? *Brit. Med. J.*, **306**, 1722–25.

Bougneres, P.F., Landais, P., Boisson, C. *et al.* (1990) Limited duration of remission of insulin dependency in children with recent overt type I diabetes treated with low-dose cyclosporine. *Diabetes*, **39**, 1264–72.

Boulton, A.J.M., Levin, S. and Comstock, J. (1990) A multicenter trial of the aldose-reductase inhibitor, tolrestat, in patients with symptomatic diabetic neuropathy. *Diabetologia*, **33**, 431–37.

Burger, W., Hovener, G., Dusterhus, R. *et al.* (1986) Prevalence and development of retinopathy in children and adolescents with type 1 (insulin dependent) diabetes mellitus. A longitudinal study. *Diabetologia*, **29**, 17–22.

Cambon-Thomsen, A., Briant, L., Dugoujon, J.M. *et al.* (1992) 'Genetic susceptibility to insulin-dependent diabetes mellitus: Population studies for HLA and non-HLA markers', in Z. Laron and M. Karp (eds). *Genetic and Environmental Risk Factors for Type I Diabetes (IDDM) Including a Discussion on the Autoimmune Basis*, pp. 1–16. Freund Publishing House; London, Tel Aviv.

Chase, H.P. (1992) *Understanding Insulin Dependent Diabetes*, 7th edn. The Guild of the Children's Diabetes Foundation, Denver.

The DCCT Research Group. (1988a) Factors in development of diabetic neuropathy. Baseline analysis of neuropathy in feasibility phase of Diabetes Control and Complications Trial (DCCT). *Diabetes*, **37**, 476–81.

The DCCT Research Group. (1988b) Are continuing studies on metabolic control and microvascular complications in insulin dependent diabetes mellitus justified? *N. Eng. J. Med.*, **318**, 246–49.

The DCCT Research Group. (1990) Diabetes Control and Complications Trial (DCCT) update. *Diabetes Care*, **13**, 427–33.

The DCCT Research Group. (1991) Epidemiology of severe hypoglycemia in the Diabetes Control and Complications Trial. *Am. J. Med.*, **90**, 450–59.

The DCCT Research Group. (1993) The effect of intensive treatment of diabetes on the development and progression of long-term complications in insulin-dependent diabetes mellitus. *N. Eng. J. Med.*, **329**, 977–86.

Dean, H.J., Mundy, R.L. and Moffatt, M. (1992) Non-insulin-dependent diabetes mellitus in Indian children in Manitoba. *Can. Med. Assoc. J.*, **147**, 52–57.

Elving, L.D., Wetzler, J.F.M., deNobel, E. *et al.* (1991) Erythrocyte sodium-lithium countertransport is not different in type 1 (insulin-dependent) diabetic patients with and without diabetic nephropathy. *Diabetologia*, **34**, 126–28.

Faiman, G., Flexer, Z., Karp, M. *et al.* (1979) 'Nutritional pattern of diabetic children in Israel – a cross sectional and longitudinal study', in Z. Laron and M. Karp (eds). *Nutrition and the Diabetic Child, Pediatric and Adolescent Endocrinology*, Vol. 7, pp. 51–55. Karger, Basel.

Fajans, S.S., Bell, G.I. and Bowden, D.W. (1992) 'Can we recognize prediabetes in NIDDM? Genetic markers in the RW MODY pedigree', in Z. Laron and M. Karp (eds). *Genetic and Environmental Risk Factors for Type I Diabetes (IDDM) Including a Discussion on the Autoimmune Basis*, pp. 33–40. Freund Publishing House; London, Tel Aviv.

Florkowski, C.M., Rowe, B.R., Nightingale, S. *et al.* (1991) Clinical and neurophysiological studies of aldose reductase inhibitor ponalrestat in chronic symptomatic diabetic peripheral neuropathy. *Diabetes*, **40**, 129–33.

Försblom, C.M., Groop, P.H., Ekstrand, A. *et al.* (1992) Predictive value of microalbuminuria in patients with insulin dependent diabetes of long duration. *Brit. Med. J.*, **305**, 1051–53.

Frank, R.N., Hoffman, W.H., Podgar, M.Y. *et al.* (1982) Retinopathy in juvenile onset type 1 diabetes of short duration. *Diabetes*, **31**, 874–82.

Galatzer, A., Amir, S., Gil, R. *et al.* (1982) Crisis intervention program in newly diagnosed diabetic children. *Diabetes Care*, **5**, 414–19.

Gil, R., Galatzer, A., Karp, M. *et al.* (1993) 'Attitude of nonaffected and affected siblings to juvenile diabetes: A retrospective study in multidiabetic families, in Z. Laron and M. Karp (eds). *Prediabetes – Are We Ready to Intervene? Pediatric and Adolescent Endocrinology*, Vol. 23, pp. 171–74. Karger, Basel.

Green, D.A., Sima, A.A.F., Albers, J.W. *et al.* (1990) Diabetic neuropathy, in H. Rifkin (ed.). *Diabetes Mellitus: Theory and Practice*, 4th edn, pp. 710–55. Elsevier, New York.

Green, D.A., Lattimer, S.A. and Sima, A.A.F. (1987) Sorbitol, phosphoinositides and sodium-potassium-atlase in the pathogenesis of diabetic complications. *N. Eng. J. Med.*, **316**, 599–606.

Guthrie, D.W. (1993) 'Parents' and siblings' responses to prediabetes', in Z. Laron and M. Karp (eds). *Prediabetes – Are We Ready to Intervene? Pediatric and Adolescent Endocrinology*, Vol. 23, pp. 165–70. Karger, Basel.

Halloran, J.D. (1992) The effectiveness of the mass media in health education. *International Diabetes Federation Bulletin*, **37** (Suppl.), 8–10.

Hansen, K.W., Pedersen, M.M., Marshall, S.M. *et al.* (1992) Circadian variation of blood pressure in patients with diabetic nephropathy. *Diabetologia*, **35**, 1074–79.

Holdaas, H., Hartmann, L., Lien, M.G. *et al.* (1991) Contrasting effects of lisinopril and nifedipine on albuminuria and tubular transport functions in insulin dependent diabetics with nephropathy. *J. Int. Med.*, **229**, 163–70.

Hurter, P. and Travis, L.B. (eds). (1991) *Introductory Course for Insulin-Dependent Diabetics*, 6th edn, Gerhards Verlagsund Vetriebs-GmbH, Frankfurt.

Jackson, R.L., Ide, C.H., Guthrie, R.A. *et al.* (1982) Retinopathy in adolescents and young adults with onset of insulin dependent diabetes in childhood. *Ophthalmology*, **89**, 7–13.

Javitt, J.C., Aiello, L.P., Bassi, L.J. *et al.* (1991) Detecting and treating retinopathy in patients with type 1 diabetes mellitus. *Ophthalmology*, **98**, 1565–74.

Jenkins, H.R., Hinton, J.L., Williams, H. *et al.* (1989) A study of metabolic control and patient acceptability in adolescent diabetics using NovoPen. *Prac. Diabetes*, **6**, 14–20.

Joner, G., Brinchmann-Hansen, O., Torres, G.G. *et al.* (1992) A nationwide cross-sectional study of retinopathy and microalbuminuria in young Norwegian type 1 (insulin dependent) diabetic patients. *Diabetologia*, **35**, 1049–54.

Kalter-Leibovici, O., Van Dyk, D.J., Leibovici, L. *et al.* (1991) Risk factors for development of diabetic nephropathy and retinopathy in Jewish IDDM patients. *Diabetes*, **40**, 201–10.

Kennedy, W.R., Navarro, X., Goetz, F.C. *et al.* (1990) Effect of pancreatic transplantation on diabetic neuropathy. *N. Eng. J. Med.*, **322**, 1031–37.

Kitagawa, T., Urakami, T., Fujita, H. *et al.* (1993) 'Glucosuria is a marker for prediabetes of slowly progressing IDDM', in Z. Laron and M. Karp (eds). *Prediabetes – Are We Ready to Intervene? Pediatric and Adolescent Endocrinology*, Vol. 23, pp. 84–89. Karger, Basel.

Klein, R., Klein, B.E.K., Moss, S.E. *et al.* (1984) The Wisconsin epidemiologic study of diabetic retinopathy. II. Prevalence and risk of diabetic retinopathy when age at diagnosis is less than 30 years. *Acta Ophthalmologica*, **102**, 520–26.

Klein, R., Klein, B.E.K., Moss, S.E. *et al.* (1985) Retinopathy in young onset diabetic patients. *Diabetes Care*, **8**, 311–15.

Klein, R., Klein, B.E.K. and Moss, S.E. (1991) The incidence of gross proteinuria in people with insulin-dependent diabetes mellitus. *Arch. Int. Med.*, **151**, 1344–48.

Klein, R., Klein, B.E.K., Linton, K.L.P. *et al.* (1992) Microalbuminuria in a population-based study of diabetes. *Arch. Int. Med.*, **152**, 153–58.

Knip, M., Vahasalo, P., Karjalainen, J. *et al.* (1993) 'Characterization of the prediabetic phase in siblings of children with newly diagnosed IDDM', in Z. Laron and M. Karp (eds). *Prediabetes – Are We Ready to Intervene? Pediatric and Adolescent Endocrinology*, Vol. 23, pp. 56–64. Karger, Basel.

Koletzko, S., Burgin-Wolff, A., Koletzko, E. *et al.* (1988) Prevalence of coeliac disease in diabetic children and adolescents: a multicentre study. *Eur. J. Pediatr.*, **148**, 113–17.

Kouri, T.T., Vikari, J.S.A., Mattila, K.S. *et al.* (1991) Microalbuminuria. Invalidity of simple concentration-based screening tests for early nephropathy due to urinary volumes of diabetic patients. *Diabetes Care*, **14**, 591–93.

Krolewski, A.S., Warram, J.H., Christlieb, A.R. *et al.* (1985) The changing natural history of nephropathy in type 1 diabetes. *Am. J. Med.*, **78**, 783–94.

Krolewski, A.S., Warram, J.H., Rand, L.I. *et al.* (1986) Risk of proliferative diabetic retinopathy in juvenile-onset type 1 diabetes: A 40-year follow-up study. *Diabetes Care*, **9**, 443–52.

Krolewski, A.S., Canessa, M., Warram, J.H. *et al.* (1988) Predisposition to hypertension and susceptibility to renal disease in insulin-dependent diabetes mellitus. *N. Eng. J. Med.*, **318**, 140–45.

Lane, P.H., Steffes, M.W. and Mauer, S.M. (1992) Glomerular fracture in IDDM women with low glomerular filtration rate and normal urinary albumin excretion. *Diabetes*, **41**, 581–86.

Laron, Z. (1981) The role of education in the treatment of diabetic children. *International Diabetes Federation Bulletin*, **26**, 20–21.

Laron, Z. (1984) Psycho-social problems of diabetic children and adolescents. *Acta Diabetologica Latina*, **21**, 35–46.

Laron, Z. (1993) Ethical issues in preventive intervention trials in relatives of IDDM patients. *Diabetes Prevention & Therapy*, **7**, 3–4.

Laron, Z. and Galatzer, A. (eds). (1982) *Psychological Aspects of Diabetes in Children and Adolescents, Pediatric and Adolescent Endocrinology*, Vol. 10. Karger, Basel.

Laron, Z. and Karp, M. (1988) 'Diabetes in the young', in L.P. Krall, K.G.M.M. Alberti and J.R. Turtle (eds). *World Book of Diabetes in Practice*, Vol. 3, pp. 297–301. Elservier Science Publ. B.V., Amsterdam.

Laron, Z., Galatzer, A., Amir, S. *et al.* (1979) A multidisciplinary comprehensive, ambulatory treatment scheme for diabetes mellitus in children. *Diabetes Care*, **2**, 343–48.

Laron, Z., Galatzer, A., Faimesser, P. *et al.* (1990) Four years experience with the microcompute system 'Diacon' in the treatment and education of diabetes. International Symposium on Computers and Quantitative Approaches to Diabetes, November 1988, Sydney, Australia. *Horm. Metab. Res.*, (suppl. 24), 129–40.

Laron, Z. and Karp, M. (1990) 'Diabetes in the young', in K.G.M.M. Alberti and L.P. Krall (eds). *The Diabetes Annual/5*, pp. 215–44. Elsevier Science Publishers, B.V., Amsterdam.

Lernmark, A. (1992) Immune intervention yes, but for what reason, for whom, when and how? *Diabetologia*, **35**, 1096–98.

Ludvigsson, J. (1993) 'Ethical aspects on clinical studies of prediabetes', in Z. Laron and M. Karp (eds). *Prediabetes – Are We Ready to Intervene? Pediatric and Adolescent Endocrinology*, Vol. 23, pp. 175–79. Karger, Basel.

Lund-Andersen, C., Frost-Larsen, K. and Starup, K. (1987) Natural history of diabetic retinopathy in insulin-dependent juvenile diabetics. A longitudinal study. *Acta Ophthalmologica*, **65**, 481–86.

Magilli, R., Bending, J.J., Scott, G. *et al.* (1988) Increased sodium-lithium countertransport activity in red cells of patients with insulin-dependent diabetes and nephropathy. *N. Eng. J. Med.*, **318**, 146–50.

Marre, M., Chatellier, G., Leblanc, H. *et al.* (1988) Prevention of diabetic nephropathy with enalapril in normotensive diabetics with microalbuminuria. *Brit. Med. J.*, **297**, 1092–95.

Massent, J.W.C., Elliott, T.G., Hill, R.D. *et al.* (1992) Prognostic significance of microalbuminuria in insulin dependent diabetes mellitus: A twenty-three year follow-up study. *Kidney International*, **41**, 836–39.

Mathiesen, E.R., Oxenboll, R., Johansen, K. *et al.* (1984) Incipient nephropathy in type 1 (insulin-dependent) diabetes. *Diabetologia*, **26**, 406–410.

Mathiesen, E.R., Hommel, E., Giesc, J. *et al.* (1991) Efficacy of captoprin in postponing nephropathy in normotensive insulin-dependent diabetic patients with microalbuminuria. *Brit. Med. J.*, **303**, 81–87.

McCance, D.R., Atkinson, A.B., Hadden, D.R. *et al.* (1989) Long-term glycemic control and diabetic retinopathy. *Lancet*, **ii**, 824–28.

McNally, P.G., Swift, P.G.F., Burden, A.C. *et al.* (1991) Where to treat newly diagnosed diabetes. *Lancet*, **337**, 1046–47.

Melbourne Diabetic Nephropathy Study Group. (1991) Comparison between perindopril and nifedipine in hypertensive and normotensive diabetic patients with microalbuminuria. *Brit. Med. J.*, **302**, 210–16.

Mogensen, C.E. (1987) Microalbuminuria as a predictor of clinical diabetic nephropathy. *Kidney International*, **31**, 673–89.

Mogensen, C.E. and Christensen, C.K. (1984)

Predicting diabetic nephropathy in insulin-dependent patients. *N. Eng. J. Med.*, **311**, 89–93.

Mogensen, C.E., Christensen, C.K. and Vittinghus, E. (1983) The stages in diabetic renal disease with emphasis on the stage of incipient diabetic nephropathy. *Diabetes*, **32** (suppl. 2), 64–78.

Mogensen, C.E., Hansen, K.W., Pedersen, M.M. *et al.* (1991) Renal factors influencing blood pressure threshold and choice of treatment for hypertension in IDDM. *Diabetes Care*, **14** (suppl. 4), 13–26.

Morelli, E., Loon, N., Meyer, T. *et al.* (1990) Effects of converting-enzyme inhibition on barrier function in diabetic glomerulopathy. *Diabetes*, **39**, 76–82.

Mozin, M.J., Dorchy, H., De Maertelaer, V. *et al.* (1978) Food habits of 215 diabetic children in Belgium. *Acta Paed. Belgica*, **31**, 56–58.

Munoz, E., Chalfin, D., Birnbaum, E. *et al.* (1989) Hospital costs, use of resources, and dynamics of death associated with diabetes mellitus. *South Med. J.*, **82**, 300–304.

Murphy, R.P., Nanda, M., Plotnick, L. *et al.* (1990) The relationship of puberty to diabetic retinopathy. *Arch. Ophthalmol.*, **108**, 215–18.

Norgaard, K., Feldt-Rasmussen, B., Borch-Johnsen, K. *et al.* (1990) Prevalence of hypertension in type 1 (insulin-dependent) diabetes mellitus. *Diabetologia*, **33**, 407–410.

O'Hara, J.A. (1990) Proliferative retinopathy and nephropathy at presentation in young insulin dependent diabtics. *Brit. Med. J.*, **300**, 579–80.

Orchard, T.J., Dorman, J.S., Maser, R.E. *et al.* (1990) Prevalence of complications in IDDM by sex and duration. Pittsburgh Epidemiology of Diabetes Complications Study II. *Diabetes*, **39**, 1116–24.

Palmberg, P., Smith, M., Waltman, S. *et al.* (1981) The natural history of retinopathy in insulin dependent juvenile onset diabetes. *Ophthalmology*, **88**, 613–18.

Palmer, J.P. (1993) Predicting IDDM – use of humoral immune markers. *Diabetes Rev.*, **1**, 104–115.

Parving, H.H., Andersen, A.R., Smidt, U.M. *et al.* (1983) Diabetic nephropathy and acterial hypertension. The effect of anti-hypertensive treatment. *Diabetes*, **32** (suppl. 2), 83–87.

Parving, H.H., Andersen, A.R., Smith, U.M. *et al.* (1987) Effect of anti-hypertensive treatment on kidney function in diabetic nephropathy. *Brit. Med. J.*, **294**, 1443–47.

Parving, H.H., Hommel, E., Nielsen, M.D. *et al.* (1989) Effect of captopril on blood pressure and kidney function in normotensive insulin-dependent diabetics with nephropathy. *Brit. Med. J.*, **299**, 533–36.

Paton, R.C., Andrew, M. and Latham, P.J. (1991) Where to treat newly diagnosed diabetes. *Lancet*, **337**, 1046–47.

Pedersen, M.M., Christiansen, J.S. and Mogensen, C.E. (1991) Reduction of glomerular hyperfiltration in normoalbuminuric IDDM patients by 6 months of aldose reductase inhibition. *Diabetes*, **40**, 527–31.

Pinelli, L. (1993) 'Nutrition issues of insulin dependent diabetes mellitus in children and adolescence', in Z. Laron and L. Pinelli (eds). *Theoretical and Practical Aspects of the Treatment of Diabetic Children*, pp. 161–69. 4th International ISGD Course, Dolimiti, Italy, March 1993, Editoriale Bios, Cosenza.

Pociot, F., Reimers, J.I. and Andersen, H.U. (1993) Nicotinamide – biological actions and therapeutic potential in diabetes prevention. IDIG Workshop, Copenhagen, Denmark, December 1992. *Diabetologia*, **36**, 574–76.

Pozzilli, P., Signore, A. and Andreani, D. (1992) What future for therapeutic prevention of type 1 (insulin-dependent) diabetes mellitus? *Diabetologia*, **35**, 1093–95.

Ramsay, R.C., Goetz, F.C., Sutherland, D.E.R. *et al.* (1988) Progression of diabetic retinopathy after pancreas transplantation for insulin diabetes mellitus. *N. Eng. J. Med.*, **318**, 208–214.

Rimoin, D.L. (1975) 'Genetic syndromes associated with abnormal glucose tolerance in childhood and adolescence', in Z. Laron (ed.). *Diabetes in Juveniles – Medical and Rehabilitation Aspects*, pp. 403–408. Karger, Basel.

Romanelli, G., Giustino, A., Bossoni, S. *et al.* (1990) Short-term administration of captopril and nifedipine and exercise-induced albuminuria in normotensive diabetic patients with early-stage nephropathy. *Diabetes*, **39**, 1333–38.

Said, G., Coulon-Goeau, C., Slama, G. *et al.* (1992) Severe early-onset polyneuropathy in insulin dependent diabetes mellitus. A clinical and pathological study. *N. Eng. J. Med.*, **326**, 1257–63.

Shah, S.C., Malone, J.I. and Simpson, N.E. (1989)

A randomized trial of intensive insulin therapy in newly diagnosed insulin dependent mellitus. *N. Eng. J. Med.*, **320**, 550–54.

Shapira, A. (1993) 'Screening for and experimental treatment of prediabetics: Ethical and legal perspectives', in Z. Laron and M. Karp (eds). *Prediabetes – Are We Ready to Intervene? Pediatric and Adolescent Endocrinology*, Vol. 23, pp. 180–83. Karger, Basel.

Silverstein, J., Maclaren, N. and Riley, W. (1988) Immunosuppression with azathioprine and prednisone in recent onset insulin-dependent diabetes mellitus. *N. Eng. J. Med.*, **319**, 599–604.

Sima, A.A.F., Bril, V., Nathaniel, V. *et al.* (1988) Regeneration and repair of myelinated fibers in sural-nerve biopsy specimens from patients with diabetic neuropathy treated with sorbinil. *N. Eng. J. Med.*, **319**, 548–55.

Singer, D.E., Nathan, D.M., Fogel, H.A. *et al.* (1992) Screening for diabetic retinopathy. *Ann. Int. Med.*, **116**, 660–71.

Skyler, J.S. (1992) Can type I diabetes be prevented? *International Diabetes Monitor*, **4**, 1–6.

Skyler, J.S. and Marks, J.B. (1993) Immune intervention in type I diabetes mellitus. *Diabetes Rev.*, **1**, 15–42.

Sorbinil Retinopathy Trial Research Group. (1990) A randomized trial of sorbinil, an aldose reductase inhibitor, in diabetic retinopathy. *Arch. Ophthalmol.*, **108**, 1234–44.

Sosenko, J.M., Boulton, A.J.M., Kubrusky, D.B. *et al.* (1985) The vibratory perception threshold in young diabetic patients: Associations with glycemia and puberty. *Diabetes Care*, **8**, 605–607.

Stehouwer, C.D.A., Fisher, H.R.A., Hackeng, W.H.L. *et al.* (1990) Identifying patients with incipient diabetic nephropathy: Should 24-hour urine collections be used? *Arch. Int. Med.*, **150**, 313–15.

Sutton, L., Plant, A.J. and Lyle, D.M. (1990) Services and cost of hospitalization for children and adolescents with insulin-dependent diabetes mellitus in New South Wales. *Med. J. Australia*, **152**, 130–36.

Tajima, N., LaPorte, R.E. on behalf of the WHO DIAMOND Project Group. (1992) 'Incidence of insulin-dependent diabetes mellitus outside Europe', in C. Levy-Marchal and P. Czernichow (eds). *Epidemiology and Etiology of Insulin-Dependent Diabetes in the Young, Pediatric and Adolescent Endocrinology*, Vol. 21, pp. 31–41. Karger, Basel.

Viberti, G.C., Jarrett, R.J., Mahmud, U. *et al.* (1982) Microalbuminuria as a predictor of clinical nephropathy in insulin-dependent diabetes mellitus. *Lancet*, **i**, 1430–32.

Viberti, G.C., Bilous, R.W., Mackintosh, D. *et al.* (1983) Long-term correction of hyperglycemia and progression of renal failure in insulin dependent diabetes. *Brit. Med. J.*, **286**, 598–602.

Virtanen, S.M., Rasanen, L., Maenpaa, J. *et al.* (1987) Dietary survey of Finnish adolescent diabetics and non-diabetic controls. *Acta Paed. Scand.*, **76**, 801–808.

Wang, P.H., Lau, J. and Chalmers, T.C. (1993) Meta-analysis of effects of intensive blood glucose control on late complications of type 1 diabetes. *Lancet*, **341**, 1306–1309.

Wentworth, S.M. (1987) 'Camping for the child and adolescent with diabetes', in S.J. Brink (ed.). *Pediatric and Adolescent Diabetes Mellitus Year Book*, pp. 391–99. Medical Publications Inc.; Chicago, London.

Wiegmann, T.B., Herron, K.G., Chonko, A.N. *et al.* (1990) Recognition of hypertension and abnormal blood pressure burden with ambulatory blood pressure recording in type 1 diabetes mellitus. *Diabetes*, **39**, 1556–60.

Wiegmann, T.B., Herron, K.G., Chonko, A.M. *et al.* (1992) Effect of angiotensin-converting enzyme inhibition on renal function and albuminuria in normotensive type 1 diabetic patients. *Diabetes*, **41**, 62–67.

Wilkin, T.J. (1992) 'Autoantibodies as markers and mechanisms of beta-cell disease', in Z. Laron and M. Karp (eds). *Genetic and Environmental Risk Factors for Type I Diabetes (IDDM) Including a Discussion on the Autoimmune Basis*, pp. 99–118. Freund Publishing House; London, Tel Aviv.

Ziegler, D., Mayer, P., Muhler, H. *et al.* (1991) The natural history of somatosensory and autonomic nerve dysfunction in relation to glycemic control during the first 5 years after diagnosis of type 1 (insulin dependent) diabetes mellitus. *Diabetologia*, **34**, 822–29.

Appendix A

THE ST VINCENT DECLARATION

Representatives of Government Health Departments and patients' organizations from all European countries met with diabetes experts under the aegis of the Regional Offices of the World Health Organization and the International Diabetes Federation in St Vincent, Italy on 10–12 October, 1989. They unanimously agreed upon the following recommendations and urged that they should be presented in all countries throughout Europe for implementation.

Diabetes mellitus is a major and growing European health problem, a problem at all ages and in all countries. It causes prolonged ill-health and early death. It threatens at least ten million European citizens.

It is within the power of national governments and health departments to create conditions in which a major reduction in this heavy burden of disease and death can be achieved. Countries should give formal recognition to the diabetes problem and deploy resources for its solution. Plans for the prevention, identification and treatment of diabetes and particularly its complications – blindness, renal failure, gangrene and amputation, aggravated coronary heart disease and stroke – should be formulated at local, national and European regional levels. Investment now will earn great dividends in reduction of human misery and in massive savings of human and material resources.

General goals and five-year targets listed below can be achieved by the organized activities of the medical services in active partnership with diabetic citizens, their families, friends and workmates and their organizations; in the management of their own diabetes and education for it; in the planning, provision and quality audit of health care; in national, regional and international organizations for disseminating information about health maintenance; in promoting and applying research.

GENERAL GOALS FOR PEOPLE – CHILDREN AND ADULTS – WITH DIABETES

- Sustained improvement in health experience and a life approaching normal expectation in quality and quantity.
- Prevention and cure of diabetes and of its complications by intensifying research effort.

FIVE-YEAR TARGETS

Elaborate, initiate and evaluate comprehensive programmes for detection and control of diabetes and of its complications with self-care and community support as major components.

Raise awareness in the population and among health care professionals of the present opportunities and the future needs for

Childhood and Adolescent Diabetes
Published in 1994 by Chapman & Hall, London
ISBN 0 412 48610 5

prevention of the complications of diabetes and of diabetes itself.

Organize training and teaching in diabetes management and care for people of all ages with diabetes, for their families, friends and working associates and for the health care team.

Ensure that care for children with diabetes is provided by individuals and teams specialized both in the management of diabetes and of children, and that families with a diabetic child get the necessary social, economic and emotional support.

Reinforce existing centres of excellence in diabetes care, education and research. Create new centres where the need and potential exist.

Promote independence, equity and self-sufficiency for all people with diabetes – children, adolescents, those in the working years of life, and the elderly.

Remove hindrances to the fullest possible integration of the diabetic citizen into society.

Implement effective measures for the prevention of costly complications.

- Reduce new blindness due to diabetes by one third or more.
- Reduce numbers of people entering end-stage diabetic renal failure by at least one third.
- Reduce by one half the rate of limb amputations for diabetic gangrene.
- Cut morbidity and mortality from coronary heart disease in the diabetic by vigorous programmes of risk factor reduction.
- Achieve pregnancy outcome in the diabetic woman that approximates that of the non-diabetic woman.

Establish monitoring and control systems using state of the art information technology for quality assurance of diabetes health care provision and for laboratory and technical procedures in diabetes diagnosis, treatment and self-management.

Promote European and international collaboration in programmes of diabetes research and development through national, regional and WHO agencies and in active partnership with diabetes patients organizations.

Take urgent action in the spirit of the WHO programme, 'Health for All' to establish joint machinery between WHO and IDF, European Region, to initiate, accelerate and facilitate the implementation of these recommendations.

At the conclusion of the St Vincent meeting, all those attending formally pledged themselves to strong and decisive action in seeking implementation of the recommendations on their return home.

Appendix B

THE ISPAD DECLARATION

The International Study Group of Diabetes in Children and Adolescents (ISGD) was founded in 1974. At the nineteenth annual international scientific meeting (Kos, 1993), having grown to a multi-disciplinary group, the name of the society was changed to the International Society for Pediatric and Adolescent Diabetes (ISPAD).

The aim of the Society remains the promotion of the care of children and adolescents with diabetes and the encouragement and support of research on diabetes in these groups.

At the Kos meeting, the members of the Society proclaimed their commitment to implement the St Vincent Declaration to promote optimal health, social welfare and quality of life for *all* children and adolescents with diabetes around the world by the year 2000. They also pledged, in particular, to work towards the following:

(1) to make insulin available for *all* children and adolescents with diabetes
(2) to reduce the morbidity and mortality rate of acute metabolic complications or missed diagnosis related to diabetes mellitus
(3) to make age-appropriate care and education accessible to *all* children and adolescents with diabetes as well as to their families
(4) to increase the availability of appropriate urine and blood self-monitoring equipment for *all* children with diabetes
(5) to develop and encourage research on diabetes in children and adolescents around the world
(6) to prepare and disseminate written guidelines and standards for practical and realistic insulin treatment, monitoring, nutrition, psychosocial care and education of young patients with diabetes – and their families – emphasizing the crucial role of health care professionals – and not just physicians – in these tasks around the world.

Childhood and Adolescent Diabetes
Published in 1994 by Chapman & Hall, London
ISBN 0 412 48610 5

Index

Page numbers in **bold** refer to figures, and page numbers appearing in *italic* refer to tables.